FUNDAMENTALS AND DESIGN OF DRUG DELIVERY SYSTEMS

FUNDAMENTALS AND DESIGN OF DRUG DELIVERY SYSTEMS

A TEXTBOOK WITH LAB ACTIVITIES

Wujie Zhang

ELSEVIER

ACADEMIC PRESS
An imprint of Elsevier

Academic Press is an imprint of Elsevier
125 London Wall, London EC2Y 5AS, United Kingdom
50 Hampshire Street, 5th Floor, Cambridge, MA 02139, United States

ISBN: 978-0-443-23521-4

For information on all Academic Press publications visit our website at https://www.elsevier.com/books-and-journals

Publisher: Peter Linsley
Acquisition Editor: Emma Skyes
Editorial Project Manager: Ellie Barnett
Production Project Manager: Haritha Dharmarajan
Cover Designer: Vicky Pearson Esser

Printed in Great Britain
Last digit is the print number: 10 9 8 7 6 5 4 3 2 1

Typeset by TNQ Tech

Contents

Preface

Courses on drug delivery (systems) have become increasingly common in pharmacy and engineering schools. This textbook addresses the rapidly evolving pharmaceutical industry by including up-to-date content such as nanotechnology in drug delivery systems. Unlike many recent books that are primarily reference books, this one provides comprehensive coverage, including delivery systems design, which is particularly critical for engineering students. Additionally, it offers lab activities that provide valuable hands-on experiences, enhancing the learning process.

With more than 20 years of research experience and 12 years of teaching experience in drug delivery, the author undertook a 2-year-long project to write this textbook (which can also serve as a reference book), incorporating easy-to-adopt lab activities to fulfill the abovementioned needs. Additionally, this book includes sample questions and case studies. It is state-of-the-art and comprehensive yet concise, covering content from the basics of pharmacology and drug delivery to the design of drug delivery systems. Nanomaterials and nanotechnology in drug delivery systems have been incorporated into various chapters to avoid repetition. Novel drug delivery systems addressed in this book include biomimetic drug delivery systems, engineered cells as drug delivery systems, drug delivery technology based on three-dimensional printing, and more.

Although the arrangement of the content is systematic—from fundamentals to applications and design—the chapters are independent of each other. Hence, instructors have the flexibility to decide which chapters to cover in class. Considering the book's adaptability, eligible instructors can access the instructor resources, including PowerPoint presentations, the Manual for Review and Practice Questions, and the Manual for Lab Questions.

Finally, the author gratefully acknowledges his students and colleagues for their support and encouragement in undertaking this project. The author also acknowledges the support for this project from the protracted leave program of the Milwaukee School of Engineering. The author appreciates the full support and love of his family members, in both the United States and China; pays homage to his mom, Aimei Nie, who inspired him to be an educator; and recognizes his sister, Qingchun Zhang, and brother-in-law, Quanzhou Luo, for their dedication to the pharmaceutical industry.

The instructor website would be at https://educate.elsevier.com/book/details/9780443235214 and contains:

- Lecture slides
- Answers to questions
- Experimental data and its analysis

CHAPTER

1

Introduction

Wujie Zhang

LEARNING OBJECTIVES

- To define drugs, drug delivery, and drug delivery systems
- To discuss the importance of drug delivery systems in pharmaceutical development
- To describe the components and functions of the mRNA-based COVID-19 vaccine

1.1 Drug delivery and drug delivery systems

Drug delivery is the method or process of delivering drugs to specific sites within an organism (the human body, for this textbook) to achieve specific outcomes. It is worth mentioning that the delivery site is not necessarily the site of action. The U.S. Food and Drug Administration (FDA) defines a drug as:

- A substance recognized by an official pharmacopeia or formulary
- A substance intended for use in the diagnosis, cure, mitigation, treatment, or prevention of disease
- A substance (other than food) intended to affect the structure or any function of the body
- A substance intended for use as a component of a medicine but not a device or a component, part, or accessory of a device
- Biological products are included within this definition and are generally covered by the same laws and regulations, but differences exist regarding their manufacturing processes (chemical process versus biological process) [1].

The European Medicines Agency defines a drug (an alternative term used is medicinal product) as a substance or combination of substances that is intended to treat, prevent, or diagnose a disease or to restore, correct, or modify physiological functions by exerting a pharmacological, immunological, or metabolic action. The definition of a drug is evolving with time, especially as the list of biological products is ever-growing. It is also worth noting that drugs are for the diagnosis, cure, mitigation, treatment, or prevention of a disease, rather than only for therapeutic effects [2].

A drug delivery system (DDS) is a formulation or a device that enables the delivery of drugs to specific sites within an organism. The focus of this textbook is on nontraditional formulations and devices.

1.2 The promise of novel DDSs

The design of DDSs tends to be overlooked or only occurs during the later stages of drug development. Novel DDSs have been used by pharmaceutical companies to either retain or gain market as a patent, with exclusivity lasting for only a specific period.We have witnessed the rapid development of the vaccine (mRNA based) against

Fundamentals and Design of Drug Delivery Systems
https://doi.org/10.1016/B978-0-443-23521-4.00001-1

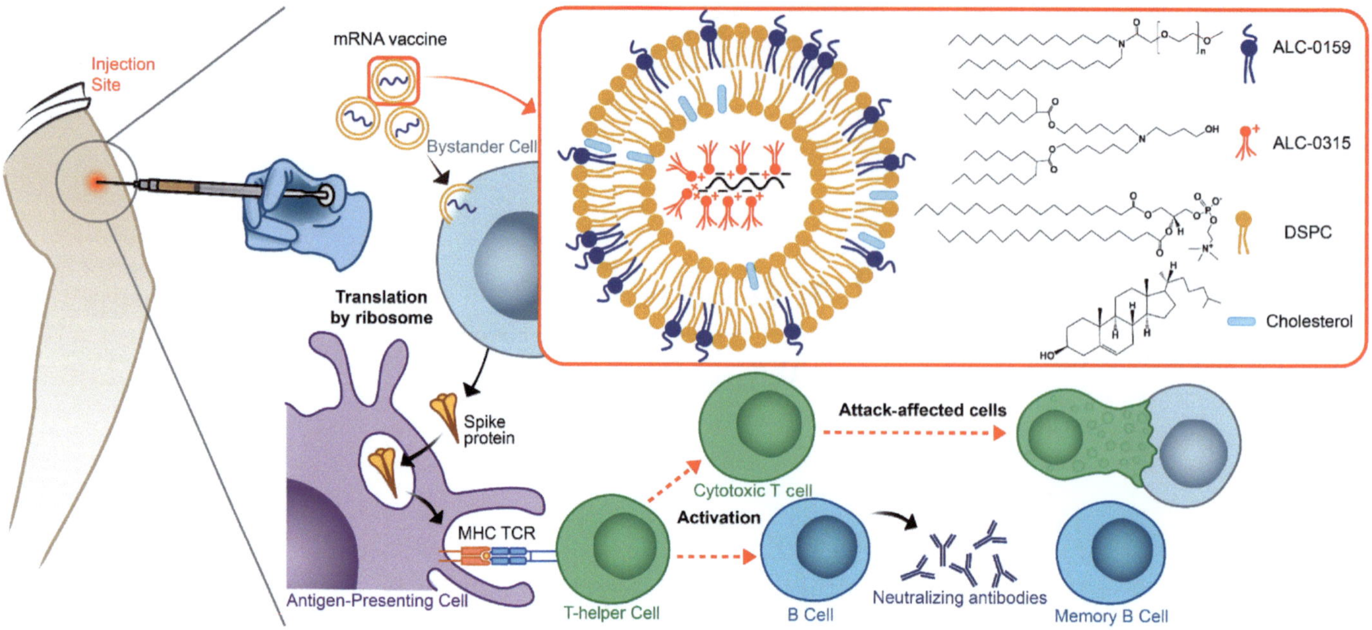

FIGURE 1.1 Pfizer-BioNTech mRNA vaccine composition and working mechanism. *MHC*, Major histocompatibility complex; *TCR*, T-cell receptor. The graph is generated using the information from Dolgin [3] and Fendler et al. [7]. *Adapted from* BioRender.com. Immune responses induced by COVID-19 vaccines. 2023. Available from: https://app.biorender.com/biorender-templates *[10]*.

the SARS-CoV-2, which caused the COVID-19 pandemic. The DDS significantly contributed to the development process. mRNA-based vaccine research and development are not recent, as the first mRNA influenza vaccine was tested in mice in the 1990s. Moreover, back in 1978, liposomes were used to transport mRNA into mammalian cells to induce protein expression [3]. mRNA, which is very unstable, cannot easily enter mammalian cells, creating a major hurdle for mRNA-based treatments, like vaccines. This explains why it was not until the coronavirus pandemic necessitated it that a breakthrough was made. Take Pfizer-BioNTech COVID-19 vaccines, for example—the mRNA that encodes the presence of small fragments (harmless) of the SARS-CoV-2 virus is encapsulated in a lipid nanoparticle. The lipid nanoparticles help deliver the mRNA into cells for expression while protecting the mRNA (Fig. 1.1). The lipid nanoparticles used are developed by the company Acuitas and contain four components: ALC-0315 ([(4-hydroxybutyl)azanediyl]di(hexane-6,1-diyl)bis(2-hexyldecanoate); a synthetic lipid, ALC-0159 (2-[(polyethylene glycol)-2000]-*N*,*N*-ditetradecylacetamide; a PEGylated lipid, 1,2-distearoyl-*sn*-glycero-3-phosphocholine (DSPC); a phosphatidylcholine lipid, and cholesterol. DSPC is a common phospholipid that contributes to the lipid bilayer vesicle formation. Cholesterol is a component of the cell membrane that regulates the fluidity of the lipid bilayer. ALC-0315 is a cationic lipid that becomes protonated at a specific pH, which can interact with negatively charged mRNA (due to the phosphate groups) and assists with the encapsulation of mRNA during the lipid nanoparticle formation. Moreover, the low pH contributes to the mRNA release on entering the cells. ALC-0159 is a PEGylated lipid. PEGylation, the covalent or noncovalent attachment of PEG (polyethylene glycol) to a molecule or structure, leads to a protective hydrophilic layer that helps stabilize the lipid nanoparticles [4]. There are concerns about PEGylation as it may lead to unexpected immune responses [5]. For example, some studies have shown that PEGylated nanoparticles lead to the production of anti-PEG antibodies [5,6]. Some researchers argue that the amount of PEG in mRNA vaccines is low and that the mRNA vaccines are often given intramuscularly rather than intravenously, allowing for slow absorption rates [5]. mRNA vaccines are delivered to the bystander cells, such as muscle and dermal cells, at the site of injection. Spike proteins are then produced through translation and are taken up and processed by antigen-presenting cells, including dendritic cells, activating T cells, B cells, and antibody responses (Fig. 1.1) [7].

1.3 Layout of the textbook

This textbook is designed to start with the fundamentals and then transition into DDSs, especially novel delivery systems and their design aspects (Fig. 1.2). Drug delivery is interdisciplinary, requiring knowledge from basic

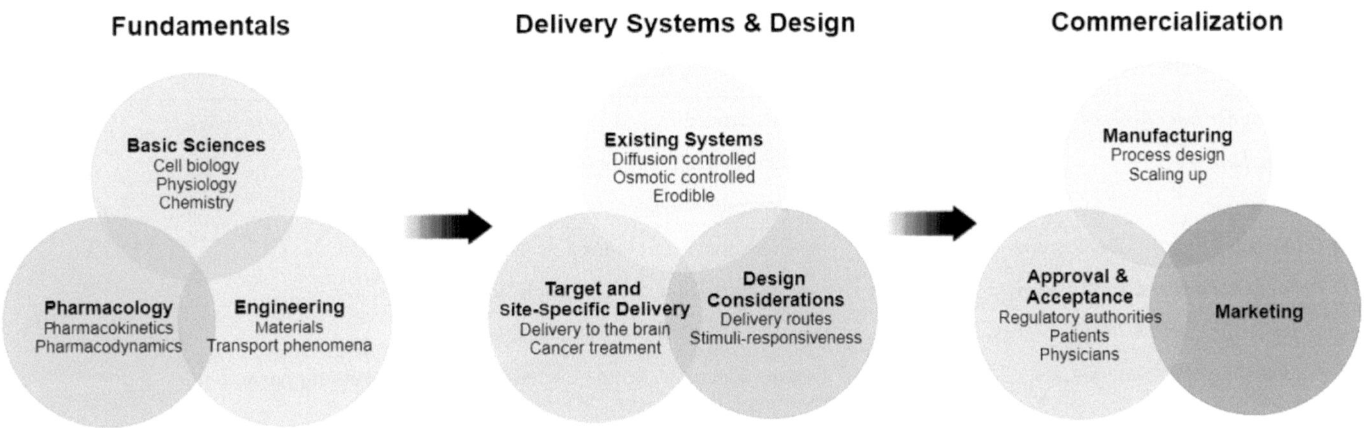

FIGURE 1.2 Content layout of the textbook.

sciences, pharmacology, and engineering. As most drugs act at the cellular level, it is critical to fully understand cellular biology, especially the mechanisms of cellular uptake, drug resistance, and so on. Pharmacology provides fundamentals on drugs (and carriers) being absorbed, distributed, and eliminated from the body. Materials (e.g., carrier design) and transport phenomena (hemodynamics, drug release mechanisms, etc.) are good examples of engineering aspects that are critical to the design of DDSs. With the fundamental knowledge and insights from existing DDSs, novel DDSs can be designed to meet the specific needs of various applications. Biomimetic DDSs are good examples, as nature is the best teacher, and we should learn from it. Regarding commercialization, the whole process should be patient-centric, as patients are the end users. Patient-focused drug development and personalized medicine are two innovative approaches. Patient-focused drug development is a systematic approach to help ensure that patient experiences, perspectives, needs, and priorities are captured and meaningfully incorporated into drug development and evaluation [8]. Instead of a one-size-fits-all for the "average patient," personalized medicine enables the tailoring of disease prevention and treatment that takes into account the differences in the genes, environments, and lifestyles of individual patients [9]. This textbook also covers manufacturing, approval and acceptance, and other topics related to commercialization.

1.4 Resources for studying drug delivery

The drug delivery field is a rapidly growing and ever-evolving field, making it necessary to use resources outside this textbook. The Controlled Release Society (CRS) is a professional society dedicated to delivery science (https://www.controlledreleasesociety.org/). They have several publications, including the CRS *Advances in Delivery Science and Technology* book series and the *Journal of Controlled Release*. There are also many journals specifically for drug delivery fields (Table 1.1). The National Institute of Biomedical Imaging and Bioengineering has a special topic on DDSs. There are many more resources that can be used to study DDSs that have not been specifically mentioned.

Lab activity I: Delivery of nucleic acids into cells using cationic lipids

Nucleic acid–based therapies are becoming more and more common, such as mRNA-based vaccines. The objectives of this lab are to:

(1) Learn how to deliver nucleic acid into mammalian cells using cationic lipids (transfection).
(2) Perform the cell transfection and analyze the transfection efficiency.

Background

There are multiple methods for transfection, such as electroporation, viral transfection, calcium phosphate precipitation, and cationic polymer/lipid transfection. Cationic lipids have been successfully used for many cell types and some intact tissues. This approach is of relatively high efficiency and low toxicity [11].

TABLE 1.1 Scientific journals related to drug delivery

Title	Website
Advanced Drug Delivery Reviews	https://www.sciencedirect.com/journal/advanced-drug-delivery-reviews
Current Drug Delivery	https://benthamscience.com/journal/18/about-journal
Drug Delivery	https://www.tandfonline.com/journals/idrd20
Drug Delivery and Translational Research	https://www.springer.com/journal/13346
Drug Development and Industrial Pharmacy	https://www.tandfonline.com/journals/iddi20
Expert Opinion on Drug Delivery	https://www.tandfonline.com/journals/iedd20
European Journal of Pharmaceutics and Biopharmaceutics	https://www.sciencedirect.com/journal/european-journal-of-pharmaceutics-and-biopharmaceutics
International Journal of Pharmaceutics	https://www.sciencedirect.com/journal/international-journal-of-pharmaceutics
Journal of Controlled Release	https://www.sciencedirect.com/journal/journal-of-controlled-release
Journal of Drug Delivery Science and Technology	https://www.sciencedirect.com/journal/journal-of-drug-delivery-science-and-technology
Journal of Drug Targeting	https://www.tandfonline.com/journals/idrt20
Pharmaceutical Development and Technology	https://www.tandfonline.com/journals/iphd20
Pharmaceutics	https://www.mdpi.com/journal/pharmaceutics

Note: This is by no means an exhaustive list and is subject to updates and additions.

Lipofectamine Transfection Reagent (cationic lipid) is used in this lab to deliver small interfering RNA (siRNA) (BLOCK-iT Alexa Fluor Red Fluorescent). The BLOCK-iT Alexa Fluor Red Fluorescent Control is an ideal indicator of lipid-mediated transfection efficiency for RNA interference (RNAi) experiments, particularly those using the Lipofectamine RNAiMAX Transfection Reagent. The sequence of the BLOCK-iT Alexa Fluor Red Fluorescent Control is not homologous to any known gene, preventing the induction of nonspecific cellular events caused by introducing the duplex into cells [12,13].

The mechanism of action of siRNA is based on post-transcriptional gene silencing. siRNA molecules are usually specific and efficient in the knockdown of disease-related genes. However, they are susceptible to nuclease-mediated degradation with low cellular uptake [14].

Materials and Instruments

Mammalian cells
6- or 24-well plates
Lipofectamine RNAiMAX Transfection Reagent (cationic lipids)
BLOCK-iT Alexa Fluor Red Fluorescent Control (siRNA)
Hoechst 33342 stain
Fluorescence microscope

Laboratory Procedure

1. Pre-lab: Seed cells to be 80% to 90% confluent at transfection using a well plate.
2. Preparation: Vent and wipe down the biosafety cabinet (BSC) with 70% ethanol. Aseptically move the items needed into the BSC.
3. Dilute Lipofectamine reagent in serum-free medium (3 μL: 50 μL for 24-well plate; 9 μL: 150 μL for 6-well plate).
4. Dilute siRNA in serum-free medium (1 μL [10 pmol]: 50 μL for 24-well plate; 3 μL [30 pmol]: 150 μL for 6-well plate).
5. Add the diluted siRNA to the diluted Lipofectamine reagent (1:1 ratio).
6. Incubate for 5 minutes at room temperature.
7. Aspirate the old medium, and then rinse the cells with Dulbecco phosphate-buffered saline (DPBS).
8. Add serum-free medium to each well (typical cell culture amount, e.g., 0.4 mL per well for a 24-well plate).
9. Add siRNA-lipid complex to cells of experimental wells (Table LI.1; the amount is enough for two wells).

Q: How many types of negative controls are needed? What are they?

TABLE LI.1 Amount of siRNA and siRNA-lipid complex per well.

Component	6 Wells	24 Wells
Final siRNA used per well	25 pmol	5 pmol
siRNA-lipid complex per well	250 μL	50 μL

10. Incubate for 12 to 24 hours and then remove the medium and rinse the cells with DPBS.
11. Add DPBS to each well.
12. Add Hoechst 33342 stain into each well (final concentration: 5 μmol/L) and incubate for 10 minutes at room temperature.
13. Visualize/analyze transfected cells under a fluorescence microscope.
14. Calculate the transfection efficiency (t.e.%):

$$t.e.\% = \frac{transfected\ cells}{total\ number\ of\ cells} \times 100\%$$

Review and practice questions

1. What is drug delivery? What is a drug delivery system?
2. How can a cationic lipid assist the delivery of nucleic acids (mRNA, siRNA, etc.)?
3. Write a short essay on a novel drug delivery system after conducting a literature search.

References

[1] U.S. Food and Drug Administration. Drugs@FDA glossary of terms. Available from: https://www.fda.gov/drugs/drug-approvals-and-databases/drugsfda-glossary-terms.

[2] European Medicines Agency. Medicinal product. Available from: https://www.ema.europa.eu/en/glossary/medicinal-product#:~:text=Medicinal%20product%20%7C%20European%20Medicines%20Agency%20Medicinal%20product,by%20exerting%20a%20pharmacological%2C%20immunological%20or%20metabolic%20action.

[3] Dolgin E. The tangled history of mRNA vaccines. Nature 2021;597(7876):318–24.

[4] Public assessment report authorisation for temporary supply COVID-19 mRNA vaccine BNT162B2 (BNT162B2 RNA), M.H.p.R. Agency, Editor.

[5] de Vrieze J. Pfizer's vaccine raises allergy concerns. Science 2021;371(6524):10–1.

[6] Mohamed M, et al. PEGylated liposomes: immunological responses. Sci Technol Adv Mater 2019;20(1):710–24.

[7] Fendler A, et al. COVID-19 vaccines in patients with cancer: immunogenicity, efficacy and safety. Nat Rev Clin Oncol 2022;19(6):385–401.

[8] U.S. Food and Drug Administration. CDER patient-focused drug development. Available from: https://www.fda.gov/drugs/development-approval-process-drugs/cder-patient-focused-drug-development

[9] U.S. Food and Drug Administration. Precision medicine. Available from: https://www.fda.gov/medical-devices/in-vitro-diagnostics/precision-medicine.

[10] BioRender.com. Immune responses induced by COVID-19 vaccines. 2023. Available from: https://app.biorender.com/biorender-templates.

[11] Capes-Davis A, Freshney RI. Chapter 22-Genetic modification and immortalization. In: Freshney, editor. Freshney's culture of animal cells: a manual of basic technique and specialized applications. 8th ed. John Wiley & Sons; 2021. p. 509–33.

[12] Thermo Fisher Scientific Inc. Lipofectamine 2000 transfection reagent protocol. Available from: https://www.thermofisher.com/document-connect/document-connect.html?url=https://assets.thermofisher.com/TFS-Assets%2FLSG%2Fmanuals%2FLipofectamine_2000_Reag_protocol.pdf.

[13] Thermo Fisher Scientific Inc. Protocol: BLOCK-iT™ alexa fluor® red fluorescent oligo. Available from: https://www.thermofisher.com/document-connect/document-connect.html?url=https://assets.thermofisher.com/TFS-Assets%2FLSG%2Fmanuals%2FBLOCK_IT_AF_RedFluorOligo_man.pdf.

[14] Alshaer W, et al. siRNA: mechanism of action, challenges, and therapeutic approaches. Eur J Pharmacol 2021;905:174178.

CHAPTER

2

Historical aspects of drugs and drug delivery

Wujie Zhang

LEARNING OBJECTIVES

- To discuss the history of drugs
- To discuss the history of drug delivery systems
- To give examples of traditional and novel delivery systems/formulations
- To describe the working mechanism of drug-eluting stents

2.1 Historical aspects of drugs, pharmacy, and pharmacy education

Dating back to the early days of human civilization, humans have attempted to improve their health through the administration of drugs. Traditional Chinese medicine (TCM) is believed to have originated in China more than 2500 years ago. According to Chinese mythology, the legendary Sheng Nong (the Fire Emperor) taught not only basic agriculture but also the use of herbal drugs. In the 16th century, *Ben Cao Gang Mu (Compendium Material Medica)* was published; it lists the plants (Fig. 2.1), minerals, and other entities that were thought to have medicinal properties [1]. Other countries, such as India and Egypt, were also early practitioners of herbal medicine.

Pharmacy emerged as a component of medicine during ancient times; around 1240, Frederick II of Hohenstaufen issued the first European edict separating the responsibilities of pharmacy from those of medicine [2]. Advances in physiology and chemistry significantly contributed to the rise and development of pharmacy, especially pharmacology. Galen, a Greek physician-surgeon and philosopher, was the first physician to use the pulse as a sign of illness and improved the science and use of drugs in therapeutics [3]. Paracelsus (real name: Philippus Theophrastus Bomastus von Hohenheim) was a German-Swiss physician and alchemist and is credited as the grandfather of pharmacology and father of toxicology. Paracelsus introduced a treatment of syphilis using carefully measured doses of mercury taken internally (recognizing the relationship between the amount of drug administered (dose) and the beneficial or harmful effects produced) [4,5]. Variolation (intentionally exposing healthy people to smallpox) was practiced in different parts of the world as early as the 15th century to prevent the spread of the illness [6]. Friedrich Sertürner (1783-1841), a German pharmacist, isolated morphine from opium in the early 19th century (Fig. 2.2A), which is generally believed to be the first isolation of an active compound (alkaloid) from a plant. Then, atropine and cocaine were isolated in 1833 and 1860, respectively [7,8]. More recently, Youyou Tu, a Chinese pharmaceutical chemist and malariologist, was awarded the 2015 Nobel Prize for Physiology or Medicine for her contribution to the isolation (from *Artemisia annua L.*; Fig. 2.2B) and study of the antimalarial substance artemisinin (*qinghaosu*), which has been the frontline treatment since the late 1990s [9].

In the early years of pharmaceutical education, the Department of Pharmacy and Materia Medica was established at the Jagiellonian University in 1783, with Professor Jan Szaster as the founder of the first pharmaceutical

Fundamentals and Design of Drug Delivery Systems
https://doi.org/10.1016/B978-0-443-23521-4.00002-3

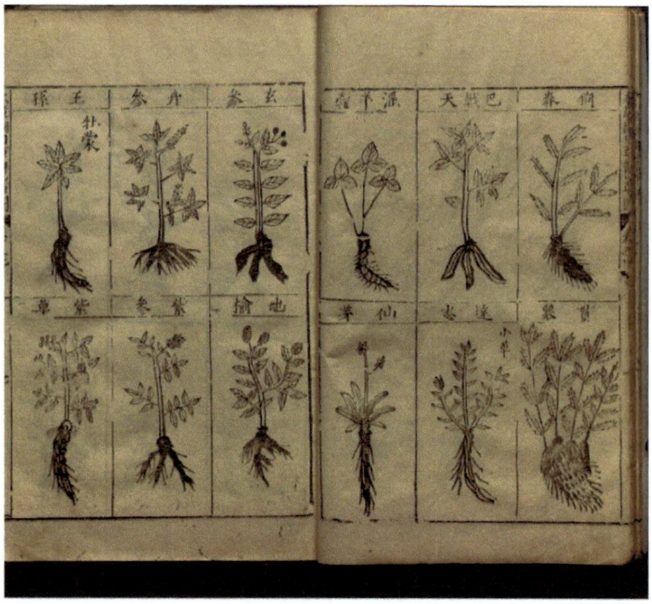

FIGURE 2.1 Pages from *Ben Cao Gang Mu* printed during the Wanli Era of the Ming Dynasty. *From the Library of Congress. https://www.loc.gov/item/2012402161/.*

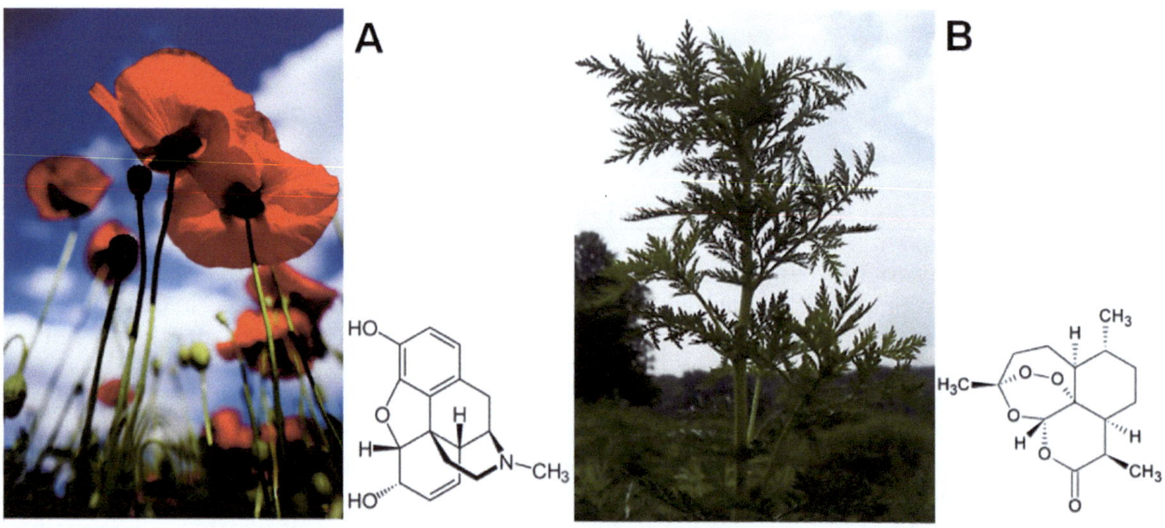

FIGURE 2.2 Images of medicinal plants and corresponding drugs isolated from them. (A) Opium poppy (photo by KS Kyungon Unsplash) and chemical structure of morphine. (B) *Artemisia annua L.* (photo by Jorge Ferreira) and chemical structure of artemisinin.

department in Poland. Twenty-four years later the first obligatory 3-year course was established in Bavaria, Germany [10]. The first two pharmacy schools established in the United States were the Philadelphia College of Pharmacy (1821) and the Massachusetts College of Pharmacy (1823) [11]. The first pharmacy school in the Eastern Mediterranean region was initiated in 1824 in Cairo, Egypt [12]. The Pharmaceutical Society of Great Britain founded the first British School of Pharmacy, the College of the Pharmaceutical Society (now University College London School of Pharmacy), in 1842. Goa, at Escola Medica de Goa, was the first in pharmacy education in Asia in 1842 [13]. John Jacob Abel, the father of American pharmacology, played a key role in developing the first pharmacology department in North America at the University of Michigan in 1891 and was offered the first full professorship of pharmacology in the United States [14,15]. Established in 1883, The University of Wisconsin-Madison School of Pharmacy was the first school of pharmacy to award a baccalaureate degree in pharmacy [11].

Regarding the medicine quality standards, the United States Pharmacopeia (USP) was formed in 1820 by a group of physicians concerned about the inconsistent and poor quality of medical preparations at the time, and the first edition of the *US Pharmacopeia* (the second national pharmacopeia ever published; a national French pharmacopeia appeared in 1818) was also published in 1820 [16]. This is recorded as the first milestone in the history of food and drug regulation in the United States on the US FDA webpage [17]. The *US Pharmacopeia* was first officially recognized with the Drug Importance Act of 1848, and the US Congress declared in the 1938 Federal Food, Drug, and Cosmetic Act that all medicines sold in the United States must meet applicable USP quality standards [18]. The National Formulary (NF) was originally published in 1888 with the name *National Formulary of Unofficial Preparations*. Later, the NF was limited to pharmaceutical ingredients; currently, the NF is published together with the USP as USP-NF [4,19]. Besides the USP, the other large pharmacopeias in the world are the European Pharmacopoeia (EP), The British Pharmacopoeia (BP), the Japanese Pharmacopoeia (JP), and the Pharmacopoeia of the People's Republic of China (PPRC) (or the Chinese Pharmacopoeia [ChP]).

2.2 Historical aspects of drug delivery

Oral drug delivery is one of the most commonly used administration routes. Over time, different delivery methods/systems have been developed to increase efficacy, decrease systemic/local toxicity, and access the target sites, which are generally difficult to reach. In 1836, French physician G.V. Lafargue conceived the idea of introducing morphine under the skin using a vaccination lancet; during administration, the lancet tip was dipped in morphine and then forced nearly horizontally under the skin [20]. Due to the various limitations of using syringes at the time, Lafargue proposed using a darning needle to pierce the skin, then inserting the drug using fingers or tweezers, and last, covering the puncture with a piece of stamp paper or such [20]. The hypodermic syringe and needle was invented in 1853 with Dr. Alexander Wood as a coinventor (Fig. 2.3). Wood published a paper in the *Edinburgh Medical and Surgical Journal* in 1855, the first on the subcutaneous injection of drugs [21].

The French pharmacist Joseph Gérard Auguste Dublanc and his student, François Achille Barnabe Mothes, filed the first patent for what came to be known as a capsule in 1833. Their invention, "bladders made of gelatin," was produced by dipping a small leather bag filled with mercury into a gelatin solution. After the gelatin dried, it was stripped off of the leather bag and filled with liquid medicine introduced by a pipette and then sealed with a drop of gelatin [22]. The two-piece hard capsules, consisting of an overlapping cap and a body piece, were invented by the Parisian pharmacist Jules Lehuby. There are now two types of capsules: hard and soft capsules. The hard capsules (two-piece) are mostly used to encapsulate solid and semisolid substances, while the soft capsules are used for liquids [23]. Generally, the capsule shell is made of gelatin, but one of the major drawbacks of using gelatin capsules is that the coating can become brittle or sticky due to the change of storage conditions or the moisture transfer between the capsule and its contents [24].

The introduction of Spansule sustained-release capsule technology marked the beginning of modern drug delivery technology. The Spansule technology is based on the coating barrier (variable layers of natural waxes) of drug granules (particles and such) within a capsule that modifies the drug dissolution by limiting its access to gastrointestinal (GI) fluids once the capsule has been ingested [25]. It was first used for the 12-hour delivery of dextroamphetamine sulfate (Dexedrine). The thickness of the Spansule layer can be adjusted to control the release profile for the encapsulated drug. Enteric-coating materials, such as cellulose acetate phthalate, were introduced in the 1950s, and they have been used to resist the early release of the drug in the acidic fluids in the stomach. The Eudragit brand was

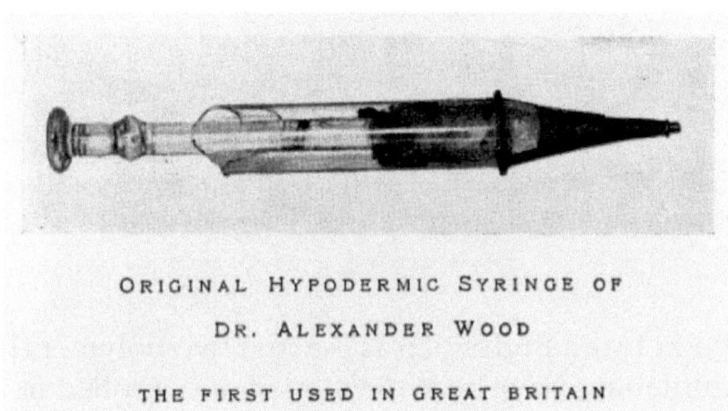

FIGURE 2.3 Image of the original hypodermic syringe of Dr. Alexander Wood. *From Comrie, J.D.* History of Scottish Medicine to 1860. *Wellcome Collection. Attribution 4.0 International (CC BY 4.0).*

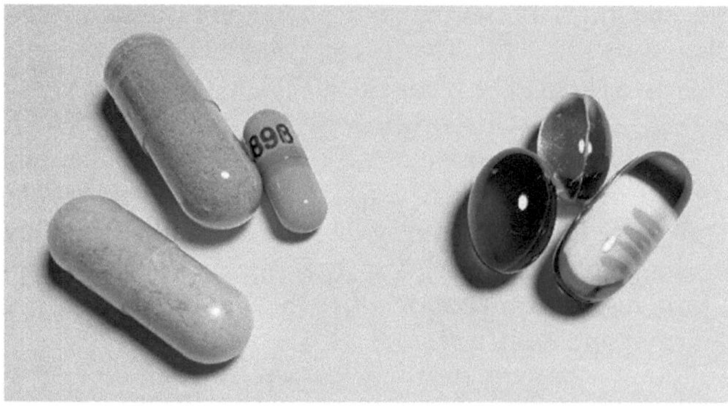

FIGURE 2.4 Examples of hard (*left*) and soft (*right*) shell capsules.

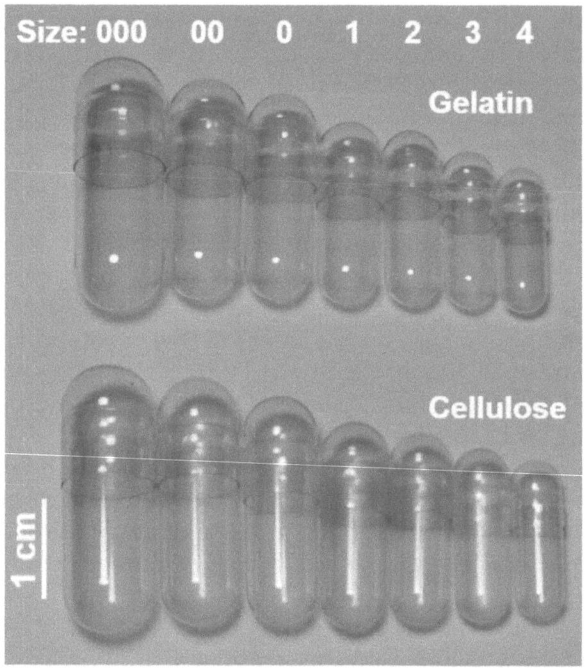

FIGURE 2.5 Hard capsules of different sizes (000 to 4). *(Top panel)*, gelatin capsules. *(Bottom panel)*, vegetable cellulose capsules. Scale bar: 1 cm.

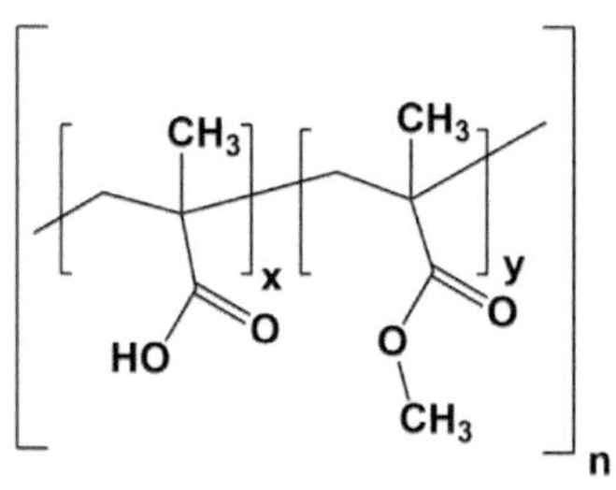

FIGURE 2.6 Chemical structure of the Eudragrit L100 and S100 for enteric coating. L100: x:y ≈ 1:1 and S100: x:y ≈1:2. The molecular mass for each is about 125,000 g/mol. The balance between the hydrophilic and pH-responsive carboxyl and hydrophobic groups, such as methyl groups, is the key.

officially released in 1954 with Eudragit L and Eudragit S as the first two polymers [poly(meth)acrylate] launched for enteric coating. Eudragit-based formulations have been developed and applied in today's methods of delivery [25].

Tablets are another commonly used drug dosage form. The modern tablet compression was believed to have been conceived in England by William Brockedon. In 1843, Brockedon invented and patented "a mode of manufacturing pills and medicated lozenges by causing the materials, when in a state of powder, granulation, or dust, by pressure in

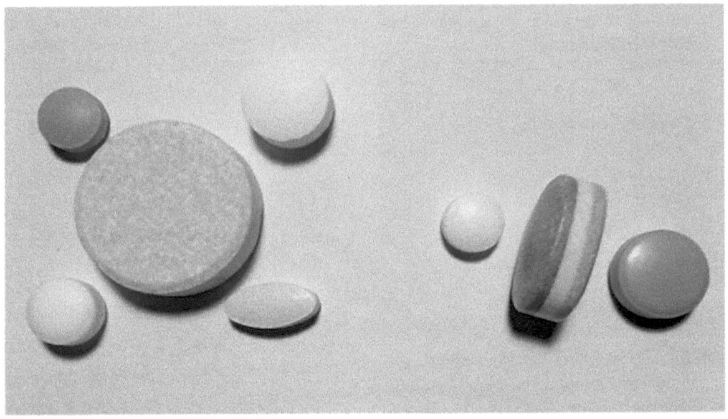

FIGURE 2.7 Examples of drug tablets of various colors, sizes, and shapes. *(Left)* Traditional tablets, including a chewable tablet *(large, orange-colored one)*. *(Right side, from left to right)* Controlled-release tablets—enteric-coated, triple-layered, and delayed-release *(from left to right)*.

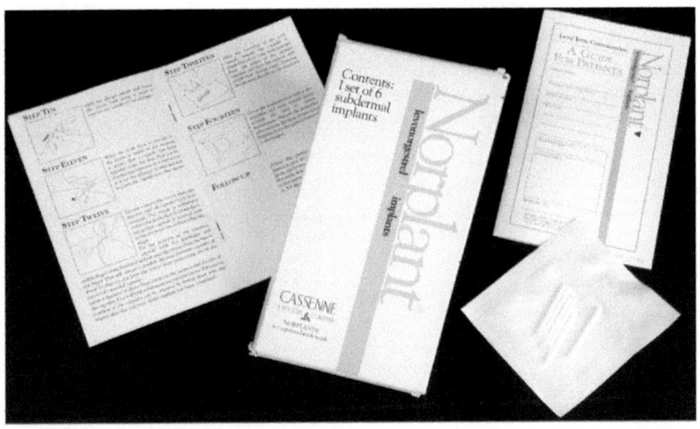

FIGURE 2.8 Packet of Norplant contraceptive implants made by Roussel Laboratories Limited. *Packet from Science Museum, London, Middlesex, England. Attribution 4.0 International (CC BY 4.0). Adapted from the Science Museum, London (https://collection.sciencemuseumgroup.org.uk/objects/co96805/packet-of-norplant-contraceptive-implants-middlesex-england-1993-contraceptive-implant).*

dies, so as to solidify the same." The first tablets produced with Brockedon's procedures contained water-soluble salts [26,27].

Liposomes, the first closed bilayer phospholipid system mimicking cell membrane structure, were described in 1965, and early pioneers, such as Gregory Gregoriadis, proposed the use of liposomes as drug carrier systems [28]. After this discovery, many other types of carriers have been developed, especially those at nano scales with the rapid development of nanotechnology.

Gale and Berggren developed the first transdermal patch (nitroglycerin patch) using a vinyl acetate rate-controlling membrane for the cessation of smoking in 1985 [29]. Around the same time, the implantable drug delivery system Norplant was developed. The first generation of Norplant delivered a daily dose of 30 μg levonorgestrel for up to 60 months for contraceptive applications [29]. Norplant was eventually removed from the U.S. market as a result of issues associated with implantation and retrieval due to operator inexperience [30].

Coronary stents were developed in the mid-1980s, and the FDA approved the use of stents to treat acute and threatened vessel closure after failed balloon angioplasties in 1994. In 1999, the first drug (sirolimus)-eluting stent was implanted in a human coronary artery [31]. The application process of drug-eluting stents is shown in Fig. 2.9. Drug-eluting stents have been found to decrease the chances of narrowing for up to a few years after initial stent implantation [32]. A long-term study indicated there were no significant differences between drug-eluting and bare-metal stents in the composite outcome of death from any cause and nonfatal spontaneous myocardial infarction, but the rates of repeat revascularization were lower in the drug-eluting stent group [33]. A more recent collaborative meta-analysis showed that the use of drug-eluting stents reduces the risk of cardiac death or myocardial infarction [34]. In particular, new-generation drug-eluting stents with increased biocompatibility and durability have shown higher efficacy and safety [35]. Drug-eluting/coated balloons delivering drugs homogeneously to the vessel wall for a short period upon inflation also show great promise [35-37].

We are witnessing the rapid development of novel drug delivery systems, such as microneedles [38], micro/nano-robotics [39], and red blood cell–based drug delivery systems [40]. Fig. 2.11 shows a few of the aforementioned novel

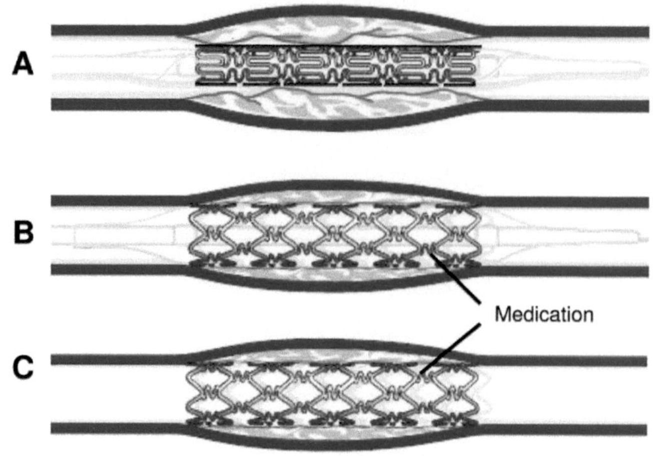

FIGURE 2.9 The application process of a drug-eluting stent. (A) The stent is mounted on a balloon catheter and advanced to the diseased, narrowed portion of the heart artery. (B) The balloon is inflated, and the stent is expanded, which opens the narrowed section of the artery. (C) The balloon is deflated and removed; the stent is embedded into the wall of the artery and stays in position. *From Maisel, W.H., and W.K. Laskey,* Drug-eluting stents. *Circulation, 2007.* ***115****(17): p. e426-427, with permission from Wolters Kluwer Health, Inc.*

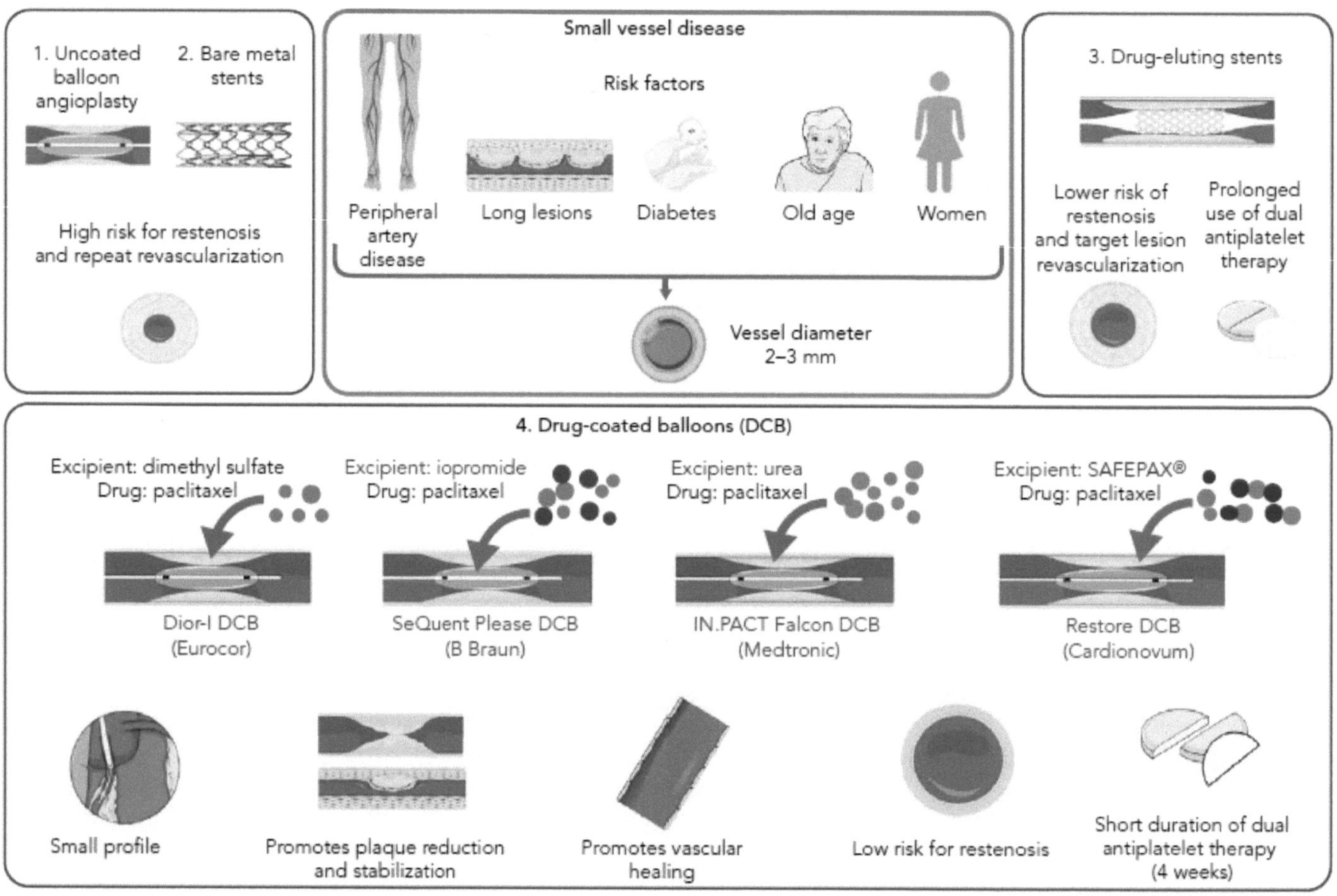

FIGURE 2.10 Percutaneous treatment of small-vessel coronary artery disease. Comparison between uncoated balloon angioplasty, bare-metal stents, drug-eluting stents, and drug-coated balloons. *From Megaly, M., M. Saad, and E.S. Brilakis,* Role of drug-coated balloons in small-vessel coronary artery disease. *US Cardiol Rev, 2019.* ***13****(1): p. 16-20, with permission from Radcliffe Cardiology.*

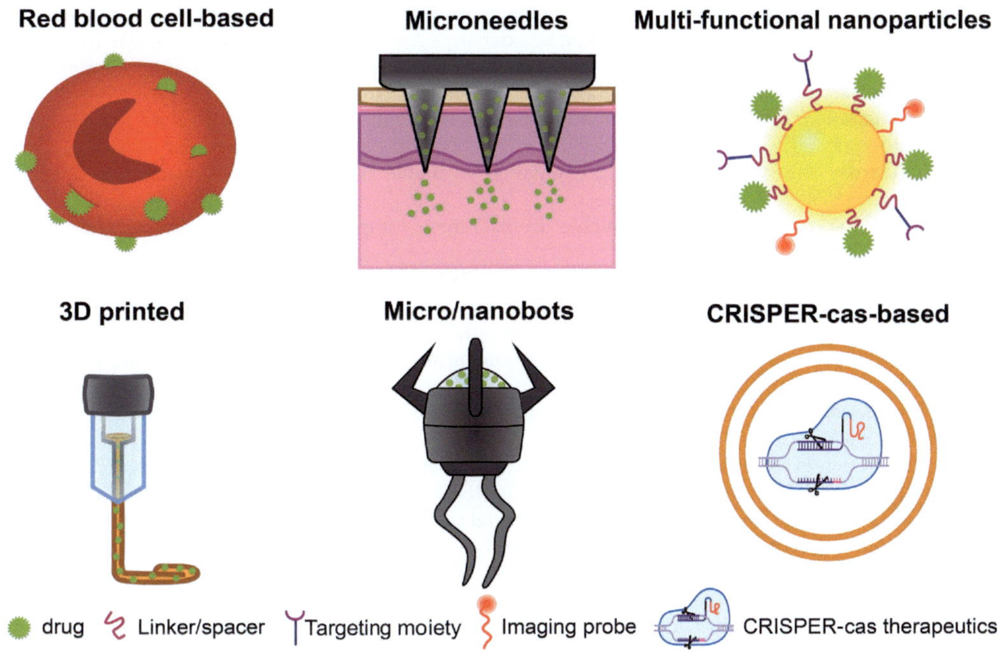

FIGURE 2.11 Examples of novel drug delivery systems.

drug delivery systems. We expect to see intelligent materials, micro/nanofluidics, additive manufacturing, CRISPR-cas gene-editing, and other advanced technologies further transform the drug delivery system development to be more personalized and intelligent [41,42].

Review and practice questions

1. Write a short essay, including a brief history, chemical structure, and working mechanism, on an active compound isolated from a medicinal plant.
2. Why are Eudragit polymers pH responsive?
3. Why are drug-eluting stents safer compared to bare-metal stents in the risk of cardiac death or myocardial infarction?

References

[1] Yuqun L. Ben Cao Gang Mu. In: Selin H, editor. Encyclopaedia of the history of science, Technology, and medicine in non-Western cultures. Dordrecht: Springer Netherlands; 2008. p. 399–400.
[2] Barrett JS. The history of drug development. In: Fundamentals of drug development; 2022. p. 5–27.
[3] Pasipoularides A. Galen, father of systematic medicine. An essay on the evolution of modern medicine and cardiology. Int J Cardiol 2014; 172(1):47–58.
[4] Levine RR, Walsh CT, Schwartz-Bloom RD. Levine's pharmacology: drug actions and reactions. Taylor & Francis e-Library; 2005.
[5] Grandjean P. Paracelsus revisited: the dose concept in a complex world. Basic Clin Pharmacol Toxicol 2016;119(2):126–32.
[6] World Health Organization. A brief history of vaccination. Available from: https://www.who.int/news-room/spotlight/history-of-vaccination/a-brief-history-of-vaccination#:~:text=From%20at%20least%20the%2015th,as%20early%20as%20200%20BCE.
[7] Isolation and Synthesis of Compounds. Available from: https://www.britannica.com/technology/pharmaceutical-industry/Isolation-and-synthesis-of-compounds.
[8] Krishnamurti C, Rao SC. The isolation of morphine by serturner. Indian J Anaesth 2016;60(11):861–2.
[9] Su XZ, Miller LH. The discovery of artemisinin and the Nobel prize in physiology or medicine. Sci China Life Sci 2015;58(11):1175–9.
[10] Zalai K. Pharmaceutical education in Central Europe: a historical view. Pharm Hist 1986;28(3):138–45.
[11] Teaching history of pharmacy according to the AIHP guidelines: D. Pharmacy Education. Available from: https://aihp.org/wp-content/uploads/2018/12/AACP-D.pdf.
[12] Alefan Q, et al. Pharmacoeconomics education in WHO Eastern mediterranean region. Curr Pharm Teach Learn 2015;7(6):819–25.
[13] About Us. Available from: https://gcp.goa.gov.in/about-us.

[14] Pohar M, Hansson N. Between two stools? Pharmacologists nominated for Nobel prizes in "physiology or medicine" and "chemistry" 1901-1950 with a focus on John Jacob Abel (1857-1938). Naunyn-Schmiedeberg's Arch Pharmacol 2021;394(3):503–13.
[15] Happy Birthday, John Jacob Abel! Available from: https://www.aspet.org/aspet/news/news/2022/05/19/happy-birthday-john-jacob-abel!
[16] Cook EF. History of the pharmacopoeia. Food, drug, cosmetic law Q 1946;1(4):518–31.
[17] U.S. Food and Drug Administration. Milestones in US Food and Drug Law. Available from: https://www.fda.gov/about-fda/fda-history/milestones-us-food-and-drug-law.
[18] From Guesswork to Standards: The History of Medicine Quality. Available from: https://www.usp.org/200-anniversary/history-of-medicine-quality.
[19] McCarthy R. Evolution of the pharmacopoeia. Available from: https://aihp.org/wp-content/uploads/2018/08/8-Evolution-of-the-Pharmacopoeia.pdf.
[20] Howard-Jones N. The origins of hypodermic medication. Sci Am 1971;224(1):96–103.
[21] Lawrence G. The hypodermic syringe. Lancet 2002;359(9311):1074.
[22] Pharmaceutical dosage forms: capsules. 1st ed. London: CRC Press; 2017.
[23] Hoag SW. Chapter 27: capsules dosage form: formulation and manufacturing considerations. In: Qiu Y, et al., editors. Developing solid oral dosage forms. 2nd ed. Boston: Academic Press; 2017. p. 723–47.
[24] Chang R-K, Raghavan KS, Hussain MA. A study on gelatin capsule brittleness: moisture transfer between the capsule shell and its content. J Pharmaceut Sci 1998;87(5):556–8.
[25] Park H, Otte A, Park K. Evolution of drug delivery systems: from 1950 to 2020 and beyond. J Control Release 2022;342:53–65.
[26] Wilkinson L, Jones RV, Paton WDM. William Brockedon, F.R.S. (1787-1854). Notes Rec R Soc Lond 1971;26(1):65–72.
[27] Skaftason JF, Jóhannesson T. [Tablets and tablet production - with special reference to Icelandic conditions]. Laeknabladid 2013;99(4):197–202.
[28] Allen TM, Cullis PR. Liposomal drug delivery systems: from concept to clinical applications. Adv Drug Deliv Rev 2013;65(1):36–48.
[29] Hashmi MP, Koester TM. Applications of synthetically produced materials in clinical medicine. In: Reference module in materials science and materials engineering. Elsevier; 2018.
[30] Major I, et al. 5 - Implantable drug delivery systems. In: Seyfoddin A, Dezfooli SM, Greene CA, editors. Engineering drug delivery systems. Woodhead Publishing; 2020. p. 111–46.
[31] Iqbal J, Gunn J, Serruys PW. Coronary stents: historical development, current status and future directions. Br Med Bull 2013;106(1):193–211.
[32] Maisel WH, Laskey WK. Drug-eluting stents. Circulation 2007;115(17):e426–7.
[33] Bønaa KH, et al. Drug-eluting or bare-metal stents for coronary artery disease. N Engl J Med 2016;375(13):1242–52.
[34] Piccolo R, et al. Drug-eluting or bare-metal stents for percutaneous coronary intervention: a systematic review and individual patient data meta-analysis of randomised clinical trials. Lancet 2019;393(10190):2503–10.
[35] Liu L, et al. Comparison of drug-eluting balloon versus drug-eluting stent for treatment of coronary artery disease: a meta-analysis of randomized controlled trials. BMC Cardiovasc Disord 2018;18(1):46.
[36] Rykowska I, Nowak I, Nowak R. Drug-eluting stents and balloons—materials, structure designs, and coating techniques: a review. Molecules 2020;25(20):4624.
[37] Megaly M, Saad M, Brilakis ES. Role of drug-coated balloons in small-vessel coronary artery disease. US Cardiol Rev 2019;13(1):16–20. 2019.
[38] Avcil M, Çelik A. Microneedles in drug delivery: progress and challenges. Micromachines 2021;12(11).
[39] Li J, et al. Micro/nanorobots for biomedicine: delivery, surgery, sensing, and detoxification. Sci Robot 2017;2(4):eaam6431.
[40] Muzykantov VR. Drug delivery by red blood cells: vascular carriers designed by mother nature. Exp Opin Drug Deliv 2010;7(4):403–27.
[41] Yi W, et al. Recent advances in developing active targeting and multi-functional drug delivery systems via bioorthogonal chemistry. Signal Transduct Target Ther 2022;7(1):386.
[42] Adepu S, Ramakrishna S. Controlled drug delivery systems: current status and future directions. Molecules 2021;26(19):5905.

CHAPTER

3

Basics of pharmacology, pharmacokinetics, and pharmacodynamics

Wujie Zhang

LEARNING OBJECTIVES

- To discuss the differences and connections between pharmacokinetics and pharmacodynamics
- To interpret a C_p-vs.-time curve and analyze the curve for a bioavailability assessment
- To describe the renal excretion process and perform related calculations
- To identify different types of phase II (conjugation) reactions
- To discuss the differences between the compartment and physiological pharmacokinetic modeling systems
- To solve zero- and first-order pharmacokinetic problems
- To differentiate between competitive and noncompetitive antagonists and distinguish between various drug antagonism mechanisms

3.1 Introduction to pharmacology, pharmacokinetics, and pharmacodynamics

Let's start with definitions. Pharmacology, from the Greek words *pharmakon* (drug, poison) and *-logia* (study of, knowledge of), is the unified study of the properties of drugs and living organisms and all aspects of their interactions [1]. The related fields of pharmacokinetics and pharmacodynamics are two of the main divisions of pharmacology (Fig. 3.1). Pharmacokinetics (in Greek *kinetikos* meaning "putting in motion" and the study of time dependency) is the science and study of the factors that determine the amount of drug at sites of biological effect at various times after applications of an agent to a biological system. It deals with the quantification of drug absorption, distribution, metabolism, and excretion (ADME) [1,2]. Pharmacodynamics (in Greek *dynamikos* means power) is the study of the actions and effects of drugs at all levels of organization of living material and the handling of the drugs by the organism [1]. Two key concepts and terms related to pharmacodynamics are E_{max} and EC_{50}. E_{max} describes the maximal effect of a drug on a parameter being measured (e.g., lower blood pressure). EC_{50} is

Fundamentals and Design of Drug Delivery Systems
https://doi.org/10.1016/B978-0-443-23521-4.00003-5

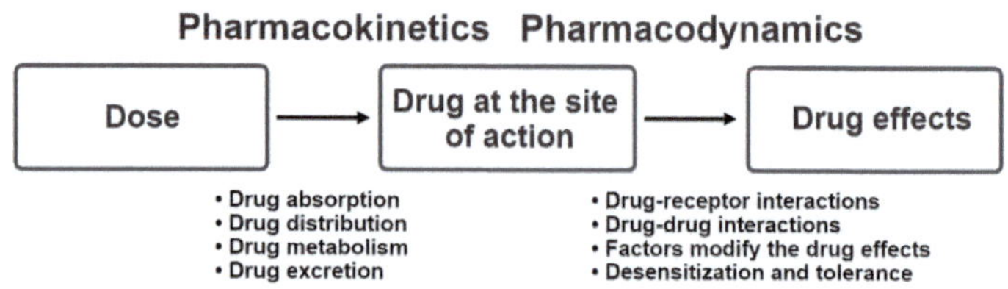

FIGURE 3.1 Relationship between pharmacokinetics and pharmacodynamics.

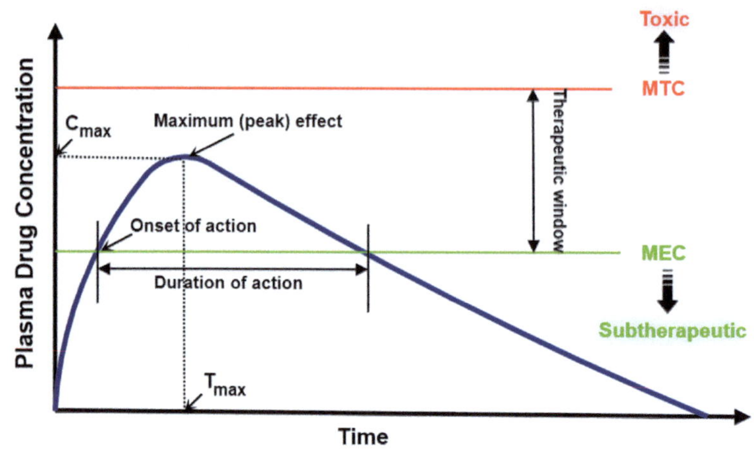

FIGURE 3.2 A typical plasma drug concentration (C_p)-vs.-time curve.

the concentration of the drug at a steady state that produces half of the maximum effect [3]. Pharmacokinetics can be simplified as studying what the body does to the drug, while pharmacodynamics answers what the drug does to the body.

In pharmacokinetics, a plasma drug concentration (C_p)-vs.-time curve is commonly used, which can be obtained by measuring the drug concentration in plasma samples at different time points. Fig. 3.2 shows a typical C_p-vs.-time curve for a drug given orally. In the beginning, the increased C_p demonstrates that absorption is the dominant process (over metabolism and excretion), followed by a decrease of C_p as the drug is eliminated due to the metabolism and excretion processes.

The area under the C_p-time curve (AUC) is a commonly used parameter as it indicates the amount of the drug that has entered systemic circulation (e.g., through absorption for oral administration) upon administration. Other terms that can be defined by using the C_p-time curve (Fig. 3.2): therapeutic window, minimum effect concentration (MEC; the lowest concentration that leads to the desired pharmacological effects), minimum toxic concentration (MTC; the lowest concentration that results in toxic effect), onset of effect, duration of action, and time of maximum (peak) concentration (T_{max}). Ideally, the C_p should be above the MEC but below the MTC (this is how we define the therapeutic window) at all times to achieve therapeutic effects without a toxic response [4]. The onset of action is the beginning of the pharmacological effect or response produced by the drug, which occurs when the C_p exceeds the MEC. The duration of action is the period for which pharmacological response is produced by the drug, which corresponds to the duration that the C_p remains above the MEC and below the MTC [5]. The T_{max} is the time required for a drug to reach its peak C_p (C_{max}). C_{max} can be estimated using the volume of distribution (V_d). V_d is an apparent (theoretical) volume that can be calculated using the dose and initial C_p (C_{p0}): $V_d = \text{dose}/C_{p0}$. For drugs given through an intravenous (IV) injection, C_{max} equals dose/V_d; otherwise, bioavailability should be considered [6].

Bioequivalence (BE) is also an important term. According to the Food and Drug Administration (FDA), two products are considered to be bioequivalent when they are equal in the rate and extent to which the active pharmaceutical ingredient (API) becomes available at the site of drug action. BE studies have been used in various situations, such as generic version manufacturing [7]. Both the European Union and the United States require the $AUC_{0\text{-}t}$ (AUC from administration to last observed concentration at time t)/$AUC_{0\text{-}\infty}$ (AUC extrapolated to infinite time), C_{max}, and such pharmacokinetic parameters for BE investigations [8,9]. The FDA considers drug products to be pharmaceutical equivalents if they meet the following three criteria: (1) they contain the same active ingredient(s); (2) they are of the same dosage form (e.g., capsule, tablet) and route of administration; and (3) they are identical in strength (amount of the active ingredient present in each dosage) or concentration. Pharmaceutically equivalent drug products may differ in characteristics such as shape, release mechanism (modified-release products include

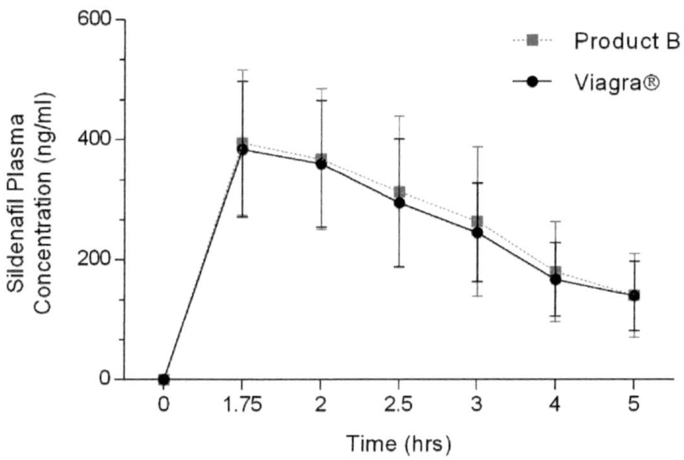

FIGURE 3.3 Comparative C_p-vs.-time curve of Viagra 100 mg and a sildenafil generic 100 mg product (product B) as a single oral dose. *From Alwhaibi, A., Alsanea, S., Alrabiah, Z. et al.,* Pharmacokinetic profile of sildenafil citrate in healthy Middle Eastern Males: Comparison with other ethnicities, 1498-1505, *Saudi Pharm J,* **29***(12), Copyright (2021), with permission from Elsevier.*

delayed-release and extended-release products), labeling (to some extent), and excipients (including colors, flavors, and preservatives) [10]. Fig. 3.3 shows an example of pharmaceutical equivalence. Drug products are considered therapeutically equivalent only if they are pharmaceutical equivalents; they are assigned by the FDA the same therapeutic equivalence codes, starting with the letter "A." To receive a letter "A," the FDA designates a brand name drug or a generic drug to be the Reference Listed Drug (RLD) and assigns therapeutic equivalence codes based on data that a drug sponsor submits in an Abbreviated New Drug Application (ANDA) to scientifically demonstrate that the product is bioequivalent (i.e., performs in the same manner as the RLD) [10]. A simple way to connect these three terms is therapeutic equivalence = pharmaceutical equivalence + BE.

Bioavailability is defined as the rate and extent to which the active ingredient or active moiety is absorbed from a drug product into the bloodstream and becomes available at the site of drug action. For drug products that are not intended to be absorbed into the bloodstream, bioavailability may be assessed by scientifically valid measurements intended to reflect the rate and extent to which the active ingredient or active moiety becomes available at the site of drug action [11]. It is a critical parameter for assessing bioequivalence. Bioavailability is measured by using three main pharmacokinetic variables: AUC, C_{max}, and T_{max}.

Sample question 3.1

A drug was given orally, and plasma drug concentrations were determined at different time points. The (C_p)-vs.-time curve is shown in Fig. 3.4A. Please show the potential curves for the same drug and the same dose given through bolus IV injection and infusion on the same curve.

Answer: Because the drug is given through bolus IV injection, the drug enters the bloodstream directly and quickly reaches the C_{max}. It takes a short time to reach C_{max} through IV infusion depending on the infusion length. The C_p decreases with time due to drug distribution, biotransformation, and excretion processes. In general, it is expected that the C_p of IV routes reaches 0 faster than the oral route since the drug elimination process becomes dominant very early on. The curves for IV injection *(red)* and infusion *(purple)* are shown in Fig. 3.4B. An example is shown in Fig. 3.5 comparing IV infusion and oral administration.

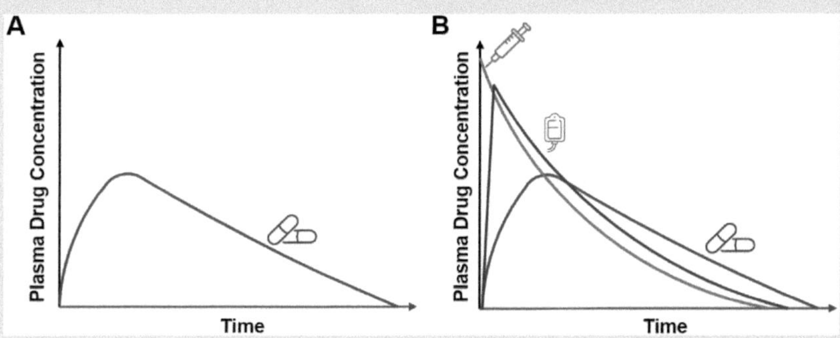

FIGURE 3.4 Comparison of C_p-vs.-time curves for the same drug (same doses) given orally and through IV injection and infusion.

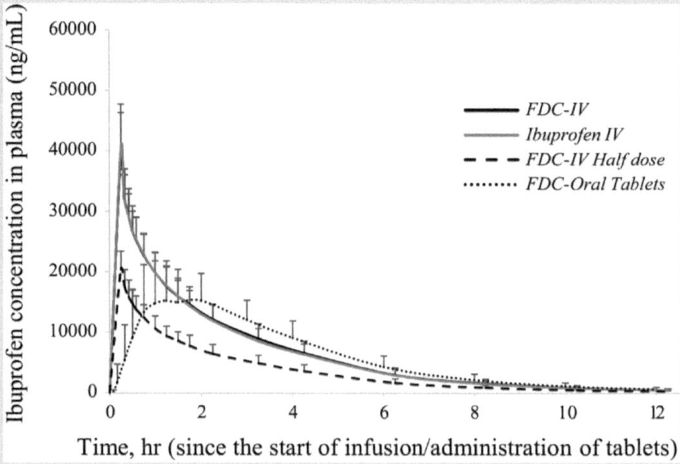

FIGURE 3.5 Plasma ibuprofen concentrations change with time. FDC-IV (3 mg/mL ibuprofen + 10 mg/mL paracetamol, 100 mL, 15 min IV infusion); FDC-IV half dose (1.5 mg/mL ibuprofen + 5 mg/mL paracetamol, 100 mL, 15 min IV infusion); and FDC-oral (ibuprofen 300 mg + paracetamol 1000 mg, 2 tablets). *From Atkinson, H.C., Stanescu, I., Frampton, C. et al.* Pharmacokinetics and bioavailability of a fixed-dose combination of ibuprofen and paracetamol after intravenous and oral administration. *Clin Drug Investig* **35**, *625–632 (2015). Available from: https://doi.org/10.1007/s40261-015-0320-8.*

Sample question 3.2

Bioavailability comparison: compare the following two C_p-vs.-time curves (Fig. 3.6A) in both C_{max} and T_{max}. Which formulation is better? I or II? Assume the same dose, administration route, and similar AUC.

Answer: It depends. First scenario (Fig. 3.6B): Formula I is preferred as II is not going to be effective (C_p below MEC). Second scenario (Fig. 3.6C): Formula II is preferred as I is going to produce toxic effects (C_p can be above MTC). Third scenario (Fig. 3.6D): Formula I is preferred for a faster onset of action.

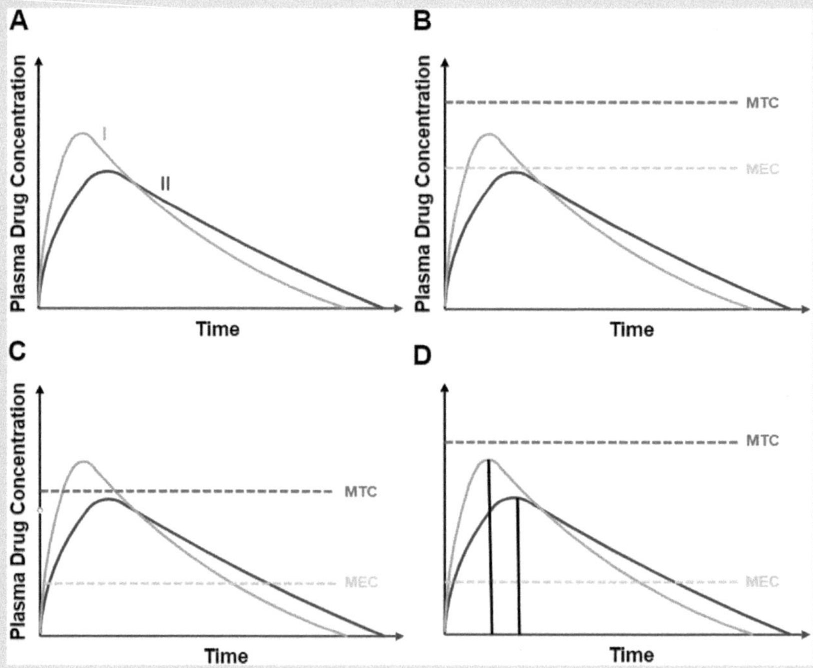

FIGURE 3.6 C_p-vs.-time curves for the same drug (same dose and same administration route) but different formulations. *MEC*, Minimum effect concentration; *MTC*, minimum toxic concentration.

3.2 Drug actions on living organisms

A drug's site of action is defined as the part of the body (organ, tissue, or cell) where a drug acts to initiate the chain of events to an effect [1]. The site of action is not always the effector site, which can be quite distant from the actual site of action. A classic example is that both atropine and morphine affect the pupillary diameter, but their sites of action are different (Fig. 3.7).

Drugs can produce their effects at extracellular, cell surface, and intracellular sites. Antacids work at extracellular sites by neutralizing gastric acid. Sodium bicarbonate and calcium carbonate are two common ingredients in antacids; they react with gastric acid (HCl) to produce H_2O, CO_2, and other substances:

$$NaHCO_3 + HCl \rightarrow NaCl + H_2O + CO_2$$

$$CaCO_3 + HCl \rightarrow CaCl_2 + H_2O + CO_2$$

Most drugs act at cellular sites, either at the cell's surface or inside the cell, and drug-receptor interaction is generally involved. The interaction requires selectivity, specificity, and reversibility. To account for the specificity, both physicochemical properties and shape are critical [1]. There are various intermolecular forces involved in drug-receptor interactions, such as electrostatic interactions, hydrophobic interactions, and van der Waals force (Fig. 3.8).

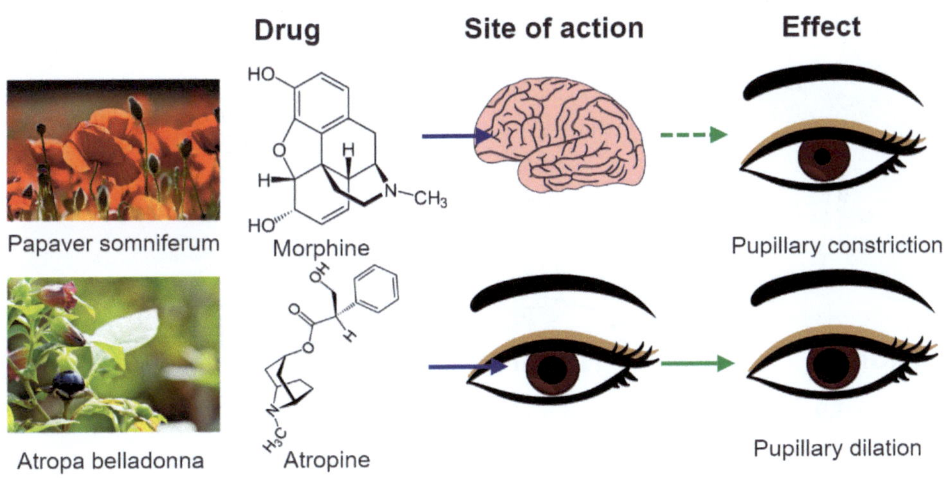

FIGURE 3.7 Sites of action of morphine and atropine on pupillary diameter. Morphine is isolated from *Papaver somniferum* (opium poppy) and atropine is extracted from *Atropa belladonna* (deadly nightshade).

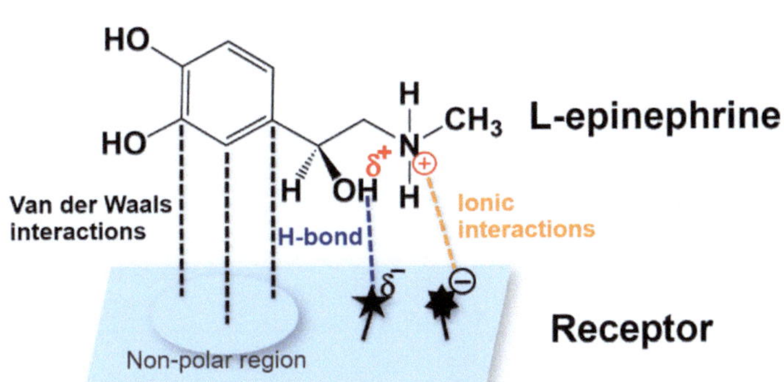

FIGURE 3.8 A model for the interactions between L-epinephrine and its receptor. The benzene ring may interact with the receptor through the van der Waals interactions, while H-bond and ionic interactions potentially account for the interaction of the hydroxyl group and the positively charged N with the receptor individually.

3.3 Termination of drug actions: excretion and metabolism

Excretion and biotransformation are the two major processes for terminating drug actions (together called elimination). Drug excretion is the removal of drugs from the body, as either a metabolite or unchanged drug. There are many different routes of excretion, including urine, bile, sweat, saliva, tears, milk, and stool [12]. The two most significant excretory organs for drugs are the kidney and liver. It is worth noting that the lungs are an important organ for excretion of gaseous substances. The liver excretes many drugs and drug metabolites into bile, such as non-steroidal anti-inflammatory drugs (NSAIDs). The bile then reaches the digestive tract and is eliminated in feces or reabsorbed through the enterohepatic cycle [13].

The basic functional unit of the kidney is the nephron (Fig. 3.9). During secretion, the drug is first filtered from the blood into the tubular lumen. The filtration rate (F; unit: mg/min) depends on the size and plasma concentration of drug molecules. Upon filtration, certain types of drug molecules can be reabsorbed (R) from the renal tubule to blood vessels, while certain types of molecules can be secreted (S) from blood directly into the renal tubules. In the end, the remaining drug molecules are excreted (E) through urine (Fig. 3.10). Hence, the excretion rate can be expressed as: $E = F - R + S$ (unit: mg/min).

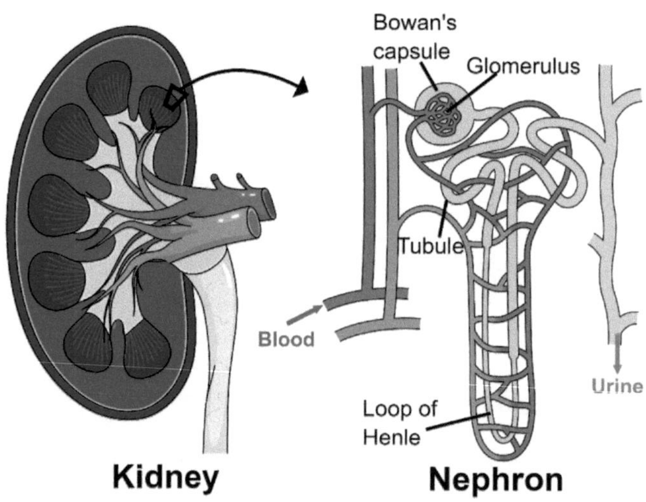

FIGURE 3.9 Structure of kidney and nephron.

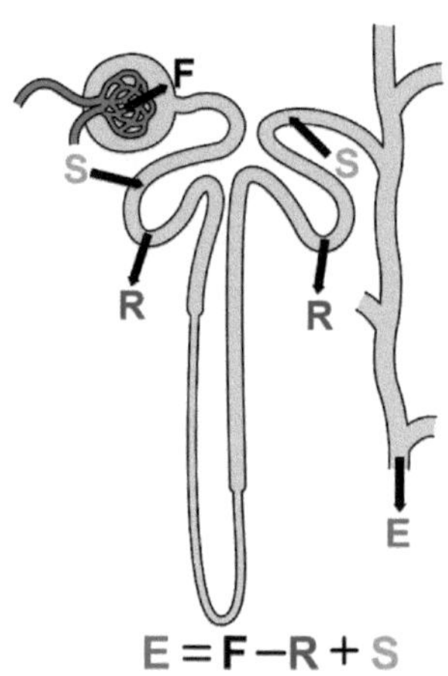

FIGURE 3.10 Relationship among filtration (F), reabsorption (R), secretion (S), and excretion (E).

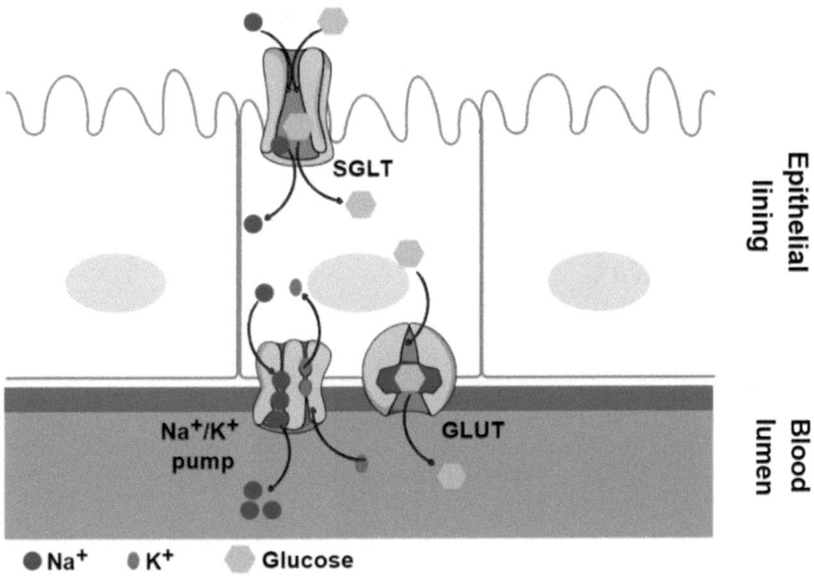

FIGURE 3.11 Glucose reabsorption mechanism in the renal tubule. *SGLT*, Sodium-glucose cotransporter; *GLUT*, glucose transport. SGLT working mechanism: Na^+ goes down its concentration gradient and generates energy to transport glucose against its concentration gradient. GLUT working mechanism: glucose goes down its concentration gradient through the carrier. The Na^+/K^+ pump helps maintain the Na^+ concentration gradient across the cell membrane for SGLT to function properly by pumping 3 Na^+ out of the cell while bringing in 2 K^+ per cycle consuming 1 ATP.

The absorption process can be extremely complex. Take glucose, for example. All the glucose molecules that are filtered are reabsorbed ($E = 0$). However, if the plasma glucose concentration is high, not all of the glucose molecules can be reabsorbed, resulting in glucose molecules being present in urine ($E > 0$). Glucose in the urine is a symptom of diabetes. The Chinese word for diabetes can be directly translated into "sweet urine disease." As far back as 1500 BCE, diabetes was documented—insects were attracted to the urine of certain individuals [14]. Examining the glucose reabsorption mechanism, sodium-glucose cotransporters (SGLTs) are involved in glucose reabsorption, while the glucose transports (GLUTs) facilitate the transportation of glucose molecules into the bloodstream. Na^+/K^+ pumps are essential as they establish the Na^+ gradient to ensure the SGLT works properly (Fig. 3.11) [15].

Renal clearance (Cl_R) is a related term to the excretion rate (E), which is defined as E/C_p (unit: mL/min). The corresponding term for the filtration rate (F) to the Cl_R is the glomerular filtration rate (GFR; $GFR = F/C_p$). GFR is a critical parameter for assessing kidney function. Inulin (polysaccharide) renal clearance can be used to determine GFR as inulin is neither reabsorbed nor secreted (i.e., $E = F$). E can be calculated using the drug concentration in urine (C_u) and the urine volumetric rate (V_u; unit: mL/min): $E = C_u \times V_u$.

Sample question 3.3

Creatinine, a breakdown product of phosphocreatine, is easily filtered but not reabsorbed and secreted during the excretion process. If the creatinine C_p and C_u are 2.0 mg/100 mL and 0.5 mg/mL urine, respectively, and the V_u is determined to be 0.75 mL/min, what is the creatinine clearance? What is its GFR?

Answer: Because $R = S = 0$, $E = F$.
Hence, Cl_R equals GFR.
$Cl_R = GFR = (C_u \times V_u)/C_p$
$= (0.5\ mg/mL \times 0.75\ mL/min)/2.0\ mg/100\ mL$
$= 18.75\ mL/min$

The liver is the most important organ in metabolism. Metabolism is a biotransformation process where endogenous (internal) and exogenous (external) compounds are converted to more polar products to facilitate their

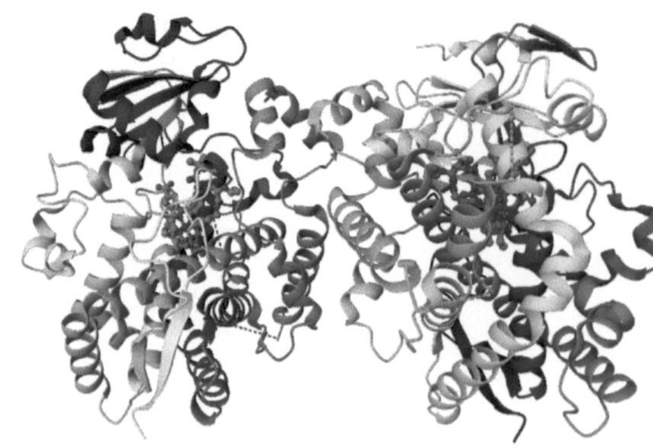

FIGURE 3.12 Crystal structure of human CYP3A4 bound to an inhibitor. Heme and inhibitors are shown in the ball-and-stick style structure. *Created with the PDB ID 6BD7 and associated publication (From Samuels, E. R., & Sevrioukova, I. (2018).* Inhibition of human CYP3A4 by rationally designed ritonavir-like compounds: impact and interplay of the side group functionalities. *Mol. Pharm,* ***15****(1), 279–288. Available from: https://doi.org/10.1021/acs.molpharmaceut.7b00957), NGL Viewer (AS Rose et al. (2018)* NGL viewer: web-based molecular graphics for large complexes. *Bioinformatics doi:10.1093/bioinformatics/bty419), and RCSB PDB.*

elimination from the body [16]. Drug metabolism involves the chemical biotransformation of drug molecules by enzymes in the body and drug transporters facilitate the movement of drugs and metabolites in and out of cells/organs [16]. Drug metabolism occurs in two phases for most drugs: phases I (modification) and II (conjugation). In some instances, phase III (additional modification and excretion) is involved [17]. These reactions can occur simultaneously or sequentially [16]. During phase I, the drug molecule is altered through oxidation, reduction, hydrolysis, or a combination of these processes. Oxidation catalyzed by the cytochrome P450 (CYP450) family is the most common phase I reaction. The name CYP450 is derived from the location where they bind to membranes within a cell (cyto) and contain a heme pigment (chrome and P) that absorbs light at a wavelength of 450 nm when exposed to carbon monoxide [18]. CYP450 enzymes are assigned a family number, a subfamily letter, and then a number for the isoform or individual enzyme, such as CYP3A4 [19]. CYP3A4 is the most abundantly expressed human CYP enzyme and metabolizes between 30% and 50% of marketed drugs [20].

Phase II reactions (conjugation reactions) mainly involve transferases. Here, glucuronide conjugation, sulfoconjugation, amino acid conjugation, acetylation, and methylation are discussed. In humans, about 40% to 70% of clinically used drugs are subjected to glucuronide conjugation (glucuronidation) [21]. Glucuronidation involves the UDP-glucuronyltransferases (UGTs) transferring a glucuronic acid from the cofactor, uridine diphosphate-glucuronic acid (UDPGA), to the substrate with functional groups, such as -OH, -COOH, and -NH_2 [22]. The glucuronidation of morphine to morphine-3-glucuronide (M3G) is shown as an example (Fig. 3.13A). Sulfoconjugation (sulfonation) is mediated by sulfotransferases (SULTs). These enzymes catalyze the transfer of sulfonate (SO_3^-) from 3′-phosphoadenosine 5′-phosphosulfate (PAPS) to the hydroxyl or amino groups of a drug [21]. A good example of sulfoconjugation is the chemical reaction of the drug minoxidil (for the treatment of male pattern baldness) shown in Fig. 3.13B. Amino acid conjugation was the first conjugation demonstrated in humans. Amino acid conjugation involves the initial formation of a xenobiotic acyl-CoA thioester, that is then conjugated principally with glycine in humans [23]. Amino acid conjugation is the most important route of detoxification, not only for many xenobiotic carboxylic acids but for endogenous acids as well [21]. Amino acid conjugation of salicylic acid is shown in Fig. 3.13C. Acetylation of amino (most common), hydroxyl, or sulfhydryl groups is catalyzed by *N*-acetyltransferases (NATs), with the acetyl group being transferred from acetyl-coenzyme A (acetyl-CoA) [24]. *N*-acetylprocainamide (NAPA) is the metabolite of procainamide (an antiarrhythmic drug) (Fig. 3.13). Methylation does not significantly change the solubility of substances. The co-factor needed for methylation is *S*-adenosyl-L-methionine (SAM; formed through the condensation of ATP and L-methionine), which becomes *S*-adenosyl-L-homocysteine (SAH) [21]. Methyl groups are generally transferred to phenol, sulfhydryl, and various amines. For example, histamine *N*-methyltransferase (HNMT) methylates the imidazole ring of histamine (Fig. 3.13E).

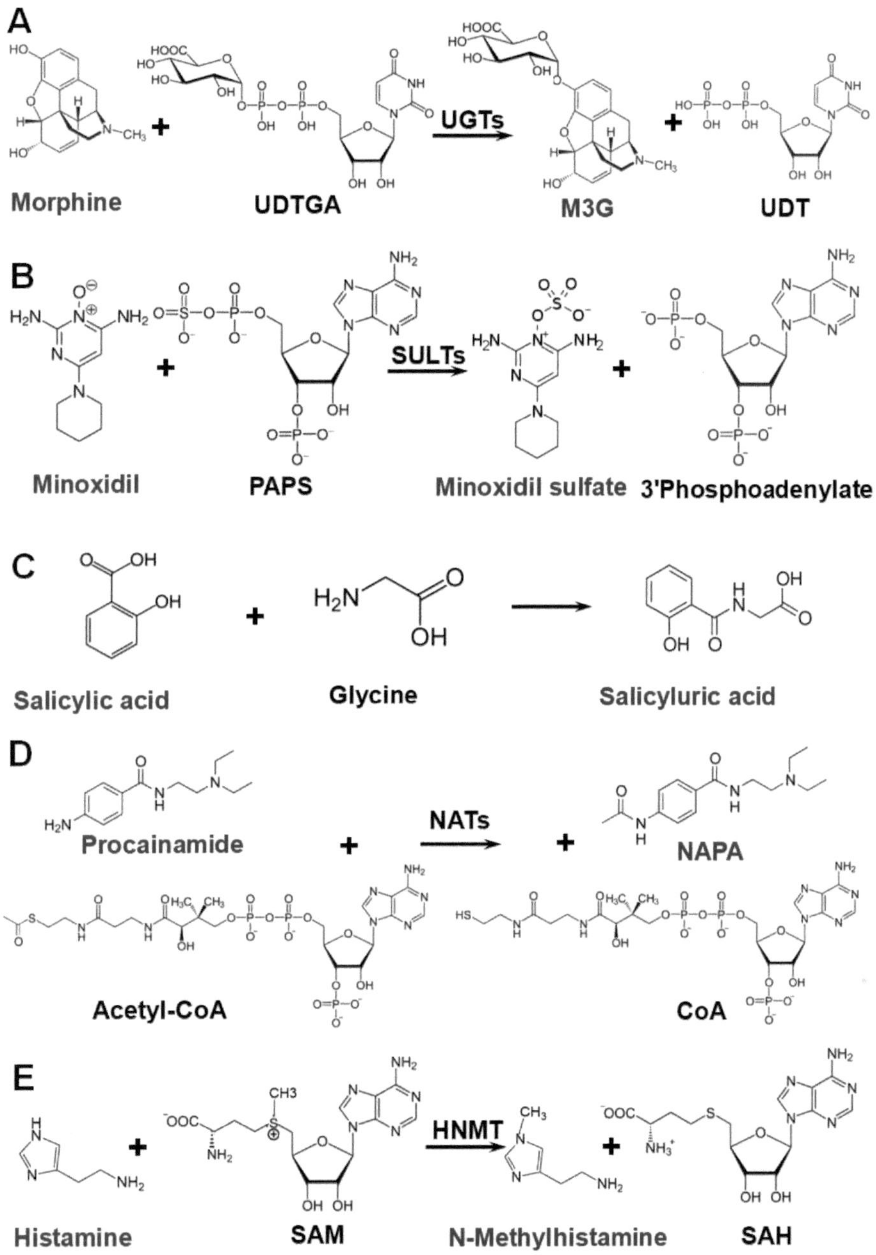

FIGURE 3.13 Examples of phase II conjugation reactions: (A) glucuronide conjugation, (B) sulfoconjugation, (C) amino acid conjugation, (D) acetylation, and (E) methylation. *UDP,* Uridine diphosphate; *UDPGA,* uridine diphosphate-glucuronic acid; *UGTs,* UDP-glucuronyltransferases; *M3G,* morphine-3-glucuronide; *SULTs,* sulfotransferases; *PAPS,* 3′-phosphoadenosine 5′-phosphosulfate; *NATs,* *N*-acetyltransferases; *CoA,* coenzyme A; *NAPA,* *N*-acetylprocainamide; *HNMT,* histamine *N*-methyltransferase; *SAM,* *S*-adenosyl-L-methionine; *SAH,* *S*-adenosyl-L-homocysteine.

3.4 Pharmacokinetics

As discussed in 3.1, pharmacokinetics focuses on the relationship between the dose and concentration of the drug-vs.-time profile at the site of action. Absorption, distribution, metabolism, and excretion processes influence the pharmacokinetics of a drug (i.e., ADME scheme; Fig. 3.14). Pharmacokinetic modeling can help describe the behavior of a drug in the body. There are different modeling systems; here, we will cover compartmental modeling and physiological modeling systems. Compartmental modeling is data-based modeling. Data (e.g., C_P vs. time) are required to determine the number of compartments needed to describe the drug's behavior in the body [25]. A one-compartment model is the simplest as it considers the whole body (tissue and fluids) as one compartment

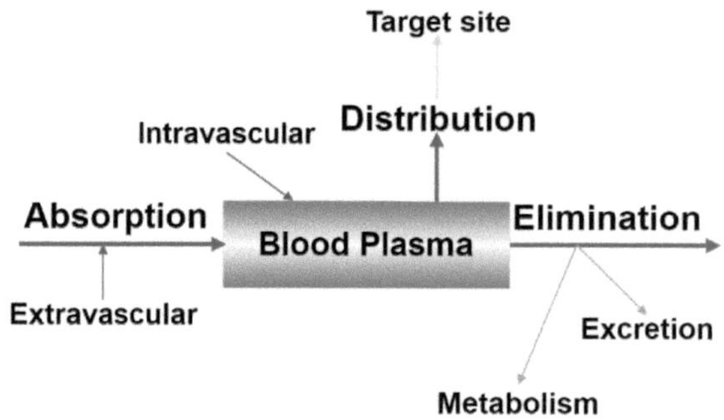

FIGURE 3.14 ADME scheme. *A*, Absorption; *D*, distribution; *M*, metabolism; *E*, excretion.

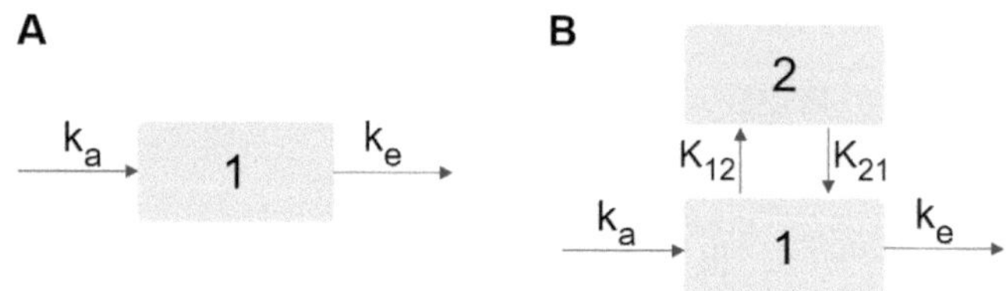

FIGURE 3.15 Comparison between one- and two-compartment models with absorption (1, central compartment; 2, peripheral compartment). k_a = absorption rate constant, and k_e = elimination rate constant.

(Fig. 3.15A). To use this model, the drug is assumed to be instantaneously distributed to the whole body upon administration and the drug equilibrates instantaneously between tissues. This does not mean $C_p = C_{tissues}$, but changes in the C_p reflect the proportional changes in $C_{tissues}$ [26, 27]. Not all drugs are distributed to all parts of the body instantaneously. Take IV injections, for example; drug distribution to the bloodstream and highly perfused organs, such as the liver and kidneys, is faster compared to other tissues/organs. A two-compartment model (Fig. 3.15B) is more appropriate as the body behaves as two different compartments: central and peripheral (or tissue) compartments. Drug elimination occurs at the central compartment because the liver and kidneys are within this compartment.

For many drugs, the absorption, distribution, metabolism, and transformation processes are either zero- or first-order processes. Hence, it is critical to discuss zero- and first-order process kinetics:

Zero-order kinetics: The rate of change of drug concentration/amount is a constant $-k$ (independent of the drug concentration/amount). Using concentration, the rate can be expressed as:

$$k = -\frac{dC}{dt}$$

$$dC = -kdt.$$

Integrating

$$\int_0^t dC = -k\int_0^t dt$$

$$C_t - C_0 = -kt$$

$$C_t = C_0 - kt.$$

A plot of C vs. time is linear, with the slope being $-k$ (k in the end is always positive) (Fig. 3.16). The unit for k is the concentration unit/time unit (e.g., mg/(mL×hr)).

It is also beneficial to express $t_{1/2}$ (half-life; the time it takes for C to decrease to half of the C_0) and t_{90} (shelf life; the time it takes for the C to decrease to 90% of the C_0).

At $t_{1/2}$ and t_{90}, $C_t = 0.5\ C_0$ and $0.9\ C_0$, respectively. Using the equation given above, we can get $t_{1/2} = \frac{0.5C_0}{k}$ and $t_{90} = \frac{0.1C_0}{k}$.

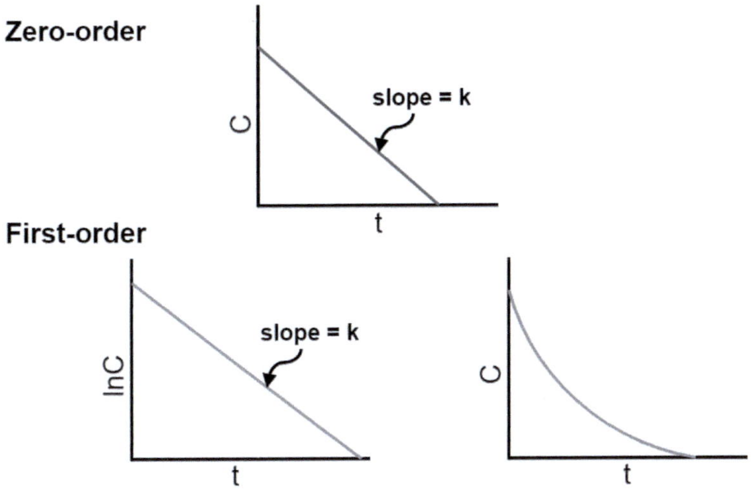

FIGURE 3.16 Plots of zero- and first-order kinetics. *C*, Concentration; *t*, time.

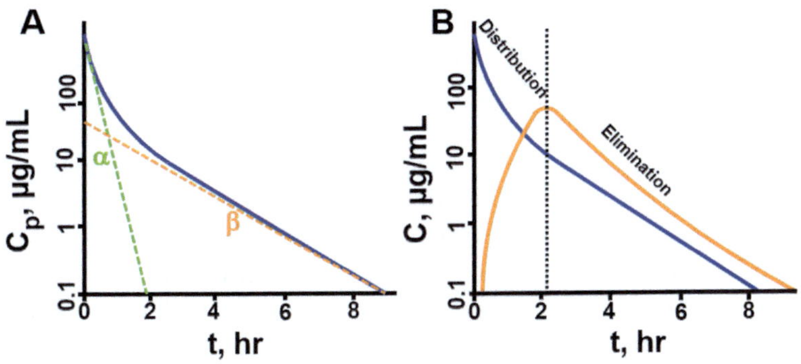

FIGURE 3.17 C_p change with time (A) and correlation (B) between C_p (*blue line*) and $C_{tissues}$ (*orange line*) for a two-compartment model (single intravenous injection). Both graphs are in a semilogarithm scale. α and β are the slopes of the *two dashed lines*. The *dashed line* in B indicates the distribution equilibrium.

First-order kinetics: The rate of change of the drug concentration/amount is proportional to the drug concentration/amount. Using concentration as an example, the first-order kinetics can be expressed as:

$$-\frac{dC}{dt} = kC$$

$$-dC/C = kdt.$$

Integrating

$$\int_0^t dC/C = -k\int_0^t dt$$

$$lnC_t - lnC_0 = -kt$$

$$lnC_t = lnC_0 - kt.$$

A plot of $\ln_{Ct}$ vs. time is linear, with the slope being $-k$ (k at the end is always positive) (Fig. 3.16). The unit for k is 1/time (e.g., 1/hr). The exponential form is also commonly used: $C_t = C_0e^{-kt}$. And the plot of C_t vs. time is exponential. Similarly, we can get $t_{1/2} = \frac{ln_2}{k} = \frac{0.693}{k}$ and $t_{90} = \frac{1n_{10/9}}{k} = \frac{0.105}{k}$.

Sample question 3.4

If the plasma $C_p = 10$ mg/L for a drug right after the IV injection. If the elimination rate of this drug is $0.15/\text{hr}^1$ (first-order process) within the patient. What would be the C_p after 10 hours?

Answer: Use the first-order kinetics equation:

$C_t = C_0 e^{-kt}$
$C_0 = 10$ mg/L
$k = 0.15/\text{hr}$
$C_t = 10\ \text{mg/L} \times e^{-(10\ \text{hr} \times 0.15/\text{hr})} = 2.23\ \text{mg/L}$

The C_p-vs.-time curve for a drug that fits a two-compartment model can be divided into two phases: distribution and elimination. Considering a drug given through an IV injection (single dose), the initial phase represents the rapid distribution of the drug from the central compartment to the peripheral compartment, while the elimination process is not dominant. At maximum tissue concentration of the peripheral compartment, the rate at which the drug enters and exits the tissues is the same. Then, the elimination phase starts, in which the drug concentration in both the central and peripheral compartments decreases, which is generally slower than the distribution phase [27]. C_p and $C_{tissues}$ decrease in parallel, and C_p provides certain information on the change of $C_{tissues}$. Considering first-order kinetics for both phases, a C_p-vs.-time curve can be described as such in Fig. 3.17A, while the correlation between C_p and $C_{tissues}$ is shown in Fig. 3.17B. Keep in mind that the maximum $C_{tissues}$ can be either higher or lower than its corresponding C_p. The relationship between C_p and t is biexponential and can be expressed as: $C_P = Ae^{\alpha} + Be^{\beta}$. A is the y-intercept of the distribution phase of the curve extrapolated to zero, and α is the slope of the line (*green dashed line* in Fig. 3.17A); B is the y-intercept of the elimination phase of the curve extrapolated to zero (*orange dashed line* in Fig. 3.17A), and β is its slope. A and B do not have physiological significance [27]. Fig. 3.18 shows the gadolinium diethylene triamine pentaacetic acid (Gd-DTPA)'s C_p-vs.-time curves of different doses. Gd-DTPA is a common exogenous paramagnetic contrast agent for MR imaging. The model shows the $C_P = 0.4 \times C_{P0}\left(e^{-(C_{P0}\alpha \times 2 \times t)} + e^{-(0.008 \times t)}\right)$ and is both time and dose dependent [28].

Physiological modeling is based on organ blood flow and the organ spaces penetrated by the drug. A physiological pharmacokinetic model considers the drug to be blood flow limited—drugs that are carried to organs by arterial blood and leave through venous blood [27]. Body compartments in physiological modeling are shown in Fig. 3.19. Each compartment represents a specific tissue/organ in the body. The transport of drugs between tissues is also described using actual physiological processes [29]. This modeling system is more complicated as prior biology/physiology information is needed, and drug physiochemical properties, such as molecular weight and solubility, are also critical for setting up the modeling system. There are professional tools for modeling, such as PK-SIM (https://www.open-systems-pharmacology.org/).

Pharmacokinetics can be either linear or nonlinear based on the dose-dependence. When considering first-order kinetics, the dose is not a factor—i.e., linear pharmacokinetics can be applied. For many drugs, such as phenytoin,

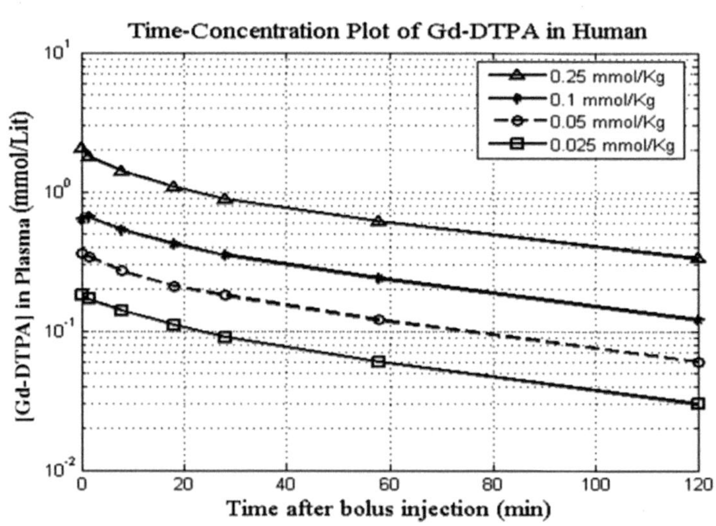

FIGURE 3.18 Gd-DTPA C_p change with time of different doses (0.025, 0.05, 0.1, and 0.25 mmol/kg) in humans. Data and *fitted curves* are for 120 min after intravenous (bolus) injection. *From Taheri, S., N.J. Shah, and G.A. Rosenberg,* Analysis of pharmacokinetics of Gd-DTPA for dynamic contrast-enhanced magnetic resonance imaging. *Magn Reson Imaging, 2016.* ***34****(7): p. 1034-1040, with permission from Elsevier.*

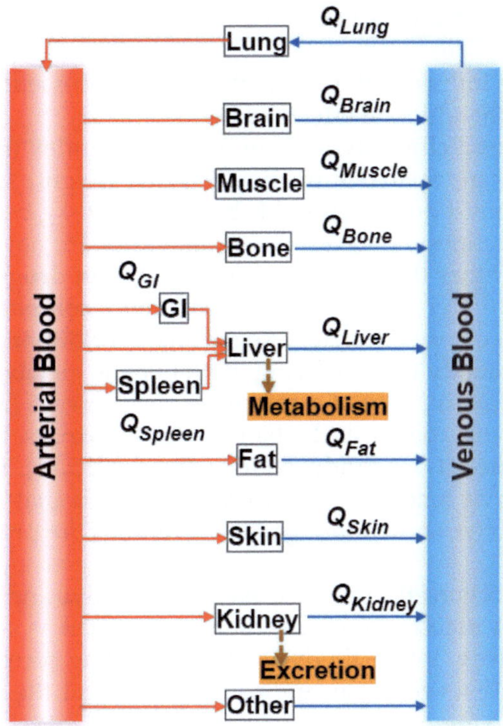

FIGURE 3.19 Blood flow to organs in a physiological model. Q, Blood flow.

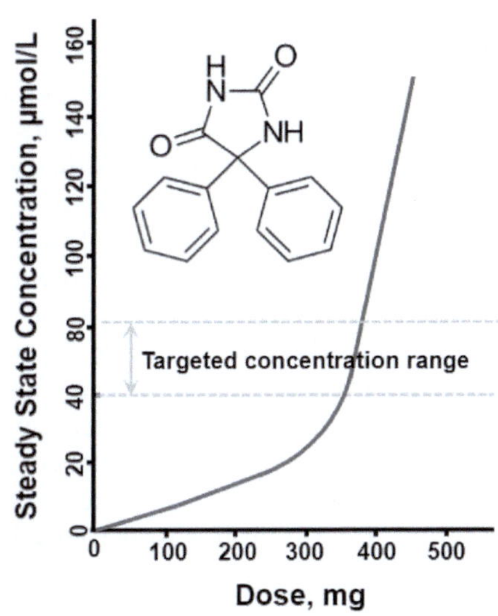

FIGURE 3.20 Steady-state phenytoin concentrations change with dose for a hypothetical patient.

nonlinear pharmacokinetics (dose-dependent) should be considered. At least one of the absorption, distribution, and elimination processes is saturable and does not follow first-order kinetics [25]. As shown in Fig. 3.20, slight increases in dosage above 300 mg can lead to great increases in the phenytoin C_p. Phenytoin is used for the management of generalized and focal seizures. The enzyme system involved in phenytoin metabolism can be saturated, resulting in a decreased elimination rate. If the enzymes are saturated, even a small increase can cause a significant rise in concentration. Individual variability may also lead to very different phenytoin concentrations, even when individuals are given the same dose. The binding of phenytoin to serum albumin is also highly variable (nonlinear). As a result, the monitoring of phenytoin dosing is critical to ensure efficacy and safety [30,31].

3.5 Factors influence the drug effects

During this section, factors that can influence the drug effects are addressed. Keep in mind that all these factors are "working" together to determine the ultimate effects of the drug.

Body size. The body size metrics used clinically include body mass index (BMI), body surface area, total body weight (TBW), lean body mass (LBM), and such (subtracting body fat weight). Generally, a higher dose is expected for a larger body size. In general, the adult dose required is based on a 70-kg body weight [1]. Some drugs, such as propofol, provide per/kg dosing guidelines; however, these guidelines are not always accurate. There are studies indicating that LBM should be used rather than TBW, at least for certain drugs, such as remifentanil. A study on remifentanil showed no appreciable difference in the pharmacokinetics comparing obese and lean subjects [32].

Age. The physiology of the body changes with aging. Regarding distribution, the volume of distribution of lipophilic drugs increases due to increased body fat with aging. Both hepatic metabolism and renal excretion are generally reduced with aging, while the bioavailability of some drugs can increase [33,34].

Gender. Gender can affect both the therapeutic and adverse effects of drugs. For example, females have a greater analgesic response but a higher incidence of drug-induced liver toxicity [35,36]. The fact is that most studies indicate females are more prone to adverse drug reactions. One of the reasons is that many clinical trials are carried out mainly on male subjects [37]. Studies have shown that gender variations are present in bioavailability, distribution, metabolism, and excretion.

Placebo and nocebo. Placebo and nocebo effects are the patients' positive and negative expectations, respectively, concerning their state of health [38]. A placebo is an inert substance (such as sugar and saline) used in controlled experiments, to test the efficacy of a drug. Interestingly, there is no strong correlation between optimism/suggestibility and placebo responsiveness. However, some studies indicated that the nocebo effect of active drug takers is more likely to happen for those who are more anxious or have greater psychological distress [38].

Genetic factors. Genetic factors can account for 20% to 95% of patient variability [39]. Genetic differences can affect drug metabolism, transport, and targets [40]. The related scientific fields are pharmacogenetics (one or more candidate genes) and pharmacogenomics (entire genome). Examining from the pharmacokinetics aspect, drug-metabolizing enzymes, such as CYP450, show very different capacities (from near absent to high activity) among different ethnic groups. Isoniazid (INH) is a common drug for tuberculosis (TB) treatment. Variations in the *N*-acetyltransferase (NAT2) affect the metabolism and disposition of isoniazid. There are three genotypes based on the molecular techniques – fast, intermediate, and slow. Slow acetylators are at risk of drug-induced adverse effects, while the fast acetylators are most likely to have reduced therapeutic effects [41]. Data from a study correlating NAT2 genotype with INH acetylation in Polish tuberculosis patients is shown in Table 3.1 (reproduced from [42]).

Abnormalities. Receptor abnormalities can also affect drug effects. Take G protein–coupled receptors (GPCRs), for example, they are the largest and most diverse group of membrane receptors and serve as the target for about one-third of the drugs on the market. Mutations can cause GPCRs to be inactive, overactive, and more [43,44] (Fig. 3.21). A study investigated the two variants of the β_1-adrenergic receptor (ADRB1; a GPCR communicating through G's alpha subunit)—ADRB1 Gly389Arg and ADRB1 Ser49Gly—and noticed that the ADRB1 Gly389Arg variant was associated with significant differences in response to therapy, but not ADRB1 Ser49Gly (Fig. 3.22). Among responders, subjects carrying the *Gly389* variant required the lowest doses of rate-controlling medications: 92 mg versus 68 mg of atenolol, 44 mg versus 20 mg of carvedilol, 80 mg versus 72 mg of metoprolol, 212 mg versus 180 mg of diltiazem, and 276 mg versus 200 mg of verapamil, respectively [45].

TABLE 3.1 Pharmacokinetic parameters of INH in plasma among fast, intermediate, and slow acetylators.

Genotype of acetylation	C_6 (μg/mL)	k_e (1/hr)	C_{max} (μg/mL)	$AUC_{0\text{-}6}$	AUC
Fast	0.27	0.51	3.39	8.60	9.20
Intermediate	0.70	0.41	5.80	15.4	17.5
Slow	2.20	0.27	7.09	24.5	35.5

C_6, Concentration of INH 6 hours after administration; k_e, elimination rate; $AUC_{0\text{-}6}$, area under the curve in the period of 0 to 6 hours.

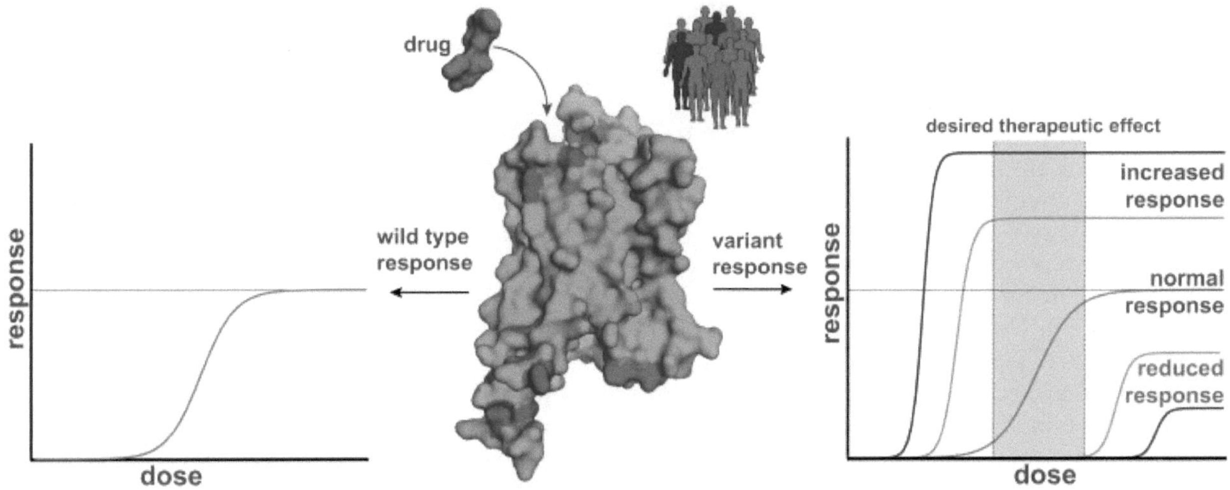

FIGURE 3.21 Differences in drug response due to different GPCR mutations between individuals in a population. *From Hauser, A.S., et al.,* Pharmacogenomics of GPCR drug targets. *Cell, 2018.* ***172****(1): p. 41-54.e19.*

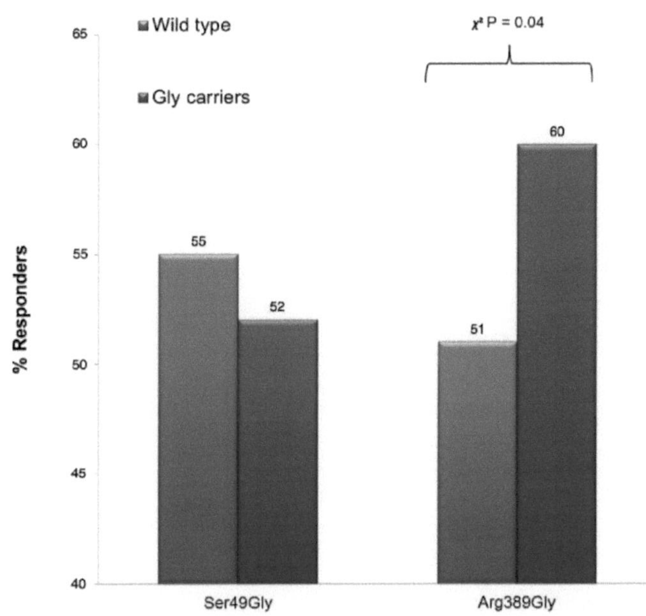

FIGURE 3.22 Percentage of patients with atrial fibrillation responded to rate-control therapy. *From Parvez, B., et al.,* A common β1-adrenergic receptor polymorphism predicts favorable response to rate-control therapy in atrial fibrillation. *J Am Coll Cardiol, 2012.* ***59****(1): p. 49-56, with permission from Elsevier.*

Drug antagonism. Drug antagonism is defined as an interaction between two or more drugs (agonist and antagonist) that have opposite effects on the body, which may block or reduce the effectiveness of one or more of the drugs. An agonist is a molecule (ligand) capable of binding to and functionally activating a target (typically a receptor) resulting in a biological response. An antagonist is a molecule that binds to a target and prevents other molecules (generally agonists) from binding [1,46,47]. Competitive antagonists are molecules (ligands) that compete with agonists for the same binding site in a receptor (or combined with adjacent sites that overlap). Noncompetitive antagonists bind to receptors and cause them to become functionally inoperative, either by preventing the agonist from binding or through some other pathways to reduce the agonist's effects, such as channel blockage (i.e., with or without any effect on the binding of the agonist to the receptor) [47,48]. A competitive antagonist's binding to the receptor is generally reversible, and it can be displaced by an excess of the agonist. The extent of the reversibility is affected by the relative concentrations of agonists to competitive antagonists, association/dissociation rate constants, and the duration of exposure. However, the effects of a noncompetitive antagonist cannot be overcome simply by increasing the concentration of the agonist. To be able to further differentiate competitive antagonists from noncompetitive antagonists, we must introduce the terms potency, maximal effect, and EC_{50} or ED_{50}. Potency is an expression of the activity of a drug, in terms of the concentration or amount (dose) needed to produce a defined effect. It is sometimes incorrectly used to indicate the maximum effect attainable. The maximal effect of an agonist is the maximal effect it can elicit in a given tissue/organ under particular conditions. EC_{50}/ED_{50} is the molar concentration/dose of an agonist that produces 50% of the maximal effect of that agonist [47]. Typically, a concentration/dose (logarithm)-effect plot is used to show the effects of antagonists (Fig. 3.23). A recent study reported a potential synthetic opioid rescue agent (compound 29). The results of the antagonism of compound 29 against oxycodone-induced antinociception are shown in Fig. 3.24 [49].

Finally, to put the mechanisms of drug antagonism into perspective. They can be classified as pharmacologic antagonism, physiologic antagonism, biochemical antagonism, and chemical antagonism [1]. As shown in Fig. 3.25, physiologic antagonism occurs when agonists and antagonists work on different sites (such as receptors), and the counteractive effects of the antagonist result in a reduced net effect of the agonist. Pharmacologic antagonism occurs when the antagonist competes with the agonist for the same binding site, preventing the binding of the agonist to its receptor. Biochemical antagonism is the reduction of the agonist's availability to its target site. Chemical reactions occur between agonist and antagonist, forming an inactive product during chemical antagonism.

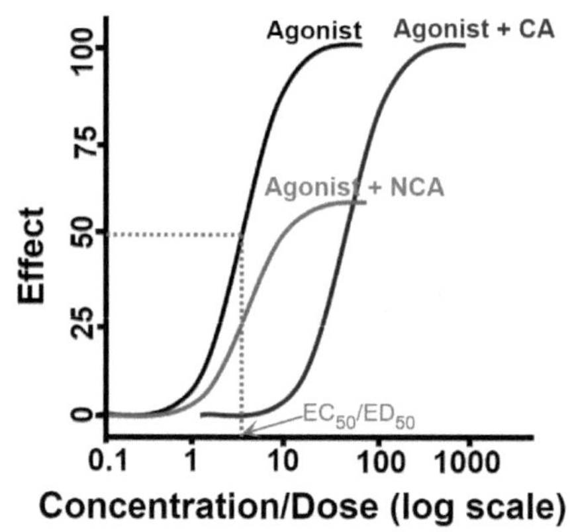

FIGURE 3.23 A typical agonist molar concentration/dose-effect plot to show the effects of antagonists. *CA*, Competitive antagonist; *NCA*, noncompetitive antagonist.

FIGURE 3.24 Dose-dependence of antagonist effects of compound 29 (0.01 to 0.1 mg/kg), administered 30 min before oxycodone (5.6 mg/kg). *PT*, Pretreatment; *MPE*, maximum possible effect. *From Hedrick, S.L., et al.,* Design, synthesis, and preliminary evaluation of a potential synthetic opioid rescue agent. *Am. J. Biomed. Sci,* 2021. *28(1): p. 62.*

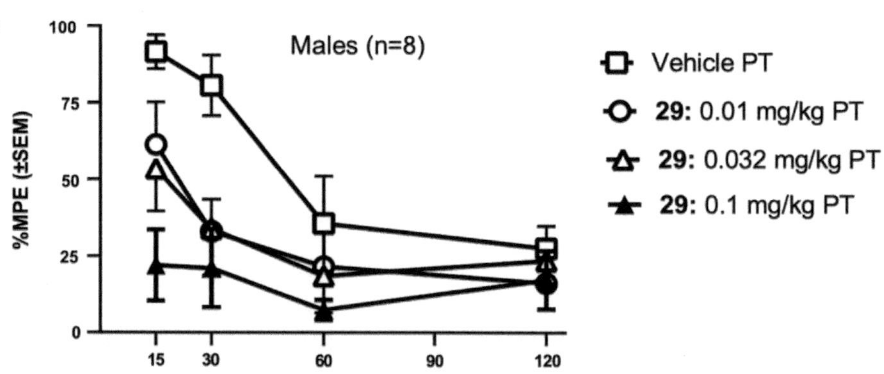

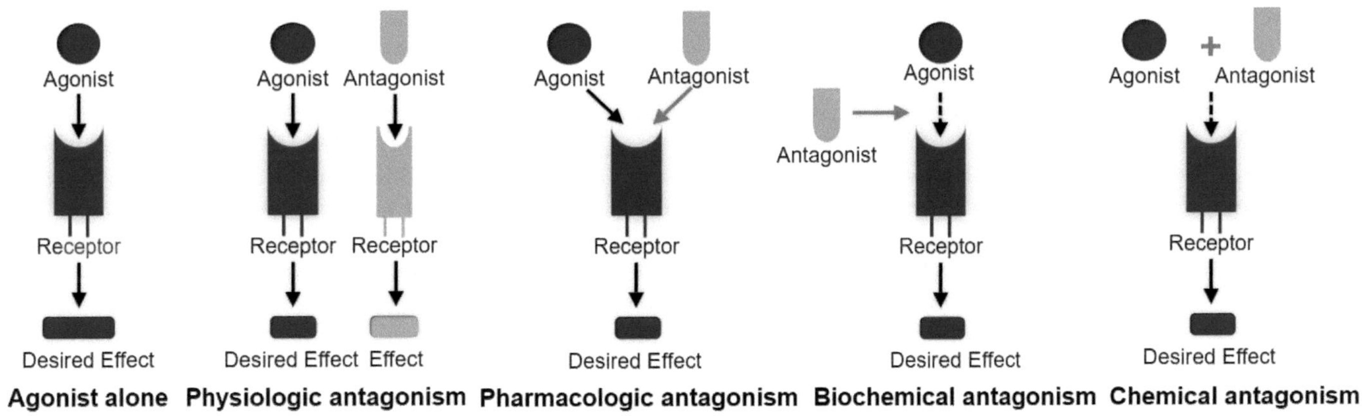

FIGURE 3.25 Mechanisms of drug antagonism. The desired effect is reduced during different types of antagonism.

Case Study I: Bioequivalence dilemma

Bioequivalent and even therapeutic equivalent drugs can have different release mechanisms. However, the parameter T_{max} (the time to maximal concentration) has been historically ignored when comparing bioequivalence [50]. A good example of this is between the antidepressant drugs Wellbutrin XL vs. Budeprion XL (generic). After switching from Wellbutrin XL to the generic Budeprion XL, patients started experiencing "headaches, anxiety, depression, and sleeplessness." As shown in Fig. CS 3.1, even having similar AUCs, the absorption rates and T_{max} for those drugs are very different, and the generic brand shows a more immediate-release formula-like profile [50]. In 2012 the FDA announced that "Budeprion XL 300 mg fails to demonstrate therapeutic equivalence to Wellbutrin XL 300 mg."

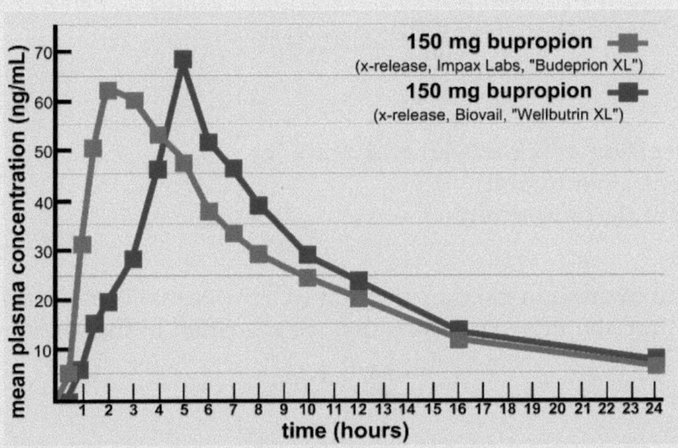

FIGURE CS 3.1 Mean bupropion (Budeprion XL and Wellbutrin XL) C_p-vs.-time curves—a "bioequivalency" profile comparing 150 mg extended-release bupropion. From CMBJ, CC BY 3.0, via Wikimedia Commons.

Lab activity II: Drug stability

The stability of a drug is of great importance. First, it becomes less effective as the drug undergoes degradation. Second, drug decomposition may yield unfavorable toxic byproducts [51]. In this experiment, aspirin's stability, which undergoes hydrolysis to form products of salicylic acid and acetic acid, will be studied. The objectives of this experiment are to:

(1) Learn how to determine drug stability and classify reactions as zero-, first-, and second-order reactions and their corresponding reaction rates.
(2) Perform the degradation study and analyze the results.

Background

Today, aspirin (acetylsalicylic acid) is one of the most widely used medications in the world. It is a salicylate drug often used as an analgesic to relieve minor aches and pains, as an antipyretic to reduce fever, and as an anti-inflammatory medication. Aspirin was first isolated by Felix Hoffmann, a chemist with the German company Bayer in 1897 [52].

Aspirin blocks the production of prostaglandins that cause inflammation, swelling, pain, and fever by inhibiting cyclooxygenase (prostaglandin H synthase; COX) [53]. Aspirin has also been used to reduce the risk of myocardial infarction and stroke [54]. Low-dose aspirin is used to decrease its gastrointestinal side effects, such as stomach bleeding. Interestingly, no significant differences were observed in the primary effectiveness or safety outcomes between 325 mg and 81 mg dosing strategies among patients with atherosclerotic cardiovascular disease [55]. Some studies have shown that long-term use of low-dose aspirin can reduce the risk of certain types of cancers [56]. Researchers have also demonstrated that aspirin use may improve bladder and breast cancer survival [57]. On the contrary, some studies did not show the benefits of aspirin. For example, a recent study reported the use of aspirin might not decrease the 5-year esophageal cancer mortality rate [58].

Aspirin hydrolyzes into salicylic acid (SA) and acetic acid (Fig. LII.1):

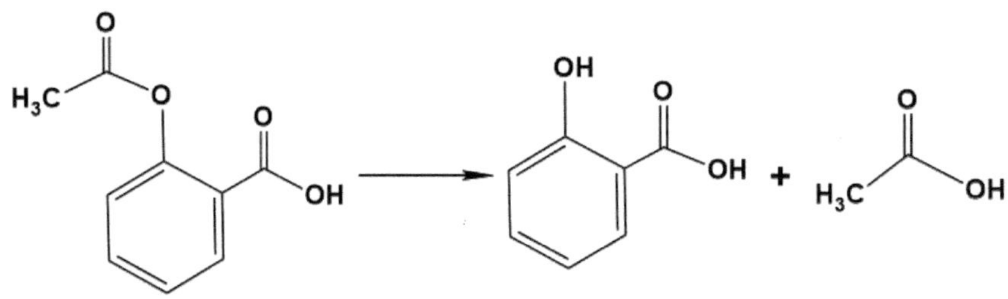

FIGURE LII.1 Hydrolysis of aspirin.

The rate of this reaction is second-order since it is dependent on both the aspirin concentration and solution pH.

$$\frac{-d[A]}{dt} = k[A][OH^-]$$

where,

[A] = the concentration of aspirin (acetylsalicylic acid) (mol/L)
$[OH^-]$ = hydroxyl ion concentration (mol/L)
k = second-order rate constant (L/(min•mol))
t = time (min).

If the solution is buffered, the hydroxyl ion concentration ($[OH^-]$) remains essentially constant. Also, replacing the concentration with the amount, the rate expression may be rewritten in the form:

$$\frac{-dA}{dt} = k'A$$

where,

A = mass of aspirin (mg)
k' (pseudo first-order rate constant; unit: min^{-1}).

From the above equation, it can be concluded that the degradation of aspirin in a buffered solution follows first-order kinetics ($k' = k[OH^-]$). Upon integration, the equation can be expressed as:

$$ln\ A_t = ln\ A_0 - k't$$

where,

A_t = mass of aspirin remaining at time t (mg)
A_0 = mass of aspirin initially present (mg).

Plotting lnA_t versus t should yield a straight line with a negative slope equal to $-k'$. To determine A_t, the amount of salicylic acid generated can be used. 1 mol aspirin (M_w = 180.16 g/mol) degrades into 1 mol salicylic acid (M_w = 138.12 g/mol) and 1 mol acetic acid. Hence, 1 mg of salicylic acid produced indicated the degradation of 1.30 mg (i.e.,

180.16/138.12 = 1.30) of aspirin. To determine the k' of aspirin at a specific temperature, the calculation process shown in Fig. LII.2 can be followed.

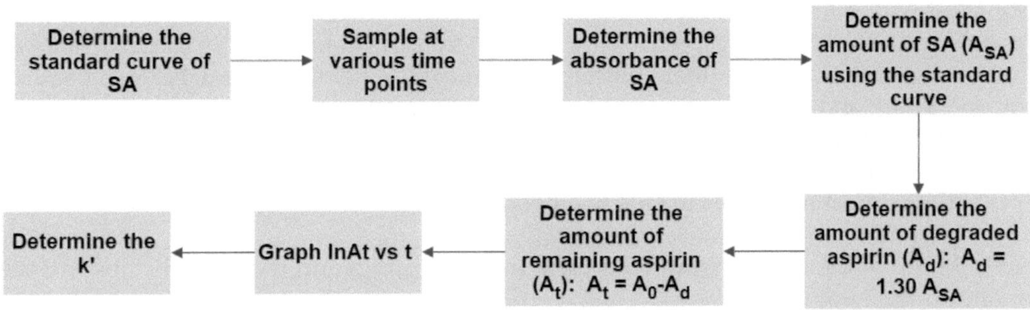

FIGURE LII.2 Calculation process for determining the k' of aspirin in a buffered solution at a specific temperature.

k' is temperature dependent. It is expected that k' increases with temperature. The famous Arrhenius equation can be used:

$$k' = \alpha e^{\frac{-E_a}{RT}}$$

where,

α = frequency constant (min^{-1})
E_a = activation energy (cal/mol)
R = gas constant (1.987 cal/(K•mol))
T = absolute temperature (K).

Upon integration, the equation can also be rewritten as seen below. There is a linear relationship between lnk′ and 1/T.

$$ln\,k' = ln\,\alpha - \frac{E_a}{R}\cdot\frac{1}{T}$$

Materials and Instruments

Aspirin
Salicylic acid
Phosphate buffer solution (pH 7.2-7.4)
Methanol
UV spectrophotometer
Hot plate

Laboratory Procedure

1. *Standard Curve*
   1. Prepare a standard curve of salicylic acid (0–0.1 mg/mL).
      Q1: What solution should be used to make the standard curve of salicylic acid?
   2. Using the UV spectrophotometer, measure the absorbance of each concentration of salicylic acid. Record the results in Table LII.1.
      Q2: What wavelength should be used to measure the absorbance? How is that determined?
   3. Make a plot of concentration vs. absorbance. Determine the slope, intercept, and R^2.

TABLE LII.1 Absorbance of SA in given concentrations.

Concentration of SA (mg/mL)	Absorbance

2. *Hydrolysis of Aspirin*

   Notes: 1. Each team performs the experiment at the temperature assigned, and data for different temperature runs are shared among teams.

   2. Since aspirin begins to degrade right after being added to water, it is important to take your initial sample quickly.

   1. Add approximately 120 mL of phosphate buffer solution (pH = 7.2–7.4) into a 125 mL flask, cover the flask opening with parafilm, and then place it on a hot plate (gently stir at 300 rpm).
      Q3: How is a constant temperature environment set up?
   2. Weigh 200 mg of aspirin and add it to a 15-mL centrifuge tube. Add 2.0 mL of methanol to dissolve the aspirin. Invert the centrifuge tube many times to ensure a good mixture. Transfer the aspirin solution to the flask when the desired temperature is reached.
   3. Pipette exactly 1.0 ml of the sample from your flask (i.e., sampling) and measure the absorbance. This sample will correspond to time point zero.
      Q4: Should the absorbance be measured directly, or does the sample need to be further diluted? What is the major factor that determines this? If dilution is needed, what solution should be used?
   4. Continue to pipette and analyze 1 mL samples from the buffer solution every 10 to 15 minutes for 60 minutes. Do not remove the flask when sampling, so the temperature remains stable. Do not forget to record your data (Table LII.2).

TABLE LII.2 Experimental data: absorbance change with time.

Temperature =	
Time (min)	**Absorbance**

   5. Obtain the results from your classmates (data obtained at different temperatures).

3. *Data Analysis*
   1. Plot $\ln A_t$ vs. time for each temperature and determine the k' for each temperature using Fig. LII.2.
   2. Construct a plot by graphing $\ln k'$ vs. $1/T$. Find the slope and intercept. The slope will be equal to $-E_\alpha/R$, and the intercept will be equal to $\ln\alpha$.
   3. Determine the E_α and α of aspirin in a buffered solution.
      Q5: At T = 300 K, how long does it take to reach $A_t = 0.1\ A_0$?

Review and practice questions

1. What are pharmacokinetics and pharmacodynamics? How are they different from each other?
2. Determine the C_{max}, T_{max}, and AUC from the figure shown below.

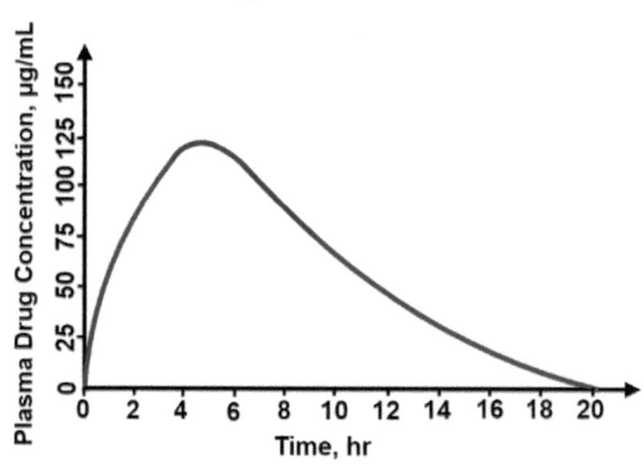

3. The C_p-vs.-time profile after a single dose (200 mg) of a drug was plotted, and the *y*-intercept was determined to be 7.5 mg/L.
   a. What is the estimated C_{max} if the drug is given through an IV injection?
   b. Calculate the dose that should achieve an initial drug concentration of 10 mg/L. Hint: Determine the V_d of this drug first.
4. How are bioequivalent, pharmaceutical equivalent, and therapeutic equivalent related?
5. Predict the potential interactions between acetylcholine (shown below; neurotransmitter) and its receptor.

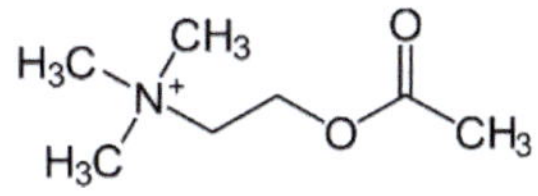

6. You are studying a newly formulated drug X and have obtained the following information relating to how it is excreted by the kidney:

$$C_p = 60\ \text{mg}/100\ \text{mL};\ R = 71\ \text{mg/min};\ V_u = 1\ \text{mL/min}$$

You also noticed that if the tubular secretion of drug X is blocked using an inhibitor (assume 100% inhibition), drug X C_u decreases from 15 mg/mL to 1 mg/mL.
   a. What is the renal clearance of drug X in the presence of its inhibitor?
   b. What is drug X's GFR?
   c. What is the secretion rate of drug X in the absence of its inhibitor?
   d. What is the renal clearance of drug X in the absence of its inhibitor?
7. What transporters are involved in glucose reabsorption, and how do they work together?
8. A mouse species has a loss-of-function mutation in the renal epithelial glucose transporter, and only half the normal number of these transport proteins are present. On the graph of the kidney function below, indicate the new filtration, reabsorption, and excretion trends for this mutant species. The filtration (blue dashed line) and reabsorption (green solid line) trends for the wild-type mice are shown.

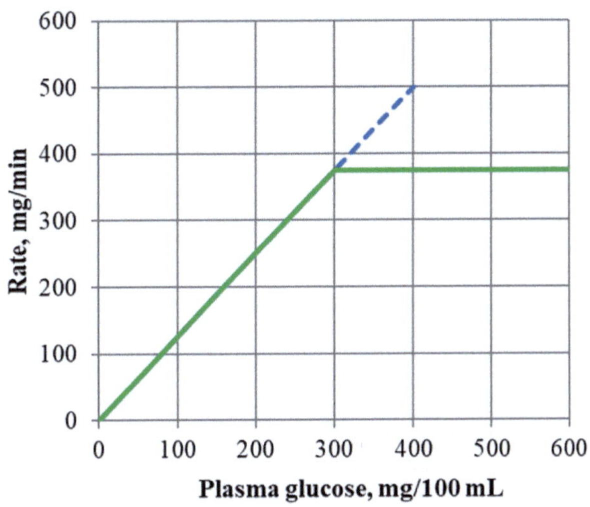

9. Show the possible structures of salicylic acid after glucuronidation.
10. Draw the structure of the metabolite of the drug structure shown below after methylation (conjugation).

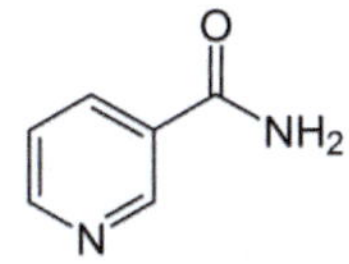

11. Why is pharmacokinetic compartment modeling a data-based modeling system?

12. A drug suspension (100 mg/mL) degrades by zero-order kinetics with a degradation rate constant of 0.1 mg/mL/hr.
   a. What is the concentration of intact drug remaining after 5 days?
   b. How long will it take for the suspension to reach 90% of its original concentration?

13. What are the factors that can influence the drug effects? List at least five of them.

14. How do G protein–coupled receptors work?

15. What are the differences between physiologic, pharmacologic, biochemical, and chemical antagonism?

References

[1] Levine RR, Walsh CT, Schwartz-Bloom RD. Levine's pharmacology: drug actions and reactions. Taylor & Francis; 2005.
[2] Wolff K. Pharmacokinetics. In: Stolerman IP, Price LH, editors. Encyclopedia of psychopharmacology. Springer Berlin Heidelberg; 2015. p. 1280–91.
[3] Marino M, Jamal Z, Zito P. Pharmacodynamics. StatPearls [Internet]. StatPearls Publishing; 2022.
[4] Boussery K, Belpaire FM, Van de Voorde J. Chapter 23: Physiological aspects determining the pharmacokinetic properties of drugs. In: Wermuth CG, et al., editors. The practice of medicinal Chemistry. 4th ed. Academic Press; 2008. p. 539–59.
[5] Gupta PK. Chapter 2 - Disposition. In: Gupta PK, editor. Illustrated toxicology: with study questions. Academic Press; 2018. p. 67–106.
[6] Lea-Henry TN, et al. Clinical pharmacokinetics in kidney disease: fundamental principles. Clin J Am Soc Nephrol 2018;13(7).
[7] U.S. Food and Drug Administration. Bioequivalence. Available from: https://www.fda.gov/animal-veterinary/abbreviated-new-animal-drug-applications/bioequivalence.
[8] Guideline on the investigation of bioequivalence. European Medicines Agency; 2010.
[9] CVM GFI #35 bioequivalence guidance. U.S. Food and Drug Administration; 2006.
[10] U.S. Food and Drug Administration. Drugs@FDA glossary of terms. Available from: https://www.fda.gov/drugs/drug-approvals-and-databases/drugsfda-glossary-terms#equivalents.
[11] U.S. Food and Drug Administration. Orange book preface. Available from: https://www.fda.gov/drugs/development-approval-process-drugs/orange-book-preface#TEC.
[12] Lu J-D, Xue J. Chapter 101: Poisoning: kinetics to therapeutics. In: Ronco C, et al., editors. Critical care nephrology. 3rd ed. Elsevier; 2019. p. 600–629.e7.
[13] Garza AZ, Park SB, Kocz R. Drug elimination. In: StatPearls [Internet]. StatPearls Publishing; 2022.
[14] Das A, Shah S. History of diabetes: from ants to analogs. J Assoc Physicians India 2011;59(Suppl. l):6–7.
[15] Jung CH, Jang JE, Park J-Y. A novel therapeutic agent for type 2 diabetes mellitus: SGLT2 inhibitor. Diabetes Metab J 2014;38(4):261–73.
[16] Almazroo OA, Miah MK, Venkataramanan R. Drug metabolism in the liver. Clin Liver Dis 2017;21(1):1–20.
[17] Susa ST, Preuss CV. Drug metabolism. In: StatPearls [Internet]. StatPearls Publishing; 2022.
[18] Lynch T, Price A. The effect of cytochrome P450 metabolism on drug response, interactions, and adverse effects. Am Fam Physician 2007; 76(3):391–6.
[19] McDonnell AM, Dang CH. Basic review of the cytochrome p450 system. J Adv Pract Oncol 2013;4(4):263–8.
[20] Urquhart BL, Nolin TD. Chapter 63: Drug metabolism in chronic kidney disease. In: Kimmel PL, Rosenberg ME, editors. Chronic renal disease. 2nd ed. Academic Press; 2020. p. 1035–51.
[21] Jančová P, Šiller M. Ch. 2 Phase II drug metabolism. In: Paxton J, editor. Topics on drug metabolism. IntechOpen; 2012.
[22] Testa B. 5.06 - Principles of drug metabolism 2: Hydrolysis and conjugation reactions. In: Taylor JB, Triggle DJ, editors. Comprehensive medicinal Chemistry II. Elsevier; 2007. p. 133–66.
[23] Knights KM, Sykes MJ, Miners JO. Amino acid conjugation: contribution to the metabolism and toxicity of xenobiotic carboxylic acids. Expert Opin Drug Metab Toxicol 2007;3(2):159–68.
[24] Rourke JL, Sinal CJ. Biotransformation/metabolism. In: Wexler P, editor. Encyclopedia of toxicology. 3rd ed. Academic Press; 2014. p. 490–502.
[25] Hedaya MA. Basic pharmacokinetics. 2nd ed. CRC Press; 2012.
[26] Dhillon S, Gill K. Basic pharmacokinetics. In: Clinical pharmacokinetics. Pharmaceutical Press; 2006.
[27] Shargel L, Yu ABC, Wu-Pong S. Applied biopharmaceutics & pharmacokinetics. Applied biopharmaceutics and pharmacokinetics. 6th ed. McGraw-Hill Medical; 2012.
[28] Taheri S, Shah NJ, Rosenberg GA. Analysis of pharmacokinetics of Gd-DTPA for dynamic contrast-enhanced magnetic resonance imaging. Magn Reson Imaging 2016;34(7):1034–40.
[29] Byers JP, Sarver JG. Chapter 10 - Pharmacokinetic modeling. In: Hacker M, Messer W, Bachmann K, editors. Pharmacology. Academic Press; 2009. p. 201–77.
[30] Wu MF, Lim WH. Phenytoin: a guide to therapeutic drug monitoring. Proceedings of Singapore Healthcare 2013;22(3):198–202.
[31] ter Heine R, et al. Nonlinear protein binding of phenytoin in clinical practice: development and validation of a mechanistic prediction model. Br J Clin Pharmacol 2019;85(10):2360–8.
[32] Egan TD, et al. Remifentanil pharmacokinetics in obese versus lean patients. Anesthesiology 1998;89(3):562–73.
[33] Shi S, Klotz U. Age-related changes in pharmacokinetics. Curr Drug Metab 2011;12(7):601–10.
[34] Midlöv P. Pharmacokinetics and pharmacodynamics in the elderly. OA Elderly Med 2013;1:1.
[35] Anderson GD. Chapter 1 Gender differences in pharmacological response. In: International review of neurobiology. Academic Press; 2008. p. 1–10.
[36] Whitley H, Lindsey W. Sex-based differences in drug activity. Am Fam Physician 2009;80(11):1254–8.
[37] Franconi F, et al. Gender differences in drug responses. Pharmacol Res 2007;55(2):81–95.

[38] Colloca L, Barsky AJ. Placebo and nocebo effects. N Engl J Med 2020;382(6):554–61.
[39] Belle DJ, Singh H. Genetic factors in drug metabolism. Am Fam Physician 2008;77(11):1553–60.
[40] Heller F. Genetics/genomics and drug effects. Acta Clin Belg 2013;68(2):77–80.
[41] Hemanth Kumar AK, et al. N-acetyltransferase gene polymorphisms & plasma isoniazid concentrations in patients with tuberculosis. Indian J Med Res 2017;145(1).
[42] Zabost A, et al. Correlation of N-acetyltransferase 2 genotype with isoniazid acetylation in Polish tuberculosis patients. BioMed Res Int 2013; 2013:853602.
[43] Zalewska M, Siara M, Sajewicz W. G protein-coupled receptors: abnormalities in signal transmission, disease states and pharmacotherapy. Acta Pol Pharm 2014;71(2):229–43.
[44] Hauser AS, et al. Pharmacogenomics of GPCR drug targets. Cell 2018;172(1). 41–54.e19.
[45] Parvez B, et al. A common β1-adrenergic receptor polymorphism predicts favorable response to rate-control therapy in atrial fibrillation. J Am Coll Cardiol 2012;59(1):49–56.
[46] Grandy DK. Chapter 10 - Amphetamines activate G-protein coupled trace amine-associated receptor 1 (TAAR1): implications for understanding and treating psychostimulant abuse. In: Preedy VR, editor. Neuropathology of drug addictions and substance misuse. Academic Press; 2016. p. 108–16.
[47] Neubig RR, et al. International union of pharmacology committee on receptor nomenclature and drug classification. XXXVIII. Update on terms and symbols in quantitative pharmacology. Pharmacol Rev 2003;55(4):597–606.
[48] Dougall IG, Unitt J. Chapter 2 - Evaluation of the biological activity of compounds: techniques and mechanism of action studies. In: Wermuth CG, et al., editors. The practice of medicinal Chemistry. 4th ed. Academic Press; 2015. p. 15–43.
[49] Hedrick SL, et al. Design, synthesis, and preliminary evaluation of a potential synthetic opioid rescue agent. J Biomed Sci 2021;28(1):62.
[50] Bate R, et al. Generics substitution, bioequivalence standards, and international oversight: complex issues facing the FDA. Trends Pharmacol Sci 2016;37(3):184–91.
[51] Farrell S. Aspirin stability lab handout. Available from: https://pharmahub.org/resources/535/download/ASA_Freshman_Lab_Handout.pdf.
[52] Sneader W. The discovery of aspirin: a reappraisal. Bmj 2000;321(7276):1591–4.
[53] Vane JR, Botting RM. The mechanism of action of aspirin. Thromb Res 2003;110(5):255–8.
[54] Davidson KW, et al. Aspirin use to prevent cardiovascular disease: US preventive services task force recommendation statement. JAMA 2022; 327(16):1577–84.
[55] Jones WS, et al. Comparative effectiveness of aspirin dosing in cardiovascular disease. N Engl J Med 2021;384(21):1981–90.
[56] Tsoi KKF, et al. Long-term use of low-dose aspirin for cancer prevention: a 10-year population cohort study in Hong Kong. Int J Cancer 2019; 145(1):267–73.
[57] Loomans-Kropp HA, Pinsky P, Umar A. Evaluation of aspirin use with cancer incidence and survival among older adults in the prostate, lung, colorectal, and ovarian cancer screening trial. JAMA Network Open 2021;4(1):e2032072–e2032072.
[58] Holmberg D, et al. Aspirin or statin use in relation to survival after surgery for esophageal cancer: a population-based cohort study. BMC Cancer 2023;23(1):375.

CHAPTER

4

Physiological and biochemical barriers to drug delivery

Wujie Zhang

LEARNING OBJECTIVES

- To differentiate transcellular and paracellular absorption pathways
- To describe various mechanisms of endocytosis
- To discuss the physiological barriers to peroral drug delivery systems
- To discuss first-pass metabolism and perform related calculations
- To discuss the advantages and disadvantages of transdermal, buccal, sublingual, pulmonary, and ocular drug delivery systems
- To discuss the two major types of biochemical barriers and explain the working mechanisms of various efflux pumps
- To discuss the potential effects of the immune system on the drug delivery systems
- To discuss the novel drug testing systems based on organoids and organ-on-a-chip

4.1 Process of drug absorption

Drug absorption is the process of transporting drugs from the site of administration to the blood circulation system for distribution. The process requires the drug to pass across semipermeable membranes, such as those of epithelial cells. Epithelial tissues cover all body surfaces exposed to the external environment and all linings along internal body cavities, which play a key role in drug absorption. Epithelial tissues are classified based on their shape (columnar, squamous, cuboidal, and columnar), layers of cells (simple, stratified, pseudostratified), and surface specialization (such as keratinization and cilia). Fig. 4.1 shows various epithelial tissues and their key functions.

Absorption can be either paracellular (*via* tight junction) or transcellular (*via* cell interior), as shown in Fig. 4.2. Transcellular pathways include passive transport, active transport, and endocytosis/exocytosis. Small hydrophobic molecules can enter cells through passive transport since the cell membrane is mainly hydrophobic. However, the

Fundamentals and Design of Drug Delivery Systems
https://doi.org/10.1016/B978-0-443-23521-4.00004-7

	Type of epithelium	Lining tissues	Key functions
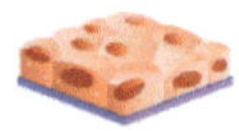	Simple squamous	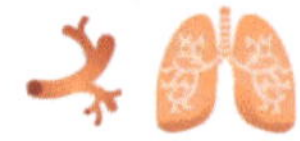	Materials exchange Secretion
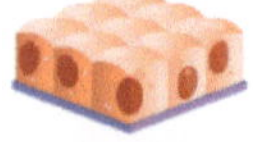	Simple cubiodal	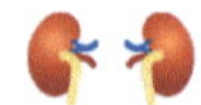	Absorption Secretion
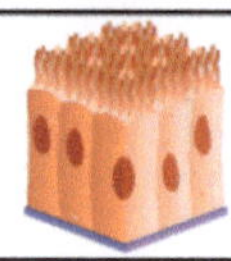	Ciliated columnar	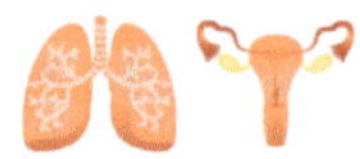	Absorption Secretion
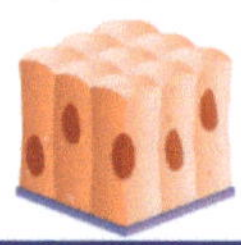	Simple columnar	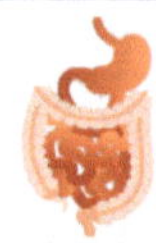	Absorption Secretion

FIGURE 4.1 Examples of epithelium associated with drug absorption/delivery.

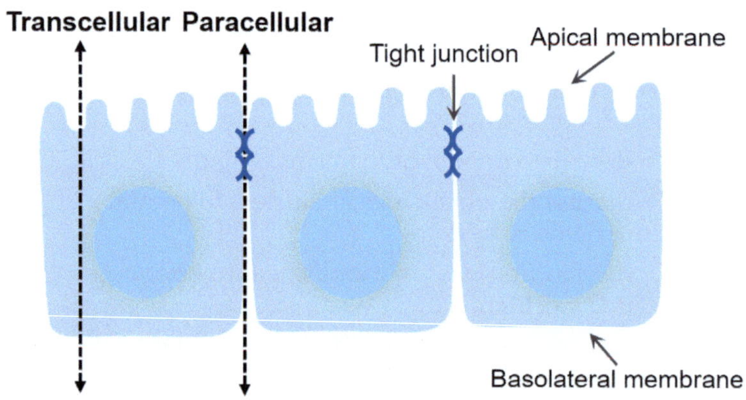

FIGURE 4.2 Paracellular and intracellular pathways of epithelium absorption.

hydrophobicity cannot be extremely high as the drug molecules may not be able to dissolve or get close to the cells because the cells are in an aqueous environment and may even remain within the cell membrane interior. The partition coefficient (logP) is commonly used for describing a molecule's lipid solubility:

$$logP = \frac{C_{oil}}{C_{water}},$$

where C_{oil} and C_{water} are the unionized drug concentrations in the organic and aqueous phases at equilibrium, respectively. For most of the drugs, logP is between 0 and 5 with the average between 3.0 and 3.5 [1,2].

Small hydrophilic molecules mostly enter cells through active transport. Some transporters can become saturated at high drug concentrations due to their capacities, unlike passive transport. As shown in Fig. 4.3, the process of passive transport, diffusion in particular, can be described by Fick's law: the rate (dm/dt) is linearly proportional to the concentration gradient (ΔC):

$$\frac{dm}{dt} = -k\Delta C = -k(C_t - C_i) \approx -kC_t,$$

when C_i (intracellular concentration) is low.

Regarding endocytosis, it becomes increasingly important due to the increase in macromolecular drugs developed compared to traditional small compounds and novel drug delivery systems; especially those at the nanoscale, such as liposomes and nanoparticles. The study of the endocytosis mechanism is still an evolving field. Endocytosis can be broadly divided into phagocytosis (cell eating) and pinocytosis (cell drinking). Phagocytosis is the process by which cells, such as macrophages, engulf large particles (bacteria, for example). Pinocytosis involves the internalization of

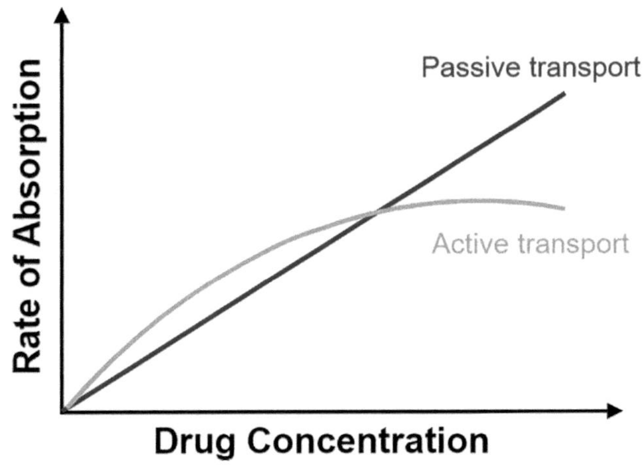

FIGURE 4.3 Comparison between passive and active transport.

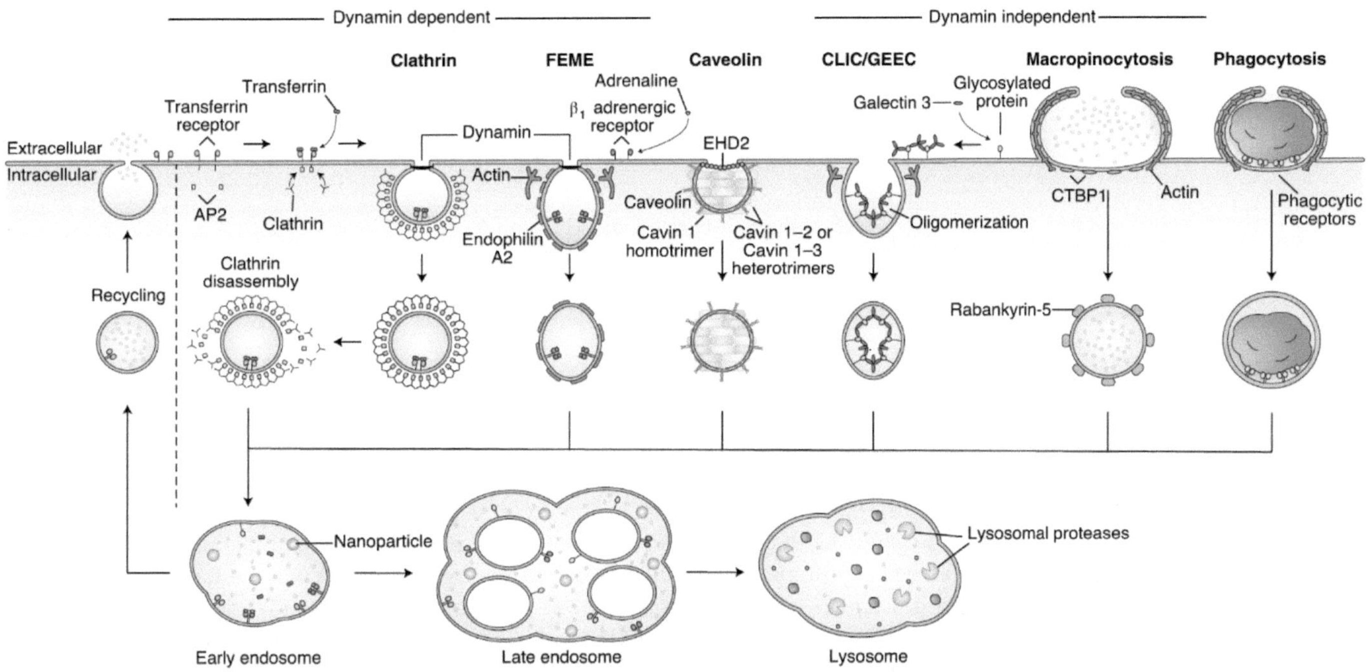

FIGURE 4.4 Summary of primary mechanisms of endocytosis. *AP2*, Assembly polypeptide 2; *CLIC/GEEC*, clathrin-independent carrier/glycosylphosphatidylinositol-anchored protein-enriched early endocytic compartment (GEEC) endocytosis; *CTBP1*, C-terminal-binding protein 1; *EHD2*, Eps15 homology domain-containing 2; *FEME*, fast endophilin-mediated endocytosis. From Rennick, J.J., A.P.R. Johnston, and R.G. Parton, *Key principles and methods for studying the endocytosis of biological and nanoparticle therapeutics.* Nat. Nanotechnol., 2021. **16**(3): p. 266-276, with permission from Springer Nature.

substances by small vesicles forming early endosomes, which then transform into late endosomes and fuse with lysosomes [3,4]. Pinocytosis can be divided into macropinocytosis, clathrin-mediated endocytosis, caveolin-mediated endocytosis, and clathrin/caveolae-independent endocytosis. Macropinocytosis is nonspecific, actin-dependent, and involves the engulfment of fluids and micro-scale particles. Both clathrin and caveolae-mediated endocytosis are specific since they involve specifically coated vesicles (specific lipid composition) [5]. A recent article [6] reviewed the primary mechanism of uptake into cells through endocytosis, shown in Fig. 4.4.

Besides hydrophobicity, molecular weight (size), carrier, and degree of ionization can also affect a drug's absorption. Many drugs are weak electrolytes and changes in pH can affect their degree of ionization. For passive transport, drugs in an ionized form tend to be more hydrophobic and remain unabsorbed, while the unionized form exhibits a higher absorption rate. The degree of ionization can be calculated using the Henderson-Hasselbalch equation:

$$pH = pKa + log_{10}\frac{[A^-]}{[HA]} \text{ (for weak acid) and } pH = pKa + log_{10}\frac{[B]}{[BH^+]} \text{ (for weak base).}$$

Sample question 4.1

Aspirin, a weak acid, has a pKa of 3.5. Which region, stomach (use pH = 2) or small intestine (use pH = 7.5), does aspirin have a higher (passive) absorption rate after oral administration?

Answer: Use the Henderson-Hasselbalch equation (weak acid):

Stomach: $2 = 3.5 + log_{10}\frac{[A^-]}{[HA]}$

$$-1.5 = log_{10}\frac{[A^-]}{[HA]}$$

$$\frac{[A^-]}{[HA]} = 10^{-1.5} = 0.03 \text{ mostly in the un – ionized form (HA).}$$

Small intestine: $7.5 = 3.5 + log_{10}\frac{[A^-]}{[HA]}$

$$4 = log_{10}\frac{[A^-]}{[HA]}$$

$$\frac{[A^-]}{[HA]} = 10^4 \text{ almost all in the ionized form } (A^-).$$

Hence, aspirin is predominantly absorbed (passive) in the stomach.

Sample question 4.2

Fig. 4.5 shows the hypothetical passive absorption curves of two drugs, aspirin and betaxolol, within the body as a function of pH. For each drug, choose the appropriate curve, I or II, that best represents the dependence of its absorption on pH.

Answer: Based on the results from question 4.1, it can be concluded that weak acids are predominately absorbed in the stomach (low pH conditions). At higher pH conditions, weak acid drugs become ionized (unabsorbable form). Weak basic drugs exhibit the opposite trend. Hence, I and II are betaxolol and aspirin, respectively. After oral administration, T_{max} has been reported to be 0.5-1.5 hours and 2-4 hours for aspirin and betaxolol, respectively. [7,8]. This indicates the overall earlier absorption (stomach vs. intestine) of aspirin within the GI tract compared to betaxolol.

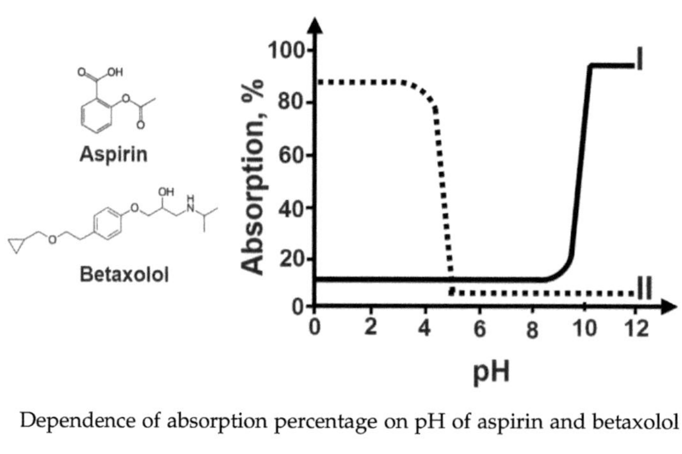

FIGURE 4.5 Dependence of absorption percentage on pH of aspirin and betaxolol (hypothetical).

4.2 Physiological barriers to peroral drug delivery

Peroral (occurring through or by way of the mouth) drug delivery is one of the most common approaches for administering drugs. Absorption of the drug given via the peroral route occurs within the gastrointestinal (GI) tract. Starting with the GI tract physiology (Fig. 4.6), it includes the mouth, esophagus, stomach, small intestine, large intestine, rectum, and anus. The liver, gallbladder, pancreas, and accessory digestive organs produce digestive fluids and enzymes. The stomach, small intestine, and large intestine are the three most important organs for drug absorption. As shown in Fig. 4.7, due to different pH, enzymes, structures, and such, drug absorption varies significantly within these organs. Age, gender, disease, food, and colonic factor variability can also greatly affect drug absorption [9]. The stomach provides a low pH environment, weak acids tend to be absorbed as discussed in Section 4.1. Aspirin, a weak acid, has a high absorption rate in the stomach. Aspirin intake can injure the gastrointestinal mucosa. One mechanism is the accumulation of aspirin (H^+) within gastric epithelial cells. Aspirin can also lead to bicarbonate production and mucus by the gastric epithelium [10].

The small intestine is the major organ within the GI tract for drug absorption due to its length and large surface area. The small intestine is very long, about 7 m for an adult [11,12]. The surface area within the small intestine is about a few hundred times that of a cylinder of the same length/diameter due to the folds of Kerckring, villi,

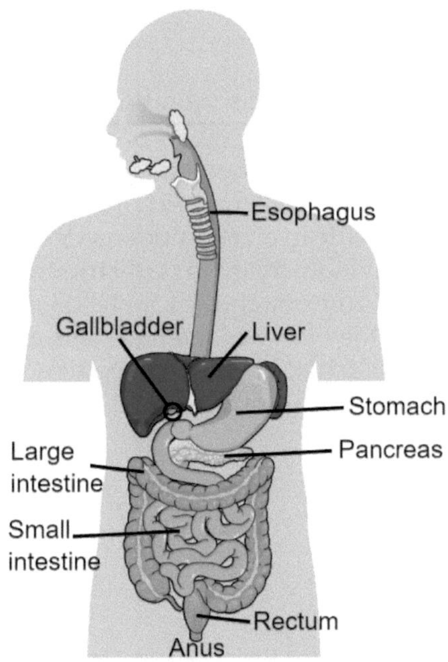

FIGURE 4.6 Human gastrointestinal tract (digestive system).

	Organ	pH	Major enzymes	Transit time	Substances absorbed
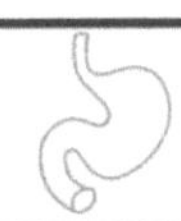	Stomach	1.0 - 2.0	Pepsin	1 - 2 hr	Weak acids, alcohol, etc
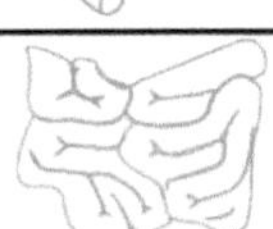	Small intestine	4.4 - 7.4	Trypsin, lipase, peptidase, maltase, lactase, aminopeptidase	2 - 4 hr	Amino acids, peptides, glucose, water, minerals, vitamins, etc
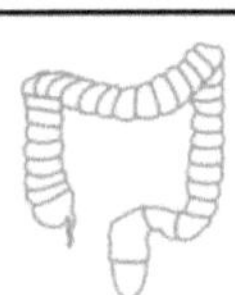	Large intestine	5.5 - 7.4	Enzymes produced by colonic microflora	10 hr - days	Ions, water, minerals, vitamins, etc

FIGURE 4.7 Physiological characteristics of the stomach, small intestine, and large intestine.

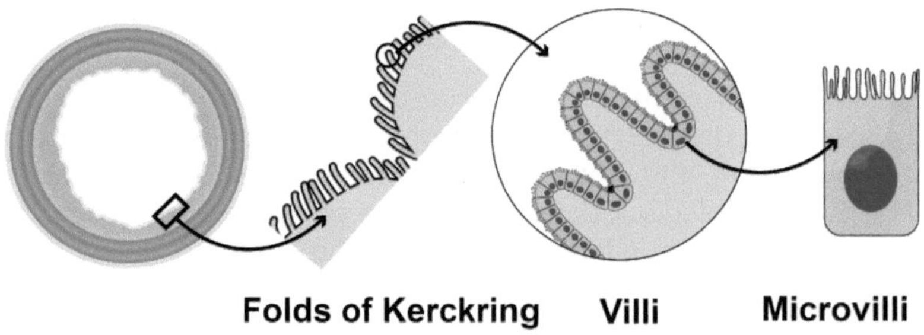

FIGURE 4.8 Three mechanisms of the small intestine's surface area.

and microvilli (Fig. 4.8) [13]. Although not a major site for absorption, the large intestine hosts the largest microbial community (bacteria, archaea, and eukarya) in the body [14]. This microbial community has a significant impact on drug delivery. The drug-microbiome interaction is bidirectional. The microbiome can affect the individual's response to a drug such as through enzymatic transformation (pharmacomicrobiomics) [15,16]. Enzymes secreted specifically by the colonic microorganisms can be used to design colon-targeted drug delivery systems, such as using pectin-based carriers [17].

4.3 First-pass metabolism

Distribution occurs after the drug is successfully absorbed into the bloodstream. However, first-pass metabolism should be considered when it comes to peroral drug delivery. First-pass metabolism is the phenomenon that occurs whenever the drug is administered orally, enters the liver, and undergoes extensive biotransformation showing sub-therapeutic action [18]. Drugs have to enter the bloodstream to be distributed. Moreover, drugs absorbed into the GI tract do not directly enter the bloodstream but go through liver metabolism *via* enterohepatic circulation (Fig. 4.9). Hence, bioavailability can be used to describe the extent of the first-pass metabolism, which can be determined by the fractions of a drug entering the systemic circulation that escape loss at each site [19,20]. Fig. 4.10 shows the method for determining the bioavailability (F). For intravenous administration, $F = 1$, as all the drug molecules directly enter the systemic circulation for distribution.

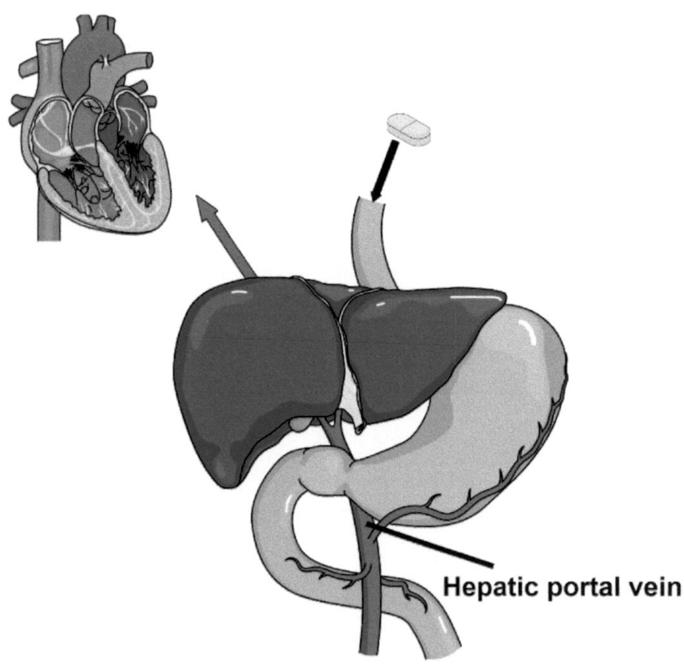

FIGURE 4.9 First-pass metabolism of a drug given orally.

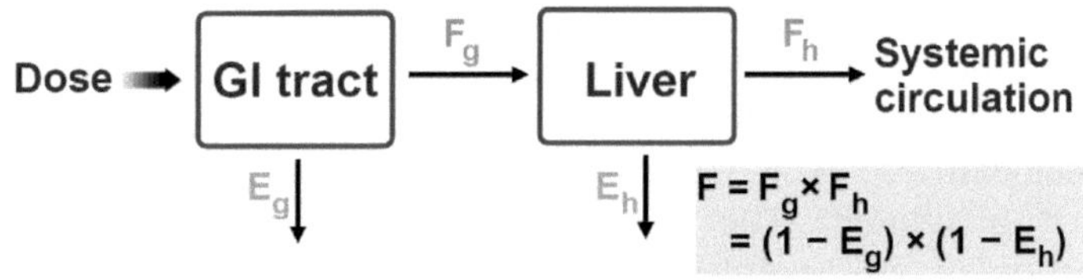

FIGURE 4.10 Barriers to drug entry into the systemic circulation after oral administration. E_g, GI tract extraction ratio; E_h, liver extraction ratio; F_g, fraction of the dose absorbed within the GI tract; F_h, fraction of the dose escaping liver metabolism.

Sample question 4.3

A drug, 100 mg, was given orally. It was 60% absorbed into the GI tract, and then 30% of the drug absorbed was eliminated through the first-pass metabolism. What was its bioavailability?

Answer:

Method I:

Keep in mind: $F_g + E_g = 1$ and $F_h + E_h = 1$

$F_g = 0.6$

$F_h = 1 - E_h = 1 - 0.3 = 0.7$

$F = F_g \times F_h = 0.6 \times 0.7 = 0.42$

Method II:

Use the amounts of the drug at different stages:

amount left after absorption: 100 mg × 60% = 60 mg

amount left after first-pass metabolism: 60 mg - 60 mg × 30% = 42 mg

last, use the definition of bioavailability: F = amount enters the systemic circulation/dose = 42 mg/100 mg = 0.42

4.4 Physiological barriers to nonperoral drug delivery

Skin. Skin is composed of the epidermis, dermis, and hypodermis (Fig. 4.11). During transdermal drug delivery, drug molecules cross the surface layers of the skin and reach blood capillaries [21]. The first transdermal product in the form of an ointment was released for angina pectoris treatment in the 1950s [22]. Dermal absorption includes

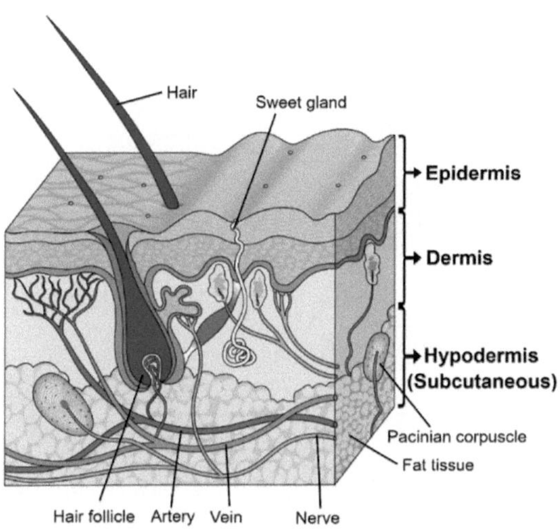

FIGURE 4.11 Structure of human skin.

three steps: entry of a substance through the skin layers (penetration), movement of a substance through one layer into another *via* hydrophobic channels (permeation), and the uptake of a substance into the vascular system (reabsorption) [23]. Drug molecules can also penetrate *via* the sweat ducts or the hair follicles with their associated sebaceous glands (transappendageal pathway) [24]. The physicochemical properties of the skin representing multiple obstacles limits transdermal drug delivery. The hydrophobic stratum corneum barrier (outermost layer of the epidermis) allows the penetration of lipid-soluble molecules more readily than water-soluble compounds [25]. Different approaches, including stratum corneum modification and stratum corneum bypassing, have been deployed for enhanced transdermal drug delivery [22]. A value of 500 Da is generally considered the molecular weight cutoff of drug molecules for efficient skin absorption [26]. The major advantages of transdermal drug delivery are stable and sustained drug releases, avoidance of first-pass metabolism, and ease of patient compliance [27]. Dermal absorption is low but can be used for sustained drug delivery.

Oral cavity. The oral cavity is rich in blood vessels, and drugs can be directly absorbed into the bloodstream (Fig. 4.12A). Buccal (between gums and cheek) and sublingual (under the tongue) administration are two approaches for delivering drugs through the mouth (Fig. 4.12B). These approaches offer various advantages: drugs enter the systemic circulation quickly, avoid first-pass metabolism, gastric acid hydrolysis, and intestinal enzymatic degradation, and the effects can be terminated by spitting the drug tablets out. These advantages are lost if accidental swallowing occurs. Rapid absorption may lead to toxic effects in some cases. Patient compliance can also be a concern.

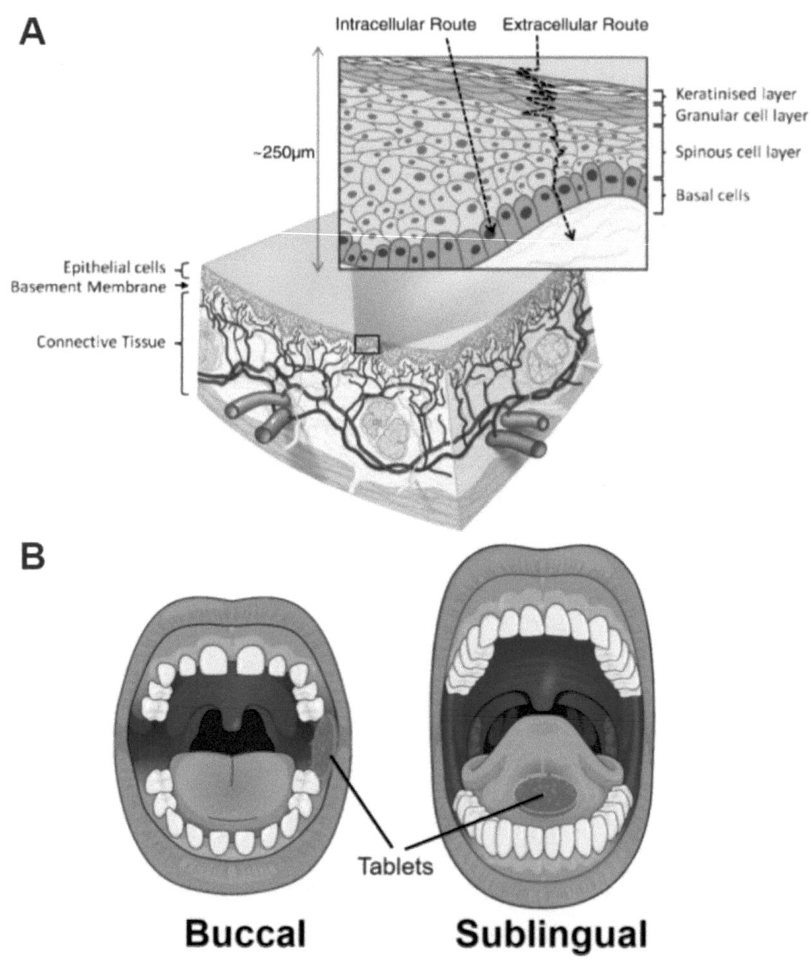

FIGURE 4.12 Structure of oral mucosa (A) and buccal and sublingual drug delivery approaches (B). (A) From Hearnden, V., et al., *New developments and opportunities in oral mucosal drug delivery for local and systemic disease.* Adv. Drug Deliv. Rev, 2012. **64**(1): p. 16-28, with permission from Elsevier.

Lung. Drugs can be delivered through the lungs for noninvasive systemic distribution. The lungs are a major part of the respiratory system (Fig. 4.13A). As shown in Fig. 4.13B, the trachea, bronchi, bronchioles, and alveoli form the tracheobronchial tree, which allows the passage of air into the lungs. The major physiological barrier of the lungs is the epithelium. The thickness is extremely thin in the deeper lungs. The lungs are more permeable to macromolecules, such as proteins, than other ports of entry into the body. The lungs are even more permeable to small molecules, especially hydrophobic substances [29]. The major advantages of drug delivery *via* the lungs are no first-pass metabolism and high bioavailability [30]. Usually, drugs delivered through the lungs are inhaled in the form of particles. There are three major forces (gravity, fluid drag, and diffusion) that affect the behavior of the particles [31]. Particle size, besides charge and shape, greatly affects regional lung deposition. The primary inhaled particle deposition mechanisms based on particle size are inertial impaction, sedimentation, and diffusion (Fig. 4.14). Inertial impaction occurs when the air stream direction changes, particles keep their trajectory and collide with the walls of the respiratory tract. Sedimentation is the settlement of particles due to gravity. Inertial impaction and sedimentation are the dominant deposition methods for coarse particles larger than 1.0 μm. Diffusion occurs when particles are small enough (< 0.1 μm) to undergo random (Brownian) motions [32,33]. In general, particles of 2 to 5 μm that are inhaled through the mouth efficiently achieve alveolar deposition. Particles of 1 to 3 μm are appropriate for

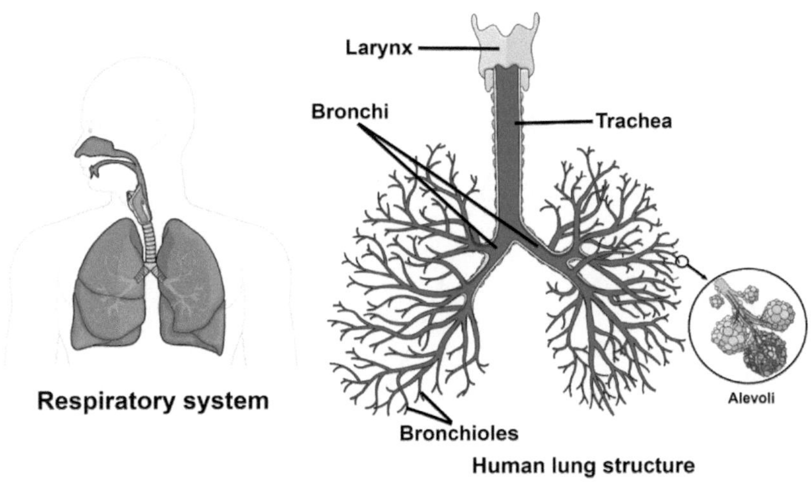

FIGURE 4.13 Structure of the human respiratory system (*left*) and lung structure (*right*).

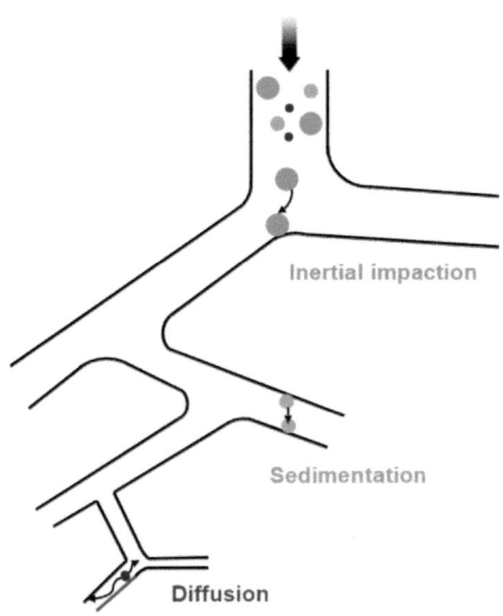

FIGURE 4.14 Primary deposition mechanisms of inhaled particles based on size.

deposition in the alveolar region via the nose [34]. Larger particles (> 10 μm) cannot easily reach the deeper lungs; while the smaller particles (< 1 μm) can be expelled during expiration. As shown in Fig. 4.15, the simulation data shows the dependence of deposition regions of the lung based on particle size. With the rapid application of nanotechnology in drug delivery, nanoformulations become increasingly common. Nanoparticles of 10 to 100 nm (primary or agglomerate size) deposit more efficiently in the alveolar region than those of 100 to 1000 nm. This may be due to a shift from impaction/sedimentation to diffusion as the dominant particle deposition mechanism [32,35]. Moreover, particles/agglomerates smaller than 100 nm are less efficiently phagocytized [35].

Eye. Ocular drug delivery has been challenging due to the unique anatomy and physiology of the eye (Fig. 4.16). The advantages of optical drug delivery are that it is self-administerable and noninvasive. Patient compliance can be an issue (Case Study 2). Structural variation of each layer of ocular tissue also displays a significant barrier [36]. Tear drainage/dilution causes significant drug loss. Moreover, the volume that can be administered is limited to about 30 μL due to the eye's anatomical constraints [37]. Conventional eye drops (make up more than 95% of the ocular drug market) have poor bioavailability and typically only 1% to 3% of a drug may reach the interior of the eye [38].

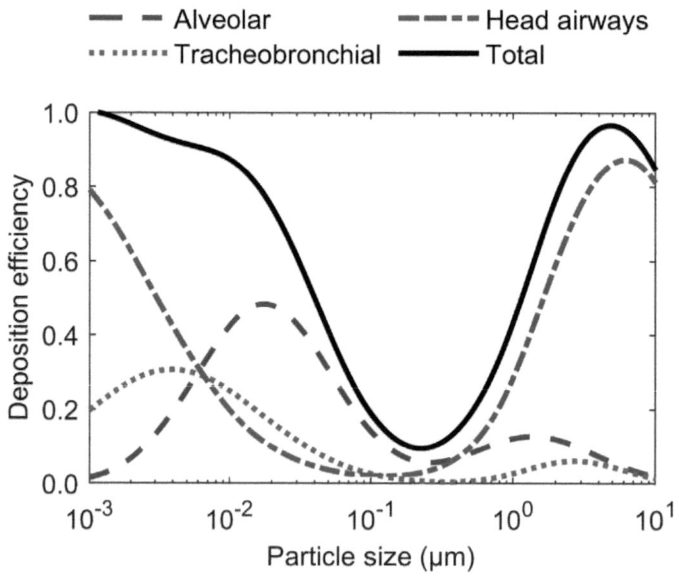

FIGURE 4.15 Deposition efficiency of particles in the human respiratory tract based on particle size. From Lepistö, T., et al., *Measurement of the human respiratory tract deposited surface area of particles with an electrical low pressure impactor.* Aerosol Sci Technol, 2020. **54**(8): p. 958-971, with permission from Taylor & Francis.

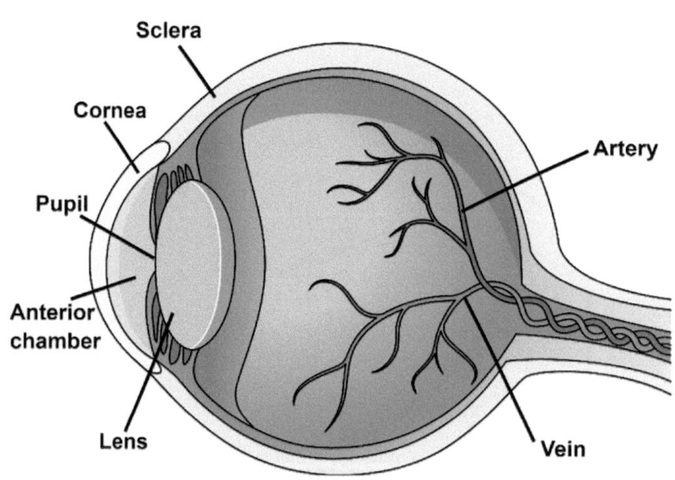

FIGURE 4.16 Structure of the human eye.

TABLE 4.1 Advantages and disadvantages of various drug delivery routes.

Route	Advantages	Disadvantages
Oral	Simple and convenient Economical Noninvasive	First-pass metabolism GI tract can be hostile to certain types of drugs (e.g., protein based) Limited targeting ability
Skin (transdermal)	Slowed and sustained release First-pass metabolism avoided Reduced dosing frequency	Skin irritations can occur Skin permeability is low
Oral cavity (buccal and sublingual)	Fast absorption First-pass metabolism avoided Quick onset of action	Low patient compliance Advantages lost if accidentally swallowed Irritation to the oral mucosa
Lung (pulmonary)	First-pass metabolism avoided Noninvasive Rapid onset of drug action	Low patient compliance Drug formulation can be challenging May stimulate cough reflex
Eye (ocular)	Easily accessible First-pass metabolism avoided	Low patient compliance Only a small volume of drugs can be delivered

4.5 Biochemical barriers to drug delivery

Metabolizing enzymes and efflux pumps are two major groups of biochemical barriers to drug delivery. As discussed in Chapter 3, the liver is the major organ in the human body for metabolism. CYPs are the most well-known drug-metabolizing enzymes and are mainly expressed in the liver [39]. Some CYPs are expressed in tissues other than the liver, such as CYP2E1 (expressed in the nose and lungs) and CYP3A4 (expressed in the stomach, lungs, small intestine, and renal tissue). Other drug-metabolizing enzymes include flavin-containing monooxygenases (FMOs), monoamine oxidases (MAOs), aldo-keto reductases (AKRs), esterases, and amidases [40].

Drug efflux pumps are membrane transporters that pump drugs out of a cell. Drug efflux pumps that recognize multiple drugs are called multidrug efflux pumps, which leads to multidrug resistance (MDR) [41]. MDR is a general health problem in cancer and infectious disease treatment. One of the major groups of efflux pumps is the ATP-binding cassette (ABC) transporter family. ABC transporters utilize the energy from ATP hydrolysis. Among the ABC family, P-glycoprotein (P-gp), multidrug resistance protein 1 (MRP1), and breast cancer resistance protein (BCRP) account for most of the reported MDR in humans [42].

P-gp (or MDR1) was the first identified ABC efflux pump [43]. P stands for "permeability" as it was thought to confer drug resistance by decreasing the membrane's permeability [44]. It prevents cellular uptake of a large number of structurally and functionally diverse compounds, including most of the cancer therapeutics. P-gp is expressed on apical membranes of hepatocytes, renal proximal tubular cells, enterocytes, brain capillary endothelial cells, and such. Its function is to limit drug absorption from the intestine to systemic circulation and the penetration of drugs across the blood-brain barrier and contributes to hepatobiliary and renal drug efflux [45]. As shown in Fig. 4.17A, P-gp contains two transmembrane domains (TMDs) and two cytoplasmic nucleotide-binding domains (NBDs). During a transport cycle, P-gp changes between inward-facing and outward-facing states (Fig. 4.17B). In the inward-facing state, P-gp can recruit substrates and then shift to the outward-facing state upon ATP binding (the NDBs dimerize and TMDs re-orientate). ATP hydrolysis resets the transporter to the inward-facing state [44]. Different models have been proposed for P-gp's MDR mechanism (Fig. 4.18). Pump models describe drugs interacting with P-gp in the cytoplasm and being pumped across the membrane and released to the extracellular space. The flippase model (most accepted) considers the drug to be flipped from the inner leaflet to the outer leaflet of the cell membrane. According to the vacuum cleaner model, drugs interact with P-gp in the lipid bilayer and are subsequently released back into the extracellular space [46,47]. P-gp is generally believed to capture drugs in the lipid membrane by attracting them *via* weak electrostatic interactions [46].

MRP1 (or ABCC1) was first identified in 1992 and has been shown to play a role in drug resistance in acute myeloblastic and lymphoblastic leukemia, breast cancer, non–small cell lung cancer, prostate cancer, and others [48-50]. MRP1 and P-gp differ significantly. P-gp recognizes hydrophobic substrates, while MRP1 mostly transports organic anions, especially those that are conjugated with glutathione, glucuronic acid, or sulfate [48,49,51]. MRP1 has three

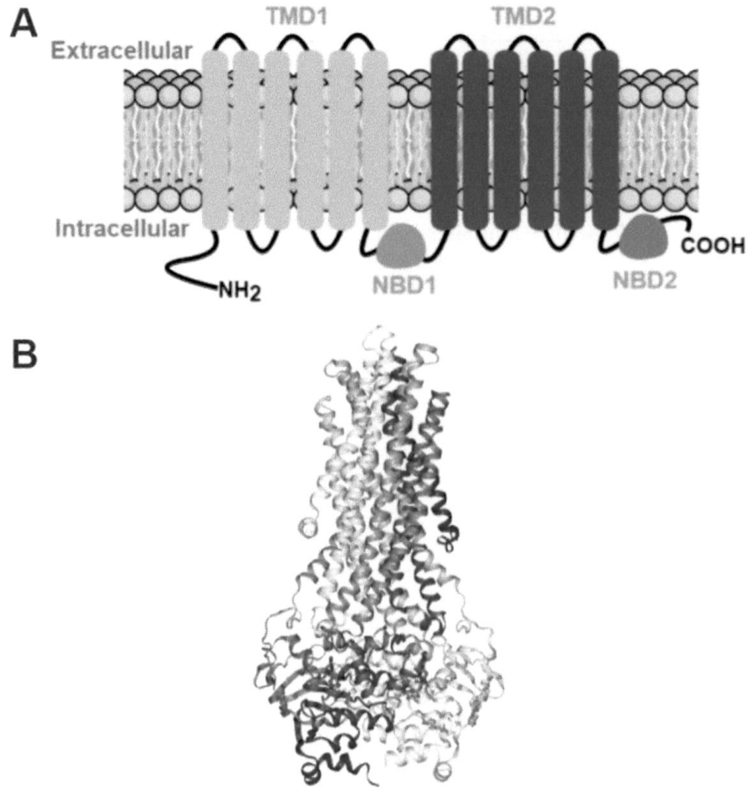

FIGURE 4.17 Predicted topological structure of P-gp (A). Molecular structure of human P-gp in the ATP-bound outward-facing configuration (B). B was created with the PDB ID 6C0V and the associated publication [44], NGL Viewer (Rose, A.S., et al., NGL viewer: web-based molecular graphics for large complexes. Bioinformatics, 2018. doi:10.1093/bioinformatics/bty419), and RCSB PDB.

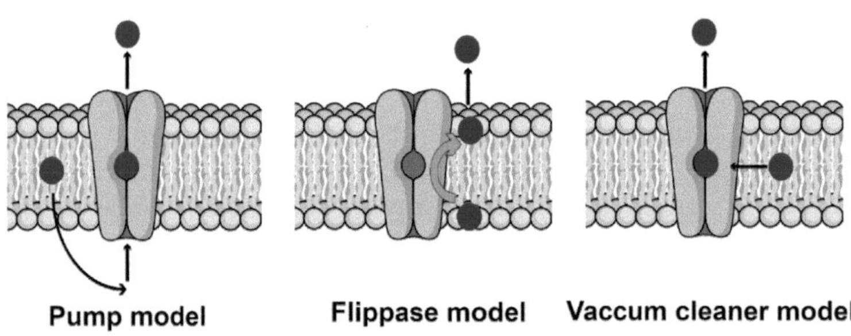

FIGURE 4.18 Different mechanism models of P-gp induced MDR.

TMDs (TMD0, TMD1, and TMD2) and two NBDs (NBD1 and NBD2) (Fig. 4.19A). It is thought that TMD0 may be critical for plasma membrane retention and that MRP1 most likely recruits its substrates directly from the cytoplasm [48]. As shown in Fig. 4.19B, ATP binding opens the transport pathway to the extracellular space and reconfigures the substrate-binding site, causing the release of the substrate (prior to ATP hydrolysis) [50].

BCRP (or ABCG2) was first discovered in multidrug-resistant breast cancer cell lines. It only has one ATP-binding cassette and is known as a half-ABC transporter [52]. The expression pattern of BCRP is similar to P-gp [53]. BCRP is also highly expressed in normal human tissues such as the small intestine and liver [52,54]. Substrates of BCRP include a wide range of chemotherapeutics, such as mitoxantrone and methotrexate, nucleoside and nucleotide analogs, and conjugated organic anions (particularly sulfated and glucuronide conjugates) [55]. The NBD in BCRP precedes the TMD in domain organization, which is opposite to that of P-gp and MRP1 (Fig. 4.20A) [55]. It has been proposed that human BCRP contains two cavities, which function like a peristaltic drug pump gated by a hydrophobic valve and a flexible lid [56,57]. BCRP is first in the apo-closed conformation with the NBDs open and the binding

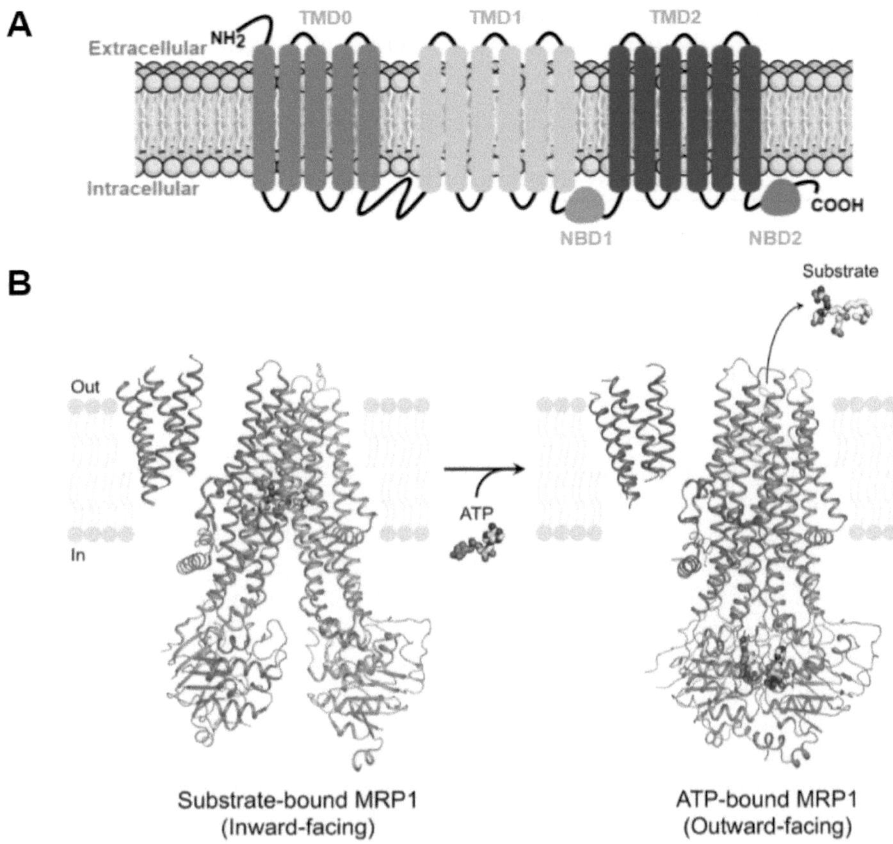

FIGURE 4.19 (A) Predicted topological structure of MRP1. (B) Bovine MRP1 in the inward-facing and outward-facing conformations. (B) From Johnson, Z.L. and J. Chen, *Structural basis of substrate recognition by the multidrug resistance protein MRP1.* Cell, 2017. **168**(6): p. 1075-1085.e9, with permission from Elsevier.

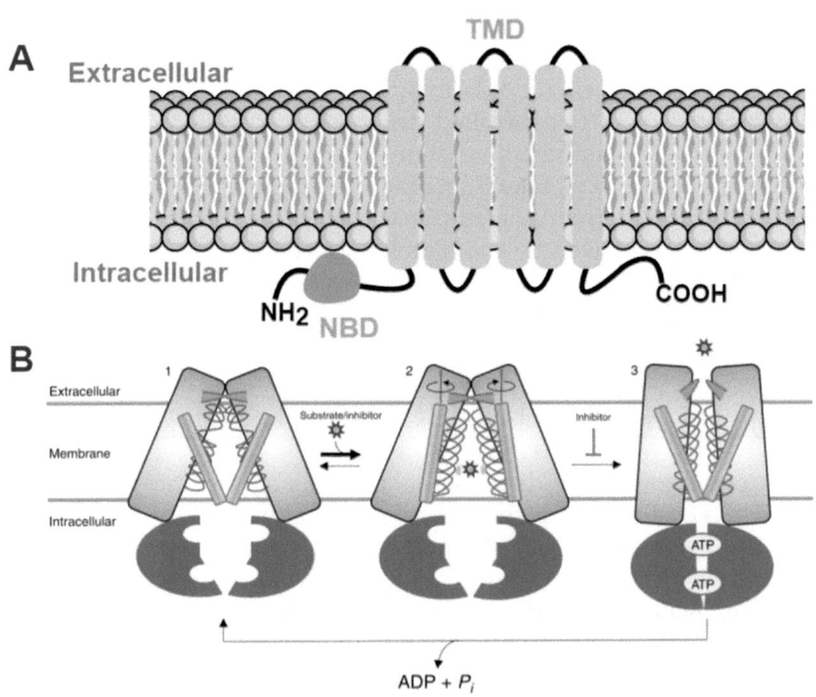

FIGURE 4.20 Predicted topological structure of BCRP (A) and drug capture and extrusion model (B). (B) From Orlando, B.J. and M. Liao, *ABCG2 transports anticancer drugs* via *a closed-to-open switch.* Nat. Commun, 2020. **11**(1): p. 2264.

of transport substrates causing the transporter to shift toward the inward-facing conformation. ATP binding promotes the efflux of the substrate to the extracellular space, while ATP hydrolysis resets the transporter to the apo-closed conformation (Fig. 4.20B) [58].

4.6 Immune system and drug delivery systems

Adverse immunological effects associated with the drug delivery system, especially those that directly enter the bloodstream, may pose serious risks to patients. The potential immunogenicity (the potential to elicit an immune response) of drug delivery systems may lead to reduced efficacy, acute reactions, and other negative effects [59]. Unfortunately, the immune system and drug delivery systems have not been extensively investigated.

Antibodies induced by the administration of the drug delivery system may "attack" the delivery system (e.g., carrier material), drugs, and targeting ligands [59]. Take accelerated blood clearance (ABC), for example, it is a phenomenon in which certain pharmaceutical agents (e.g., PEGylated systems) are rapidly cleared from the blood upon second and subsequent administrations [60]. This phenomenon was initially observed with PEGylated liposomes and is thought to be the result of increased splenic production of anti-PEG IgM. A study showed that the PEGylated organic-inorganic hybrid particles can elicit the ABC phenomenon and can limit the passive targeting capabilities of nanoparticles to accumulate in ischemic tissues and increase liver uptake [61]. Another study reported a rapid onset of ABC for mRNA-formulated lipid nanoparticles—the production of anti-phosphorylcholine IgM by B-1 lymphocytes in response to the initial injection and production of anti-PEG IgM by B-2 lymphocytes upon repeated injections [60]. As discussed in Chapter 1, Pfizer-BioNTech's vaccine is PEGylated, which has raised allergy concerns. However, the risks are thought to be low considering the relatively low amount of PEGylated lipids and the intramuscular administration route [62].

Complement activation and opsonization of drug delivery systems may or may not be associated with antibody formation. The complement system is an essential component of innate immunity that functions primarily as a first-line host defense against pathogenetic infections. Three main pathways that can activate the complement systems are classic, lectin, and alternative. The classic pathway is triggered by antigen-antibody immune complexes. The lectin pathways use members of the collectin family of plasma proteins. The alternative pathway is constitutively active at low levels in the normal host [63]. Complement activation may induce formulation destabilization, promote opsonization, and affect the biological and therapeutic performance of drug delivery systems. Opsonization and the assembly of pore-forming membrane attack complexes (MAC) are the two main defense functions of complement activation [64]. Opsonization is the process where microorganisms and inanimate colloids (e.g., liposomes, particles) are coated with host-produced proteins and lipids (e.g., IgG, IgM, and complement factors), thus facilitating the binding of the opsonized microorganisms or colloids to specific receptor molecules present on phagocytes [65]. Opsonization is a critical biological barrier to controlled drug delivery as the opsonized substances in the bloodstream are rapidly cleared by the reticuloendothelial system *via* phagocytic uptake [66,67].

Drug delivery systems may also lead to platelet aggregation as platelets are the primary actors in hemostasis. Platelets may bridge innate and adaptive immune responses or act as innate inflammatory cells in an immune response. Platelet aggregation may be directed by the platelet-activating factor and the presence of immune complexes in the drug delivery systems [59]. Fig. 4.21 shows the interrelationship between various immunological reactions/processes.

4.7 Novel models for drug testing

In general, drug testing is done through two-dimensional (2D) cell culture and animal studies before the clinical trials. The major drawback of a 2D cell model is the lack of architecture and microenvironments present in three-dimensional (3D) models. It has been shown that 3D models are superior compared to 2D models as they better mimic the native cellular environment. Generating 3D models—especially patient-specific organoids for drug testing—has become an emerging field. Organoids are simple tissue-engineered cell-based *in vitro* models that recapitulate many aspects of the complex structure and function of the corresponding *in vivo* tissue [68]. Organoids that resemble the brain, kidneys, lungs, intestines, stomach, liver, and other organs have been developed (Fig. 4.22). As shown in Fig. 4.23, to engineer organoids, cells, soluble factors (such as growth factors), matrix (mimicking extracellular matrix), and physical cues are the major components [68]. It has been proposed that the next generation of

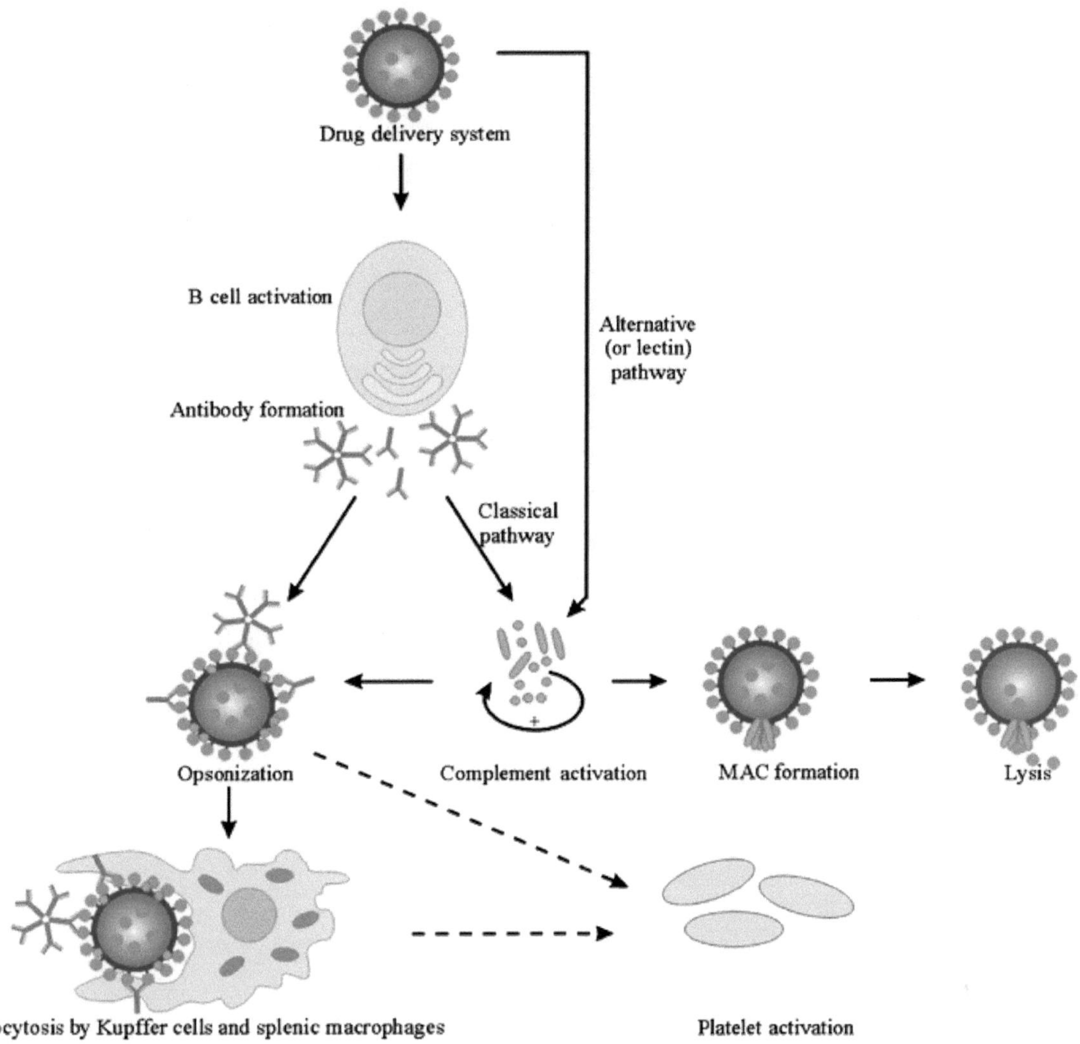

FIGURE 4.21 Interrelations of various immunological reactions/processes. *MAC*, Membrane attack complex. From Jiskoot, W., et al., *Immunological risk of injectable drug delivery systems.* Pharm Res, 2009. **26**(6): p. 1303-1314, with permission from Springer Nature.

organoids (multilayer tissue complexity and higher-order functions) can be designed with engineering-based narrative design. The three key design considerations of narrative engineering are space design (tissues designed as a spatial default for preparedness towards self-organization), biological environmental control, and synthetic environmental control [69].

Although organoids enable complexity in cellular composition, they generally lack stromal, vascular, and immunological components [68]. Moreover, precise control of organoids and their local environment remains challenging. Organs-on-a-chip have also drawn more and more attention since they are becoming more reproducible and controlled. Organs-on-a-chip are microfabricated cell culture devices designed to model the functional units of human organs *in vitro*. Organ-on-a-chip technology relies on the knowledge of human organs to engineer artificial constructs in which cells and their microenvironment are precisely controlled, whereas organoids follow intrinsic developmental programs and develop from self-organizing stem cells to reproduce the key structural and functional properties of their *in vivo* counterparts [72]. A classic example is the organ-on-a-chip model of the alveolar-capillary unit of the lung (Fig. 4.24). The microfluidic system contains two microchannels separated by a thin, porous, flexible, and fibronectin or collagen-coated poly(dimethylsiloxane) (PDMS) membrane. Human alveolar epithelial and pulmonary microvascular endothelial cells were seeded on opposite sides of the membrane. Air was introduced to the epithelial compartment to create an air-liquid interface (mimicking the lining of the alveolar air space). Pressure-

FIGURE 4.22 Examples of organoids: neuroepithelial organoids (A) and small intestine organoids (B). (A) Retinoic acid (RA) treatment had a substantial influence on the geometry and topology of organoids. (B) Acute *Chlamydia trachomatis* infection at 34 and 96 hours postinfection showing a change in the localization of the bacteria (Ctr, *red*) from the inclusions within the primarily infected host cells (*left*) to the lumen of the organoid (*right*) (β-catenin, *green*). *PODXL,* Podocalyxin-like protein; *ZO-1,* Zonula occludens protein-1. (A) Reproduced from Ishihara, K., et al., *Topological morphogenesis of neuroepithelial organoids.* Nat Phys, 2023. **19**(2): p. 177–183. (B) Reproduced from Kessler, M., et al., *Chronic Chlamydia infection in human organoids increases stemness and promotes age-dependent CpG methylation.* Nat Commun, 2019. **10**(1): p. 1194.

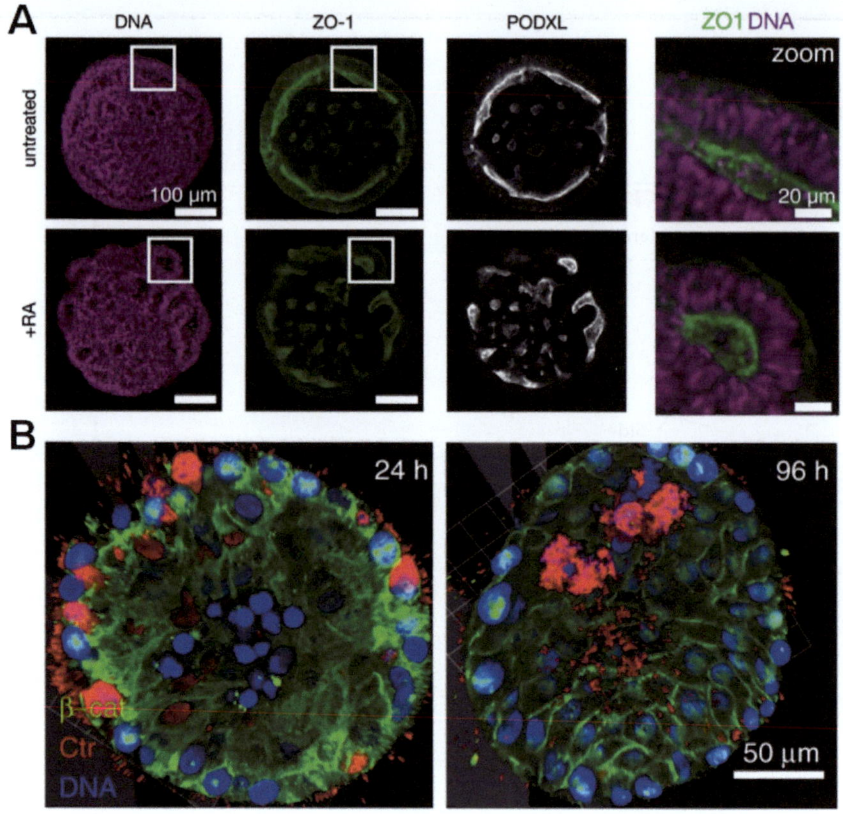

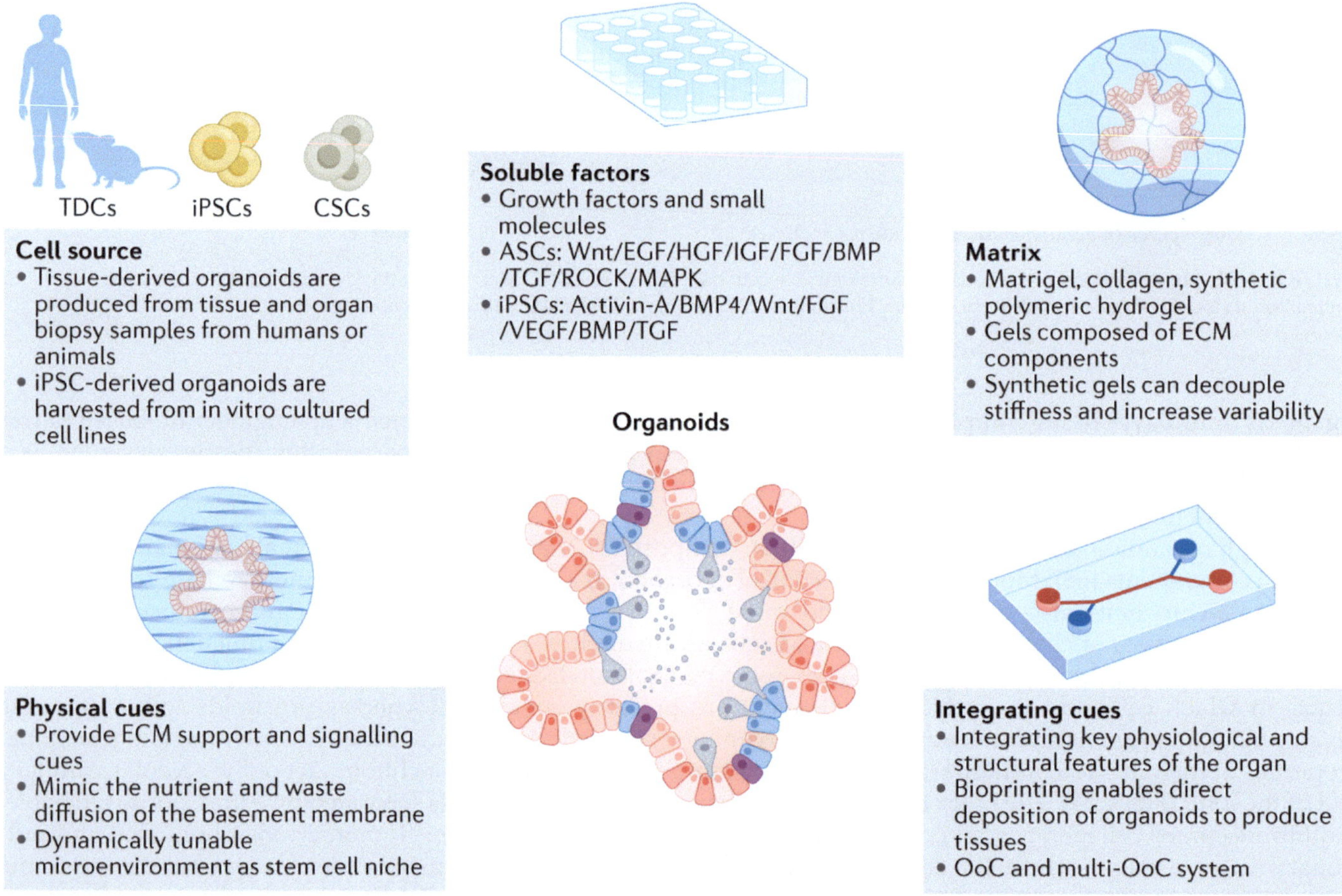

FIGURE 4.23 Components of organoid engineering. *ASCs,* Adult stem cells; *CSCs,* cancer stem cells; *ECM,* extracellular matrix; *FGF,* fibroblast growth factor; *iPSCs,* induced pluripotent stem cells; *OoC,* organ-on-a-chip; *TDCs,* tissue-derived cells. From Zhao, Z., et al., *Organoids.* Nat Rev Methods Primers, 2022. **2**(1): p. 94, with permission from Springer Nature.

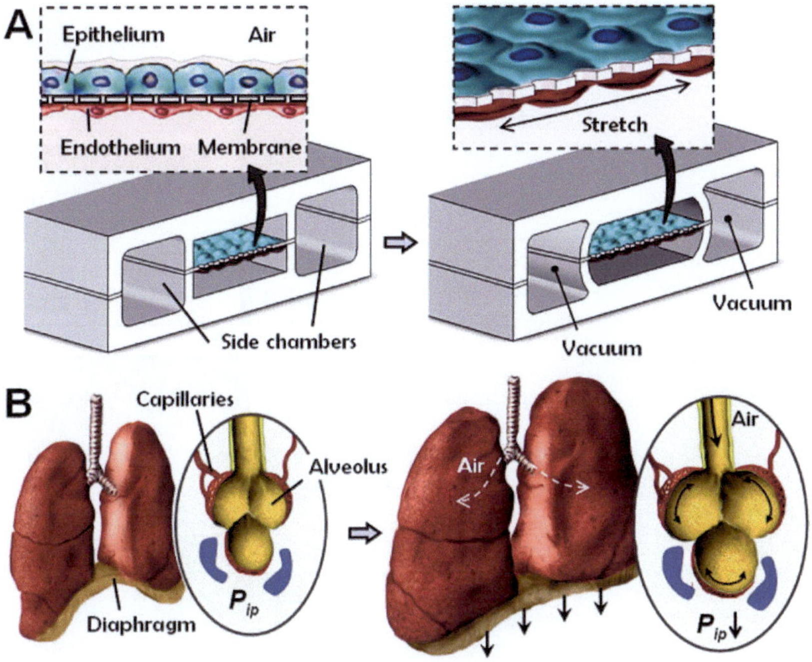

FIGURE 4.24 Design of a human breathing lung-on-a-chip microsystem. The system uses compartmentalized PDMS microchannels to form an alveolar-capillary barrier. (A) The physiological breathing movements were recreated by applying a vacuum to the side chambers and causing mechanical stretching of the membrane. (B) The contraction of the diaphragm causes a reduction in intrapleural pressure (Pip) during inhalation, leading to distension of the alveoli and physical stretching of the alveolar-capillary interface. From Huh, D., et al., *Reconstituting organ-level lung functions on a chip.* Science, 2010. **328**(5986): p. 1662-1668, with permission from The American Association for the Advancement of Science.

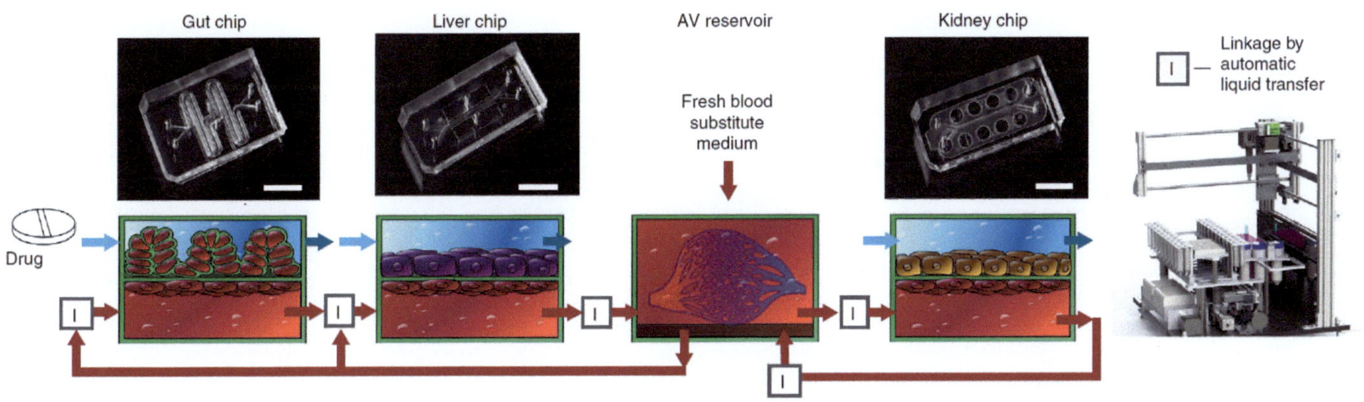

FIGURE 4.25 A multiorgan-chip first-pass metabolism model. *Top,* Photograph of organ chips. *Bottom,* Diagram indicating all the chips are fluidically linked to each other and to the arteriovenous reservoir. Scale bars: 5 mm. From Herland, A., et al., *Quantitative prediction of human pharmacokinetic responses to drugs* via *fluidically coupled vascularized organ chips.* Nat Biomed Eng, 2020. **4**(4): p. 421-436, with permission from Springer Nature.

driven stretching was replicated by incorporating two larger lateral microchambers and applying/releasing a vacuum [73].

Various organ-on-a-chip devices can be linked fluidically to generate human body-on-a-chip systems recapitulating the interactions between different tissues. Human body-on-a-chip systems can be defined as multiorgan systems and are often designed to emulate human physiological responses to drugs [74]. For example, a multiorgan-chip first-pass metabolism model (Fig. 4.25) has been developed by coupling vascularized organ chips of the gut, liver, and kidneys [75]. Similarly, a body-on-a-chip was created, shown in Fig. 4.26, by linking eight vital organs—the gut, liver, heart, kidneys, lungs, heart, blood-brain barrier, and skin [76]. To summarize, significant progress has been made in the fields of organoids and organ/body chips. However, they are complementary, rather than replacements (at least at the current stage) to animal and other *in vivo* drug testing approaches.

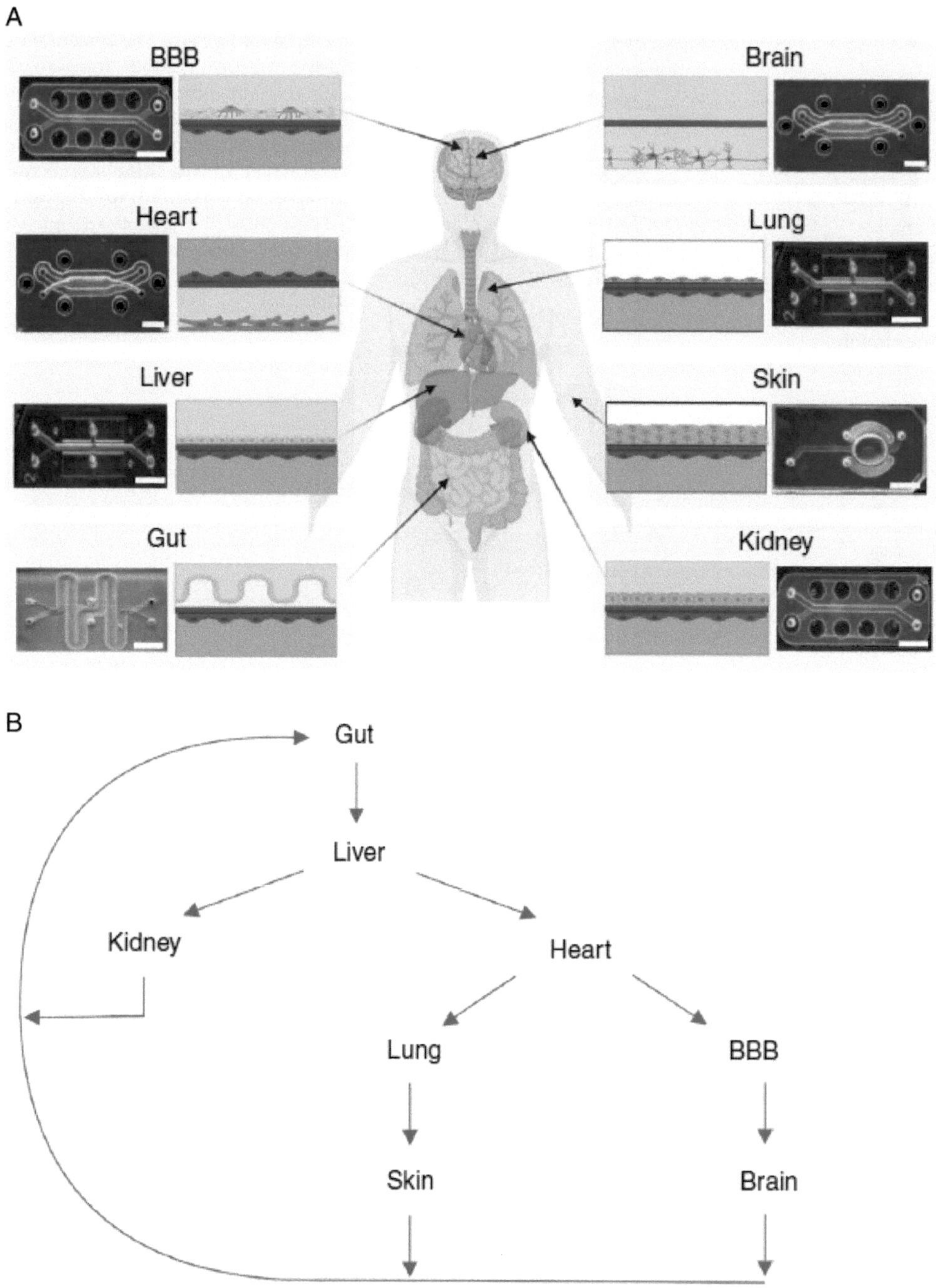

FIGURE 4.26 Linking scheme of eight organ chips to build a body-on-a-chip. (A) Photographs and diagrams of each organ chip. (B) Linking scheme of eight organs through vascular endothelial channels. Scale bars: 5 mm. From Novak, R., et al., *Robotic fluidic coupling and interrogation of multiple vascularized organ chips.* Nat Biomed Eng, 2020. **4**(4): p. 407-420, with permission from Springer Nature.

Case Study II Evolution of ophthalmic drug delivery systems

The occurrence of chronic fundus oculi diseases and age-related macular degeneration is continuously increasing due to the prolonged wearing of contact lenses, diabetes mellitus, and the increased older population [77]. Eyedrops are the most commonly noninvasive treatments for eye diseases.

As discussed in Section 4.4, only small volumes can be applied to the eyes. The maximum volume that the palpebral fissure can hold is estimated to be 30 μL under normal conditions when the patient is upright and not blinking. Although most dropper bottles are designed to deliver 25 to 70 μL drops, smaller volumes of 5 to 15 μL should

CASE STUDY II EVOLUTION OF OPHTHALMIC DRUG DELIVERY SYSTEMS (*cont'd*)

be instilled from a biopharmaceutical and economic point of view [78]. There are engineered designs, such as Nanodropper, to generate smaller drops. Also, various adapters have been developed, such as Precision Dropper.

The patient's handling of the dropper bottle significantly affects the size of the drops and the amount of drugs entering the eyes. Hence, patient compliance is another big concern, especially for the elderly population. Some good examples of patient-centric designs are Zeteo Biomedical LLC's ophthalmic drug delivery systems. These systems are designed to simplify patient usage and reduce administration errors and drug waste. For example, the credit card-size AquilaMR multidose delivery system (Fig. CS 4.1) utilizes a reloadable cartridge for precision dosing (ranging from 5 to 26 μL) based on engineered blisters (Fig. CS 4.1) and operates in any physical orientation without required priming. Moreover, it allows for one- or two-handed operation with adjustable actuation force [79].

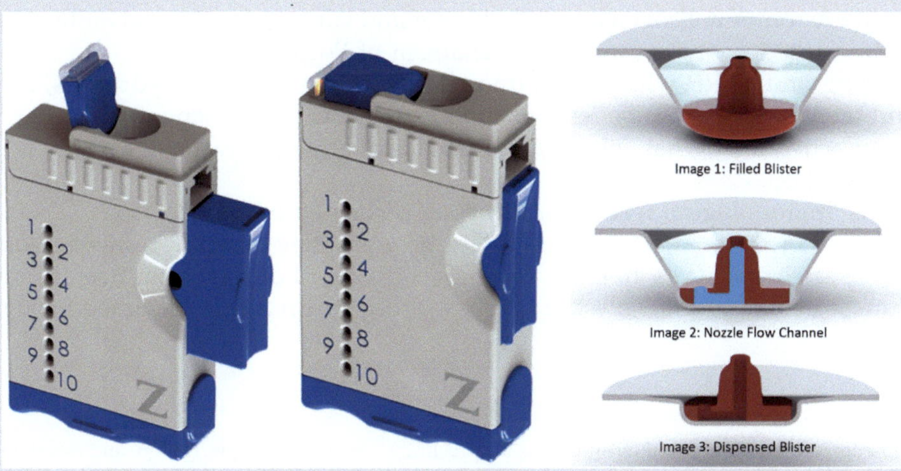

FIGURE CS 4.1 AquilaMR multidose delivery system (*left*) and working mechanism of the engineered blister (*right*). From Zeteo Biomedical LLC (Austin, Texas).

Review and practice questions

1. What are other types of cell-cell junctions besides tight junctions?
2. What type of drug molecules can easily enter cells through passive transport?
3. What is the general process of pinocytosis?
4. Hypothetical passive absorption curves of two drugs, spironolactone and glycopyrronium bromide, within the body as a function of pH are shown below. For each drug, choose the appropriate curve (I or II), that best represents the dependence of its absorption on pH and explain why.

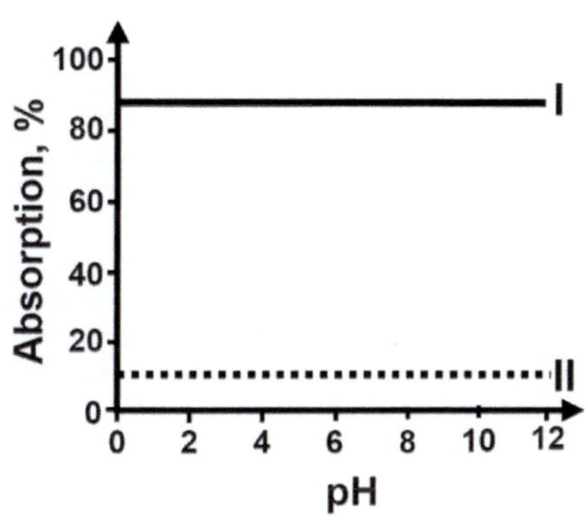

5. Trimethoprim is an antibiotic used to treat bacterial infections and has a pKa of about 7.1. Which region, stomach (use pH = 2) or small intestine (use pH = 7.5), does trimethoprim have a higher (passive) absorption rate after oral administration?
6. Why is the small intestine the primary site for drug absorption within the GI tract?
7. If you desire to study the liver biotransformation of a novel drug directly, where should the drug be administered?
8. A 200-mg dose of a drug was given orally, and 90 mg entered the systemic circulation. What was the E_h, if E_g was 0.3? Use two different approaches.
9. What are the advantages of peroral drug delivery?
10. What are the advantages and disadvantages of nonperoral routes?
    a. Skin (transdermal)
    b. Oral cavity (buccal and sublingual)
    c. Lung (pulmonary)
    d. Eye (ocular)
11. Study two drug delivery routes not covered in this chapter and summarize their advantages and disadvantages.
12. What are the three models describing the MDR mechanism of P-gp?
13. Regarding P-gp, MRP1, and BCRP, what occurs upon ATP binding and ATP hydrolysis, respectively?
14. What is ABC? And what is thought to be responsible for the ABC phenomenon?
15. What is complement activation? What are the three main activation pathways?
16. What is opsonization?
17. What are the various immunological reactions/processes discussed in this chapter?
18. What are organoids and organ-on-a-chip devices? And how are they different from each other?
19. Conduct a literature search and write an essay on a novel organoid designed for drug testing.
20. Conduct a literature search and write an essay on a novel organs-on-a-chip designed for drug testing.

References

[1] Gao Y, Gesenberg C, Zheng W. Chapter 17 - oral formulations for preclinical studies: principle, design, and development considerations. In: Qiu Y, et al., editors. Developing solid oral dosage forms. 2nd ed. Academic Press; 2017. p. 455–95.
[2] Berger TA, Berger BK, Kogelman K. Supercritical fluid chromatography for chiral analysis and semi-preparative purification. In: Reference module in chemistry, molecular sciences and chemical engineering. Elsevier; 2022.
[3] Salatin S, Yari Khosroushahi A. Overviews on the cellular uptake mechanism of polysaccharide colloidal nanoparticles. J Cell Mol Med 2017; 21(9):1668–86.
[4] Hu Y-B, et al. The endosomal-lysosomal system: from acidification and cargo sorting to neurodegeneration. Transl Neurodegener 2015; 4(1):18.
[5] Sousa de Almeida M, et al. Understanding nanoparticle endocytosis to improve targeting strategies in nanomedicine. Chem Soc Rev 2021; 50(9):5397–434.
[6] Rennick JJ, Johnston APR, Parton RG. Key principles and methods for studying the endocytosis of biological and nanoparticle therapeutics. Nat Nanotechnol 2021;16(3):266–76.
[7] Al-wadei MJ, et al. Chapter three - Betaxolol: A comprehensive profile. In: Al-Majed AA, editor. Profiles of Drug substances, excipients and related methodology. Academic Press; 2021. p. 91–136.
[8] Dei Cas M, et al. In-vitro and in-vivo metabolism of different aspirin formulations studied by a validated liquid chromatography tandem mass spectrometry method. Sci Rep 2021;11(1):10370.
[9] Vinarov Z, et al. Impact of gastrointestinal tract variability on oral drug absorption and pharmacokinetics: an UNGAP review. Eur J Pharm Sci 2021;162:105812.
[10] Lavie CJ, et al. Upper gastrointestinal toxicity associated with long-term aspirin therapy: consequences and prevention. Curr Probl Cardiol 2017;42(5):146–64.
[11] Weaver LT, Austin S, Cole TJ. Small intestinal length: a factor essential for gut adaptation. Gut 1991;32(11):1321–3.
[12] Hounnou G, et al. Anatomical study of the length of the human intestine. Surg Radiol Anat 2002;24(5):290–4.
[13] Levine RR, Walsh CT, Schwartz-Bloom RD. Levine's pharmacology: drug actions and reactions. Taylor & Francis; 2005.
[14] Possemiers S, et al. The intestinal microbiome: a separate organ inside the body with the metabolic potential to influence the bioactivity of botanicals. Fitoterapia 2011;82(1):53–66.
[15] Weersma RK, Zhernakova A, Fu J. Interaction between drugs and the gut microbiome. Gut 2020;69(8):1510–9.
[16] Sun C, Chen L, Shen Z. Mechanisms of gastrointestinal microflora on drug metabolism in clinical practice. Saudi Pharm J 2019;27(8):1146–56.
[17] Stealey S, et al. Calcium-oligochitosan-pectin microcarrier for colonic drug delivery. Pharm Dev Technol 2020;25(2):260–5.
[18] Maheshwari R, et al. Chapter 20 - manipulation of physiological processes for pharmaceutical product development. In: Tekade RK, editor. Dosage form design considerations. Academic Press; 2018. p. 701–29.
[19] Pond SM, Tozer TN. First-pass elimination. Basic concepts and clinical consequences. Clin Pharmacokinet 1984;9(1):1–25.

[20] Mehvar R. Clearance concepts: fundamentals and application to pharmacokinetic behavior of drugs. J Pharm Pharm Sci 2018;21(1s): 88s–102s.
[21] 4 - Biomechanics for pathology and treatment. In: Yamaguchi T, Ishikawa T, Imai Y, editors. Integrated nano-biomechanics. Elsevier; 2018. p. 101–46.
[22] Ramadon D, et al. Enhancement strategies for transdermal drug delivery systems: current trends and applications. Drug Deliv Transl Res 2022;12(4):758–91.
[23] Singh AK. Chapter 6 - Nanoparticle pharmacokinetics and toxicokinetics. In: Singh AK, editor. Engineered nanoparticles. Academic Press; 2016. p. 229–93.
[24] Homayun B, Lin X, Choi H-J. Challenges and recent progress in oral drug delivery systems for biopharmaceuticals. Pharmaceutics 2019; 11(3):129.
[25] Jeong WY, et al. Recent advances in transdermal drug delivery systems: a review. Biomater Res 2021;25(1):24.
[26] Bos JD, Meinardi MM. The 500 Dalton rule for the skin penetration of chemical compounds and drugs. Exp Dermatol 2000;9(3):165–9.
[27] Ventre M, et al. Chapter 2 - nanotechnologies for tissue engineering and regeneration. In: Uskoković V, Uskoković DP, editors. Nanotechnologies in preventive and regenerative medicine. Elsevier; 2018. p. 93–206.
[28] Hearnden V, et al. New developments and opportunities in oral mucosal drug delivery for local and systemic disease. Adv Drug Deliv Rev 2012;64(1):16–28.
[29] Patton JS, Fishburn CS, Weers JG. The lungs as a portal of entry for systemic drug delivery. Proc Am Thorac Soc 2004;1(4):338–44.
[30] He S, et al. A roadmap to pulmonary delivery strategies for the treatment of infectious lung diseases. J Nanobiotechnology 2022;20(1):101.
[31] Sonnenberg AH, et al. A Markov chain model of particle deposition in the lung. Scientific Reports 2020;10(1):13573.
[32] Carvalho TC, Peters JI, Williams RO. Influence of particle size on regional lung deposition: what evidence is there? Int J Pharm 2011;406(1): 1–10.
[33] Lepistö T, et al. Measurement of the human respiratory tract deposited surface area of particles with an electrical low pressure impactor. AS&T 2020;54(8):958–71.
[34] Hanes J, et al. Gene delivery to the lung. In: Hickey AJ, editor. Pharmaceutical inhalation aerosol technology. Marcel Dekker Inc.; 2003. p. 489–539.
[35] Braakhuis HM, et al. Physicochemical characteristics of nanomaterials that affect pulmonary inflammation. Part Fibre Toxicol 2014;11(1):18.
[36] Chen VSK, Penm JH-D. Management of eye disorders and the pharmacist's role: eye infections. In: Babar Z-U-D, editor. Encyclopedia of pharmacy practice and clinical pharmacy. Elsevier; 2019. p. 580–97.
[37] Davies NM. Biopharmaceutical considerations in topical ocular drug delivery. Clin Exp Pharmacol Physiol 2000;27(7):558–62.
[38] Maulvi FA, et al. Recent advances in ophthalmic preparations: ocular barriers, dosage forms and routes of administration. Int J Pharm 2021; 608:121105.
[39] Zhao M, et al. Cytochrome P450 enzymes and drug metabolism in humans. Int J Mol Sci 2021;22(23).
[40] Penner N, Woodward C, Prakash C. Appendix: Drug metabolizing enzymes and biotransformation reactions. In: Zhang D, Surapaneni S, editors. ADME-enabling technologies in drug design and development. 1st ed. John Wiley & Sons; 2012. p. 545–65.
[41] Nishino K, et al. Function and inhibitory mechanisms of multidrug efflux pumps. Front Microbiol 2021;12:737288.
[42] Sun YL, et al. Role of ABC transporters in cancer chemotherapy. Chin J Cancer 2012;31(2):51–7.
[43] Ambudkar SV, et al. P-glycoprotein: from genomics to mechanism. Oncogene 2003;22(47):7468–85.
[44] Kim Y, Chen J. Molecular structure of human P-glycoprotein in the ATP-bound, outward-facing conformation. Science 2018;359(6378):915–9.
[45] Elmeliegy M, et al. Effect of P-glycoprotein (P-gp) inducers on exposure of P-gp substrates: review of clinical drug–drug interaction studies. Clin Pharmacokinet 2020;59(6):699–714.
[46] Seelig A. P-glycoprotein: one mechanism, many tasks and the consequences for pharmacotherapy of cancers. Front Oncol 2020;10:576559.
[47] Dewanjee S, et al. Natural products as alternative choices for p-glycoprotein (P-gp) Inhibition. Molecules 2017;22(6):871.
[48] Johnson ZL, Chen J. Structural basis of substrate recognition by the multidrug resistance protein MRP1. Cell 2017;168(6):1075–1085.e9.
[49] Lu JF, Pokharel D, Bebawy M. MRP1 and its role in anticancer drug resistance. Drug Metab Rev 2015;47(4):406–19.
[50] Johnson ZL, Chen J. ATP binding enables substrate release from multidrug resistance protein 1. Cell 2018;172(1):81–89.e10.
[51] Wang J-Q, et al. Multidrug resistance proteins (MRPs): structure, function and the overcoming of cancer multidrug resistance. Drug Resist Updat 2021;54:100743.
[52] Kawahara I, et al. The impact of breast cancer resistance protein (BCRP/ABCG2) on drug transport across Caco-2 cell monolayers. Drug Metab Dispos 2020;48(6):491–8.
[53] Lai Y. 4 - Breast cancer resistance protein (BCRP)/ABCG2. In: Lai Y, editor. Transporters in Drug discovery and development. Woodhead Publishing; 2013. p. 295–326.
[54] Ni Z, et al. Structure and function of the human breast cancer resistance protein (BCRP/ABCG2). Curr Drug Metab 2010;11(7):603–17.
[55] Mao Q, Unadkat JD. Role of the breast cancer resistance protein (BCRP/ABCG2) in drug transport–an update. AAPS J 2015;17(1):65–82.
[56] Khunweeraphong N, et al. The ABCG2 multidrug transporter is a pump gated by a valve and an extracellular lid. Nat Commun 2019;10(1): 5433.
[57] Taylor NMI, et al. Structure of the human multidrug transporter ABCG2. Nature 2017;546:504–9.
[58] Orlando BJ, Liao M. ABCG2 transports anticancer drugs via a closed-to-open switch. Nat Commun 2020;11(1):2264.
[59] Jiskoot W, et al. Immunological risk of injectable drug delivery systems. Pharm Res 2009;26(6):1303–14.
[60] Besin G, et al. Accelerated blood clearance of lipid nanoparticles entails a biphasic humoral response of B-1 followed by B-2 lymphocytes to distinct antigenic moieties. ImmunoHorizons 2019;3(7):282–93.
[61] Im H-J, et al. Accelerated blood clearance phenomenon reduces the passive targeting of PEGylated nanoparticles in peripheral arterial disease. ACS Appl Mater Interfaces 2016;8(28):17955–63.
[62] de Vrieze J. Pfizer's vaccine raises allergy concerns. Science 2021;371(6524):10–1.
[63] Noris M, Remuzzi G. Overview of complement activation and regulation. Semin Nephrol 2013;33(6):479–92.
[64] Moghimi SM, et al. Complement activation by drug carriers and particulate pharmaceuticals: principles, challenges and opportunities. Adv Drug Deliv Rev 2020;157:83–95.

[65] Bryers JD, Woodrow KA. 4.21 Engineering interfaces for infection immunity. In: Ducheyne P, editor. Comprehensive biomaterials II. Elsevier; 2017. p. 381–403.
[66] Owens DE, Peppas NA. Opsonization, biodistribution, and pharmacokinetics of polymeric nanoparticles. Int J Pharm 2006;307(1):93–102.
[67] Nelemans L, Gurevich L. Drug delivery with polymeric nanocarriers—cellular uptake mechanisms. Materials 2020;13:366.
[68] Zhao Z, et al. Organoids. Nat Rev Methods Primers 2022;2(1):94.
[69] Takebe T, Wells JM. Organoids by design. Science 2019;364(6444):956–9.
[70] Ishihara K, et al. Topological morphogenesis of neuroepithelial organoids. Nature Physics 2023;19(2):177–83.
[71] Kessler M, et al. Chronic Chlamydia infection in human organoids increases stemness and promotes age-dependent CpG methylation. Nat Commun 2019;10(1):1194.
[72] Park SE, Georgescu A, Huh D. Organoids-on-a-chip. Science 2019;364(6444):960–5.
[73] Huh D, et al. Reconstituting organ-level lung functions on a chip. Science 2010;328(5986):1662–8.
[74] Sung JH, et al. Recent advances in body-on-a-chip systems. Anal Chem 2019;91(1):330–51.
[75] Herland A, et al. Quantitative prediction of human pharmacokinetic responses to drugs via fluidically coupled vascularized organ chips. Nat Biomed Eng 2020;4(4):421–36.
[76] Novak R, et al. Robotic fluidic coupling and interrogation of multiple vascularized organ chips. Nat Biomed Eng 2020;4(4):407–20.
[77] Shen J, et al. Eyedrop-based macromolecular ophthalmic drug delivery for ocular fundus disease treatment. Science Advances 2023;9(4): eabq3104.
[78] Van Santvliet L, Ludwig A. Determinants of eye drop size. Surv Ophthalmol 2004;49(2):197–213.
[79] Ophthalmic drug delivery systems. Available from: https://zeteobiomed.com/ophthalmic-drug-delivery/.

CHAPTER

5

Prodrugs as drug delivery systems

Wujie Zhang

LEARNING OBJECTIVES

- To interpret the basic working mechanism of prodrugs for drug delivery
- To understand and explain the benefits associated with prodrugs for drug delivery
- To differentiate different types of prodrug systems
- To understand and apply prodrug design principles
- To identify and design ester-based and salt-based prodrugs
- To understand, explain, and compare novel prodrug systems (ADEPT, GDEPT/VDEPT) and suicide gene therapy
- To provide examples of prodrugs in therapy

5.1 Introduction to prodrugs

Prodrugs, with little or no pharmacological activity, are reversible derivatives of drug molecules that undergo an enzymatic and/or chemical transformation *in vivo* to release active parent drugs, which can then exert the desired pharmacological effect. Around 5% to 7% of drugs approved worldwide can be classified as prodrugs [1,2]. The term prodrug was first introduced in medicinal chemistry by Adrien Albert in 1951 [3]. As shown in Fig. 5.1, regardless of the site of action, prodrugs have to be activated to liberate the parent drugs. The activation can be either chemical (e.g., redox) or enzyme-mediated (e.g., cytochrome P450) [4]. There are various benefits associated with prodrug systems, including higher solubility, enhanced permeability, improved stability, and prolonged systemic circulation. Moreover, prodrugs have been used for site-selective drug delivery with reduced side effects and presystemic drug metabolism [1].

There are essentially two types of prodrugs: bioprecursor and carrier-linked prodrugs. Bioprecursor prodrugs are activated by transformation *in vivo* upon administration. A carrier-linked prodrug contains a carrier moiety that is temporarily covalently linked to the drug. Cleavage of the carrier moiety releases the drug. The carrier may serve as a targeting moiety or biologically inert. For example, polyethylene glycol (PEG) is commonly used as a carrier (i.e., PEGylation) [3]. PEGylation can increase the circulating half-life by avoiding phagocytosis of the reticuloendothelial system, decreasing the surface adsorption of proteins, and reducing renal

Fundamentals and Design of Drug Delivery Systems
https://doi.org/10.1016/B978-0-443-23521-4.00005-9

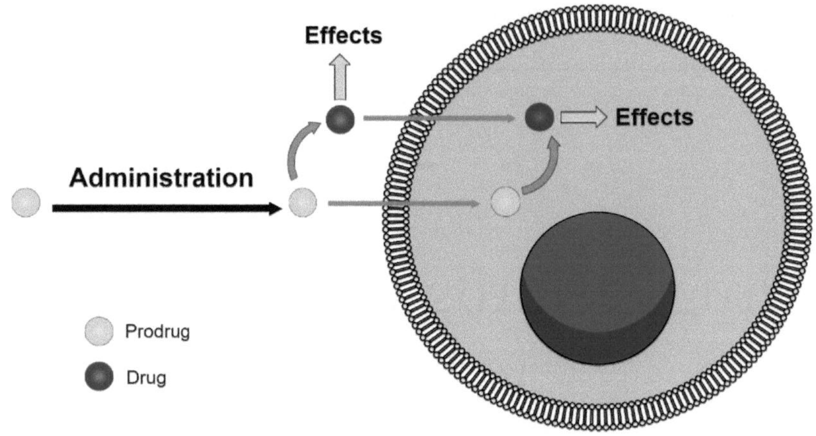

FIGURE 5.1 Working mechanism of prodrugs as drug delivery systems. Prodrugs can be activated either extracellularly or intracellularly.

clearance, enzymatic degradation, and immunogenicity by increasing the hydrodynamic volume and shielding recognition sites [5,6].

5.2 Principles of prodrug design

To engineer a prodrug, pharmaceutical, pharmacokinetic, and pharmacodynamic aspects should be considered (as summarized in Fig. 5.2).

Ester-based prodrugs. Ester-based prodrugs are more hydrophobic compared to their parental drug. They are generally designed for improved drug absorption/bioavailability and stability. Ester moieties are often used to mask alkyl hydroxyl groups, aryl hydroxyl groups, carboxyl groups, and even amines. Ester-based prodrugs can be activated *in vivo* through either enzyme catalysis (esterases) or hydrolysis [7]. In general, esterases catalyze the conversion of an ester to a carboxylic acid and an alcohol [8]. The diversity and complexity of esterases should not be overlooked. Moreover, the collection of esterases in biology is heterogeneous, and small changes in ester-masked compounds may lead to significant changes in biological activity [7].

Quinapril is a prodrug for quinaprilat (Fig. 5.3), which is used for the treatment of hypertension and congestive heart failure. Quinapril is metabolized into quinaprilat in the liver and enters the systemic circulation [9]. A study performed a pharmacodynamic and pharmacokinetic comparison of intravenous quinaprilat and oral quinapril. The results showed that the oral quinapril, at about half dose, produced a pharmacodynamic comparable to that of intravenous quinaprilat [10].

Salt-based prodrugs. Salt-based prodrugs, such as phosphates, sulfamate salts, and pyridinium salts, can be designed for improved aqueous solubility and stability. Phosphate groups are commonly used to enhance the solubility of poorly soluble compounds. A phosphoric moiety can be directly linked to the parental drug (e.g., through the hydroxyl group) or *via* a chemical linker [11]. The bioconversion can be done through phosphatases *in vivo*.

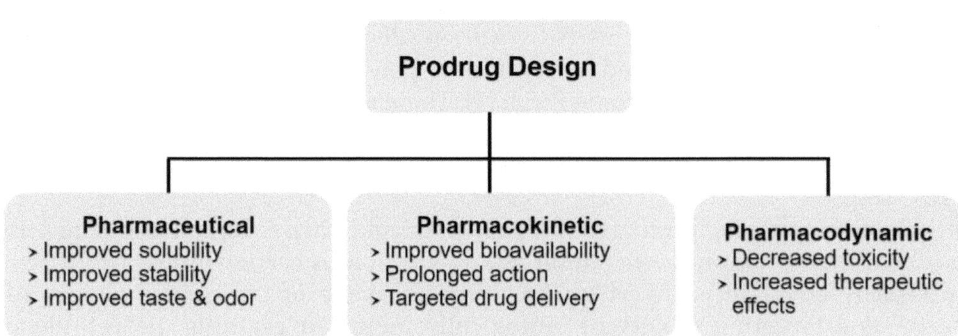

FIGURE 5.2 Prodrug design considerations.

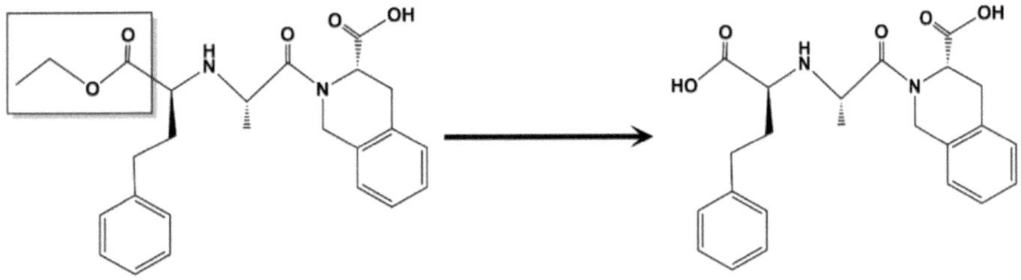

FIGURE 5.3 The structure of quinapril and quinaprilat.

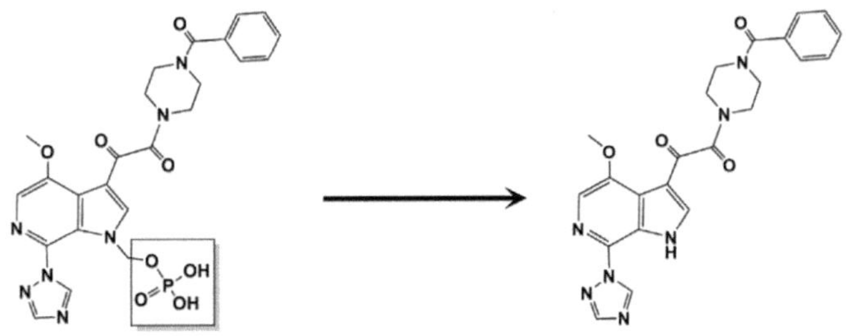

FIGURE 5.4 The structures of fostemsavir and temsavir.

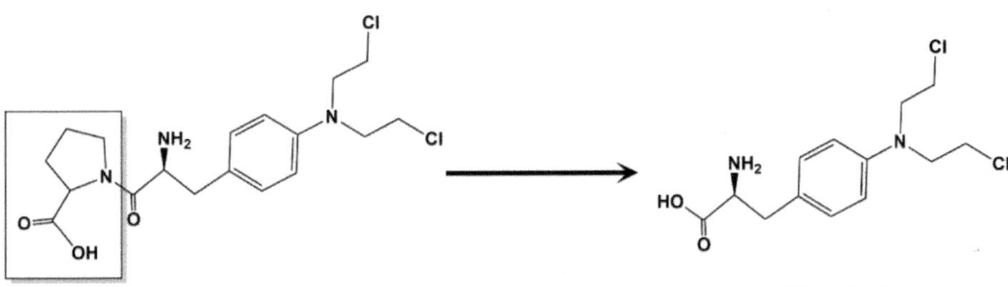

FIGURE 5.5 The structure of Mel-pro and melphalan.

Fostemsavir is a salt-based prodrug of temsavir (Fig. 5.4). It is developed specifically for use in patients with human immunodeficiency virus type I infection who have undergone multiple therapies [12]. The phosphate moiety enhanced the solubility by 500-fold and increased the bioavailability from 40% to 80–122% [11].

Amino acids/peptides in prodrug design. Amino acids/peptides have been used in prodrug design to improve drug solubility and permeability, especially in oral drug delivery. α-Amine or α-carboxyl groups of an amino acid/peptide can be linked to the parent drug's functional groups, such as hydroxyl, amine, and carboxyl groups, forming an ester or amide. α-Amine and α-carboxyl groups can also be linked to parent drugs through carbonate and carbamate links [13]. Amino acids/peptides can be used to target certain transporters that are overexpressed in certain organs, such as L-type amino acid transporters (LAT1) at the blood-brain barrier [14].

The proline prodrug of melphalan (Mel-pro) showed increased efficacy against cancer cell line MDA-MB-231. The possible mechanisms were improved transport across cell membranes and higher prolidase activity in MDA-MB-231 cells [14,15].

5.3 Advances in prodrugs as drug delivery systems

One of the major advances in prodrugs as drug delivery systems is the directed enzyme prodrug therapy. These prodrugs can be used to target specific tissues/cells. These systems generally require the delivery of both prodrugs and enzymes. Prodrugs are converted to drugs under specific enzymatic activity. This strategy includes antibody-directed enzyme prodrug therapy (ADEPT), gene-directed enzyme prodrug therapy (GDEPT), viral-directed enzyme prodrug therapy (VDEPT), polymer-directed enzyme prodrug therapy (PDEPT), and clostridia-directed enzyme prodrug therapy (CDEPT) [4].

Regarding ADEPT, an antibody is conjugated to an enzyme that is not normally present within the human body. The antibody-enzyme conjugate and prodrugs are co-administered, then antibodies bind to its antigen and convert the prodrug to the drug *in situ* (Fig. 5.6A). Besides antibodies, low molecular weight ligands can also be used. Folate derivatives are promising ligands that bind to the folate receptor (highly overexpressed in many epithelial cancers) [2].

Both GDEPT (using nonviral vectors) and VDEPT (using viral vectors) deliver the specific enzyme-producing gene into cells. Through gene expression, the specific enzyme is produced to convert a prodrug to its parental drug (Fig. 5.6B). In particular, GDEPT is a suicide gene therapy approach. As shown in Fig. 5.7, the suicide gene is first introduced into cancer cells. Through gene expression, the suicide gene leads to specific enzyme production—which converts the prodrug to a toxic drug and destroys the transfected cells. Then, drug molecules enter surrounding cancer cells (nontransduced) through gap junction or diffusion and kill them (bystander effect) [16–18]. It has also shown that suicide gene therapy can cause a release of damage-associated molecular patterns and/or induce a display of neoantigens leading to immunogenic cell death [17].

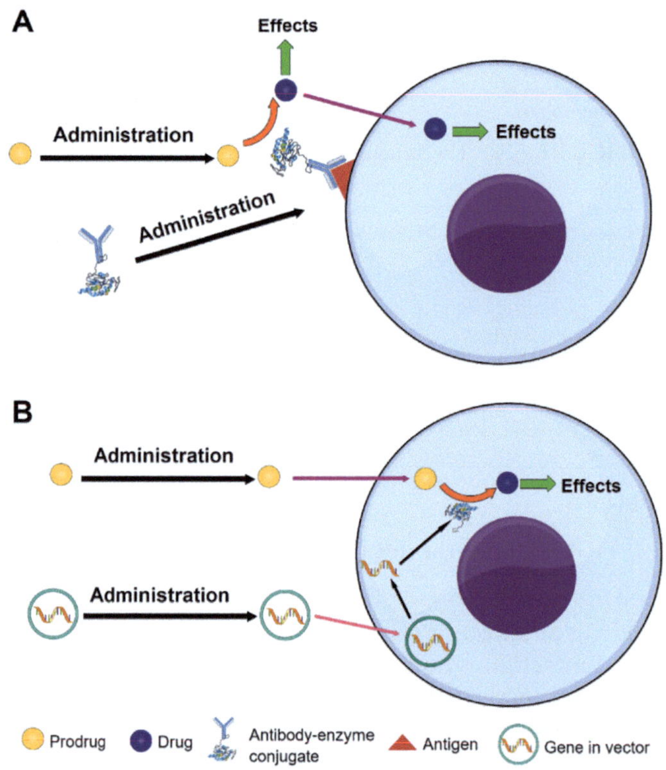

FIGURE 5.6 Working mechanisms of ADEPT (A) and GDEPT/VDEPT (B).

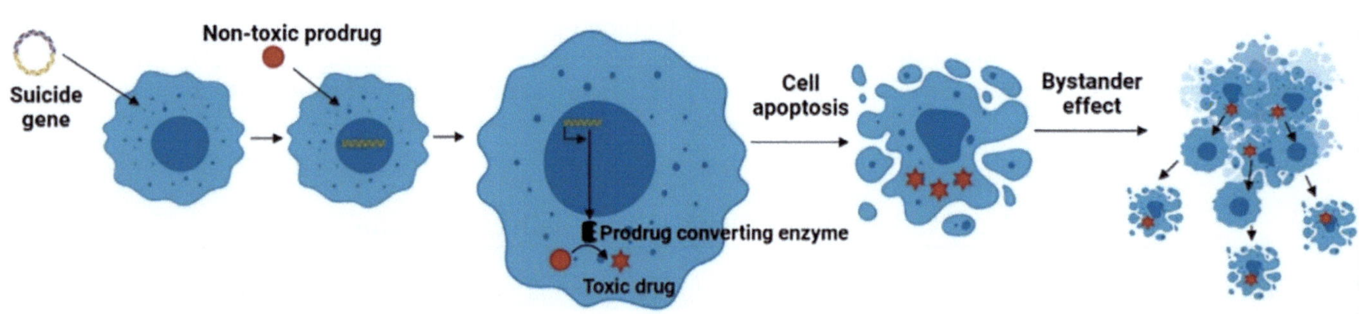

FIGURE 5.7 Working mechanisms of suicide gene therapy. From Saeb, S. et al., *Suicide gene therapy in cancer and HIV-1 infection: an alternative to conventional treatments*. Biochem. Pharmacol, 2022. **197**: p. 114893, with permission from Elsevier.

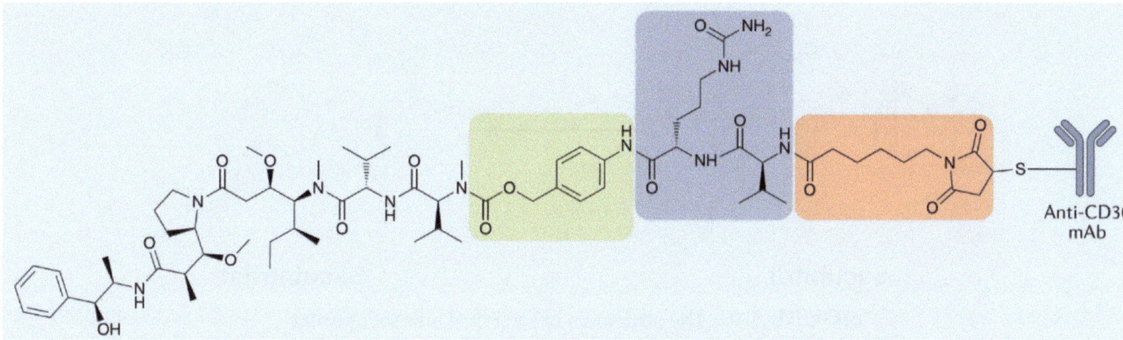

FIGURE 5.8 The structure of the prodrug brentuximab vedotin. Linker (*blue*): dipeptide valine-citrulline and Spacer (*orange*): maleimidocaproyl. Dipeptide valine-citrulline and *para*-amino benzyloxycarbonyl (*green*) moieties are cleaved by cathepsin B. From Rautio, J. et al., *The expanding role of prodrugs in contemporary drug design and development.* Nat. Rev. Drug Discov, 2018. **17**(8): p. 559-587, with permission from Springer Nature.

When it comes to carrier-linked prodrugs, linkers and/or spacers are also incorporated to improve the drug's efficacy. A good example is brentuximab vedotin (Adcetris). This antibody-drug conjugate, the structure shown in Fig. 5.8 (prodrug), is in clinical use for stage III and IV classic Hodgkin lymphoma. A recent study showed that the treatment with brentuximab vedotin plus doxorubicin, vinblastine, and decarbazine ($A_{+}AVD$) resulted in an improvement in both progression-free survival and overall survival [19]. A promising case report on the efficacy and safety of extended courses of brentuximab vedotin monotherapy in a hemodialysis patient with classic Hodgkin lymphoma was recently published [20]. The monoclonal antibody that brentuximab targets, CD30, is a defining marker of Hodgkin lymphoma and systemic anaplastic large-cell lymphoma [2,21]. The drug, vedotin (auristatin E), is an antimitotic agent that inhibits cell division by blocking tubulin polymerization. The linker, dipeptide valine-citrulline, is designed to be site-selectively cleaved by the proteolytic enzyme, cathepsin B, to release vedotin upon the endocytosis of the conjugate by tumor cells. At the same time, the maleimidocaproyl spacer provides space for cathepsin B's access and cleavage action [2].

5.4 New prodrugs in therapy

In recent years, a large number of prodrugs have been approved, including those that were granted priority review by the U.S. Food and Drug Administration (FDA), such as Entresto (sacubitril/valsartan) and Xofluza (baloxavir marboxil). Entresto, approved by the FDA and European Union in 2015, is a combination of a neprilysin inhibitor and an angiotensin II receptor blocker for the reduction of risk of cardiovascular death and hospitalization in adult patients with chronic heart failure. Sacubitril is a prodrug that undergoes de-ethylation *via* esterases and activation into sacubitrilat (Fig. 5.9), which acts as an inhibitor of the enzyme endopeptidase neprilysin, inducing vasodilation [22]. Baloxavir marboxil, approved by the FDA and Japan in 2018, is the prodrug of baloxavir acid for the treatment of acute uncomplicated influenza (flu) in patients 12 years of age and older who have been symptomatic for more than 48 hours [23]. Baloxavir marboxil was developed by the addition of a phenolic hydroxyl group (Fig. 5.10), resulting in improved oral absorption [24,25]. Baloxavir acts within the polymerase acidic protein subunit of the influenza A and B viruses' polymerase complex and inhibits the cap-dependent endonuclease (an essential protein involved in the initiation of viral transcription) [24,26].

Nexletol (bempedoic acid), an adenosine triphosphate-citrate lyase inhibitor, was approved in 2020 for the treatment of high low-density lipoprotein cholesterol by the FDA (first-in-class). Bempedoic acid is a prodrug, which is converted to the active metabolite bempedoyl–CoA (Fig. 5.11) by endogenous liver acyl-coenzyme A (CoA) synthetase activity [27–29].

Azstarys (dexmethylphenidate chloride and dexmethylphenidate hydrochloride) was approved by the FDA in 2021 for the treatment of attention deficit hyperactivity disorder in patients 6 years of age and older. Serdexmethylphenidate chloride is an inactive prodrug of dexmethylphenidate hydrochloride (Fig. 5.12). Immediate release of the formulation of dexmethylphenidate hydrochloride provides an early onset of the pharmacological effect. More than 97% of an oral dose of serdexmethylphenidate chloride stays within the GI tract and slowly converts to dexmethylphenidate hydrochloride in the lower intestine, prolonging the duration of effects [30].

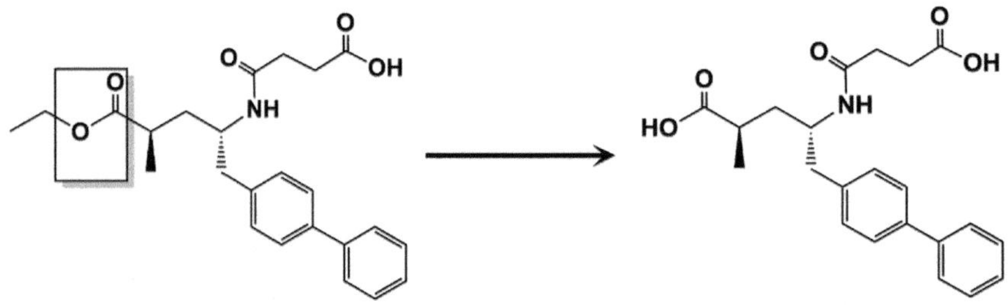

Sacubitril Sacubitrilat

FIGURE 5.9 The structures of sacubitril and sacubitrilat.

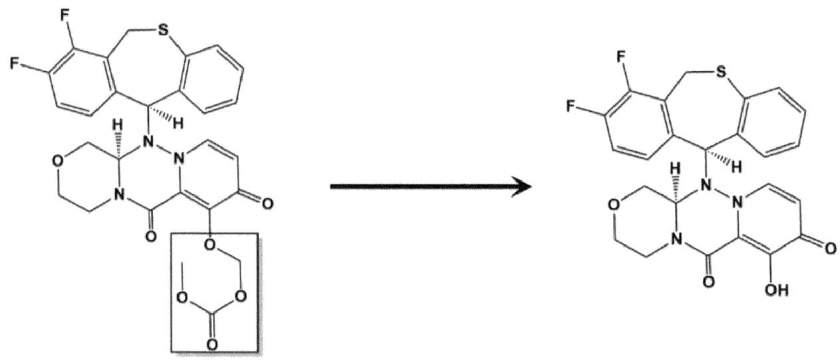

Baloxavir marboxil Baloxavir acid

FIGURE 5.10 The structures of baloxavir marboxil and baloxavir acid.

Bempedoic acid

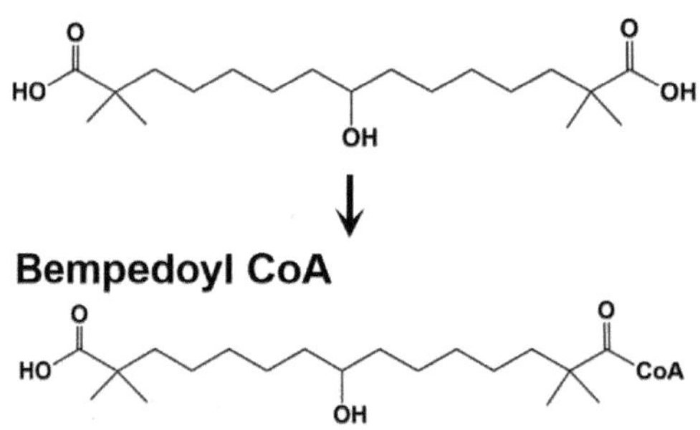

Bempedoyl CoA

FIGURE 5.11 The structures of bempedoic acid and bempedoyl-CoA.

Serdexmethylphenidate chloride

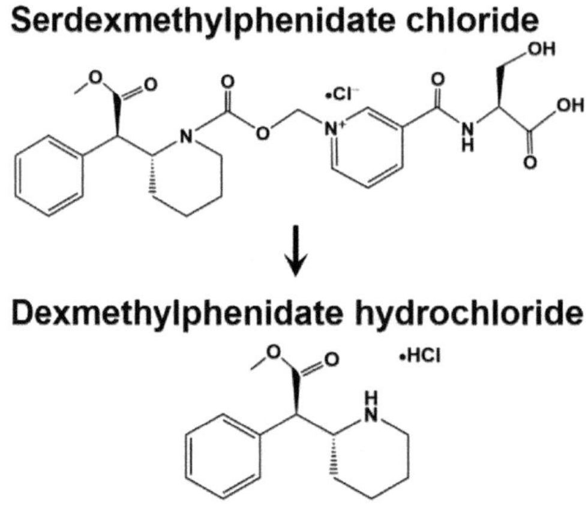

Dexmethylphenidate hydrochloride

FIGURE 5.12 The structures of serdexmethylphenidate chloride and dexmethylphenidate hydrochloride.

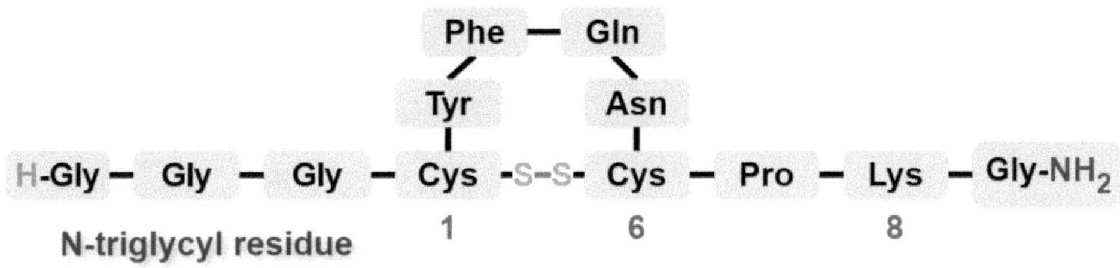

FIGURE 5.13 The structure of terlipressin. Lysine is at position 8 of the lysine-vasopressin. The *N*-triglycyl residue is cleaved by peptidases.

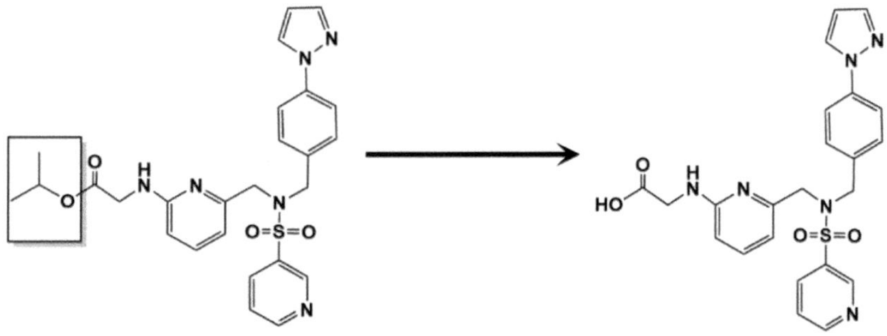

Omidenepag isopropyl **Omidenepag**

FIGURE 5.14 The structures of omidenepag isopropyl and omidenepag.

Terlivaz (terlipressin) was approved in 2022 by the FDA (received priority review and fast track status and orphan drug designation) for the improvement of kidney function in adults with hepatorenal syndrome with rapid reduction in kidney function. Terlipressin, a vasopressin analog, serves as a prodrug for lysine-vasopressin while exhibiting pharmacological activity. Terlipressin is a synthetic peptide composed of one molecule of lysine-vasopressin and three additional glycine residues and is then metabolized *via* exopeptidases into lysine-vasopressin (Fig. 5.13) [31,32]. It is believed to decrease portal hypertension and blood circulation in portal vessels and increase effective arterial volume and mean arterial pressure [33]. Omlonti (omidenepag isopropyl ophthalmic solution) was also approved in 2022 for the reduction of elevated intraocular pressure in patients with open-angle glaucoma or ocular hypertension. Omidenepag isopropyl is a relatively selective prostaglandin E2 receptor agonist. It is an ester prodrug of omidenepag (Fig. 5.14) [34].

Case Study III: Acyclovir "goes pro"

Acyclovir, a synthetic acyclic purine nucleoside analog, was the first agent to be licensed for the prevention and treatment of viral infections such as herpes simplex virus (HSV). However, acyclovir has low water solubility and absorption (membrane permeability), resulting in an oral bioavailability of only 10% to 20% [35].

Valacyclovir, an ester-based prodrug of acyclovir, shows much greater bioavailability (threefold to fivefold higher), and it converts to acyclovir by the valacyclovir hydrolase in the digestive tract and liver [36,37].

Phosphorylation is critical for acyclovir to function. Production of acyclovir monophosphate is catalyzed by thymidine kinase, caused by cells infected by HSV [37]. Considering the importance of the phosphate group, the prodrug, acyclovir ProTides, was developed to be nucleoside kinase-independent. It is a monophosphorylated acyclovir with the phosphate group masked by a lipophilic group. The lipophilic group is introduced to increase cellular uptake by improving membrane permeability. This prodrug shows great potential in suppressing both human immunodeficiency virus type I (HIV-1) and HSV-2. The acyclovir ProTides suppresses HIV reverse transcriptase and inhibits HSV-2, which is a known copathogen of HIV-1 [38,39].

Continued

Case Study III: Acyclovir "goes pro" *(cont'd)*

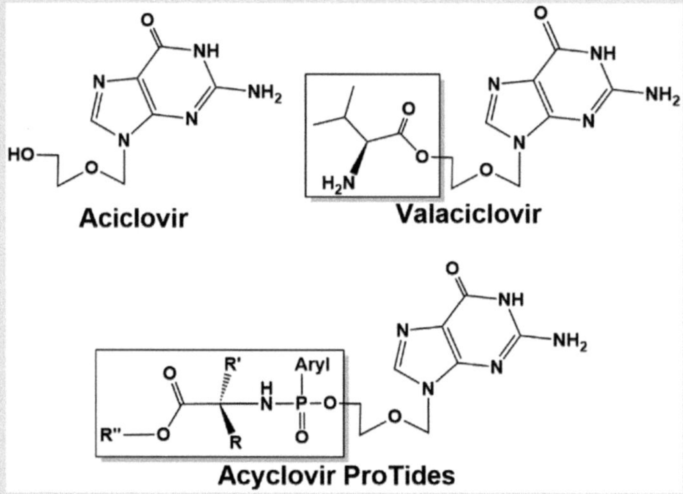

FIGURE CS 5.1 The structures of acyclovir and its prodrugs.

Review and practice questions

1. What are prodrugs? And what are the two types of prodrugs?
2. What are the benefits of using prodrugs as drug delivery systems?
3. What are the benefits associated with PEGylation?
4. What aspects are considered for prodrug design?
5. Show the chemical structure of levodopa based on the structure of its ester-based prodrug melevodopa (shown below).

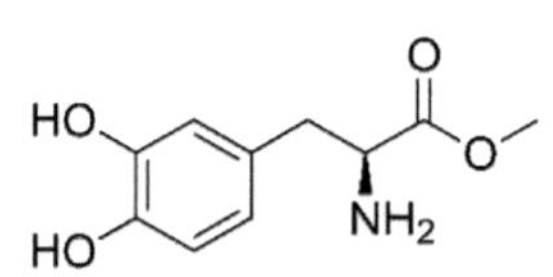

6. Show the chemical structure of phenytoin based on the structure of its phosphate prodrug fosphenytoin (shown below).

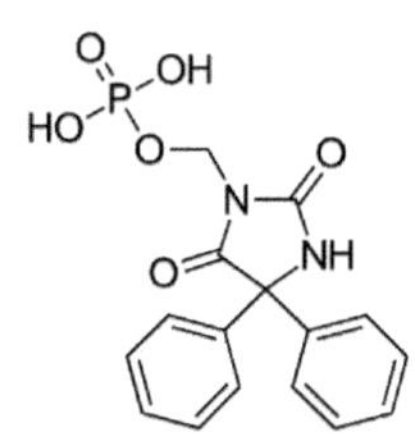

7. Show the chemical structure of brivanib based on the structure of its prodrug brivanib alaninate (shown below).

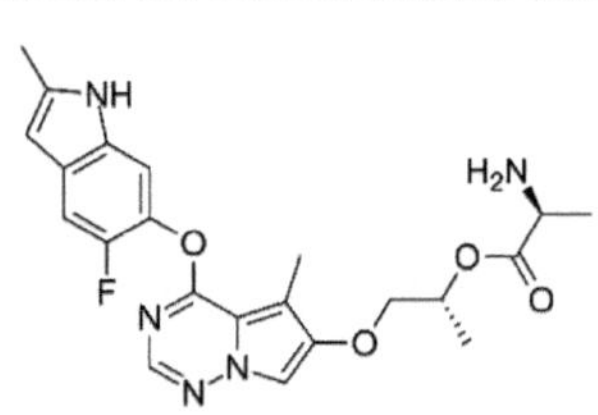

8. What is the working mechanism of ADEPT?
9. What is the working mechanism of GDEPT/VDEPT?
10. Describe the function of each component of the prodrug brentuximab vedotin.
11. Conduct a literature search on a prodrug that is not discussed in this chapter and write a short essay. Include the structures of both the drug and prodrug, clinical application(s) of the drug/prodrug, and benefits of the prodrug.

References

[1] Rautio J, et al. Prodrugs: design and clinical applications. Nat Rev Drug Discov 2008;7(3):255–70.
[2] Rautio J, et al. The expanding role of prodrugs in contemporary drug design and development. Nat Rev Drug Discov 2018;17(8):559–87.
[3] Abet V, et al. Prodrug approach: an overview of recent cases. Eur J Med Chem 2017;127:810–27.
[4] Markovic M, Ben-Shabat S, Dahan A. Prodrugs for improved drug delivery: lessons learned from recently developed and marketed products. Pharmaceutics 2020;12(11).
[5] Li Y, et al. Impact of the amount of PEG on prodrug nanoassemblies for efficient cancer therapy. Asian J Pharm Sci 2022;17(2):241–52.
[6] Böttger R, Knappe D, Hoffmann R. PEGylated prodrugs of antidiabetic peptides amylin and GLP-1. J Control Release 2018;292:58–66.
[7] Lavis LD. Ester bonds in prodrugs. ACS Chem Biol 2008;3(4):203–6.
[8] Larsen EM, Johnson RJ. Microbial esterases and ester prodrugs: an unlikely marriage for combating antibiotic resistance. Drug Dev Res 2019; 80(1):33–47.
[9] Tandan N, Patel P, Cassagnol M. Quinapril. StatPearls [Internet] 2022. Available from: https://www.ncbi.nlm.nih.gov/books/NBK557398/.
[10] Breslin E, et al. A pharmacodynamic and pharmacokinetic comparison of intravenous quinaprilat and oral quinapril. J Clin Pharmacol 1996; 36(5):414–21.
[11] Sanches BMA, Ferreira EI. Is prodrug design an approach to increase water solubility? Int J Pharm 2019;568:118498.
[12] Kozal M, et al. Fostemsavir in adults with multidrug-resistant HIV-1 infection. N Engl J Med 2020;382(13):1232–43.
[13] Vig BS, et al. Amino acids as promoieties in prodrug design and development. Adv Drug Deliv Rev 2013;65(10):1370–85.
[14] Vale N, et al. Amino acids in the development of prodrugs. Molecules 2018;23(9):2318.
[15] Chrzanowski K, Bielawska A, Pałka J. Proline analogue of melphalan as a prodrug susceptible to the action of prolidase in breast cancer MDA-MB 231 cells. Il Farmaco 2003;58(11):1113–9.
[16] Alekseenko I, et al. Step-by-step immune activation for suicide gene therapy reinforcement. Int J Mol Sci 2021;22(17):9376.
[17] Hossain JA, et al. Suicide gene therapy for the treatment of high-grade glioma: past lessons, present trends, and future prospects. Neurooncol Adv 2020;2(1):vdaa013.
[18] Saeb S, et al. Suicide gene therapy in cancer and HIV-1 infection: an alternative to conventional treatments. Biochem Pharmacol 2022;197: 114893.
[19] Ansell SM, et al. Overall survival with brentuximab vedotin in stage III or IV Hodgkin's lymphoma. N Engl J Med 2022;387(4):310–20.
[20] Uchimura A, et al. Hodgkin lymphoma on hemodialysis successfully treated with extended courses of brentuximab vedotin. Case Rep Oncol 2022;15(1):263–6.
[21] Scott LJ. Brentuximab vedotin: a review in CD30-positive hodgkin lymphoma. Drugs 2017;77(4):435–45.
[22] Nussinovitch U, et al. Chapter 6: Novel treatments for diastolic heart failure. In: Nussinovitch U, editor. Emerging technologies for heart diseases. Academic Press; 2020. p. 95–127.
[23] U.S. Food and Drug Administration. FDA approves new drug to treat influenza. Available from: https://www.fda.gov/news-events/press-announcements/fda-approves-new-drug-treat-influenza.
[24] Abraham GM, Morton JB, Saravolatz LD. Baloxavir: a novel antiviral agent in the treatment of influenza. Clin Infect Dis 2020;71(7):1790–4.
[25] Omoto S, et al. Characterization of influenza virus variants induced by treatment with the endonuclease inhibitor baloxavir marboxil. Sci Rep 2018;8(1):9633.
[26] Ikematsu H, et al. Baloxavir marboxil for prophylaxis against influenza in household contacts. N Engl J Med 2020;383(4):309–20.
[27] Bilen O, Ballantyne CM. Bempedoic Acid (ETC-1002): an investigational inhibitor of ATP citrate lyase. Curr Atheroscler Rep 2016;18(10):61.
[28] Goldberg AC, et al. Effect of bempedoic acid vs placebo added to maximally tolerated statins on low-density lipoprotein cholesterol in patients at high risk for cardiovascular disease: the CLEAR Wisdom Randomized Clinical Trial. JAMA 2019;322(18):1780–8.
[29] Pinkosky SL, et al. Liver-specific ATP-citrate lyase inhibition by bempedoic acid decreases LDL-C and attenuates atherosclerosis. Nat Commun 2016;7(1):13457.
[30] U.S. Food and Drug Administration. Drug approval package: AZSTARYS. Available from: https://www.accessdata.fda.gov/drugsatfda_docs/nda/2021/212994Orig1s000TOC.cfm.
[31] Colson PH, et al. Terlipressin, a vasoactive prodrug recommended in hepatorenal syndrome, is an agonist of human V1, V2 and V1B receptors: implications for its safety profile. Pharmacol Res 2016;113:257–64.
[32] Pichler RH, et al. Terlipressin: hopes fulfilled or dashed? Clin J Am Soc Nephrol 2022;17(1):140–2.
[33] U.S. Food and Drug Administration. FDA approves treatment to improve kidney function in adults with hepatorenal syndrome. Available from: https://www.fda.gov/drugs/news-events-human-drugs/fda-approves-treatment-improve-kidney-function-adults-hepatorenal-syndrome.
[34] Omidenepag isopropyl. Am J Health Syst Pharm 2022;80(3):93–5.
[35] Karaman R, et al. Prodrugs of acyclovir–a computational approach. Chem Biol Drug Des 2012;79(5):819–34.
[36] Paintsil E, Cheng Y-C. Antiviral agents. In: Schaechter M, editor. Encyclopedia of microbiology. 3rd ed. Academic Press; 2009. p. 223–57.
[37] Kausar S, et al. A review: mechanism of action of antiviral drugs. Int J Immunopathol Pharmacol 2021;35:20587384211002621.
[38] Vanpouille C, et al. A new class of dual-targeted antivirals: monophosphorylated acyclovir prodrug derivatives suppress both human immunodeficiency virus type 1 and herpes simplex virus type 2. J Infect Dis 2010;201(4):635–43.
[39] Derudas M, et al. The application of phosphoramidate protide technology to acyclovir confers anti-HIV inhibition. J Med Chem 2009;52(17): 5520–30.

CHAPTER

6

Engineered carriers in drug delivery

Wujie Zhang

LEARNING OBJECTIVES

- To identify different types of polymers
- To provide examples of both natural and synthetic polymers in drug delivery
- To discuss and compare different types of microscale drug carriers and their fabrication approaches
- To discuss and compare different types of nanoscale drug carriers and their fabrication approaches
- To apply the drug carrier design considerations for drug carrier design
- To understand and evaluate different drug carrier modification methods and design the process for modifying drug carriers

6.1 Materials for drug carriers

Both hard and soft materials have been used in developing drug delivery systems. Hard materials that have been used include metals [1], ceramics [2], and glass [3]; soft materials that are used are generally polymeric materials. This section focuses on polymers as they are of great property diversity and have been commonly used in almost all major dosage forms, such as tablets and capsules, as well as novel drug delivery systems [4,5]. Particularly, biodegradable and bioabsorbable polymers are of great interest [6].

The term polymer (Greek) means many parts. The building blocks (parts) of polymers are monomers. Based on the number of types of monomers, polymers can be classified into homopolymers (one type of monomer/polymer) and copolymers (two or more types of monomers/polymer). Copolymers are block copolymers if one or more types of monomers form "blocks" within the polymer chain. Polymers can also be linear, branched, or crosslinked. Based on their sources, polymers can be natural or synthetic.

Polymers can be produced through direct biosynthesis (i.e., natural polymers, such as alginate and collagen), chemical synthesis of biofeedstock (e.g., chemical synthesis of lactic acid produced through fermentation to manufacture polylactide), and chemical synthesis of petrochemical raw materials. Alongside social, economic, and environmental aspects, natural polymers have advantages over synthetic polymers such as high biocompatibility and specific interactions with biomolecules (such as enzymes) within the body [7,8]. Both natural polysaccharides and proteins have been widely used in drug delivery.

Fundamentals and Design of Drug Delivery Systems
https://doi.org/10.1016/B978-0-443-23521-4.00006-0

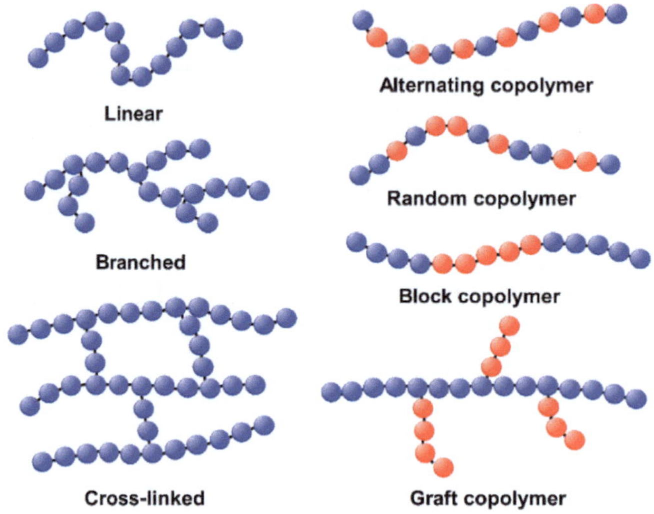

FIGURE 6.1 Different polymer structures.

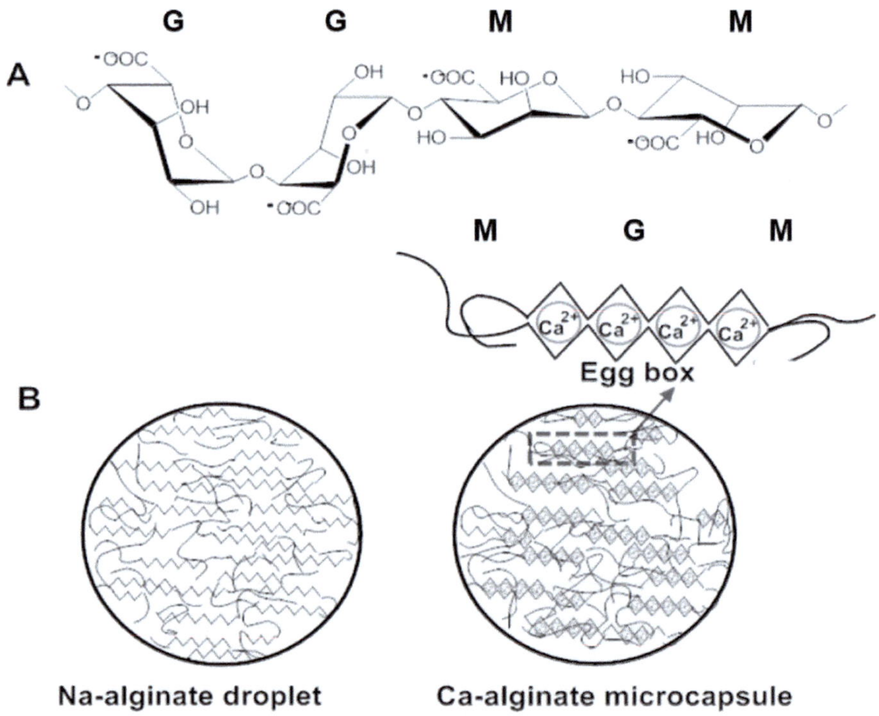

FIGURE 6.2 Chemical structure of alginate (A) and alginate-based hydrogel formation mechanism (B). *From W. Zhang, Encapsulation of transgenic cells for gene therapy,* in Gene Therapy, D. Hashad, Editor. 2015, IntechOpen. p. Ch. 8.

Alginate. Alginates are linear polysaccharides consisting of α-L-guluronic acid (G) and β-D-mannuronic acid (M) blocks (Fig. 6.2A). They are mostly present in the cell walls of brown algae as different salt forms of alginic acid, such as sodium salts [9,10]. Divalent and polyvalent cations, such as Ca^{2+} and Ba^{2+}, can crosslink alginate molecules, forming hydrogels through carboxyl groups (i.e., egg-box model; Fig. 6.2B). The G and M contents of alginate molecules can affect the gel's properties, including mechanical strength and biocompatibility [10].

Pectin. Pectin is a polysaccharide found in the cell walls of plants and is primarily comprised of α-(1-4)-linked D-galacturonic acid residues with interspersed 1,2-linked L-rhamnose residues. About 80% of the acid groups are in the form of methyl esters (Fig. 6.3). There are two types of pectin based on the degree of esterification (DE): high DE and low DE pectin. Very similar to alginate, pectin forms a gel when exposed to divalent cations, low DE pectin in particular [11,12]. The shifted "egg-box" model can be used to describe the structure due to a pronounced shift of the galacturonate chain in relation to the other chain in chain-chain association [13]. Besides cationic ions, oligochitosan (or chitosan oligosaccharide or chitooligosaccharide) has also been shown to serve as a crosslinker for pectin. Interestingly, red blood cell–shaped hydrogels can be formed using oligochitosan (molecular weight ~ 3 kD) as a crosslinker (Fig. 6.4) [14–16]. The system shows great potential for developing oxygen therapeutics mimicking natural red blood cells. However, no red blood cell–shaped hydrogel can be formed when using different types of alginate with oligochitosan as a crosslinker [17].

Hyaluronic acid. Hyaluronic acid (HA) is a nonsulfated glycosaminoglycan and is composed of repeating polymeric disaccharides of D-glucuronic acid and *N*-acetyl-D-glucosamine linked by interchanging β-(1-4) and β-(1-3) glycosidic bond (Fig. 6.5). It is most abundant in the skin of humans [18]. The features that make HA attractive in drug delivery are cellular permeability, site-specific functionalization of molecules, tunable chemical structure, biocompatibility, and responsiveness to external stimuli. HA has been used to make different formulations such as creams, gels, and sera [19].

Chitin and chitosan. Chitin, β-(1-4)-poly-*N*-acetyl-D-glucosamine, is the second most abundant polysaccharide after cellulose and the most abundant aminopolysaccharide in nature. It is the major structural component of the exoskeletons of crustaceans, insects, and the cell walls of fungi [20]. Chitosan is the deacetylated derivative of chitin, with the conversion of a fraction of the *N*-acetyl-D-glucosamine to D-glucosamine, and is more commonly used in

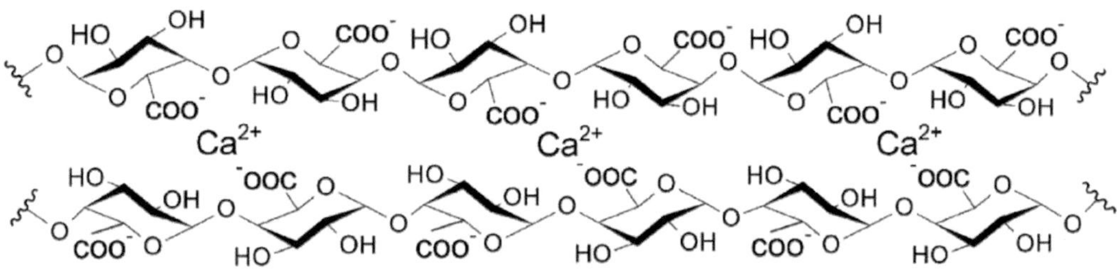

FIGURE 6.3 Ca-pectin hydrogel structural model. *From Gawkowska, D., J. Cybulska, and A. Zdunek,* Structure-related gelling of pectins and linking with other natural compounds: a review. *Polymers, 2018.* ***10****(7): p. 762.*

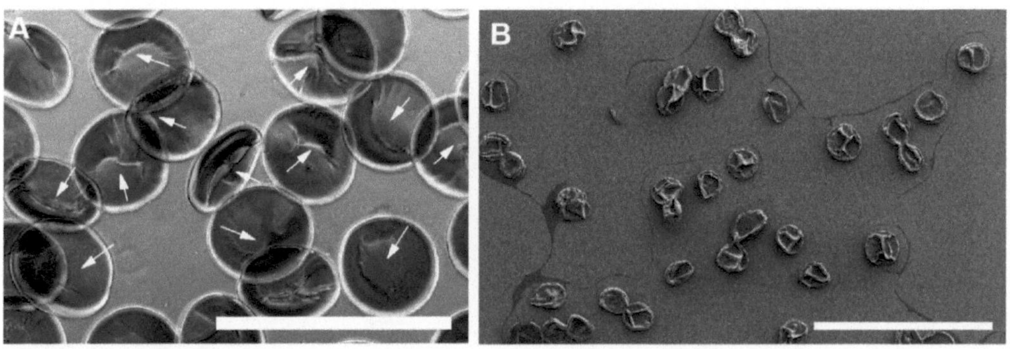

FIGURE 6.4 Optical (A) and SEM (B) images of micro-scale pectin oligochitosan hydrogels (microcapsules). The *arrows* indicate the concave red blood cell–like shape. Scale bars: 1000 μm. *From Crouse, J.Z., et al.,* Development of a microscale red blood cell-shaped pectin-oligochitosan hydrogel system using an electrospray-vibration method: preparation and characterization. *J Appl Biomater Funct Mater, 2015.* ***13****(4): p. e326-31.*

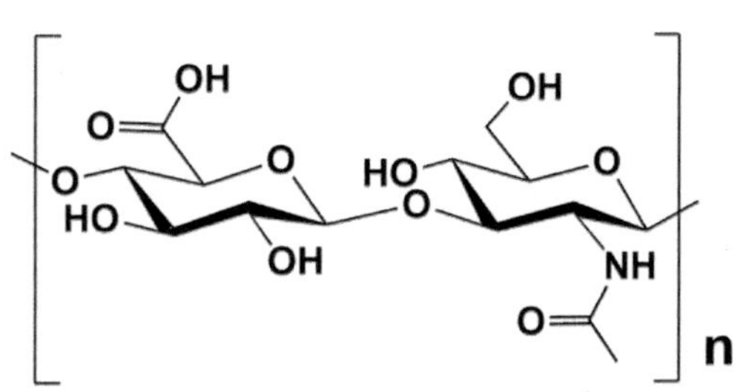

FIGURE 6.5 Structure of hyaluronic acid.

biomedical fields due to the amino groups (Fig. 6.6) [21]. The polycationic surface of chitosan, contributed by the amino groups, can lead to the formation of hydrogen and ionic bonds with drug molecules, including nucleic acids [22]. These amino groups also enable mucoadhesion, permeation enhancement, and efflux pump inhibitory properties regarding drug delivery applications [23]. However, chitosan is only soluble in aqueous acids, which limits its applications. Oligochitosan is water-soluble due to its shorter chain length and free amino groups [24]. Hence, it can be used as a crosslinker to replace cations, e.g., the formation of pectin-based hydrogel and nanoparticle/capsule surface coating [25,26].

Collagen and gelatin. Collagen is the most abundant protein in the human body (about 25% to 35% of the total protein body mass). Collagen forms a triple-helix structure. Moreover, it interacts with a large number of molecules, such as cell surface receptors, which leads to biological interactions [27]. Gelatin is derived from collagen through partial acid-, alkaline-, or heat-based hydrolysis (Fig. 6.7). Gelatin has a higher number of accessible functional groups, which is favorable in developing a drug delivery system [28]. Gelatin is more soluble when compared to collagen and goes through a sol-gel (colloid to nonfluid colloidal/polymer network) transition at temperatures around 20 to 30°C [29,30]. Because collagen and gelatin exhibit different properties, they are generally used in

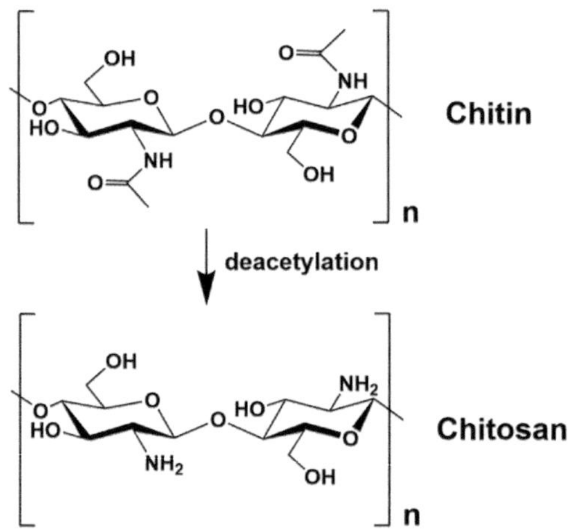

FIGURE 6.6 Structure of chitin and chitosan.

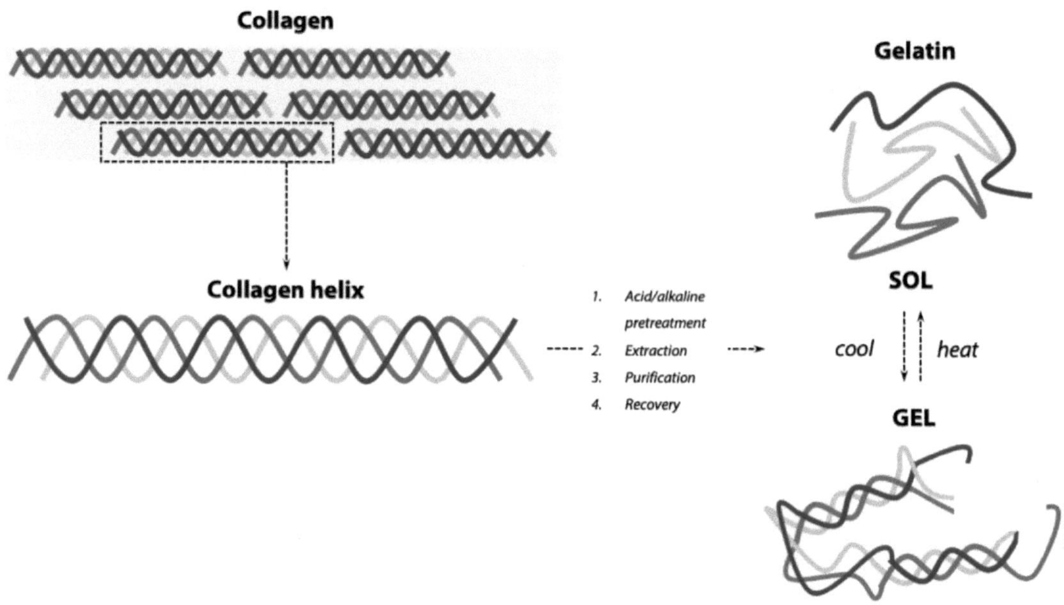

FIGURE 6.7 Processing of collagen for gelatin extraction. *From Campiglio, C.E. et al.,* Cross-linking strategies for electrospun gelatin scaffolds. *Materials, 2019.* ***12****(15): p. 2476.*

distinctive drug delivery applications. Generally, collagen has been applied as hydrogels, films, sponges, or coatings in drug delivery. Gelatin is more commonly used for generating micro- and nano-scale drug delivery system.

Silk fibroin. Fibroin is a dominant silk protein and has been widely used in drug delivery due to its solubility, biocompatibility, controllable degradability, and tunable drug-release properties [30,31]. The primary structure of silk fibroin consists of repetitive blocks of hydrophobic heavy chains and hydrophilic light chains, linked together through disulfide bonds (Fig. 6.8). The secondary structure of silk can be classified into different crystalline forms: silk I (partially ordered structure), II (β-sheet crystalline structure), and III (mostly trifold helical chain conformation) [32]. The silk fibroin–based drug delivery systems developed include hydrogels, films, sponges, fibers, and particles [33].

PLGA. Poly(lactic-*co*-glycolic) acid (PLGA) is a linear copolymer of lactic and glycolic acids (Fig. 6.9). PLGA is biodegradable, which makes it attractive for drug delivery and other biomedical applications. PLGA degrades through the hydrolysis of ester linkages in aqueous environments. PLGA's properties can be easily controlled by

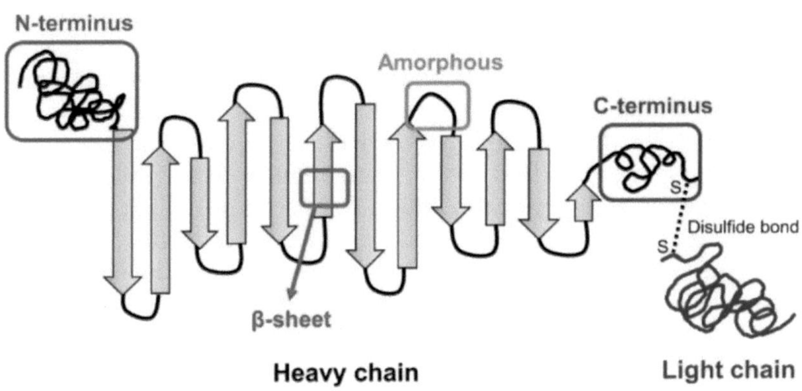

FIGURE 6.8 Structure of heavy and light chains of silk fibroin. *From Tomeh, M.A., R. Hadianamrei, and X. Zhao, Silk fibroin as a functional biomaterial for drug and gene delivery. Pharmaceutics, 2019.* ***11****(10): p. 494.*

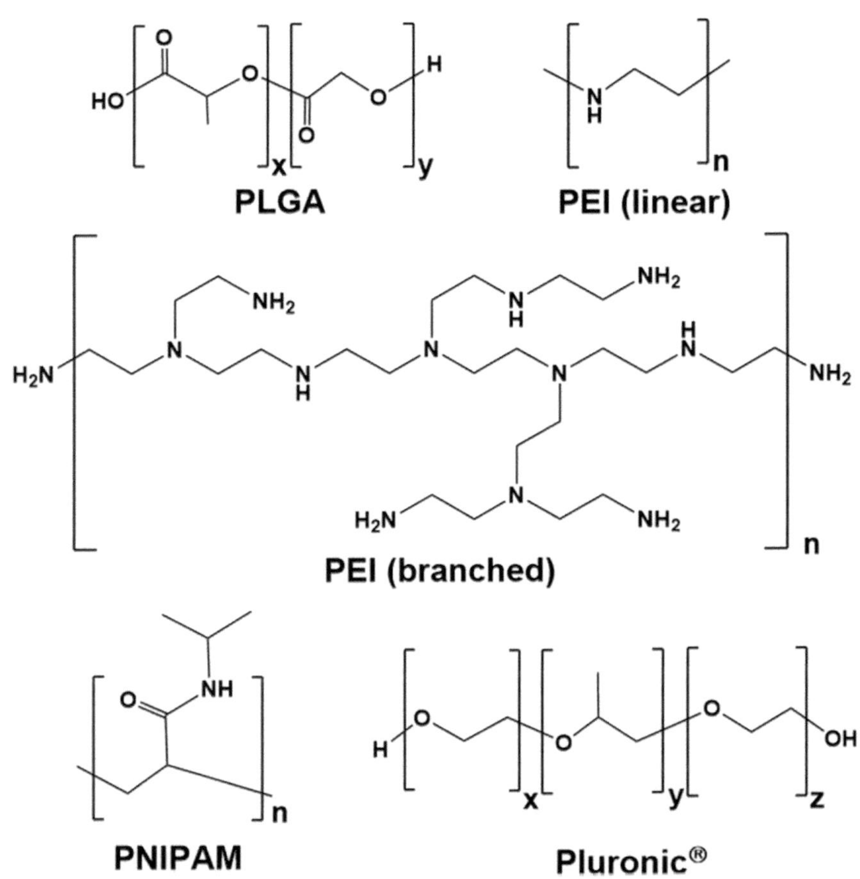

FIGURE 6.9 Common synthetic polymers used in drug delivery systems.

adjusting the molecular weight, lactic acid—to—glycolic acid ratio, mixtures of D— and L—lactic acid monomers, and end-group functionalization [34]. PLGA has been widely used to prepare microspheres for drug encapsulation and delivery. PLGA microspheres produced through the single emulsification method are typically for hydrophobic drug molecule encapsulation. The double emulsification approach is a strategy for hydrophilic drug molecule encapsulation but with low encapsulation efficiency. Other technologies, such as electrospray, have been developed to improve the PLGA microsphere production process [35].

PEI. Poly(ethylenimine) (PEI) is a cationic polymer composed of abundant amine groups (primary, secondary, and tertiary amino groups). It can be synthesized as a linear or branched polymer (Fig. 6.9) [36]. Due to its positive charge, it is attractive for intracellular drug delivery, especially nucleic acids (negatively charged due to phosphate groups). Moreover, it can facilitate drug release including with nucleic acids from endosomes/lysosomes through the "proton sponge effect." The traditional review of a proton sponge is that amine groups sequester protons, acidifying endosomal/lysosomal compartments. The "proton pump" results in the retention of one Cl^- ion and one water molecule, leading to endosomal/lysosomal swelling and rupture (Fig. 6.10) [37,38]. Membrane destabilization and polymer swelling are additional factors influencing endosomal/lysosomal escape [39]. Currently, no consensus has been reached about the validity of this hypothesis. The safety of PEI also remains a concern for its clinical translation as it could induce necrotic cell death and apoptosis [40].

PNIPAM and Pluronic. Poly(*N*-isopropylacrylamide) (PNIPAM) is a thermal-responsive polymer that contains both hydrophobic isopropyl and hydrophilic amide groups (Fig. 6.9). It is soluble (solvation of hydrophilic amide groups) but becomes hydrophobic and insoluble in water above a critical solution temperature (LCST; ~ 32 to 35°C) [41,42]. Because its LCST is close to body temperature, it is a promising material for the development of targeted drug delivery systems [43]. Another class of commonly used thermal-responsive polymers is Pluronic, developed by BASF. Pluronic polymers are nonionic triblock copolymers of polyethylene oxide-polypropylene oxide-polyethylene

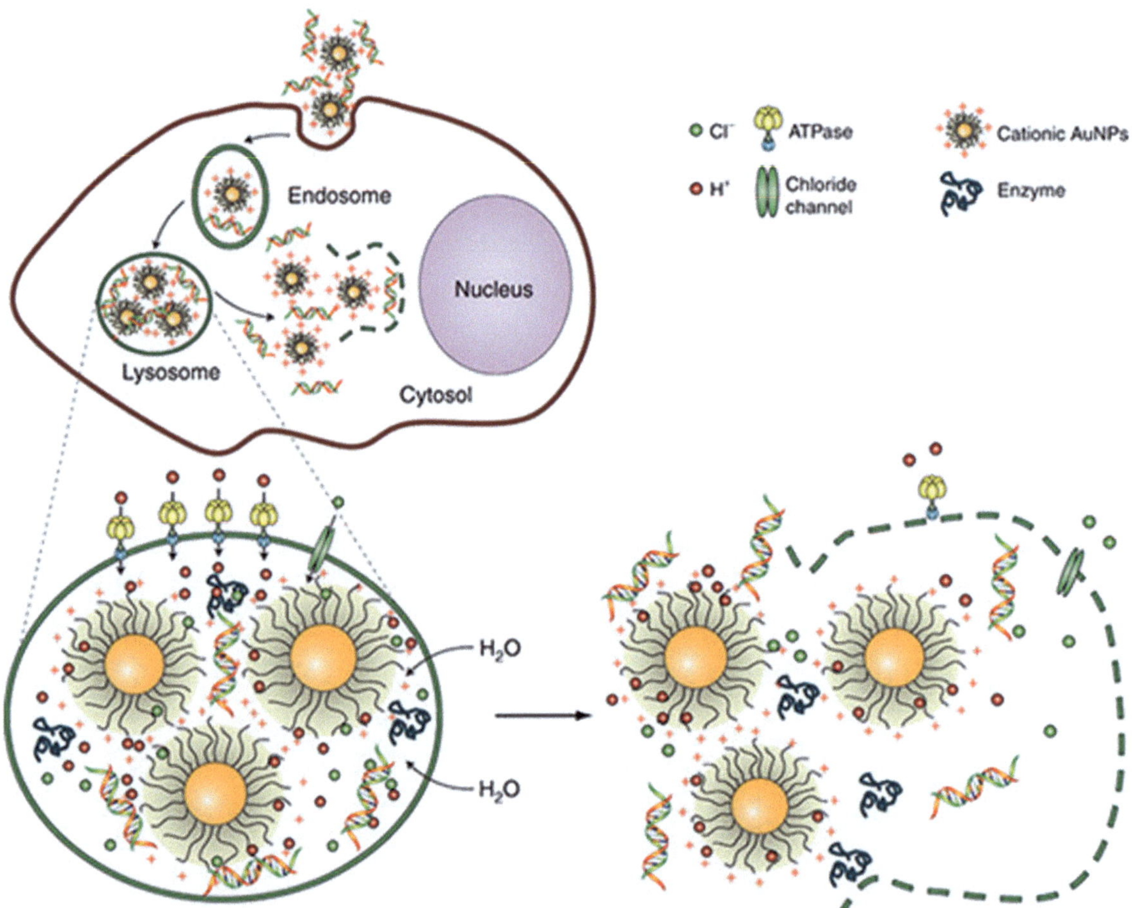

FIGURE 6.10 Schematic of the possible mechanism of the proton sponge effect leading to lysosomal damage and the induction of cytotoxicity by cationic nanoparticles. *From Nel, A.E. et al.,* Understanding biophysicochemical interactions at the nano—bio interface. *Nat Mater,* 2009. **8***(7): p. 543-557, with permission from Springer Nature.*

oxide (PEO-PPO-PEO), with the length of each block being modifiable [44]. For example, Pluronic F-127 (PEO_{100}-PPO_{65}-PEO_{100}) has an LCST lower than 40°C. The sol-gel transition is thought to be the dehydration of PPO blocks [25]. In an aqueous solution, when the Pluronic concentration is high enough (> critical micelle concentration (CMC)), the polymer molecules self-assemble to form micelles with a PPO core bounded by PEO coronas. Pluronic-based micelles are promising drug carriers [45]. Various Pluronic-based nanocarriers, Pluronic-PEI and Pluronic-oligochitosan nanocapsules, have been developed [25,46].

Drug loading can be either passive or active. During passive loading, drug molecules are encapsulated before or during the carrier formation. For active loading (remote loading), drugs are loaded into the preformed carriers [47].

6.2 Microscale drug carriers

Common microscale drug carriers are microspheres, microcapsules, and microneedles. There are also novel microscale systems such as microrobots and red blood cell–based carriers that are discussed in Chapter 15.

Microspheres and Microcapsules. Although these two terms are used interchangeably, they do have distinct differences. Microcapsules are core-shell structured microscale particles (mostly spherical), whereas microspheres are microscale spherical particles that are generally homogeneous. To fabricate microspheres and microcapsules, commonly used approaches include polymerization, coacervation, double-emulsion, electrospray, microfluidic chips, and spray-drying techniques. The electrospray and microfluidic chip methods are discussed in Chapter 7 as they are commonly employed for cell microencapsulation.

Regarding the polymerization approach for microsphere formation, monomers (and initiators if necessary) are dispersed in water with a stabilizer. Then under vigorous agitation and specific conditions (heat or irradiation), polymerization starts, and microspheres are formed. Last, the microspheres are separated and dried (Fig. 6.11).

Coacervation is defined as the associative phase separation process induced by modification of the media environment (such as T, pH, and ionic strength) under controlled conditions [48]. Coacervation can be divided into two types: simple (use of one colloidal solute/polymer and coacervation occurs due to dehydration or salting out) and complex coacervation (coacervation and phase separation from the interaction of two or more oppositely charged colloids/polymers, usually polysaccharides and proteins) [48–50]. Coacervation has been widely used to produce drug-loaded microcapsules. As shown in Fig. 6.12, the coacervation process, in general, consists of four steps: (1) prepare a polymer-containing aqueous solution; (2) disperse the hydrophobic phase (with drug; core) into the aqueous solution, forming a stable emulsion; (3) modify the pH, temperature, ionic strength, or other conditions which induces coacervation and phase separation; and (4) hardening/crosslinking the polymer matrices (shell) [48,50].

Double emulsion (water-in-oil-in-water emulsion; W/O/W) has been used for encapsulating hydrophilic drugs to sustain their releases, although with low encapsulation efficiencies. In general, double emulsions are prepared through a two-step process: (1) prepare the W/O emulsion; (2) use the former W/O emulsion as the oil phase for the second emulsion [(W/O)/W] (Fig. 6.13) [51]. Surfactants are needed to stabilize the structure of emulsions (Fig. 6.14). Surfactants with hydrophilic lipophilic balance (HLB) values lower than 7 (commonly around 3 to 4; higher oil affinity) should be used for preparing W/O emulsions. Surfactants with HLB values higher than 10 (water solubility) are needed to stabilize the W/O/W emulsions [51,52].

Spray drying is an effective method to prepare particles (Fig. 6.15). Due to the elevated temperature, this method is not suitable for heat-sensitive drugs [53,54]. A typical spray drying process involves four stages: (1) atomization of the liquid feed (a drug with carrier materials) into small droplets; (2) injection of small droplets into a drying chamber containing hot air; (3) drying of droplets into solid particles; and (4) collection of particles [55].

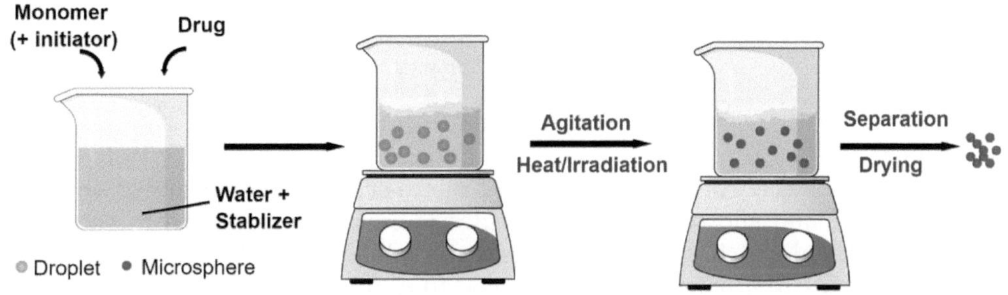

FIGURE 6.11 Polymerization method for microsphere formation.

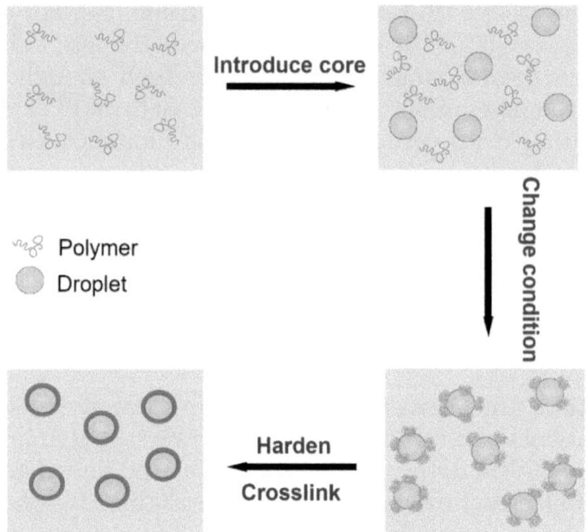

FIGURE 6.12 Coacervation process for microcapsule formation.

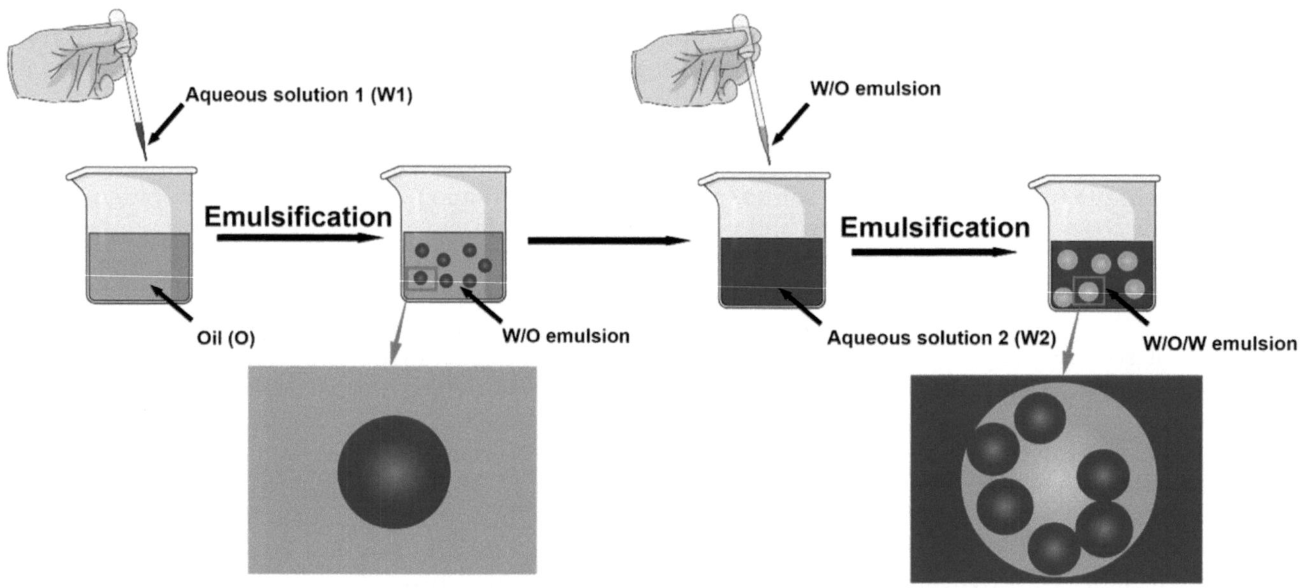

FIGURE 6.13 Mechanism of the two-step process of producing double emulsions.

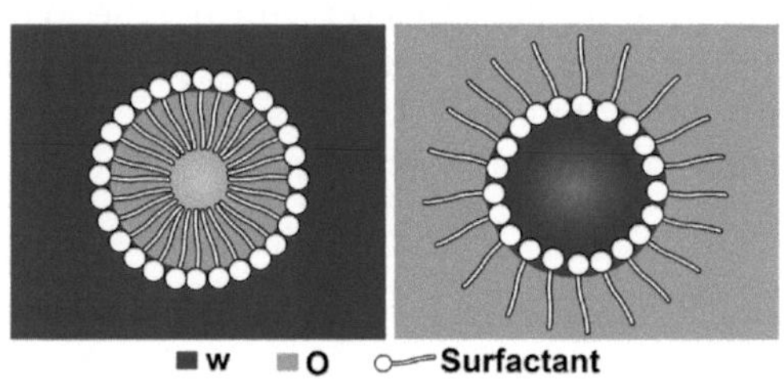

FIGURE 6.14 Surfactant arrangement at the water-oil interface in O/W *(left)* and W/O *(right)* emulsions.

Microneedles. Microneedle devices consist of needles at a micro-scale that are arranged on a small patch. Microneedles are minimally invasive and allow the drug molecules to cross the stratum corneum, improving bioavailability compared to transdermal patches. Microneedles can deliver large hydrophilic molecules, which are difficult to penetrate the skin [56]. Microneedles are fabricated in different geometries and with different materials,

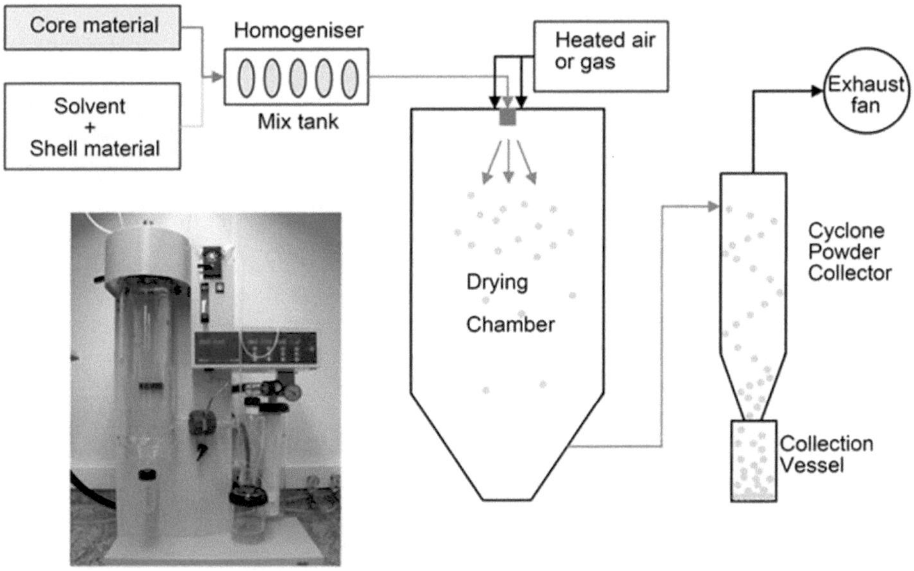

FIGURE 6.15 Schematic of microcapsule/sphere production using spray drying techniques. *From Andrea, T. et al.,* Microencapsulation of lipase and savinase enzymes by spray drying using Arabic gum as wall material. *JEAS, 2016.* ***06****: p. 161-173.*

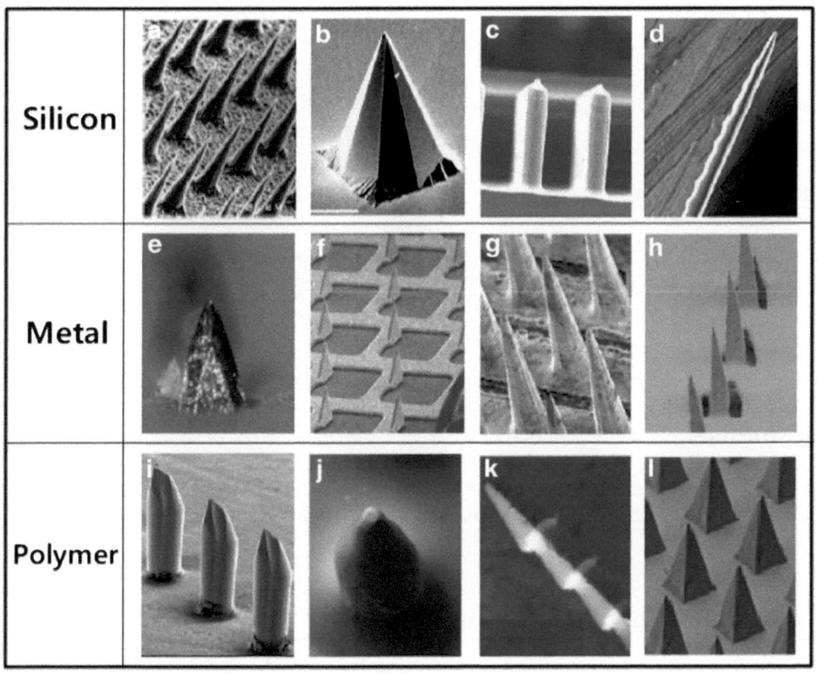

FIGURE 6.16 Microneedles made of different types of materials and with different geometries. *From Kim, Y.-C., J.-H. Park, and M.R. Prausnitz,* Microneedles for drug and vaccine delivery. *Adv. Drug Deliv. Rev, 2012.* ***64****(14): p. 1547-1568, with permission from Elsevier.*

such as metals, polymers, and silicones (Fig. 6.16) [57,58]. There are different types of microneedles: solid, coated, dissolving, hollow, and hydrogel-forming (Fig. 6.17). Solid microneedles are used as a skin pretreatment to form micropores on the skin's surface. After micropores are formed, the drug can then be applied. Drug delivery through hollow microneedles is done *via* a pressure-driven flow of a liquid formulation upon the application of the microneedles. Dissolving microneedles are made using biodegradable materials, causing the drug release by the dissolution of the needles upon application. Coated microneedles consist of solid microneedles coated with drug molecules (either a drug solution or a drug dispersion layer). Upon application, coated drug molecules are detained within the skin [56,57]. Hydrogel-forming microneedles, composed of nondissolving hydrogels, are the newest type of microneedle. Upon application, microneedles swell due to the hydrophilic nature of the hydrogel facilitating drug delivery [59,60]. There are multiple methods for fabricating the microneedles and the most common approaches are laser ablation, micro-molding, additive manufacturing, injection molding, and surface/bulk micromachining [61].

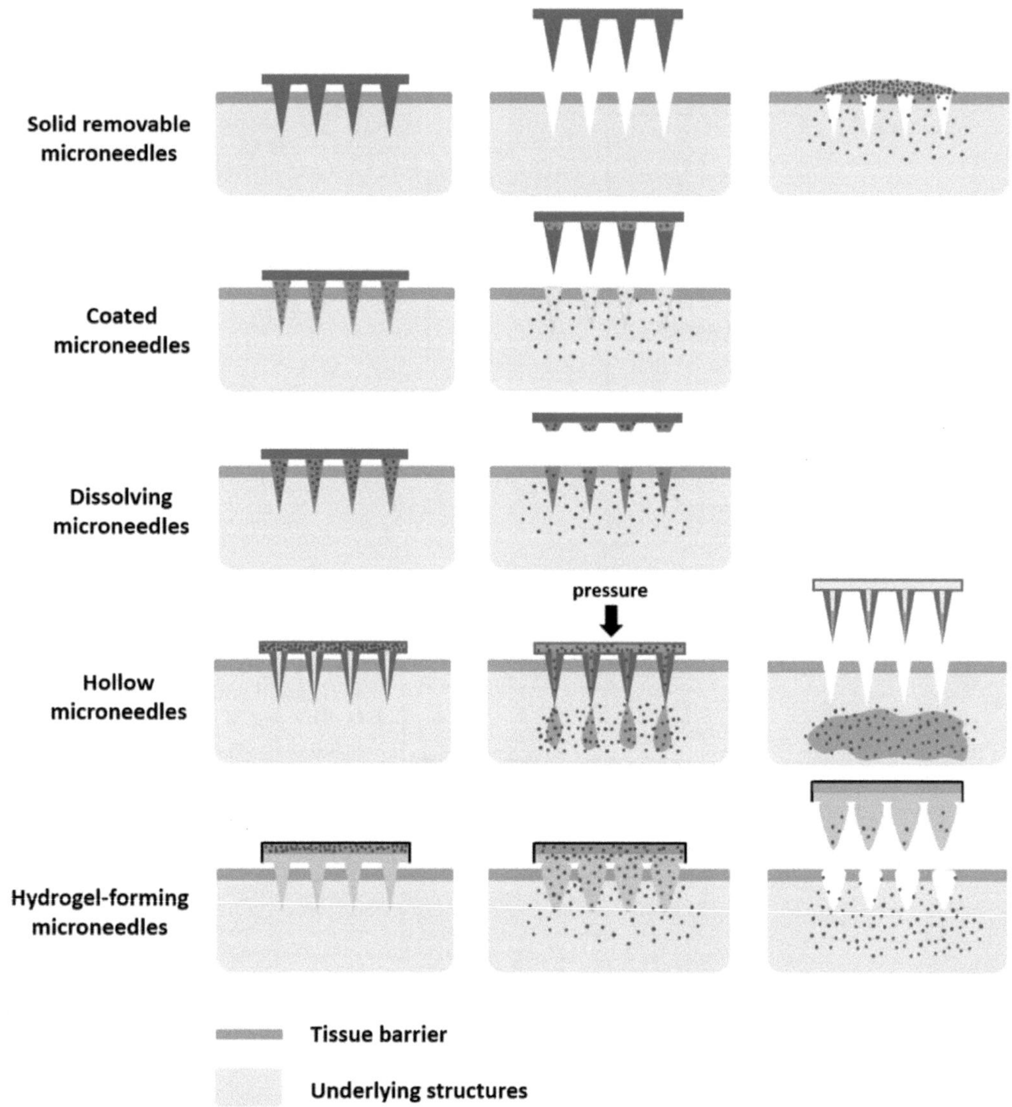

FIGURE 6.17 Different types of microneedles and their working mechanisms. *From Rzhevskiy, A.S. et al.,* Microneedles as the technique of drug delivery enhancement in diverse organs and tissues. *JCR, 2018.* ***270****: p. 184-202, with permission from Elsevier.*

6.3 Nanoscale drug carriers

It is generally agreed upon that the nanoscale is from 1 to 100 nm. There are different nanomaterials/systems/structures: 0D, 1D, and 2D, based on how many dimensions are not at the nanoscale. Typical 0D nanomaterials are nanoparticles, nanocapsules, and quantum dots as none of the dimensions (0) are not at the nanoscale. Nanofibers and nanotubes are considered 1D, while nanofilm and graphene are 2D. With the rapid development of nanoscience and nanotechnology, a large spectrum of nanoscale drug carriers have been designed and developed, such as liposomes, nanoparticles, nanocapsules, nanofibers, and nanotubes (Fig. 6.18).

Liposomes and Micelles. Both liposome and micelle formations are classic examples of self-assembly. Self-assembly is the spontaneous molecular arrangement of the disordered entities of molecules into ordered structures, resulting from specific local interactions among the components themselves [62]. To form liposomes or micelles, amphiphilic molecules, such as phospholipids and surfactants, are needed. They are molecules characterized by spatially distinguishable polar and nonpolar regions [63]. Self-assembly usually involves hydrophobic interactions, H-bonds, and other intermolecular forces. The hydrophobic interaction that derivates *via* aliphatic lipid chains is the driving force of the self-assembly of liposomes [64].

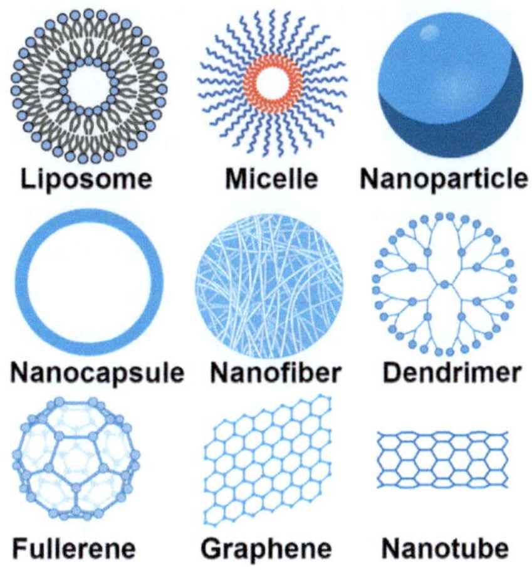

FIGURE 6.18 Different types of nanoscale drug carriers.

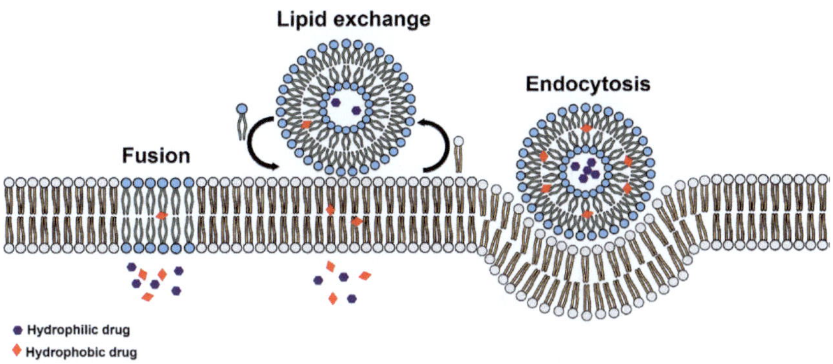

FIGURE 6.19 Different pathways of liposome uptake and drug release.

In 1961, British hematologist Dr. Alec. D. Bangham was the first person to introduce the term "liposomes." G. Gregoriadis was the first to suggest that liposomes can be used as drug carriers in the 1970s, and the first liposome drug formulations came into the market in the 1990s [65]. As drug vehicles, liposomes have multiple advantages: protection of the encapsulated drug molecules, an extension of the half-life of the drug, and biocompatibility [66]. Liposomes can also be used for encapsulating both hydrophilic (in the core) and hydrophobic (within the lipid bilayer) drugs. Liposomes can easily deliver drugs into cells by mimicking the cell membrane and can enter cells *via* multiple routes (Fig. 6.19). During fusion, liposomal lipids are integrated into the cell membrane. During the lipids exchange between liposomes and the cell membrane, the stability of the liposomes decreases, resulting in the release of the encapsulated drug molecules. Endocytosis is the uptake of intact liposomes through endocytotic vesicles [67].

Various natural and synthetic lipids have been used for liposome production, such as phosphatidic acid (PA), phosphatidylcholine (PC), phosphatidylethanolamine (PE), phosphatidylglycerol (PG), phosphatidylinositol (PI), 1,2-dioleoyl-*sn*-glycero-3-phospho-L-serine (DOPS), 1,2-dioleoyl-3-trimethylammonium-propane (DOTAP), and 1,2-distearoyl-*sn*-glycero-3-phosphocholine (DSPC). The hydrophilic group of the lipid can be negatively or positively charged, or zwitterionic. The hydrophobic groups can vary in length, saturation, and symmetry. Both groups determine the final liposome size, stability, drug encapsulation efficiency, and more. Cholesterol is also commonly incorporated to modify the liposome's fluidity, membrane permeability, and stability [68]. The conventional methods for preparing liposomes include (1) dissolution of lipids in an organic solvent; (2) removal of the organic solvent to form a lipid film/cake; and (3) hydration of the lipid film/cake with agitation. During hydration, the lipid molecules form multilamellar vesicles (MLVs), which are highly heterogeneous in both size and lamellarity [69]. Extrusion is commonly used to reduce the liposome's size, while a liposome suspension is forced to pass through a membrane filter of a defined pore size [70].

Active loading of drugs into liposomes can be done through the driven force generated by the transmembrane gradient of pH or ion concentrations [66]. A recent study utilized click reaction for active drug loading into liposomes. The general principle is that drug molecules have relatively high permeability across liposome membranes. Upon entering the liposomes, the drug molecules change their properties such as through ionization or chemical reactions (Fig. 6.21).

Micelles are amphiphilic colloidal structures having particle diameters ranging from 5 to 100 nm. Micelles are made of amphiphilic molecules (having two regions of different affinities for water). Critical micelle concentrations and temperatures have to be reached for micelle formation. Micelles can be used for hydrophobic drug encapsulation (within the core) and delivery. The differences between liposomes and micelles are summarized in Table 6.1.

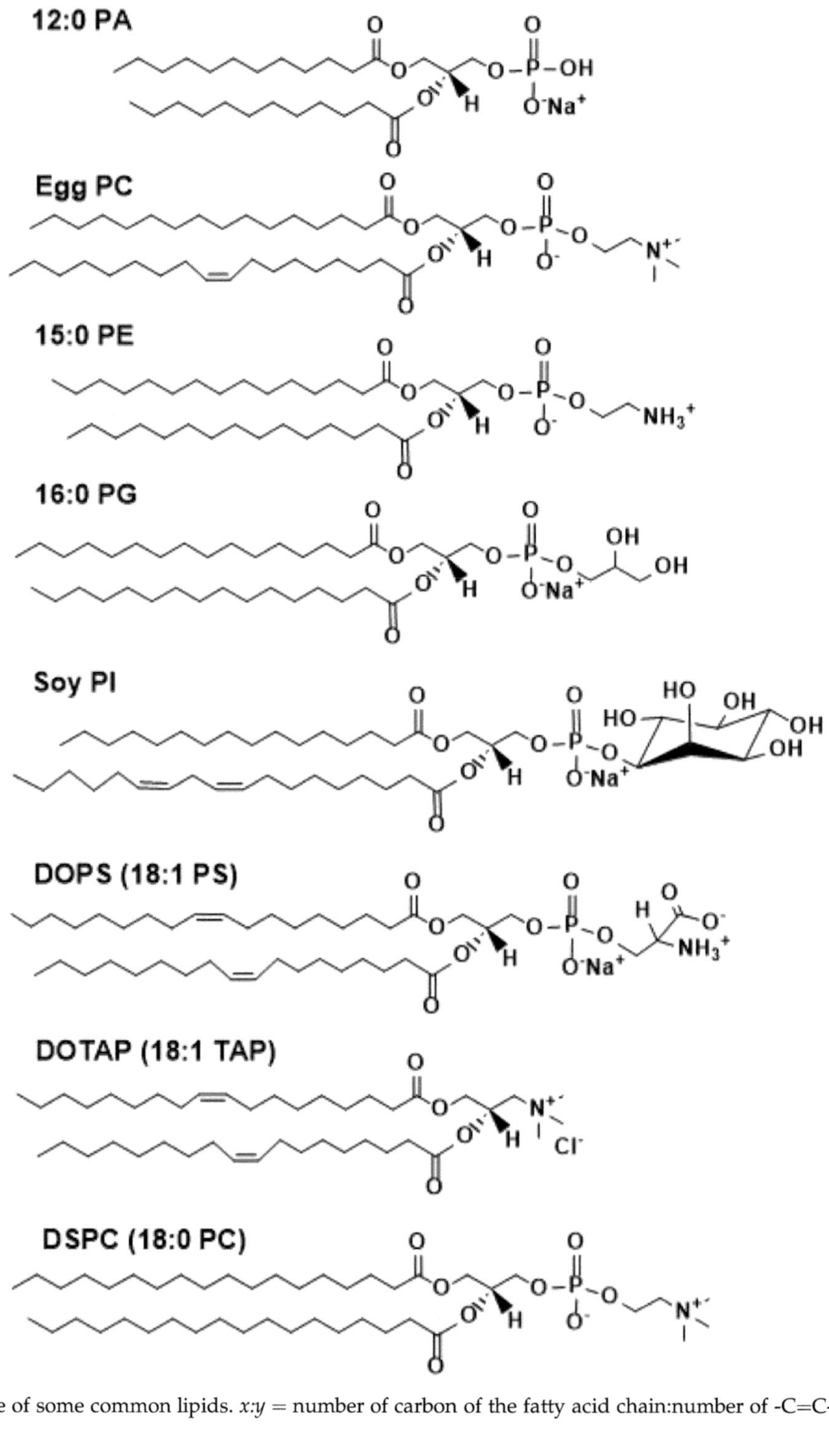

FIGURE 6.20 Structure of some common lipids. x:y = number of carbon of the fatty acid chain:number of -C=C-.

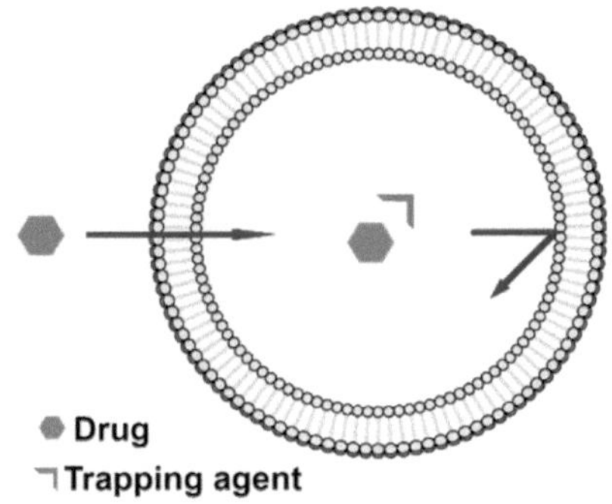

FIGURE 6.21 General mechanism of active drug loading into liposomes.

TABLE 6.1 Differences between liposomes and micelles.

	Liposomes	Micelles
Structure	Bilayer	Monolayer
Constituents	Lipids (phospholipids mostly)	Surfactants
Formation	The hydration of dry lipid films/cakes with agitation	The aggregation of surfactant molecules in a polar solvent
Drug delivery	Hydrophilic drug molecules in the core and hydrophobic drug molecules in the lipid bilayer	Hydrophobic drug molecules in the core

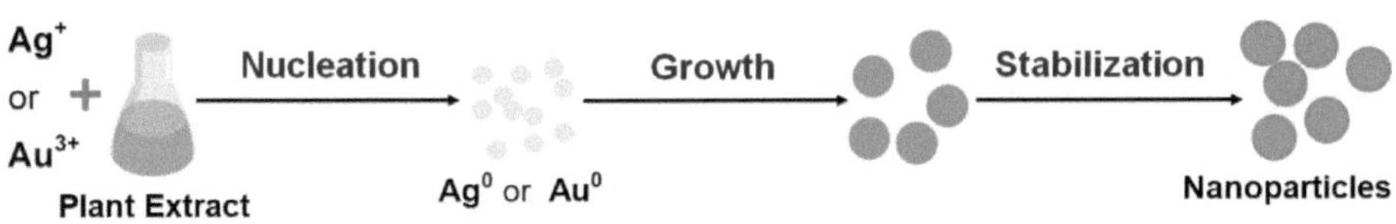

FIGURE 6.22 Green synthesis route of colloidal Ag and Au nanoparticles.

Polymeric nanoparticles/nanocapsules can be produced through the polymerization of monomers and the dispersion of preformed polymers (such as solvent evaporation, spontaneous emulsification, and nonaqueous phase separation) [68]. Metallic nanoparticles can be prepared physically (such as milling), chemically (such as chemical reduction), or biochemically (such as biosynthesis and green synthesis). Green synthesis, such as using plant extract, is of particular interest for metallic nanoparticle synthesis as it is environmentally conscious and cost-effective [71]. As shown in Fig. 6.22, different compounds within the extracts serve as reducing and/or stabilizing/capping agents when it comes to plant-mediated green synthesis [72].

Electrospun nanofibers (fibers from electrospinning) have been widely explored for drug delivery *via* a range of routes including oral, transdermal, ocular, and implantation [73]. The benefits of using electrospun nanofibers for drug delivery are (1) favorable surface chemical properties for drug absorption; (2) high drug-loading efficiency and fast stimuli-responsiveness due to the high porosity and large surface area-to-volume ratio; and (3) the extracellular matrix–like morphology promotes cellular drug uptake [74]. Electrospinning is an electrohydrodynamic process and utilizes viscous solutions or melts to produce micro-/nano-scale fibers. As shown in Fig. 6.23, an electrospinning setup involves a high-voltage supply, a syringe pump with a spinneret (mostly a blunt metallic needle), and a collector. When a high voltage is applied on viscous solutions/melts, a pendant droplet forms at the tip of the spinneret. With the increase in the electrostatic repulsion to overcome the surface tension and viscous force, the droplet deforms into a conical shape (i.e., Taylor cone). At the critical voltage value, a fine and charged jet erupts from the tip of the spinneret and the jet is stretched and solidified during the fly, and eventually deposits onto the collector [75–77].

Dendrimers are nano-sized, radially symmetric molecules with well-defined, homogeneous, and monodispersed structures consisting of tree-like arms or branches (Fig. 6.24) [78]. They have polymer-like repetitive structures (representing a novel class of polymers) [79]. The two approaches for dendrimer synthesis are divergent and convergent.

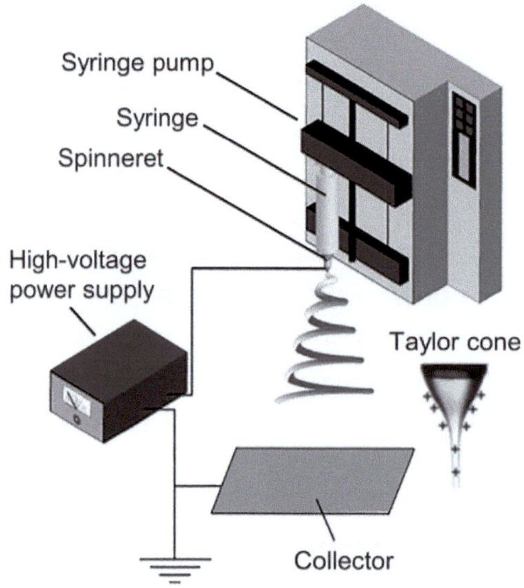

FIGURE 6.23 Typical electrospinning setup. Adapted *from Xue, J. et al.,* Electrospinning and electrospun nanofibers: methods, materials, and applications. *Chem Rev, 2019.* ***119****(8): p. 5298-5415. Copyright (2019) American Chemical Society.*

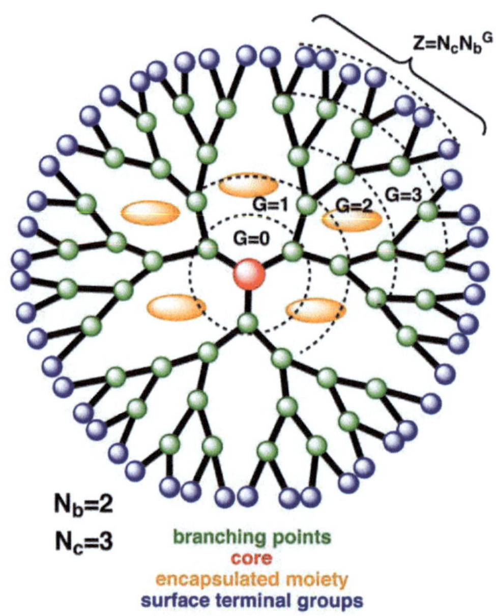

FIGURE 6.24 Structure of a dendrimer. The *dotted spherical lines* indicate each generation (G). N_c represents the number of branches in the core, N_b is the branch cell multiplicity, and Z gives the total number of surface terminal groups ($= 3 \times 2^4 = 48$ for this case). *From Ray, S. et al.,* Dendrimer- and copolymer-based nanoparticles for magnetic resonance cancer theranostics. *Theranostics, 2018.* ***8****(22): p. 6322-6349.*

During the divergent approach, the synthesis starts from the core of the dendrimer to which the arms are attached by adding building blocks (generation by generation). The convergent approach starts with the synthesis of dendrons (dendrimer segments), and they are eventually coupled to a multivalent core (Fig. 6.25) [78,80]. The use of dendrimers for drug delivery applications started in the 1990s due to their structural diversity and adaptability. Drugs can be either physically entrapped or covalently coupled on dendrimers [81,82].

Fullerenes (such as C_{60}), carbon nanotubes (CNTs), and graphene are 0D, 1D, and 2D nanomaterials, respectively (Fig. 6.18). Fullerenes consist of sp^2 carbons that present unique chemical and physical properties and a highly symmetrical cage with different sizes [83]. Fullerenes can penetrate the plasma membrane through passive entry rather than endo-/phagocytosis [84,85]. Fullerenes can have direct bioactivity with functionalized surfaces and/or serve as

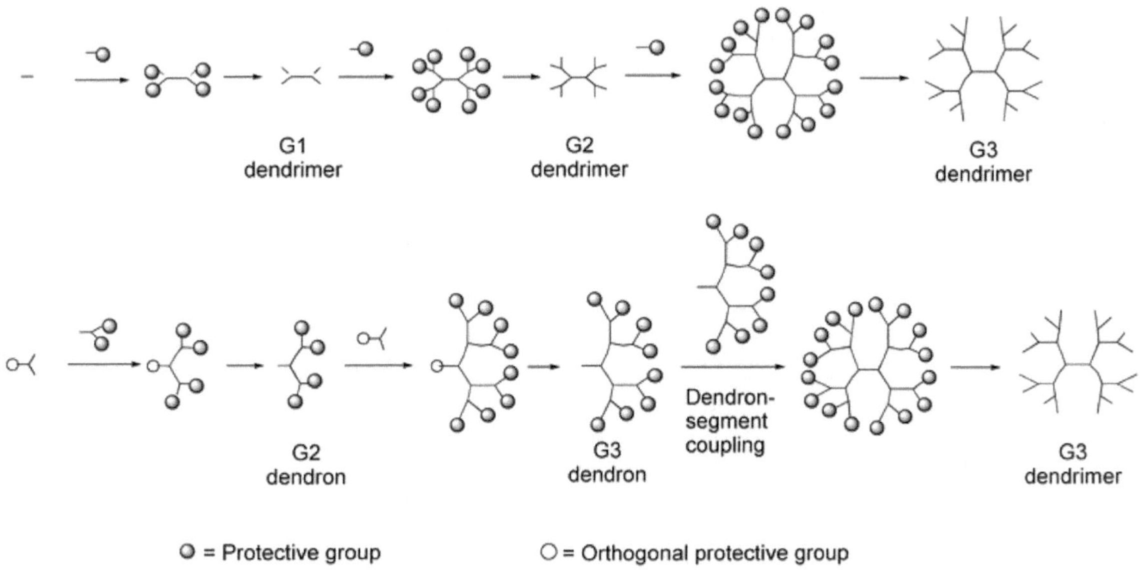

FIGURE 6.25 Dendrimer synthesis approaches. *Top*, divergent. *Bottom*, convergent. *From Boas, U. and P.M.H. Heegaard,* Dendrimers in drug research. *Chem Soc Rev, 2004.* ***33****(1): p. 43-63,* with permission from the Royal Society of Chemistry.

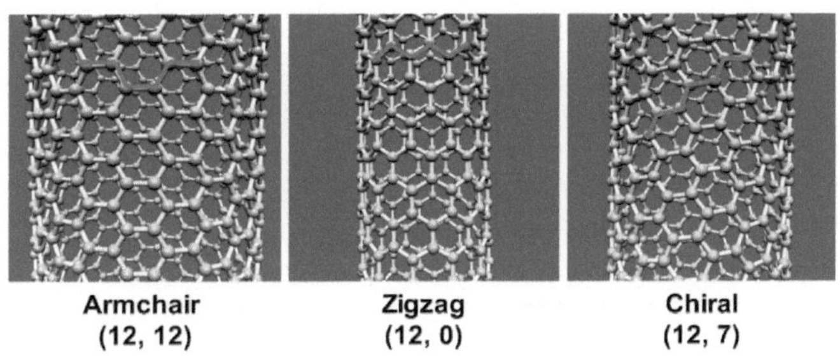

FIGURE 6.26 Different nanotube structures: armchair, zigzag, and chiral. All the structures are generated using the Nanotube Modeler (Version 1.8.0 © 2005–2018 JCrystalSoft).

a drug carrier [86]. In some cases, C_{60} can be used for photodynamic therapy due to its ability to produce reactive oxygen species (ROS). On the contrary, it can also serve as a neuroprotective agent downregulating ROS. The mechanism is still not fully understood [83].

Graphene is a single layer of carbon atoms that are bound together by overlapping sp^2 hybrid bonds [87]. The graphene family includes graphene, graphene oxide (GO), reduced graphene oxide (rGO), and others [88]. The graphene family materials were first used as carriers for anticancer drugs in biomedical fields due to their high drug-load capacity. In particular, GO can have excellent water solubility, which has been used to improve the hydrophilicity of insoluble drugs [88]. The surface modification and functionalization of graphene are commonly performed to improve its biocompatibility and drug delivery performance [89].

CNTs can be considered as rolled graphene [77,89]. CNTs can be single and multiwalled. CNTs can be indicated by their chirality using two integers (n, m) and can be classified as an armchair ($m = n$), chiral ($m = 0$), or zigzag ($m \neq n$), based on how they are "rolled" (Fig. 6.26) [90]. Different types of nanotubes have different physical, chemical, and biochemical properties. Similar to fullerene and graphene, surface modification and functionalization of CNTs are performed for drug delivery applications. CNTs can enter cells *via* diffusion (needle-like penetration) or endocytosis [91]. Drugs can be either trapped or linked to the surface of CNTs.

Although fullerenes, graphene, and CNTs are promising drug delivery carriers, their potential toxicity cannot be overlooked. They can cause acute and long-term tissue injuries by penetrating different tissue barriers, such as the blood-brain barrier, and by accumulating in the lung, liver, and spleen, similar to other nanomaterials. The toxic effects include inflammatory response, DNA damage, apoptosis/necrosis, and such [92]. The overall performance of these nanocarriers is determined by their purity, size, geometry, and surface properties.

6.4 Design and modify drug carriers

There are various factors that affect the design of drug carriers, including the administration route and the drug molecule's properties. Regarding the administration route, nanoscale carriers are more appropriate for intravenous drug delivery because most capillaries are less than 10 μm. However, nanoscale carriers are generally cleared rapidly within the body, so it is necessary to modify the carriers to increase their circulation time.

When designing the carriers, multiple aspects of the drug molecule properties should be considered including size, solubility, and the nature of the molecules. Drug substances are categorized into four classes based on their aqueous solubility and intestinal permeability (combined with the dissolution of the drug product) according to the Biopharmaceutical Classification System (BCS) (Fig. 6.27). In 2000, the FDA announced the BCS system as an approach to allow waiver of *in vivo* bioavailability and bioequivalence testing of immediate-release solid oral dosage forms for class I drugs exhibiting rapid dissolution [93]. Carriers can be designed to increase the solubility and permeability of class II-IV drugs. For example, liposomes can be used to increase the solubility of poorly water-soluble drugs and enhance the permeability of the epithelial cell membrane [94].

Pharmacokinetic and pharmacodynamic aspects are also critical players in drug carrier design. Take the absorption, biodistribution, and clearance of nanocarriers, for example; these processes are size-dependent. Nanoparticles, smaller than 5 nm, quickly undergo renal clearance upon intravenous administration, and larger particles (> 200 nm) tend to accumulate in the liver and spleen [95–97]. As shown in Fig. 6.28, the charge and shape (such as curvature

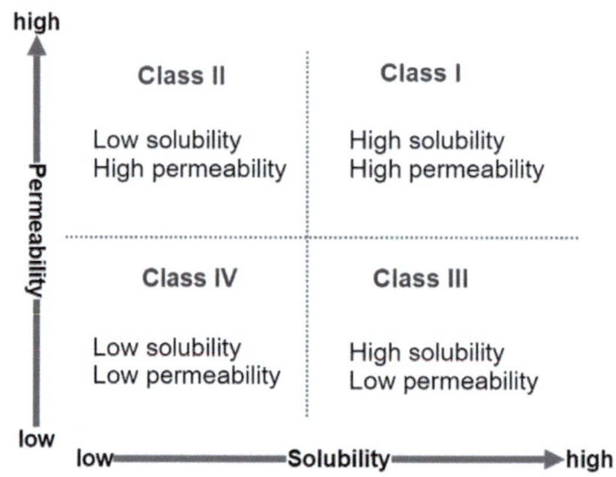

FIGURE 6.27 The Biopharmaceutical Classification System of the drug substances.

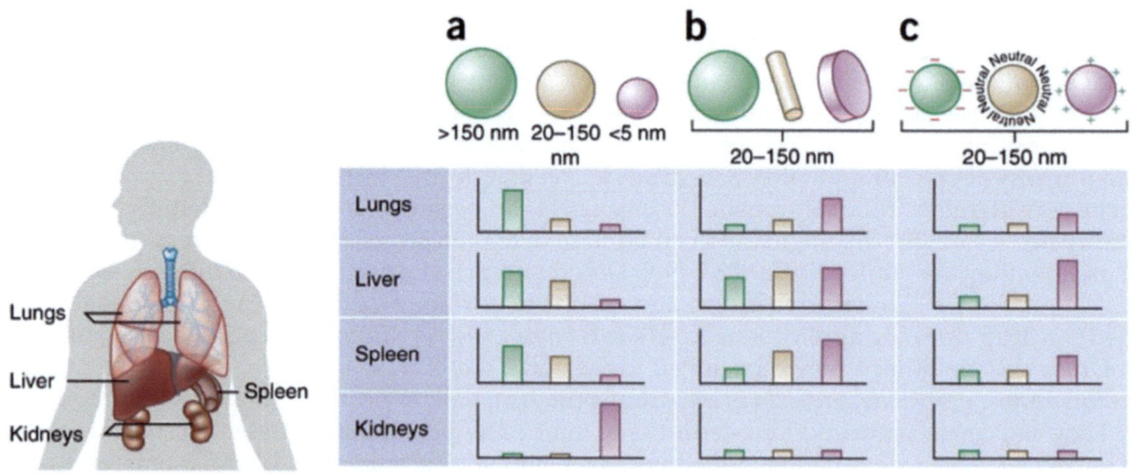

FIGURE 6.28 (a) Size, (b) shape, and (c) surface charge affect the biodistributions of nanoparticles in the lungs, liver, spleen, and kidneys. *From Blanco, E., H. Shen, and M. Ferrari,* Principles of nanoparticle design for overcoming biological barriers to drug delivery. *Nat Biotechnol, 2015. 33(9): p. 941-951, with permission from Springer Nature.*

and aspect ratio) of the carriers also affect their biodistribution. The interactions with cells and flow characteristics of nanoparticles can be affected by their shape and morphology. The surface charge of nanoparticles influences their opsonization, circulation times, and interactions with macrophages [95].

The modification of drug carriers can be either covalent or noncovalent. Noncovalent approaches mostly employ electrostatic interactions, hydrophobic interactions, and affinity interactions. For example, the streptavidin-biotin complex has one of the strongest noncovalent interactions found in nature [98].

Covalent approaches mostly focus on functional groups. Reactions between carboxylates and primary amines can be done through (1-ethyl-3-(3-dimethylaminopropyl)carbodiimide hydrochloride) (EDC) crosslinking. *N*-Hydroxysuccinimide (NHS) or sulfo-NHS can be added to increase the crosslinking efficiency (Fig. 6.29). EDC is a zero-length crosslinker, as it does not become part of the final amide-bond crosslink. Crosslinkers can be either homobifunctional or heterobifunctional, depending on whether the end reactive groups are identical or different.

Sulfhydryls (-SH) and disulfide bonds (can be reduced to sulfhydryls) can exist in cystine-containing proteins/peptides. Sulfhydryls are reactive toward maleimides, haloacetyls, and pyridyl disulfides (Fig. 6.30). Aldehydes can be produced in glycoproteins or other reducing-sugar-containing molecules through mild oxidation, and then the conjugations can be done using hydrazides (forming stable hydrazone bonds) [99]. Photoreactive crosslinkers are also commonly used. They are activated by different light sources, such as ultraviolet (UV) light. Aryl azide and diazirine are two of the most used photoreactive chemical groups in crosslinking (Fig. 6.31). Upon photoirradiation, aryl azide produces nitrene, which can react with neighboring C-H and heteroatom-H bonds or with a nucleophile through subsequent ring expansion. Carbene can be generated from diazirine and is very reactive. It can be inserted into neighboring C-H or heteroatom-H bonds [99,100].

Click chemistry shows great potential in drug delivery. Click chemistry was first articulated in 2001. The "click" in click chemistry conveys that if the two ends of the buckle (two groups) can reach each other, the linkage is made [101]. The types of reaction and reaction kinetics should be considered when choosing the right type of click chemistry for drug delivery applications [102]. Four of the most commonly used types of reactions in bioconjugations are strain-promoted reactions of an alkyne with an azido group (moderately fast reaction kinetics), Cu-catalyzed azido-alkyne cycloaddition (fast reaction kinetics), thiol-ene reaction, and Diels-Alder reaction (Fig. 6.32) [102,103]. One example of applying click chemistry is *in situ* one-step labeling of exosomes for diagnostics and therapeutics. As shown in Fig. 6.33, the exosome donor cells were treated to express azide groups on their surface. Then, the azide groups were labeled with Cy5-conjugated (a near-infrared fluorescent dye) dibenzylcyclooctyne (DBCO) *via* click chemistry [104].

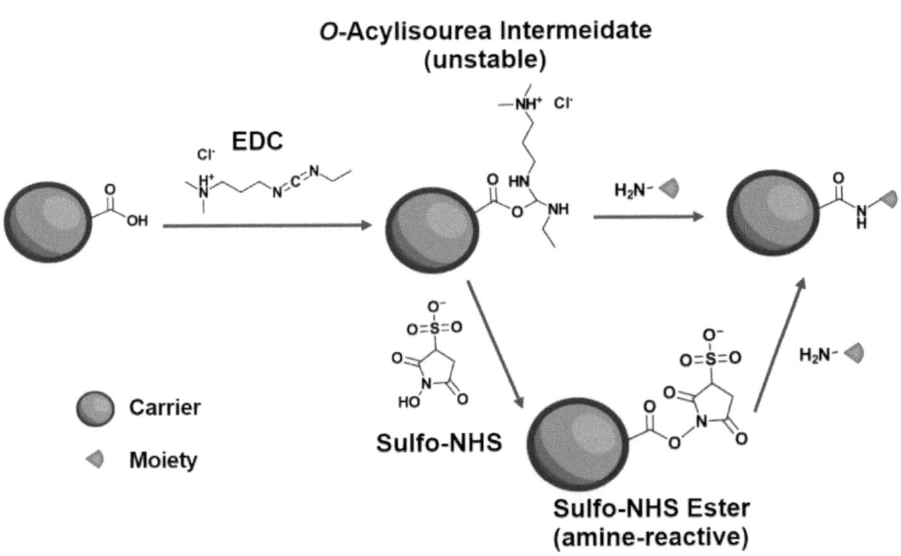

FIGURE 6.29 Reaction mechanism of EDC and EDC/sulfo-NHS crosslinking.

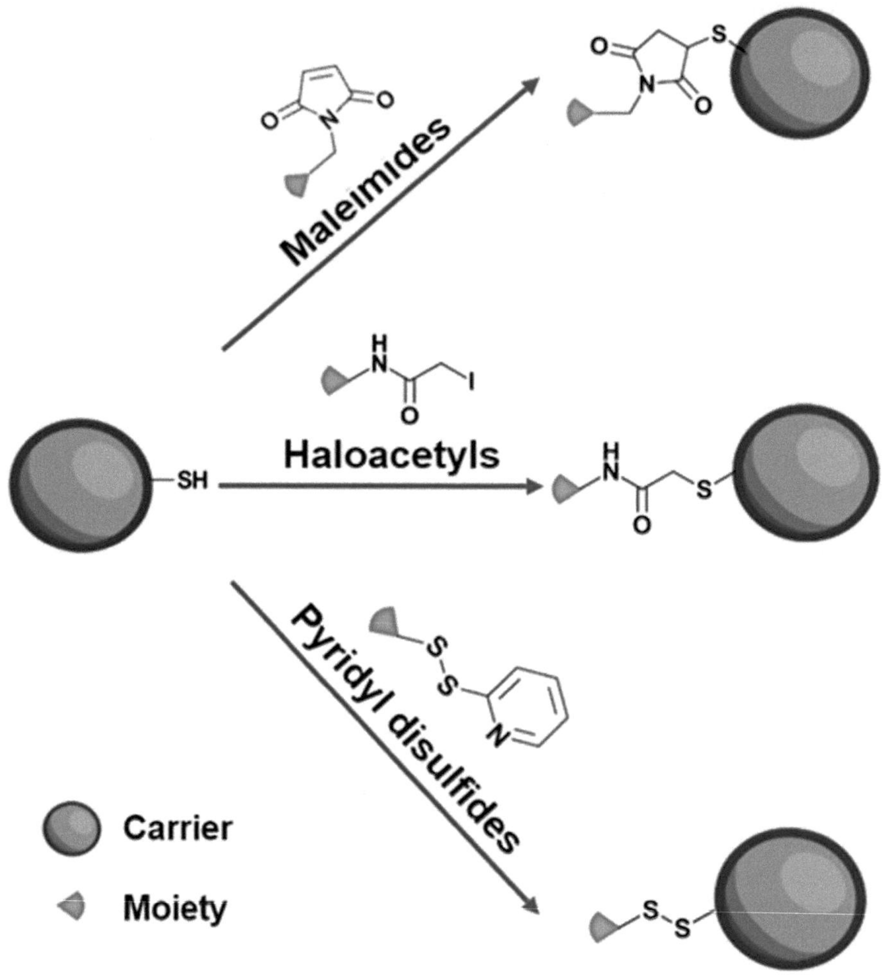

FIGURE 6.30 Reaction mechanism of various chemical conjugations to a sulfhydryl.

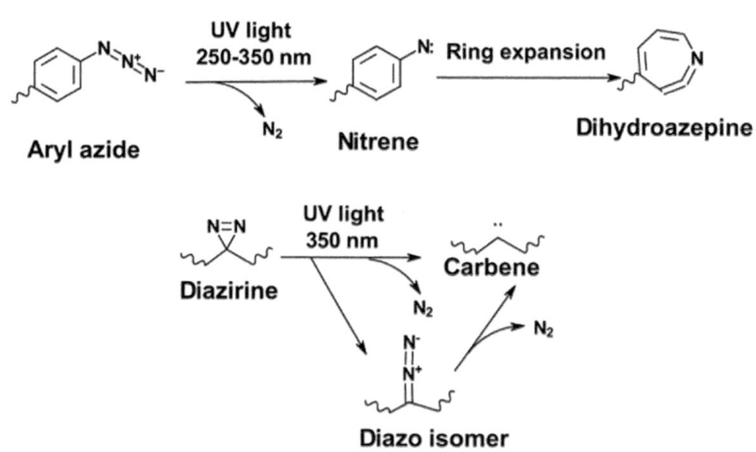

FIGURE 6.31 Mode of action of aryl azide and diazirine.

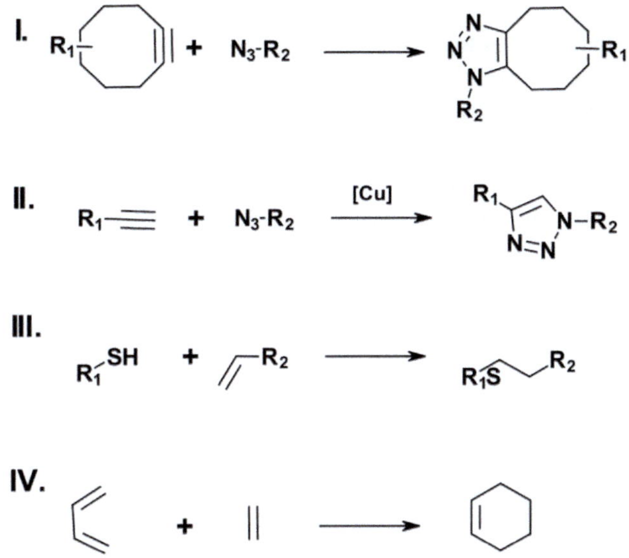

FIGURE 6.32 Click chemistry used for direct conjugation in drug delivery: (I) strain-promoted azido-alkyne cycloaddition, (II) Cu-mediated azido-alkyne cycloaddition, (III) thiol-ene reaction, and (IV) Diels-Alder reaction.

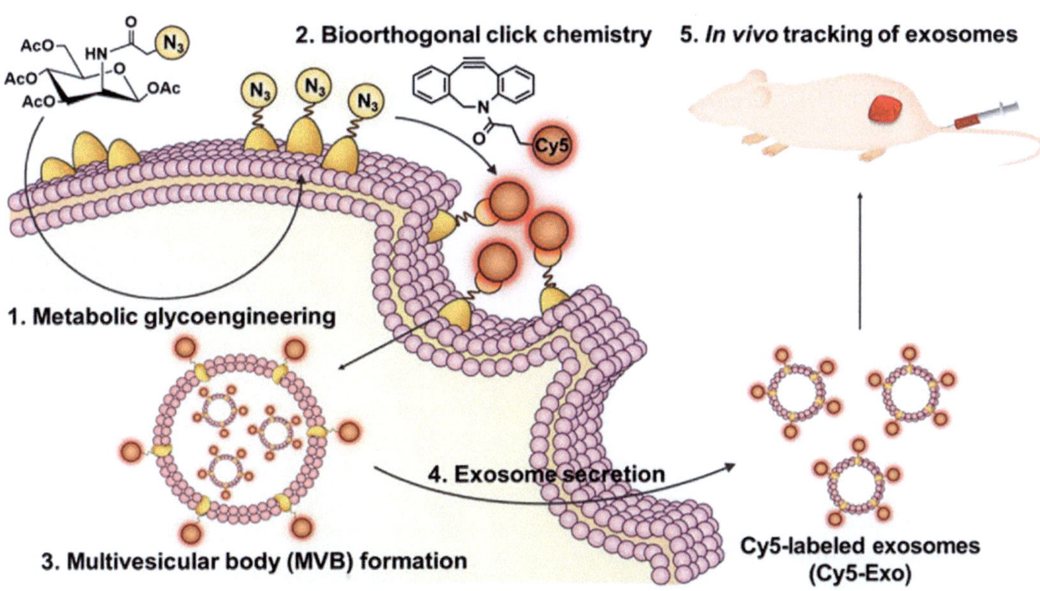

FIGURE 6.33 Strategy of *in situ* one-step fluorescence labeled exosome production *via* click chemistry. (1) Through metabolic glycoengineering, donor cells express azide group-containing molecules on their surface. (2) The azide groups are labeled with DBCO-Cy5 *via* click chemistry. (3, 4) Production and secretion of Cy5-labeled exosomes. (5) Application of Cy5—labeled exosomes. *Adapted from Song, S. et al.,* In situ one-step fluorescence labeling strategy of exosomes via bioorthogonal click chemistry for real-time exosome tracking in vitro and in vivo. *Bioconjugate Chem, 2020.* ***31****(5): p. 1562-1574. Copyright (2020) American Chemical Society.*

Lab Activity III: Natural biopolymer purification

Biopolymers have been widely used in pharmaceutical industries (e.g., controlled drug delivery and release); however, most biopolymers, especially natural biopolymers, need to be purified to achieve pharmaceutical grade before clinical applications. In this experiment, alginate will be used as an example to design and study the biopolymer purification process. The objectives of this experiment are to:

(1) Learn how to design a biopolymer purification protocol.
(2) Study the biopolymer purification processes.

Background

Most of the commercially available alginates are crude products extracted from algae, which are often contaminated with several inflammation-provoking components, such as polyphenols, impurity proteins, and endotoxins [105–107]. Hence, the raw alginate product needs to be purified to improve its biocompatibility and other properties.

The general routes of biopolymer purification are:

1. Dissolve and filter the biopolymers, to remove insoluble impurities.
2. Mix with activated charcoal and filter, for decolorization and to remove/reduce many natural and organic volatile organic chemicals, etc. [108].
3. Precipitate the biopolymers (using the unique properties of biopolymers), to remove the impurities that do not have the same unique properties as the biopolymer.
4. Rinse the biopolymers using certain solvents (making sure that the biopolymers do not dissolve in these solvents), to remove the impurities that dissolve in these solvents.

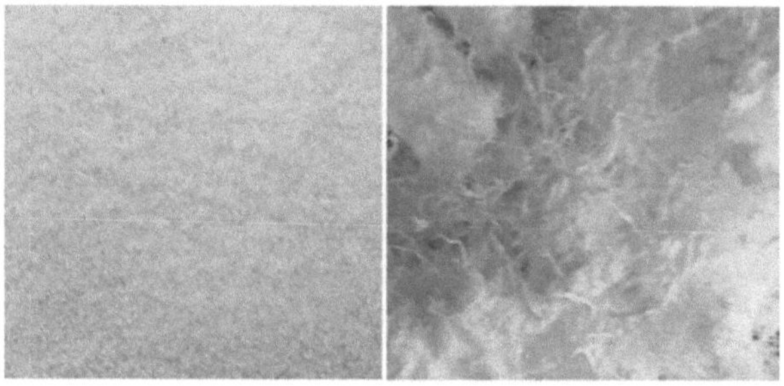

FIGURE LIII.1 Pictures of sodium alginate without *(left)* and with *(right)* purification.

Materials and Instruments

Sodium alginate (low viscosity)
Chloroform or dichloromethane
Activated charcoal (carbon)
$CaCl_2$
Ethanol (95% or higher)
Ethylenediaminetetraacetic acid (EDTA)
0.22- or 0.45-μm syringe filter
Dialysis tube

Laboratory Procedure

I. *Design the Purification Protocol*

The four properties of sodium alginate are:

a. Hydrophilic
b. Forms a gel when exposed to divalent ions, such as Ca^{2+} and Ba^{2+} (i.e., change from sodium alginate (liquid) to calcium or barium alginate (gel))
c. Gel can be dissolved in EDTA solution (i.e., change from calcium or barium alginate (gel) to sodium alginate (liquid))
d. Insoluble in ethanol

II. *Perform the Sodium Alginate Purification*

1. Incubate the alginate powder in chloroform or dichloromethane and filter under a vacuum on filter paper (this chloroform extraction is performed three times in practice).
   Q1: What is the purpose of this step?
2. Dissolve the sodium alginate in DI water (or use a prepared sodium alginate solution; 2% (w/v); about 20 mL per group is recommended).
3. Add an equivalent alginate-weight of activated charcoal (two washes in distilled water and two washes in 95% ethanol in practice) to the solution and vortex the mixture. Filter the solution using a syringe filter (multiple filters may be required as the solution is viscous).

4. Generate the alginate hydrogel (beads) using a 150 mmol/L $CaCl_2$ solution as the gelling agent (introduce the filtered sodium alginate solution into a 30 mL $CaCl_2$ solution by using a syringe dropwise).
5. Collect the hydrogel beads by removing the liquid and rinse them twice with DI water.
6. Dissolve the collected beads in a 20 mL alkaline 250 mmol/L EDTA solution (pH ~ 10).
7. Transfer the solution to a dialysis tube and proceed with the dialysis against DI water.
   Q2: How do you choose a dialysis tube?
8. Add two volumes of 95% or higher ethanol to the aqueous alginate solution to precipitate the alginate.
   Q3: How is the precipitated alginate collected?
   Q4: How is the alginate product dried?

Lab Activity IV: Microscale carrier preparation: hydrogel microspheres

Microscale drug carriers are commonly used for achieving controlled drug delivery. In this experiment, hydrogel microsphere production using either alginate or pectin will be investigated. The objectives of this experiment are to:

(1) Understand and learn how to operate the encapsulator or other setups.
(2) Understand how different factors influence the microencapsulation process.
(3) Perform the experimental design.

Background

Microsphere morphology and size greatly affect their performance as drug carriers. Factors affecting the microsphere production process should be investigated to optimize the process. The BÜCHI Encapsulator is a common system used for microsphere/microcapsule production. The encapsulator is used to generate the micro-scale size droplets, which is based on the principle that a laminar flowing liquid jet breaks up into equal-sized droplets by superimposed vibration. Droplets are then sprayed into a gelling bath (e.g., $CaCl_2$ solution for both alginate and pectin) as a result of multiple forces such as electrostatic forces (due to the electrostatic potential applied between the gelling bath and the needle), surface tension, and gravity. Other commonly used setups include electrospray/electrospinning and microfluidic devices [11,15–17,109,110].

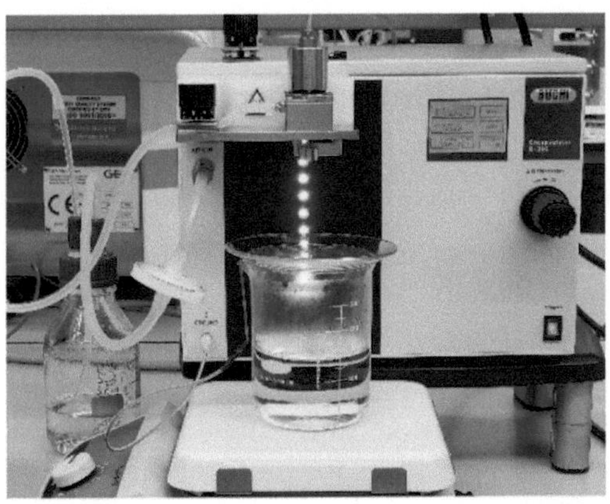

FIGURE LIV.1 Picture of BÜCHI Encapsulator setup (single-flow input).

Materials and Instruments

Sodium alginate [low viscosity; 2 % (w/v)]
LM pectin [3 % (w/v)]
150 mmol/L $CaCl_2$ solution
Encapsulator (or other setups)
Digital microscope
NIH ImageJ software

Laboratory Procedure

1. Determine the factors to study and choose three levels for each factor. Fill in Tables LIV.1 and 2. For each factor, pilot experiments may be needed to determine the parameter range.
2. Set up and run the device according to the design and system.
3. Collect the microspheres from each run and take images of the microspheres using the microscope.

4. Repeat the above process and keep all the settings the same, except the factor being studied.
5. Use the NIH ImageJ software (Appendix A) for image analysis and measure the size of at least 20 microspheres per sample. Record the results (both morphology and size of microspheres) in Table LIV.2. The morphology can be assessed by both roundness and uniformity of the size of microspheres.

Table LIV.1 Experimental design.

Factors	Level 1	Level 2	Level 3
e.g., Frequency	1000 Hz	2000 Hz	3000 Hz

Table LIV.2 Parameters for each run.

Run	Factor 1	Factor 2	Factor 3	Morphology	Size
1					
2					
3					
4					
5					
6					
7					
8					
9					

Lab Activity V: Nanoscale carrier preparation: metallic nanoparticles

Metallic nanoparticles have been widely used for drug delivery. In this experiment, the green synthesis of gold (Au) nanoparticles using upland cress will be investigated. The objectives of this experiment are to:

(1) Understand the green synthesis mechanism of metallic nanoparticles.
(2) Perform the green synthesis of metallic nanoparticles.
(3) Characterization of metallic nanoparticles.

Background

Gold nanoparticles show unique surface interactions and can be functionalized with drugs, radioisotopes, targeting moieties, PEG, and others, to offer novel approaches for medical diagnosis and treatment [71]. The leafy extracts of many plants, such as *Camellia sinensis* (green tea), *Ginkgo biloba* (ginkgo tree), *Coffee arabica* (coffee), and *Nasturtium officinale* (watercress), contain the reducing and capping agents necessary for metallic nanoparticle synthesis. Some of these agents have been identified as phenolic compounds, proteins with amine groups, etc. Upland cress (*Barbarea verna*) is a widely available biennial leafy green in the *Brassicaceae* family, which has been found to contain a high amount of phytochemicals, including ascorbic acid and carotenoids that are potentially useful for metallic nanoparticle synthesis. Phenolics within the upland cress extract mainly contribute to the reducing process, while phenolics and other plant metabolites (such as sugars and enzymes) are responsible for stabilization and capping [71,111].

Materials and Instruments

Fresh upland cress
Gold (III) chloride trihydrate ($HAuCl_4 \cdot 3H_2O$)
Red food dye
Blender
Shaker
UV spectrophotometer
Green laser pointer

Laboratory Procedure

I. *Prepare the Upland Cress Extract*
   1. Blend 10 g of upland cress in 100 mL deionized (DI) water for 15 seconds.
   2. Vacuum filter the extract twice using Whatman filter paper and centrifuge at 4000 rpm for 5 min to produce the extract (supernatant).

II. *Green Synthesis of Au Nanoparticles*
   1. Add 5 mL of the extract, 0.4 mL of 10 mmol/L gold (III) chloride trihydrate, and 35 mL of DI water into a 100-mL flask.
   2. Incubate the solution in a shaker (215 rpm) at 37°C for about 5 to 6 hours.
   3. Observe the solution color changes with time.
      Q1: Why are small gold nanoparticles red?

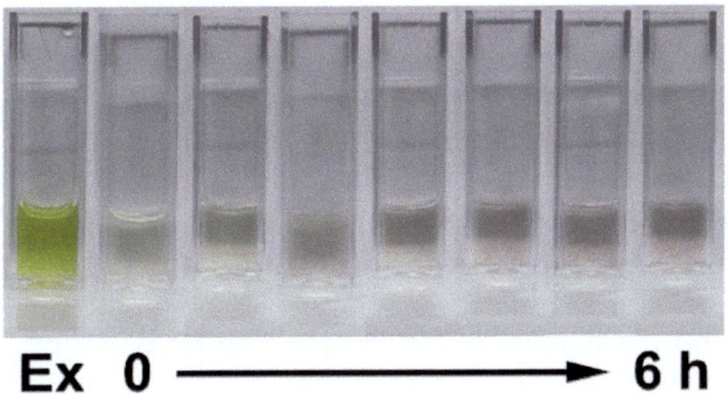

FIGURE LV.1 Solution color change of the upland cress extract and gold(III) chloride trihydrate mixture during the incubation period. *From Hutchinson, N., et al.,* Green synthesis of gold nanoparticles using upland cress and their biochemical characterization and assessment. *J Nanomater, 2022.* ***12****(1): p. 28.*

III. *Characterization of Au Nanoparticles*
   1. Place a few milliliters of DI water in a glass test tube and add a drop of red food dye.
   2. Place a few milliliters of the nanoparticle solution in a glass test tube.
   3. Shine a green laser pointer through the solution and observe the "path" of the light differences (**Q2**).
   4. Put 1 mL of the nanoparticle solution into a cuvette and run a scan (400 to 600 nm) using a UV spectrophotometer. Record the spectrum.
      Q3: Which peak is characteristic of the gold nanoparticles?

Review and practice questions

1. What are the different classifications of polymers?
2. What are the advantages of using polymers in drug delivery?
3. What are the advantages of using natural polymers over synthetic polymers in drug delivery?
4. What is the process of obtaining chitosan from chitin?
5. Why do collagen and gelatin show different sol-gel transitions even though they are from the same source?
6. What is the traditional review of the proton sponge effect?
7. Draw the Pluronic micelle structure in an aqueous solution.
8. What is the major difference between microspheres and microcapsules?
9. Describe the general process of polymerization for microsphere production.
10. Describe the general process of coacervation for microcapsule production.
11. Conduct a literature search and give an example of a surfactant used for stabilizing a W/O emulsion and one example for stabilizing an O/W emulsion.
12. Describe the general process for microparticle production using a spray dryer.
13. What are the five types of microneedles? And what are their working mechanisms?
14. What is the driving force for liposome formation?

15. Determine the x:y for these phospholipids:

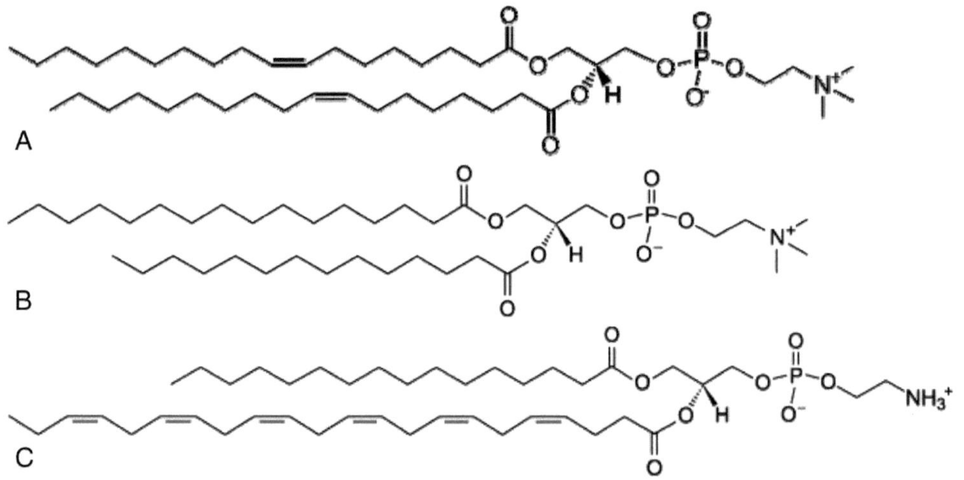

16. What is the major difference between passive and active drug loading?

17. What are the different mechanisms for the cellular uptake of liposomes and the release of encapsulated drug molecules?

18. Describe the general process and mechanism of electrospinning for nanofibers.

19. What are the two general approaches for dendrimer synthesis?

20. This shows the synthetic scheme of poly (propylene imine) dendrimers with 1,4-diaminobutane as the core. Please indicate the core, dendrons, and each generation on the graph.

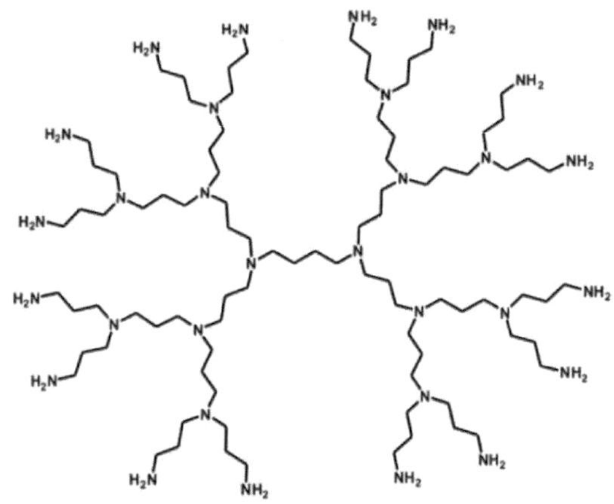

21. Based on the chirality, what are the three types of CNTs?

22. What are the toxicity concerns of using fullerenes, graphene, and CNTs as drug carriers?

23. What are some of the considerations for drug carrier design?

24. What characteristics of carriers can affect drug absorption, distribution, and elimination?

25. What are the common noncovalent approaches for drug carrier modification?

26. Explain the mechanism of EDC/EDC-sulfo-NHS crosslinking.

27. Conduct a literature search and write a short essay on an example of drug carrier modification using either a proto-reactive crosslinker or click chemistry.

References

[1] Boros E, Dyson PJ, Gasser G. Classification of metal-based drugs according to their mechanisms of action. Chem 2020;6(1):41–60.

[2] Chauhan NPS. Ceramic-based hybrid nanoparticles in drug delivery. In: Joshy KS, Thomas S, Thakur VK, editors. Nanoparticles for drug delivery. Springer Singapore; 2021. p. 109–31.

[3] Domingues ZR, et al. Bioactive glass as a drug delivery system of tetracycline and tetracycline associated with β-cyclodextrin. Biomaterials 2004;25(2):327–33.
[4] Nyamweya NN. Applications of polymer blends in drug delivery. Futur J Pharm Sci 2021;7(1):18.
[5] Ulery BD, Nair LS, Laurencin CT. Biomedical applications of biodegradable polymers. J Polym Sci B Polym Phys 2011;49(12):832–64.
[6] Sung YK, Kim SW. Recent advances in polymeric drug delivery systems. Biomater Res 2020;24(1):12.
[7] Gowthaman NSK, et al. Chapter 15 - Advantages of biopolymers over synthetic polymers: social, economic, and environmental aspects. In: Thomas S, Gopi S, Amalraj A, editors. Biopolymers and their industrial applications. Elsevier; 2021. p. 351–72.
[8] Tong X, et al. Recent advances in natural polymer-based drug delivery systems. React Funct Polym 2020;148:104501.
[9] Silva SS, et al. 2.11 Polymers of biological origin. In: Ducheyne P, editor. Comprehensive biomaterials II. Elsevier; 2017. p. 228–52.
[10] Zhang W. Encapsulation of transgenic cells for gene therapy. In: Hashad D, editor. Gene therapy. IntechOpen; 2015. Ch. 8.
[11] Kanungo M, et al. Development of gelatin-coated microspheres for novel bioink design. Polymers 2021;13(19):3339.
[12] Siew CK, Williams PA, Young NW. New insights into the mechanism of gelation of alginate and pectin: charge annihilation and reversal mechanism. Biomacromolecules 2005;6(2):963–9.
[13] Gawkowska D, Cybulska J, Zdunek A. Structure-related gelling of pectins and linking with other natural compounds: a review. Polymers 2018;10(7):762.
[14] Phakousonh D, et al. Design and stability improvement of pectin-based red blood cell-mimicking microcapsules for oxygen therapeutics. J Biomed Nanotechnol 2021;17(9):1798–805.
[15] Cherwin A, et al. Design of a novel oxygen therapeutic using polymeric hydrogel microcapsules mimicking red blood cells. Pharmaceutics 2019;11(11):583.
[16] Crouse JZ, et al. Development of a microscale red blood cell-shaped pectin-oligochitosan hydrogel system using an electrospray-vibration method: preparation and characterization. J Appl Biomater Funct Mater 2015;13(4):e326–31.
[17] Zhang W, et al. Design of artificial red blood cells using polymeric hydrogel microcapsules: hydrogel stability improvement and polymer selection. Int J Artif Organs 2016;39(10):518–23.
[18] Papakonstantinou E, Roth M, Karakiulakis G. Hyaluronic acid: a key molecule in skin aging. Dermatoendocrinol 2012;4(3):253–8.
[19] Vasvani S, Kulkarni P, Rawtani D. Hyaluronic acid: a review on its biology, aspects of drug delivery, route of administrations and a special emphasis on its approved marketed products and recent clinical studies. Int J Biol Macromol 2020;151:1012–29.
[20] Elieh-Ali-Komi D, Hamblin MR. Chitin and chitosan: production and application of versatile biomedical nanomaterials. Int J Adv Res (Indore) 2016;4(3):411–27.
[21] Kozma M, Acharya B, Bissessur R. Chitin, chitosan, and nanochitin: extraction, synthesis, and applications. Polymers 2022;14(19):3989.
[22] Baharlouei P, Rahman A. Chitin and chitosan: prospective biomedical applications in drug delivery, cancer treatment, and wound healing. Marine Drugs 2022;20(7):460.
[23] Aranaz I, et al. Chitosan: an overview of its properties and applications. Polymers 2021;13(19):3256.
[24] Naveed M, et al. Chitosan oligosaccharide (COS): an overview. Int J Biol Macromol 2019;129:827–43.
[25] Zhang W, et al. Synthesis and characterization of thermally responsive Pluronic F127-chitosan nanocapsules for controlled release and intracellular delivery of small molecules. ACS Nano 2010;4(11):6747–59.
[26] Rao W, et al. Chitosan-decorated doxorubicin-encapsulated nanoparticle targets and eliminates tumor reinitiating cancer stem-like cells. ACS Nano 2015;9(6):5725–40.
[27] An B, Lin Y-S, Brodsky B. Collagen interactions: drug design and delivery. Adv Drug Deliv Rev 2016;97:69–84.
[28] Milano F, et al. Current trends in gelatin-based drug delivery systems. Pharmaceutics 2023;15(5):1499.
[29] Innocenzi P. Understanding sol–gel transition through a picture. A short tutorial. J Solgel Sci Technol 2020;94(3):544–50.
[30] Campiglio CE, et al. Cross-linking strategies for electrospun gelatin scaffolds. Materials 2019;12(15):2476.
[31] Pham DT, Tiyaboonchai W. Fibroin nanoparticles: a promising drug delivery system. Drug Deliv 2020;27(1):431–48.
[32] Nguyen TP, et al. Silk fibroin-based biomaterials for biomedical applications: a review. Polymers 2019;11(12):1933.
[33] Tomeh MA, Hadianamrei R, Zhao X. Silk fibroin as a functional biomaterial for drug and gene delivery. Pharmaceutics 2019;11(10):494.
[34] Gentile P, et al. An overview of poly(lactic-co-glycolic) acid (PLGA)-based biomaterials for bone tissue engineering. Int J Mol Sci 2014;15(3): 3640–59.
[35] Su Y, et al. PLGA-based biodegradable microspheres in drug delivery: recent advances in research and application. Drug Delivery 2021; 28(1):1397–418.
[36] Zhao C, Zhou B. Polyethyleneimine-based drug delivery systems for cancer theranostics. J Funct Biomater 2023;14(1):12.
[37] Ding Y, et al. Gold nanoparticles for nucleic acid delivery. Mol Ther 2014;22(6):1075–83.
[38] Nel AE, et al. Understanding biophysicochemical interactions at the nano–bio interface. Nat Mater 2009;8(7):543–57.
[39] Vermeulen LMP, et al. The proton sponge hypothesis: fable or fact? Eur J Pharm Biopharm 2018;129:184–90.
[40] Yuan W, Li H. Chapter 14 - Polymer-based nanocarriers for therapeutic nucleic acids delivery. In: Andronescu E, Grumezescu AM, editors. Nanostructures for drug delivery. Elsevier; 2017. p. 445–60.
[41] Haq MA, Su Y, Wang D. Mechanical properties of PNIPAM based hydrogels: a review. Mater Sci Eng C 2017;70:842–55.
[42] Sanzari I, et al. Poly(N-isopropylacrylamide) based thin microgel films for use in cell culture applications. Sci Rep 2020;10(1):6126.
[43] Pasban S, Raissi H. PNIPAM/Hexakis as a thermosensitive drug delivery system for biomedical and pharmaceutical applications. Sci Rep 2022;12(1):14363.
[44] Cai X, et al. Chapter Three - lipid nanoparticle steric stabilization roadmap. In: Iglič A, Rappolt M, Pérez PL, editors. Advances in biomembranes and lipid self-assembly. Academic Press; 2022. p. 41–75.
[45] Prasanthan P, Kishore N. Self-assemblies of pluronic micelles in partitioning of anticancer drugs and effectiveness of this system towards target protein. RSC Advances 2021;11(36):22057–69.
[46] Zhang W, et al. The encapsulation and intracellular delivery of trehalose using a thermally responsive nanocapsule. Nanotechnology 2009; 20(27):275101.
[47] Saraf S, et al. Topotecan liposomes: a visit from molecular to therapeutic platform. Crit Rev Ther Drug Carrier Syst 2016;33(5):401–32.

[48] Timilsena YP, et al. Complex coacervation: principles, mechanisms and applications in microencapsulation. Int J Biol Macromol 2019;121: 1276–86.
[49] Salaün F. 9 - Microencapsulation technology for smart textile coatings. In: Hu J, editor. Active coatings for smart Textiles. Woodhead Publishing; 2016. p. 179–220.
[50] Napiórkowska A, Kurek M. Coacervation as a novel method of microencapsulation of essential oils: a review. Molecules 2022;27(16):5142.
[51] Ding S, et al. Double emulsions prepared by two-step emulsification: history, state-of-the-art and perspective. J Control Release 2019;295: 31–49.
[52] Rahaman SM, et al. Chapter 11 - Application of biosurfactants as emulsifiers in the processing of food products with diverse utilization in the baked goods. In: Inamuddin, Adetunji CO, editors. Applications of next generation biosurfactants in the food sector. Academic Press; 2023. p. 203–37.
[53] Díaz-Torres RDC, et al. Chapter 6 - Bioactive compounds obtained from plants, their pharmacological applications and encapsulation. In: Bhat RA, Hakeem KR, Dervash MA, editors. Phytomedicine. Academic Press; 2021. p. 181–205.
[54] Andrea T, et al. Microencapsulation of lipase and savinase enzymes by spray drying using Arabic gum as wall material. J Encapsulation Adsorption Sci 2016;06:161–73.
[55] Ferreira PA, et al. Chapter 9 - spray-drying for the formulation of oral drug delivery systems. In: Martins JP, Santos HA, editors. Nanotechnology for oral drug delivery. Academic Press; 2020. p. 253–84.
[56] Waghule T, et al. Microneedles: a smart approach and increasing potential for transdermal drug delivery system. Biomed Pharmacother 2019;109:1249–58.
[57] Menon I, et al. Microneedles: a new generation vaccine delivery system. Micromachines 2021;12(4):435.
[58] Kim Y-C, Park J-H, Prausnitz MR. Microneedles for drug and vaccine delivery. Adv Drug Deliv Rev 2012;64(14):1547–68.
[59] Turner J, et al. Hydrogel-forming microneedles: current advancements and future trends. Macromol Biosci 2020;21:2000307.
[60] Rzhevskiy AS, et al. Microneedles as the technique of drug delivery enhancement in diverse organs and tissues. J Control Release 2018;270: 184–202.
[61] Aldawood FK, Andar A, Desai S. A comprehensive review of microneedles: types, materials, processes, characterizations and applications. Polymers 2021;13(16).
[62] Yadav S, Sharma AK, Kumar P. Nanoscale self-assembly for therapeutic delivery. Front Bioeng Biotechnol 2020;8:127.
[63] Facci P. Chapter 7 - Semiconductor nanocrystals from Langmuir-blodgett films: synthesis, characterization, and applications. In: Nalwa HS, editor. Handbook of surfaces and interfaces of materials. Academic Press; 2001. p. 281–310.
[64] Parchekani J, et al. Design and simulation of the liposomal model by using a coarse-grained molecular dynamics approach towards drug delivery goals. Sci Rep 2022;12(1):2371.
[65] Sharma VK, Agrawal MK. A historical perspective of liposomes-a bio nanomaterial. Mater Today Proc 2021;45:2963–6.
[66] Liu P, Chen G, Zhang J. A review of liposomes as a drug delivery system: current status of approved products, regulatory environments, and future perspectives. Molecules 2022;27(4):1372.
[67] Liu W, et al. Research progress on liposomes: application in food, digestion behavior and absorption mechanism. Trends in Food Science & Technology 2020;104:177–89.
[68] Nsairat H, et al. Liposomes: structure, composition, types, and clinical applications. Heliyon 2022;8(5):e09394.
[69] Lombardo D, Kiselev MA. Methods of liposomes preparation: formation and control factors of versatile nanocarriers for biomedical and nanomedicine application. Pharmaceutics 2022;14(3):543.
[70] Ong SG, et al. Evaluation of extrusion technique for nanosizing liposomes. Pharmaceutics 2016;8(4):36.
[71] Hutchinson N, et al. Green synthesis of gold nanoparticles using upland cress and their biochemical characterization and assessment. Nanomaterials 2022;12(1):28.
[72] Zhang W. Nanofabrication II: biosynthesis of silver and gold nanoparticles. In: Zhang W, editor. Nanotechnology for bioengineers. Springer International Publishing; 2020. p. 15–22.
[73] Godakanda VU, et al. Electrospun fibers in drug delivery. In: Vaseashta A, Bölgen N, editors. Electrospun nanofibers: principles, technology and novel applications. Springer International Publishing; 2022. p. 159–81.
[74] Li L, et al. Electrospun fibers control drug delivery for tissue regeneration and cancer therapy. Adv Fiber Mater 2022;4(6):1375–413.
[75] Xue J, et al. Electrospun nanofibers: new concepts, materials, and applications. Acc Chem Res 2017;50(8):1976–87.
[76] Xue J, et al. Electrospinning and electrospun nanofibers: methods, materials, and applications. Chem Rev 2019;119(8):5298–415.
[77] Zhang W. Nanofabrication I: electrospinning of nanofibers. In: Nanotechnology for bioengineers. Springer International Publishing; 2020. p. 7–13.
[78] Abbasi E, et al. Dendrimers: synthesis, applications, and properties. Nanoscale Res Lett 2014;9(1):247.
[79] Ray S, et al. Dendrimer- and copolymer-based nanoparticles for magnetic resonance cancer theranostics. Theranostics 2018;8(22):6322–49.
[80] Boas U, Heegaard PMH. Dendrimers in drug research. Chem Soc Rev 2004;33(1):43–63.
[81] Chauhan AS. Dendrimers for drug delivery. Molecules 2018;23(4):938.
[82] Wang J, et al. Dendrimer-based drug delivery systems: history, challenges, and latest developments. J Biol Eng 2022;16(1):18.
[83] Kazemzadeh H, Mozafari M. Fullerene-based delivery systems. Drug Discov Today 2019;24(3):898–905.
[84] Nisoh N, et al. Fullerenes' interactions with plasma membranes: insight from the MD simulations. Biomolecules 2022;12(5):639.
[85] Russ KA, et al. C60 fullerene localization and membrane interactions in RAW 264.7 immortalized mouse macrophages. Nanoscale 2016;8(7): 4134–44.
[86] Bolskar RD. Fullerenes for drug delivery. In: Bhushan B, editor. Encyclopedia of nanotechnology. Springer Netherlands; 2016. p. 1267–81.
[87] Verma D, Goh KL. Chapter 11 - Functionalized graphene-based nanocomposites for energy applications. In: Jawaid M, Bouhfid R, Kacem Qaiss Ae, editors. Functionalized graphene nanocomposites and their derivatives. Elsevier; 2019. p. 219–43.
[88] Song S, et al. Biomedical application of graphene: from drug delivery, tumor therapy, to theranostics. Colloids Surf B Biointerfaces 2020;185: 110596.
[89] Liu J, Cui L, Losic D. Graphene and graphene oxide as new nanocarriers for drug delivery applications. Acta Biomaterialia 2013;9(12): 9243–57.

[90] Aqel A, et al. Carbon nanotubes, science and technology part (I) structure, synthesis and characterisation. Arab J Chem 2012;5(1):1–23.
[91] Ravi Kiran AVVV, Kusuma Kumari G, Krishnamurthy PT. Carbon nanotubes in drug delivery: focus on anticancer therapies. J Drug Deliv Sci Technol 2020;59:101892.
[92] Shah P, Lalan M, Jani D. Toxicological aspects of carbon nanotubes, fullerenes and graphenes. Curr Pharm Des 2021;27(4):556–64.
[93] Benet LZ. The role of BCS (biopharmaceutics classification system) and BDDCS (biopharmaceutics drug disposition classification system) in drug development. J Pharm Sci 2013;102(1):34–42.
[94] Lee M-K. Liposomes for enhanced bioavailability of water-insoluble drugs: in vivo evidence and recent approaches. Pharmaceutics 2020; 12(3):264.
[95] Blanco E, Shen H, Ferrari M. Principles of nanoparticle design for overcoming biological barriers to drug delivery. Nat Biotechnol 2015;33(9): 941–51.
[96] Zhang A, et al. Absorption, distribution, metabolism, and excretion of nanocarriers in vivo and their influences. Adv Colloid Interface Sci 2020;284:102261.
[97] Aryal S, et al. Top-down fabrication-based nano/microparticles for molecular imaging and drug delivery. Int J Nanomedicine 2019;14: 6631–44.
[98] Marangoni JM, et al. Engineering a disulfide-gated switch in streptavidin enables reversible binding without sacrificing binding affinity. Sci Rep 2020;10(1):12483.
[99] Thermo Fisher Scientific Inc. Bioconjugation and crosslinking technical handbook. Available from: Bioconjugation and crosslinking technical handbook.
[100] Murale DP, et al. Photo-affinity labeling (PAL) in chemical proteomics: a handy tool to investigate protein-protein interactions (PPIs). Proteome Science 2017;15(1):14.
[101] Devaraj NK, Finn MG. Introduction: click chemistry. Chem Rev 2021;121(12):6697–8.
[102] Kondengadan SM, et al. Click chemistry and drug delivery: a bird's-eye view. Acta Pharmaceutica Sinica B 2023;13(5):1990–2016.
[103] Li X, Xiong Y. Application of "click" chemistry in biomedical hydrogels. ACS Omega 2022;7(42):36918–28.
[104] Song S, et al. In situ one-step fluorescence labeling strategy of exosomes via bioorthogonal click chemistry for real-time exosome tracking in vitro and in vivo. Bioconjug Chem 2020;31(5):1562–74.
[105] Torres ML, et al. Purification of alginate improves its biocompatibility and eliminates cytotoxicity in matrix for bone tissue engineering. Algal Res 2019;40:101499.
[106] Zhang WJ, et al. Biocompatibility and membrane strength of C3H10T1/2 cell-loaded alginate-based microcapsules. Cytotherapy 2008;10(1): 90–7.
[107] Dusseault J, et al. Evaluation of alginate purification methods: effect on polyphenol, endotoxin, and protein contamination. J Biomed Mater Res A 2006;76(2):243–51.
[108] Johnson C. 2.4 - Advances in pretreatment and clarification technologies. In: Ahuja S, editor. Comprehensive water quality and purification. Elsevier; 2014. p. 60–74.
[109] Zieman J, et al. Development of gelatin-coated hydrogel microspheres for novel bioink design: a crosslinker study. Pharmaceutics 2023; 15(1):90.
[110] Majewski RL, et al. Bioencapsulation technologies in tissue engineering. J Appl Biomater Funct Mater 2016;14(4):395–403.
[111] Johnson DL, et al. Biosynthesis of silver nanoparticles using upland cress: purification, characterisation, and antimicrobial activity. Micro & Nano Letters 2020;15(2):110–3.

CHAPTER

7

Cell encapsulation: a living drug delivery approach

Wujie Zhang

LEARNING OBJECTIVES

- To understand the concepts of cell macro- and microencapsulation
- To explain the mechanism of using cell encapsulation as a drug delivery system
- To describe cell microencapsulation methods that use electrospray and microfluidic devices
- To provide examples and discuss the challenges and future directions
- To discuss the differences between the compartment and physiological pharmacokinetic modeling systems of cell encapsulation in therapies
- To design and modify alginate-based cell encapsulation systems

7.1 Introduction to cell encapsulation and microencapsulation

Cell encapsulation is the process of confining cells within a matrix for immunoisolation, which allows the use of both allogenic and xenogeneic cells in addition to scarcely available autologous cells [1]. Based on the system size, there are cell macroencapsulation (> 1000 μm in one dimension) and cell microencapsulation. Cell macroencapsulation systems come in different shapes, including discs, flat sheets, and hollow fibers. In microencapsulation, mostly, cell(s) are enclosed in gel-like microspheres (average < 1000 μm in diameter) [2]. Both macro- and microencapsulation systems have been used for various disease treatments including cancer and tissue engineering [3–5]. For example, as shown in Fig. 7.1, both systems can be used for islet transplantation.

The major disadvantage of cell macroencapsulation systems is the relatively low surface area-to-volume ratio [6]. The surface area/volume ratio is the amount of surface area per unit volume of an object, which largely affects its transport properties. For example, materials with large surface area-to-volume ratios allow for faster diffusion. Cell microencapsulation is the immobilization of cells in a micro-scale matrix with a semipermeable membrane, generally in a spherical shape. As shown in Fig. 7.2, the membrane protects encapsulated cells from the host's immune system and mechanical stresses while allowing the free diffusion of nutrients and metabolic waste for the cells to

Fundamentals and Design of Drug Delivery Systems
https://doi.org/10.1016/B978-0-443-23521-4.00007-2

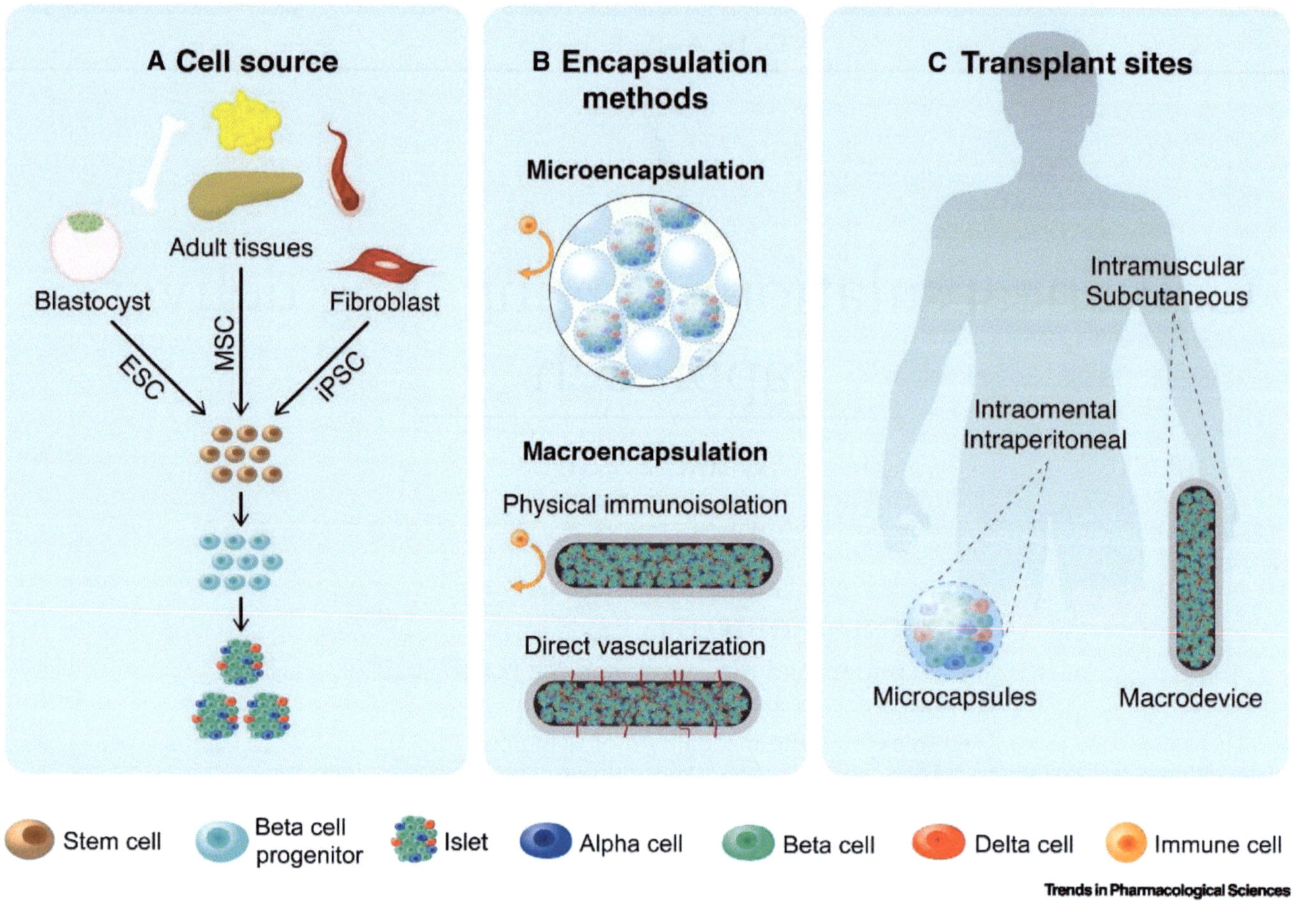

FIGURE 7.1 Strategies to address the current limitations in islet transplantation: (A) Embryonic stem cells (ESCs), mesenchymal stem cells (MSCs), and induced pluripotent stem cells (iPSCs) can be differentiated into insulin-producing cells to circumvent donor shortage. (B) To prevent immune rejection, islets may be microencapsulated or macroencapsulated in immunoisolating materials. Some macroencapsulation devices allow blood vessel penetration for direct graft vascularization to prevent hypoxia. (C) Due to large transplant volumes and to facilitate oxygen diffusion, microcapsules are typically deployed in the omentum or peritoneum. Macrodevices are commonly implanted intramuscularly or subcutaneously for ease of monitoring, refilling, and retrievability. From Paez-Mayorga, J. et al., *Emerging strategies for beta cell transplantation to treat diabetes. Trends in Pharmacological Sciences*, 2022. **43**(3): p. 221-233, with permission from Elsevier.

FIGURE 7.2 A schematic illustration of the concept of cell microencapsulation as a living drug delivery system. From Zhang, W. and X. He, *Microencapsulating and banking living cells for cell-based medicine. J. Healthc. Eng*, 2011. **2**: p. 875406.

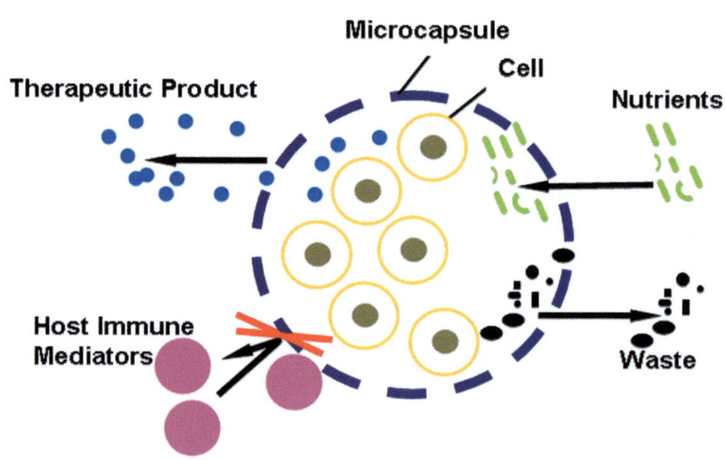

survive. Moreover, the membrane also controls the release of the therapeutic products produced by the encapsulated cells [7].

Semipermeable microcapsules for encapsulation (enzymes) and cell microencapsulation (bioartificial endocrine pancreas) were first reported in the 1960s and the 1980s, respectively [8,9]. After that, cell microencapsulation has been applied to almost all areas of disease treatment. Various studies have shown the benefits of small (< 100-μm) microcapsules, considering the size limitations of transplantation sites and the transport of oxygen and nutrients [7,10]. The intercapillary distance of the human body is around 100 μm in human tissues, which indicates the extent of oxygen and nutrient diffusion [11]. With this, small microcapsules have been shown to exhibit better mechanical properties, stability, and biocompatibility [7].

Sample question 7.1

Compare the surface area/volume ratios of 250-μm and 100-μm (diameter) microspheres.

Answer: For a sphere, surface area/volume equals $4 \times \pi \times (D/2)^2/(4/3 \times \pi \times (D/2)^3)$, which is 6/D.
For 250-μm sphere: surface area/volume = 6/(250 μm)= 0.024 μm^{-1}.
For 100-μm sphere: surface area/volume = 6/(100 μm)= 0.06 μm^{-1}.
The surface area–to–volume ratio of the 100-μm sphere is 2.5 times that of the 250-μm sphere (Fig. 7.3).

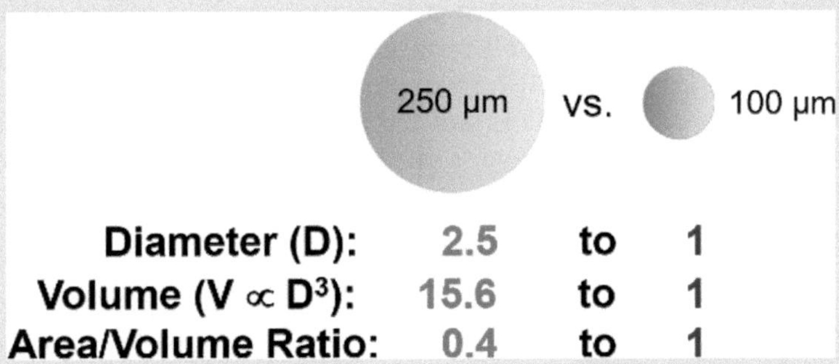

FIGURE 7.3 Comparison between 250-μm and 100-μm microspheres.

Efficacy (including biocompatibility) and biosafety are currently two of the major focuses for developing cell microencapsulation systems [6]. Regarding biocompatibility, encapsulated cells should maintain their viability and metabolic activities, the system should not trigger severe immune responses, including those that could lead to pericapsular fibrosis (Fig. 7.4), and the system should not lead to any toxic effects. It is worth noting that biocompatibility is a property of a system rather than a material, as it can only be considered in the context of the characteristics of both the material and the biological host within which it is placed [12]. Both efficacy and biosafety considerations require the precise and accurate release of the demanded drug dose and the encapsulated cells should be well protected and not released from the system [6].

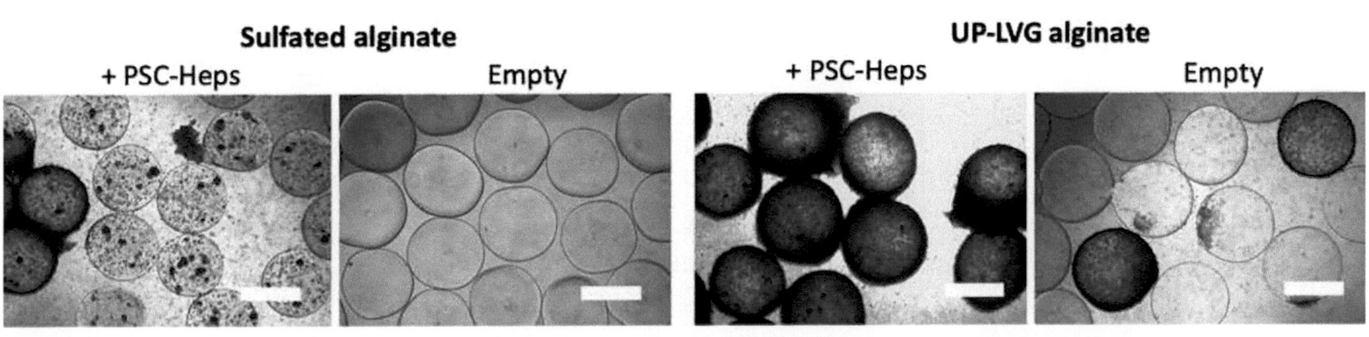

FIGURE 7.4 Microscopic images of alginate microbeads retrieved from mice 10 days after intraperitoneal implantation. Human induced pluripotent stem cell-derived hepatocyte spheroids encapsulated in sulfated alginate show a lower degree of fibrotic overgrowth compared to the spheroids encapsulated in nonmodified alginate. Empty microbeads exhibit the same trend. Scale bars: 500 μm. From Syanda, A.M. et al., *Sulfated alginate reduces pericapsular fibrotic overgrowth on encapsulated cGMP-compliant hPSC-hepatocytes in mice. Front. Bioeng. Biotechnol*, 2022. **9**.

To improve the performance of the cell microencapsulation systems, materials used for encapsulation should be extensively examined. Both natural (alginate, agarose, collagen/gelatin, and hyaluronic acid) and synthetic [poly(-vinyl alcohol), 2-hydroxyethyl methacrylate, polyethylene glycol, and poly(lactic-co-glycolic acid)] polymers have been used for cell microencapsulation. The origin, purity, and molecular weight are critical factors of the encapsulation materials. In general, such information is missing. Modification of the materials is sometimes beneficial, e.g., sulfation and zwitterion grafting. As shown in Fig. 7.4, sulfated alginate reduces pericapsular fibrotic overgrowth on encapsulated human induced pluripotent stem cell-derived hepatocytes (hPSC-Heps) in mice [13].

7.2 Cell microencapsulation methods

Various methods for cell microencapsulation have been developed including electrostatic spray, microfluidics, vibration nozzle, jet cutter, lithography, and superhydrophobic surfaces [7,14]. Electrospray and microfluidics are the two most commonly used methods for cell microencapsulation. Both methods can be used to produce cell-loaded microspheres and microcapsules with cells entrapped in the core. The method of producing core-shell structured cell-load microcapsules using an electrospray setup is shown in Fig. 7.5. Generally, a cell polymer mixture or two (a shell flow and a core flow with cells) is extruded through a nozzle. At the tip of the nozzle (metallic blunt needle mostly), droplets are broken down into smaller ones as the result of multiple forces—electrostatic force, surface tension, and gravity [10,15]. The electrospray method provides many advantages, such as easy operation and high efficiency.

Microfluidic devices can be used to produce small monodisperse microcapsules. Rapid removal of the toxic oil phase is critical to maintain high cell viability [5,16]. In general, cells are within the aqueous (core) flow, which is sheared by the oil (continuous) flow. Microdroplets are formed due to the immiscible nature of water and oil. The microdroplets solidify (e.g., gelling agents diffuse from the oil phase to the microdroplets leading to the gel formation) as they travel (Fig. 7.6).

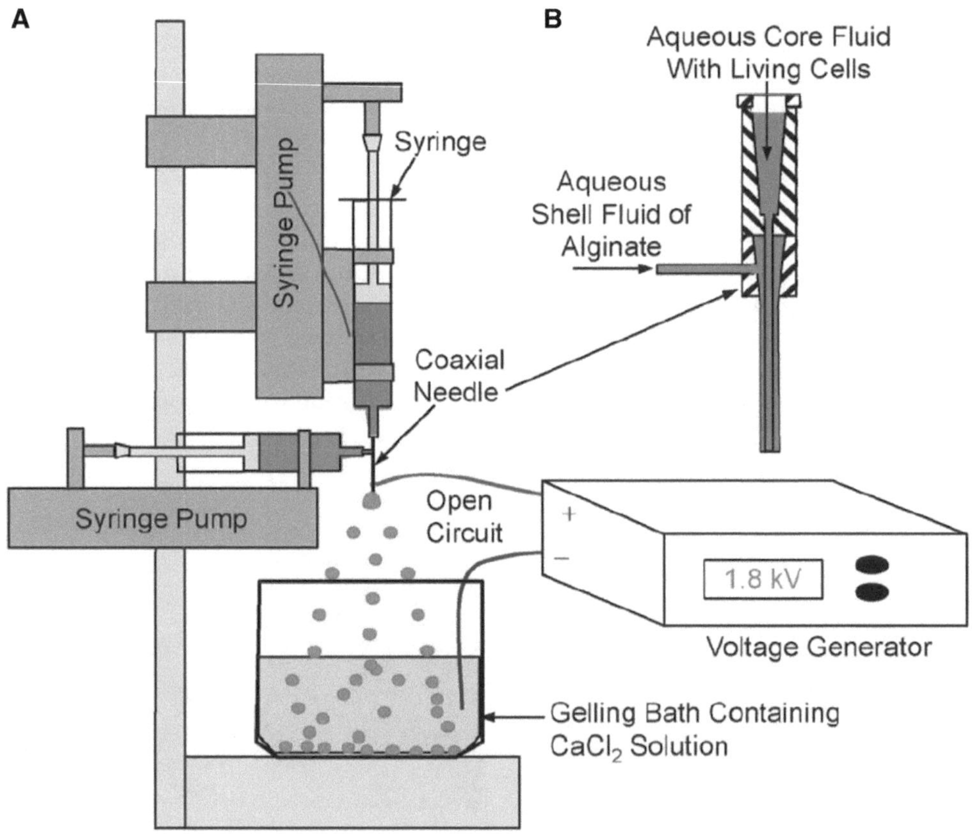

FIGURE 7.5 A schematic illustration of a coaxial electrospray system for producing core-shell microcapsules with alginate hydrogel shell in one step using two aqueous fluids: (A) an overview of the complete setup; (B) a cross-sectional view of the coaxial needle design. From Zhao, S. et al., *Coaxial electrospray of liquid core—hydrogel shell microcapsules for encapsulation and miniaturized 3D culture of pluripotent stem cells. Int. J. Integr. Biol*, 2014. **6**(9): p. 874-884, with permission from The Royal Society of Chemistry.

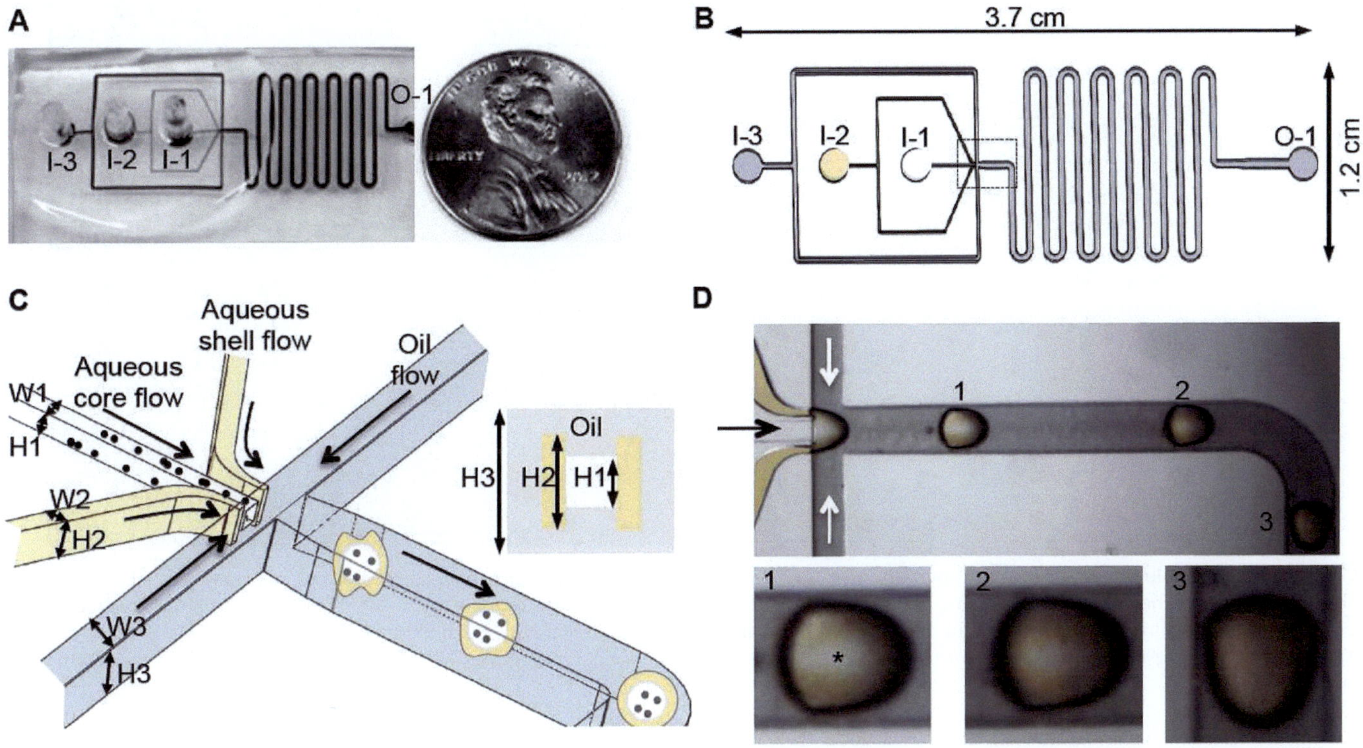

FIGURE 7.6 A microfluidic flow-focusing device for one-step generation of core-shell microcapsules: (A) a picture of the microfluidic device in comparison to a U.S. quarter; (B) a schematic view of the microchannel system: I-1, I-2, and I-3 are the inlets of core (aqueous flow 1), shell (aqueous flow 2), and oil flows, respectively, and O-1 is the outlet; (C) a zoom-in look of the nonplanar design of a flow-focusing junction (the *dashed box region* in B); and (D) typical images showing gradual coverage of the core fluid by the shell fluid that was stained yellow. From Agarwal, P. et al., *One-step microfluidic generation of pre-hatching embryo-like core-shell microcapsules for miniaturized 3D culture of pluripotent stem cells.* Lab Chip, 2013. **13**(23): p. 4525-4533, with permission from The Royal Society of Chemistry.

Alginate-based systems are the most common for cell microencapsulation. Both electrostatic spray and microfluidic setups, shown in Figs. 7.5 and 7.6, are designed for alginate-based core-shell microcapsules with the shell being Ca-alginate. Ba^{2+} has been studied to replace Ca^{2+} as a crosslinker/gelling agent for alginate due to its higher affinity for alginate compared to Ca^{2+} and radiopacity. However, the toxicity of Ba^{2+} remains a concern [17,18]. A more common approach for producing an alginate-based system is to produce the alginate microspheres first. Both electrostatic and microfluidic setups can be applied, with cells being suspended in alginate as a single flow rather than two. Due to the negative charge of the alginate, a polycation polymer is applied to coat the surface of the alginate microspheres to control its permeability. Then, an alginate solution is used to neutralize the positively charged surface. This layer further controls the permeability and also prevents or delays the immune cells from attacking the encapsulated cells (electrostatic repulsion between negatively charged immune cells and polyanionic alginate) [18]. Initially, poly-L-lysine (PLL) was used as the polycationic coating. The PLL-alginate layer can take three different structures by intramolecular hydrogen bonding: random coil formation between alginate and PLL, the α-helical structure between amide groups of PLL, and an antiparallel β-sheet structure between amide groups of PLL [19]. Due to PLL's biocompatibility concerns, other cationic polymers such as poly-L-ornithine (PLO), protamine sulfate, and chitosan are of interest [18,20,21]. A previous study showed that alginate-polyornithine microcapsules effectively protected the xenogeneic cells from the host immune system and supported their survival for 6 months or more in the brains of rats without adverse effects (Fig. 7.7) [22]. The alginate-chitosan complex was shown to be more stable than alginate-PLL [23]. A sodium citrate solution is also commonly used to "liquefy" the Ca-alginate core by removing Ca^{2+} from alginate which has been shown to be beneficial for cell proliferation [20]. The process for producing cell-loaded alginate-chitosan-alginate (ACA) microcapsules is shown in Fig. 7.8, and images of cell-loaded microspheres/capsules are shown in Fig. 7.9.

Single-cell encapsulation has also been studied and can be leveraged to advance single-cell analysis platforms and cell-based medicine [24]. There are different approaches for single-cell encapsulation: attach encapsulation materials to the cell surface (Fig. 7.10) [25], use microfluidic devices [26], and microgels [24].

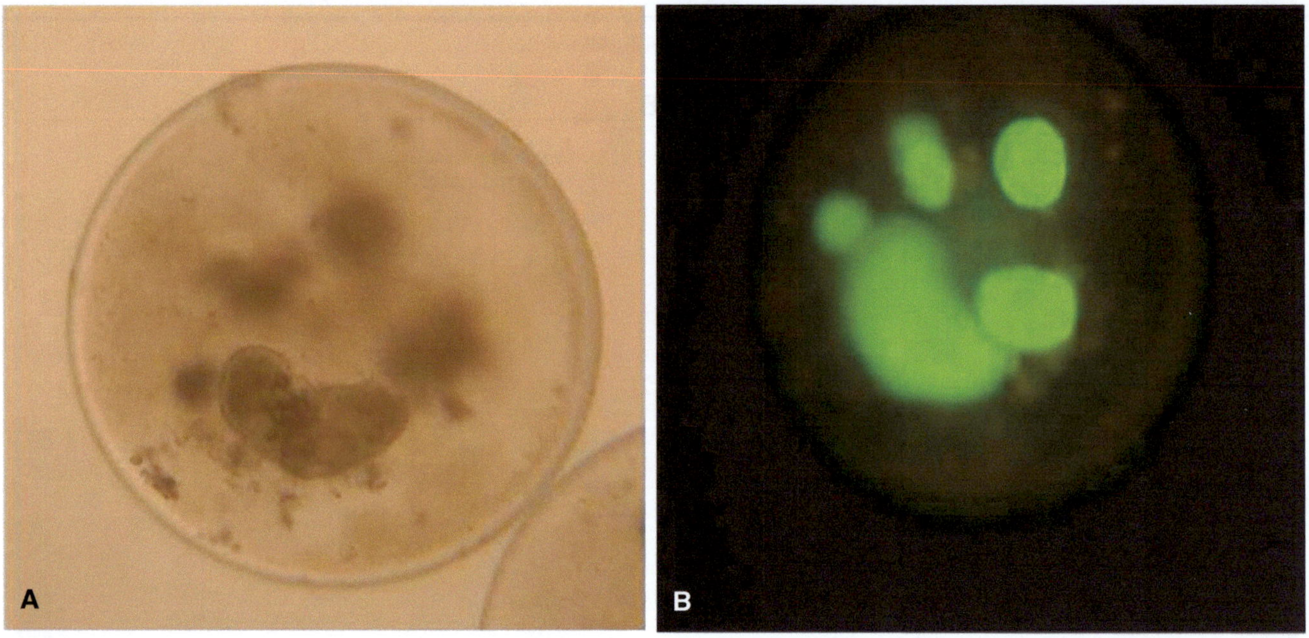

FIGURE 7.7 Capsule retrieved from rat brain after 6 months *in vivo*. (A) Phase contrast image. One large and four smaller cell clusters are visible. The surface of the capsule is free of any adherent cells. (B) The corresponding fluorescence microscopy image after viability staining. The five cell clusters are stained *green* with calcein, indicating that the majority of cells are alive. From Skinner, S.J. et al., *Encapsulated living choroid plexus cells: potential long-term treatments for central nervous system disease and trauma*. J. Neural Eng, 2009. **6**(6): p. 065001, with permission from IOP Publishing.

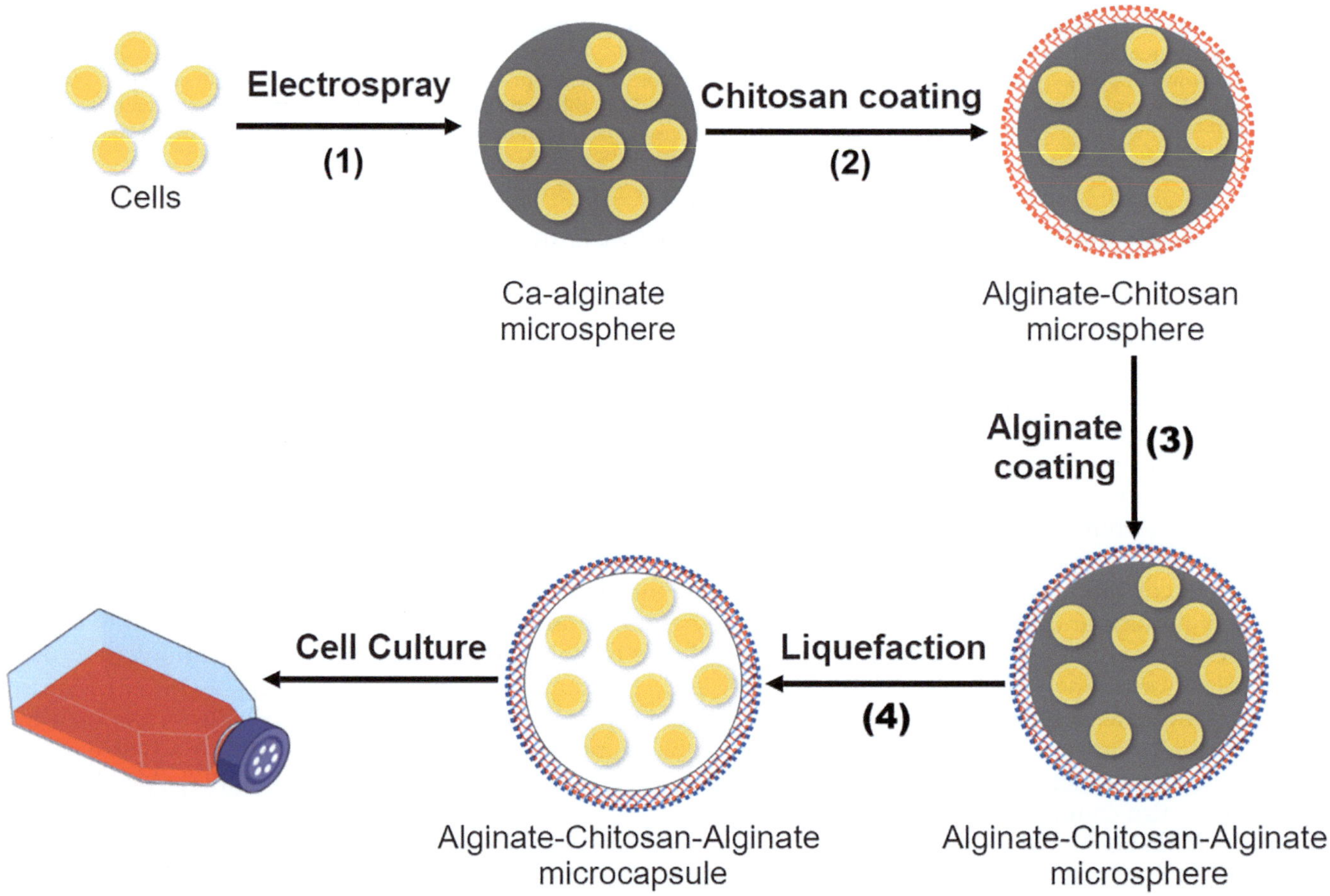

FIGURE 7.8 A schematic illustration of the procedure for preparing ACA microcapsules loaded with cells by (1) producing cell-loaded plain alginate microbeads (Ca-alginate microspheres) using electrospray (or other approaches); (2) coating the microbeads with chitosan to form alginate-chitosan microspheres; (3) coating the alginate-chitosan microcapsules with alginate to form ACA microspheres; and (4) liquefying the Ca-alginate hydrogel core to give rise to the ACA microcapsules.

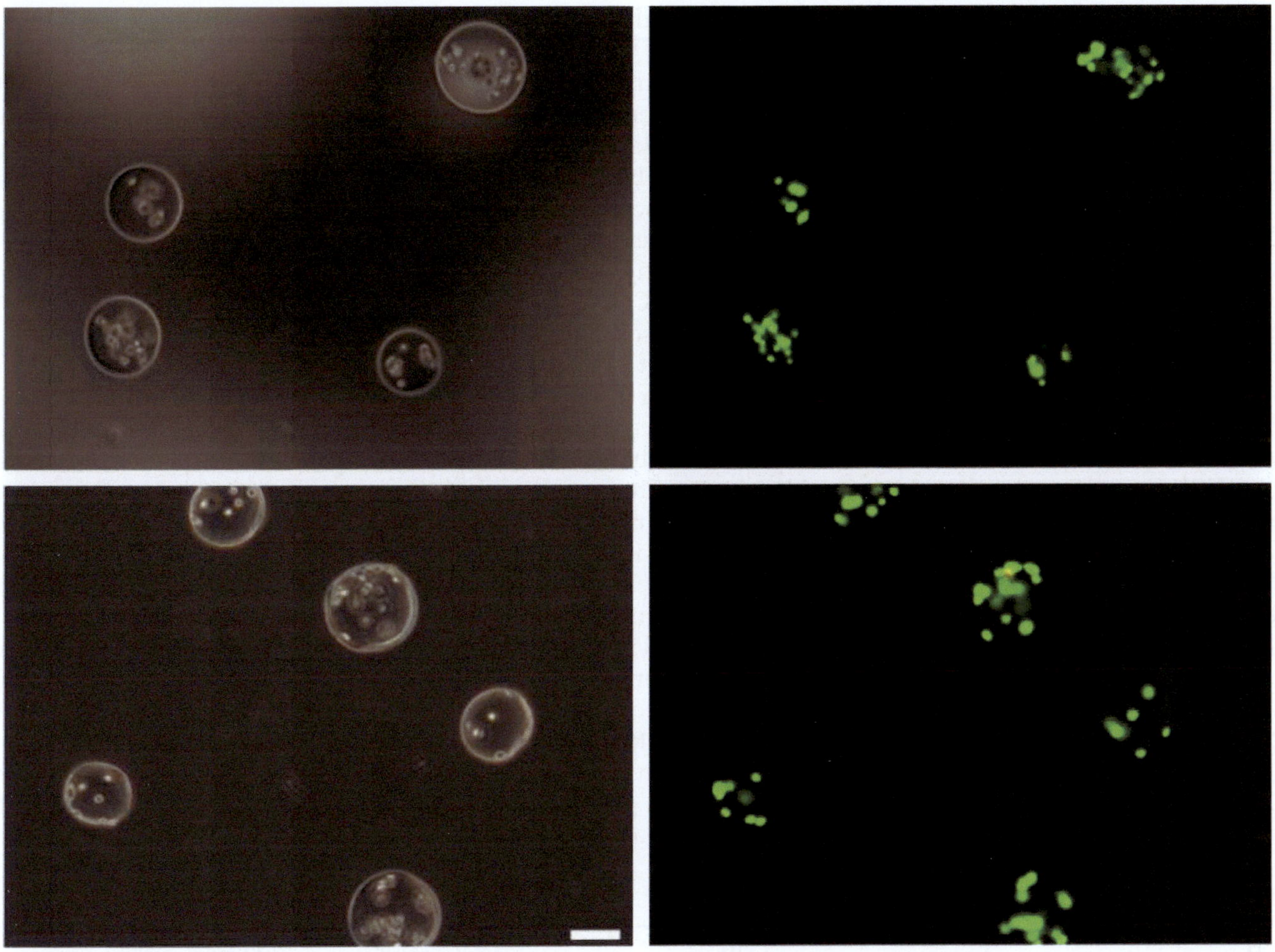

FIGURE 7.9 Microscopic images of encapsulated C3H10T1/2 cells. *Top*, Ca-alginate microspheres and *bottom*, ACA microcapsules. *Right*, the corresponding fluorescent images indicating high cell viability. *Green*, live cells; *red*, dead cells. Scale bar: 100 μm.

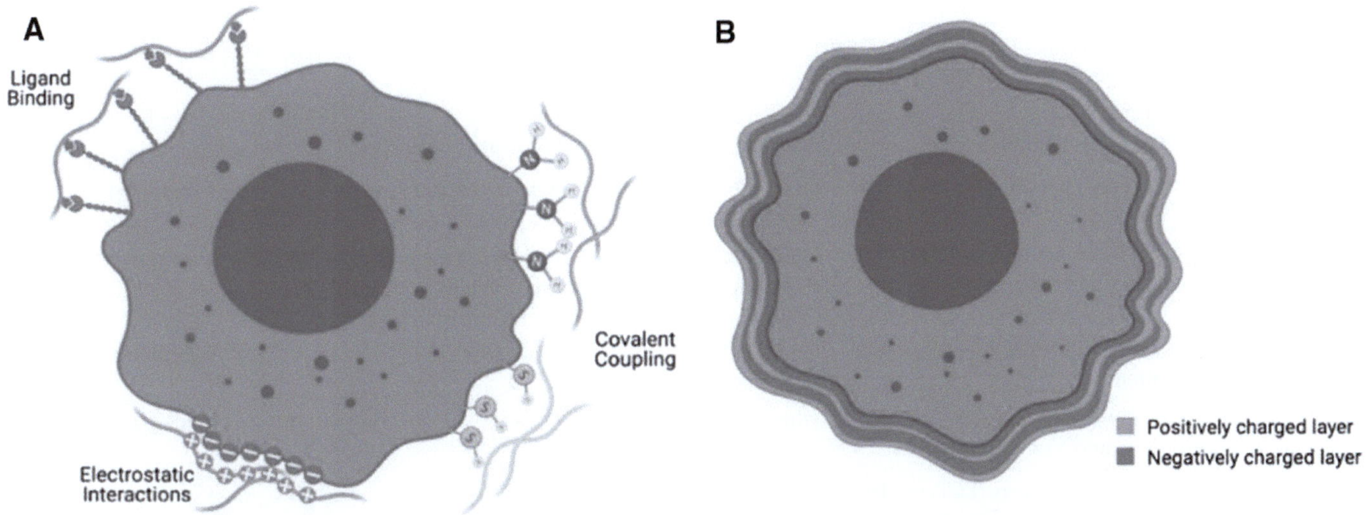

FIGURE 7.10 Schematic overview of the different methods to coat cells. (A) Various interactions to anchor encapsulation materials. (B) Layer-by-layer coating of a cell with alternating encapsulation materials. From Marikar, S.N. et al., *Microencapsulation-based cell therapies.* Cell Mol Life Sci, 2022. **79**(7): p. 351.

7.3 Cell encapsulation in therapy

Cell encapsulation has been applied for acute liver failure, Parkinson's disease, type 1 diabetes treatment, retinitis pigmentosa, cancer, and more (Table 7.1) [4,25,27]. Microencapsulated cells were first tested in humans in 1994 (islets in alginate-PLL-alginate microcapsules) [27]. Some of the leading companies in the sustained release of therapeutics from encapsulated cells are Neurotech Pharmaceuticals, Inc., Living Cell Technologies Ltd., PharmaCyte Biotech, Inc., and Sigilon Therapeutics, Inc. Neurotech Pharmaceuticals developed the Encapsulated Cell Technology (ECT) platform (NT-501 implant, Fig. 7.9) which provides an immunoisolation microenvironment optimized for cell survival and consistent drug delivery. The cells are engineered to produce therapeutic proteins, such as ciliary neurotrophic factor (CNTF) [28]. LCT's platform is NTCELL, an alginate-coated capsule containing clusters of neonatal porcine choroid plexus cells targeting Parkinson's disease. LCT has completed two clinical trials of NTCELL with a clinically relevant effect being observed at 24 months postimplant [29]. The alginate-coated capsule is an alginate-polyornithine microcapsules (600 to 660 μm in diameter) [30]. PharmaCyte Biotech develops cellular therapies for cancer and diabetes treatments using an encapsulation technology, "Cell-in-a-Box" [31]. The technology, semipermeable cellulose beads, is developed by Austrianova and uses Gel8 (a proprietary cellulose sulfate solution) [32]. Sigilon has developed the Shielded Living Therapeutics platform for non−viral cell−based products. Their dual-layer sphere is composed of an Afibromer matrix [33].

To successfully translate encapsulated cells for clinical applications, there is still a long way to go. Regarding cell microencapsulation, the major challenge is that the long-term survival of the transplanted cells is limited by a characteristic foreign body response, which leads to pericapsular fibrosis and death of the encapsulated cells. Surface modification of the microcapsules using immune-modulatory small molecules and the application of ultra-low-fouling zwitterionic biomaterials are the two popular approaches. The implantation approach and site should also be carefully examined. For example, a secondary "container" may be needed to keep the encapsulated cells in place. Regarding microencapsulation, it is challenging to ensure there is a sufficient oxygen and nutrient supply [34]. Prevascularized, vascularized, and vascularization-promoting microencapsulation systems are preferred [34,35]. Last, three-dimensional printing also shows great promise in therapies using encapsulated cells, especially to achieve personalized medicine, such as fabricating a patient-specific cell encapsulation device.

TABLE 7.1 Clinical trials involving encapsulated cells.

Project	Cells	Target disease(s)	Phase	Status
Micro-encapsulated Hepatocyte Intraperitoneal Transplantation in Liver Failure Adults	Hepatocytes	Liver failure	I	Not yet recruiting
Hepatocyte Microbeads for Acute Liver Failure (HELP)	Hepatocytes and mesenchymal stromal cells	Acute liver failure	I/II	Not yet recruiting
A Study of Encapsulated Cell Technology (ECT) Implant for Participants with Early Stage Retinitis Pigmentosa	Human NTC-201 cells releasing CNTF	Early stage retinitis pigmentosa	II/III	Completed
A Study of Encapsulated Cell Technology (ECT) Implant for Participants with Late Stage Retinitis Pigmentosa	Human NTC-201 cells releasing CNTF	Late stage retinitis pigmentosa	II/III	Completed
Evaluation of Safety of Ciliary Neurotrophic Factor Implants in the Eye	Human NTC-201 cells releasing CNTF	Retinitis pigmentosa	I	Completed
Retinal Imaging in CNTF-Releasing Encapsulated Cell Implant Treated Patients for Early-stage Retinitis Pigmentosa	Human NTC-201 cells releasing CNTF	Retinitis pigmentosa; Usher syndrome type 2; Usher syndrome type 3	II	Completed
Dual Intravitreal Implantation of NT-501 Encapsulated Cell Therapy for Glaucoma	Human NTC-201 cells releasing CNTF	Glaucoma	II	Recruiting
Study of NT-501 Encapsulated Cell Therapy for Glaucoma Neuroprotection and Vision Restoration	Human NTC-201 cells releasing CNTF	Glaucoma	II	Active, not recruiting
A Study of Encapsulated Cell Technology (ECT) Implant for Participants with Atrophic Macular Degeneration	Human NTC-201 cells releasing CNTF	Atrophic macular degeneration	II	Completed
Study of the Intravitreal Implantation of NT-503-3 Encapsulated Cell Technology (ECT) for the Treatment of Recurrent Choroidal Neovascularization (CNV)	Cells release a soluble VEGF receptor	Macular degeneration	I/II	Terminated

TABLE 7.1 Clinical trials involving encapsulated cells.—cont'd

Project	Cells	Target disease(s)	Phase	Status
Secondary to Age-Related Macular Degeneration (AMD)				
A Phase 2 Multicenter Randomized Clinical Trial of CNTF for MacTel	Human NTC-201 cells releasing CNTF	Macular telangiectasia type 2	II	Completed
Extension Study of NT-501 Ciliary Neurotrophic Factor (CNTF) Implant for Macular Telangiectasia (MacTel)	Human NTC-201 cells releasing CNTF	Macular telangiectasia	II	Completed
Open-label Investigation of the Safety and Clinical Effects of NTCELL in Patients with Parkinson's Disease	Choroid plexus cells	Parkinson's disease	I/IIa	Completed
Investigation of the Safety and Efficacy of NTCELL [Immunoprotected (Alginate-Encapsulated) Porcine Choroid Plexus Cells for Xenotransplantation] in Patients with Parkinson's Disease	Choroid plexus cells	Parkinson's disease	IIb	Completed
Encapsulated Cell Biodelivery of Nerve Growth Factor to Alzheimer's Disease Patients	NGF-producing, genetically engineered human cell line	Alzheimer's disease	I	Unknown
A Safety, Tolerability, and Efficacy Study of VC-02TM Combination Product in Subjects With Type 1 Diabetes Mellitus and Hypoglycemia Unawareness	Encapsulated PEC-01 cells	Type 1 diabetes mellitus with hypoglycemia	I/II	Active, not recruiting
A Study to Evaluate Safety, Engraftment, and Efficacy of VC-01 in Subjects with T1 Diabetes Mellitus (VC01-103)	Encapsulated PEC-01 cells	Type 1 diabetes mellitus	I/II	Active, not recruiting
Safety and Efficacy of PEG-Encapsulated Islet Allografts Implanted in Type I Diabetic Recipients	Huma allogenic cultured islet cells	Type 1 diabetes mellitus	I/II	Terminated
Safety and Efficacy Study of Encapsulated Human Islets Allotransplantation to Treat Type 1 Diabetes	Human islets	Type 1 diabetes mellitus	I	Withdraw
Open-label Investigation of the Safety and Efficacy of DIABECELL in Patients With Type 1 Diabetes Mellitus	Porcine islets	Type 1 diabetes mellitus	IIb	Completed
Long-term Function of Beta Cell Allografts in Non-uremic Type 1 Diabetic Patients	Beta-cells	Type 1 diabetes mellitus	I/II	Unknown
Safety and Efficacy Study of Encapsulated Human Islets Allotransplantation to Treat Type 1 Diabetes	Human islets	Type 1 diabetes mellitus	I	Withdrawn
Arthroscopic Autologous Chondrocyte Implantation Versus Microfractures	Autologous chondrocytes	Tear; knee, cartilage, articular	III	Completed
AuriNovo for Auricular Reconstruction	Autologous auricular cartilage cells (chondrocytes)	Microtia	I/II	Terminated
GLP-1 CellBeads for the Treatment of Stroke Patients With Space-Occupying Intracerebral Hemorrhage	Allogeneic mesenchymal cells producing GLP-1	Intracerebral hemorrhage	I/II	Terminated
A Study of Intraperitoneally Administered AVB-001 in Patients With Serous Adenocarcinoma of the Ovary	Cells produce native human interleukin-2	Neoplasm, ovarian; Fallopian tube cancer; Primary peritoneal cavity cancer; etc.	I/II	Recruiting
Pilot Immunotherapy Trial for Recurrent Malignant Gliomas	Autologous tumor cells treated with IGF-1R/AS ODN	Malignant glioma of the brain	I	Completed
Safety & Efficacy of Encapsulated Allogeneic FVIII Cell Therapy in Haemophilia A	Allogeneic cells producing BDD-hFVIII.	Hemophilia A	I/II	Terminated
Safety and Efficiency of Encapsulated Allogeneic MPS-1 Therapy	Allogeneic cells producing hIDUA	MSP I	I/II	Withdrawn

Note: This is by no means an exhaustive list and is subject to updates and additions. Data were collected from ClinicalTrials.gov (June 2023).
CNTF, *Ciliary neurotrophic factor*; NTC-201, *derived originally from the human retinal pigment epithelium cell line*.

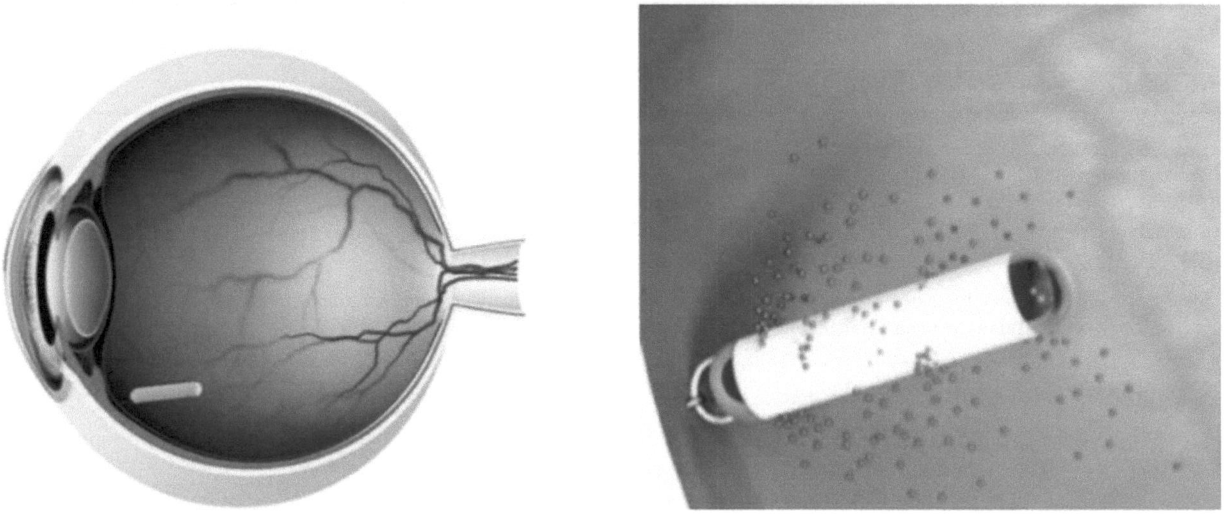

FIGURE 7.11 Neurotech Pharmaceuticals' ECT implant's working mechanism, providing constant delivery of therapeutic proteins to the back of the eye on a long-term basis with no immunogenic effect. From Delivery System. Available from: https://www.neurotechpharmaceuticals.com/delivery with permission from Neurotech Pharmaceuticals Inc.

Case Study IV: Cell encapsulation for type 1 diabetes treatment

Diabetes mellitus is a chronic metabolic disorder caused by either a relative or absolute failure of beta cells in the pancreatic islets of Langerhans, leading to insulin deficiency. Type 1 diabetes mellitus is characterized by severe insulin deficiency, usually caused by immune-mediated destruction of beta cells, while type 2 results from insulin resistance (relative insulin insufficiency) [36]. Transplantation of encapsulated islets and such (e.g., human embryonic stem cell—derived pancreatic progenitor cells) is a promising approach for type 1 diabetes treatment that avoids complications associated with daily insulin administrations and reduces the surgical risks involved with whole pancreas transplantation [37]. Moreover, the encapsulated cells produce insulin in response to food intake, which enables improved control of blood sugar levels [22,38]. Alginate is commonly used in islet encapsulation. Live alginate-encapsulated porcine islets retrieved from a patient 9.5 years after xenotransplantation have been reported [39].

Islets have been successfully macro- and microencapsulated using various platforms. Compared to macroencapsulation systems, microencapsulation offers improved diffusion, better survival of the encapsulated islets, and a less invasive implantation procedure. However, the separation of islets-loaded microcapsules from empty ones is challenging. In addition, it is difficult to control the location of every microencapsulated islet upon implantation and retrieve it completely after implantation [37]. The first successful clinical trial was in the 1990s with alginate-poly-L-lysine-alginate microencapsulated allogeneic islets transplanted into the peritoneum of a diabetic patient under immunosuppression treatment [37]. PLL may evoke fibrosis and inflammation and, as a result, other polycations have been applied to replace PLL, such as PLO. DOL's Diabecell capsules are composed of an inner core of alginate coated with PLO and are masked by an outer layer of alginate [40]. A clinical study confirmed the benefit of Diabecell transplantation without immunosuppression (Fig. CS 7.1) [41]. One of the major challenges for the clinical application of microencapsulated cells is the pericapsular fibrotic overgrowth upon implantation. Chemical modification of alginate may enable long-term islets for the correction of insulin deficiency [42]. Additionally, the incorporation of cellulose nanocrystals for improved mechanical strength and unique porous structure shows great promise for the long-term transplantation of islets [43].

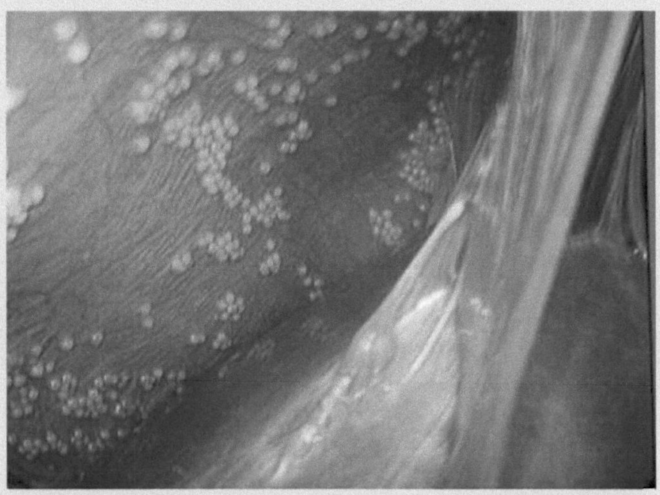

FIGURE CS 7.1 Laparoscopic observation of intraperitoneal space at the time of second transplantation. From Matsumoto, S. et al., *Clinical benefit of islet xenotransplantation for the treatment of type 1 diabetes.* eBioMedicine, 2016. **12**: p. 255-262, with permission from Elsevier.

The macroencapsulation system design is also challenging as several requirements have to be met, including an adequate number of cells, survival of cells at the site, immune evasion and fibrosis mitigation, and functionality of cells. Also, the peri-implant environment is temporally

Case Study IV: Cell encapsulation for type 1 diabetes treatment *(cont'd)*

dynamic since the processes of implant vascularization and fibrosis evolve from device implantation to early integration in parallel to the maturation of the transplanted cells (Fig. CS7.2) [44]. Two of the companies that have been developing cell macroencapsulation systems for type 1 diabetes treatment are ViaCyte (recently acquired by Vertex Pharmaceuticals Inc.) and Beta-O2 Technologies. ViaCyte (Vertex) uses PEC-01 cells (human embryonic stem cell–derived pancreatic progenitor cells) and two different types of encapsulation devices: PEC-Encap and PEC-Direct. PEC-Encap provides immunoisolation and PEC-Direct supports vascularization but not immune protection [38,45] (Fig. CS 7.3). Clinical studies showed that PEC-Direct encapsulated pluripotent stem cells may offer a scalable and renewable alternative to pancreatic islet transplants [46] and evidence of meal-regulated insulin secretion by differentiated stem cells in patients [47]. The Beta-O2 bioartificial pancreas device (βAir) consists of two islet compartments and an oxygen reservoir, which can be refilled through port connections that maintain physiological oxygen pressure without direct contact with the bloodstream (Fig. CS 7.4) [48,49].

Overall, the encapsulation of islets or other insulin-producing cells provides a promising route for type 1 diabetes treatment. To accelerate its clinical translations, more advances are needed to achieve a better islet immunoisolation while maintaining sufficient oxygen and nutrient supply. Additionally, more studies on safety and efficacy in preclinical trials with larger animal models are needed as rodent studies do not always translate to human response [36]. There are also macroencapsulation systems being developed: such as Cell Pouch and MailPan [35].

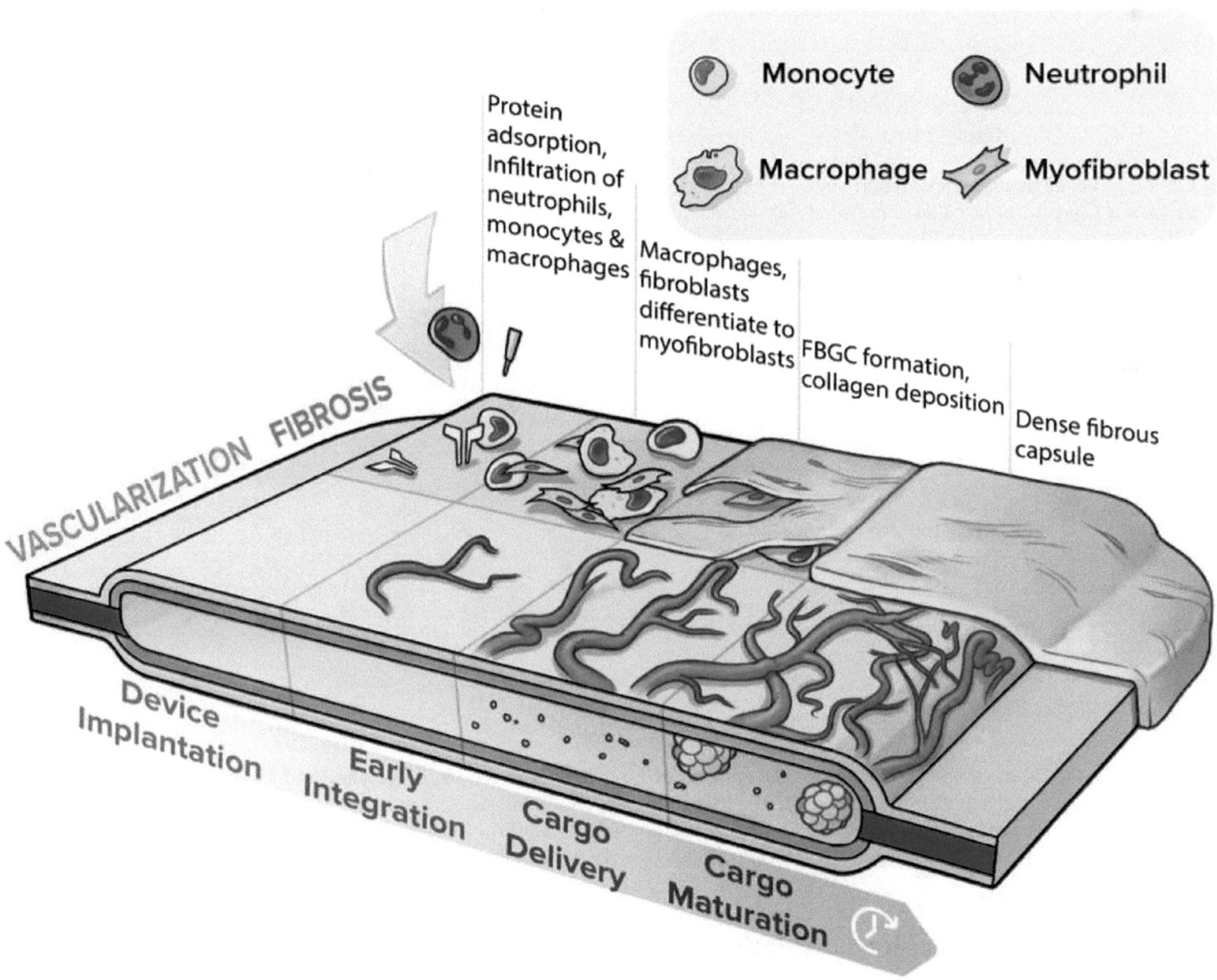

FIGURE CS 7.2 Schematic of the temporally dynamic peri-implant environment depicting how the processes of fibrosis and vascularization are both increasing with time. From Goswami, D. et al., *Design considerations for macroencapsulation devices for stem cell derived islets for the treatment of type 1 diabetes.* Advanced Science, 2021. **8**(16): p. 2100820.

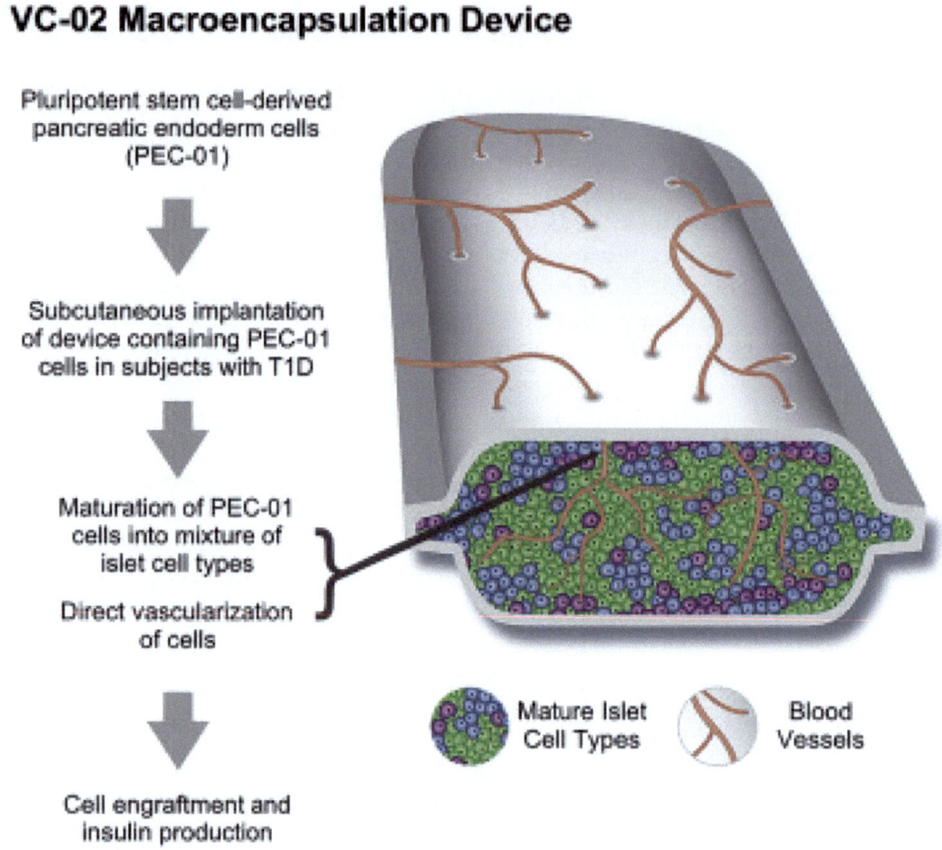

FIGURE CS 7.3 VC-02 macroencapsulation device (PEC-01 cells encapsulated in PEC-Direct) working mechanism. From Shapiro, A.M.J. et al., *Insulin expression and C-peptide in type 1 diabetes subjects implanted with stem cell-derived pancreatic endoderm cells in an encapsulation device. Cell Rep*, 2021. **2**(12): p. 100466 with permission from Elsevier.

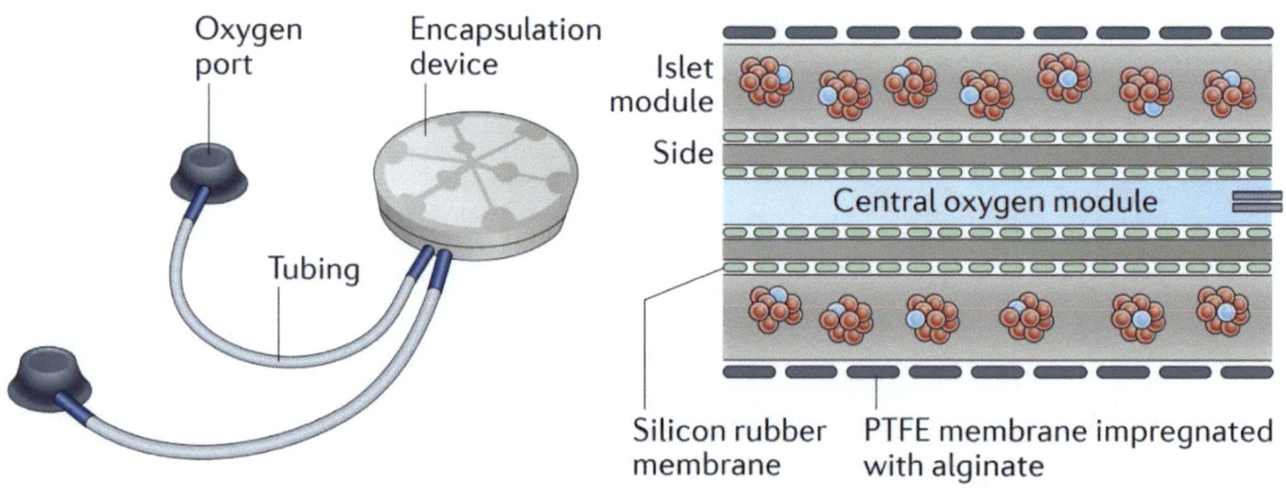

FIGURE CS 7.4 Image and schematic of the Beta-O2 device showing the ports for recharging oxygen and the encapsulation device. The central module can be filled with oxygen to diffuse outwards to the islet modules. The PTFE membrane is seeded with alginate to prevent cell infiltration but allows for nutrient and hormone transport. *PTFE*, Polytetrafluoroethylene. From Desai, T. and L.D. Shea, *Advances in islet encapsulation technologies.* Nature Reviews. Drug Discovery, 2017. **16**(5): p. 338-350, with permission from Springer Nature.

Lab Activity VI: Cell (micro)encapsulation in hydrogel

Cell encapsulation technology has shown great promise for immunoisolation and the controlled release of therapeutic products towards various biomedical applications, such as gene therapy and tissue engineering [4]. In this experiment, the (micro)encapsulation of mammalian cells into alginate-based hydrogel is investigated. The objectives of this experiment are to:

(1) Learn the process of cell microencapsulation.
(2) Perform the cell microencapsulation and assess the viability of encapsulated cells.

Background

Cell encapsulation can be classified based on the size of the system. During cell macroencapsulation, cells are immobilized in relatively large semipermeable chambers. Cell microencapsulation offers the advantage of a large surface area–to–volume ratio, which allows for efficient oxygen and nutrient transport [6].

Maintaining high cell viability is critical during cell encapsulation. Cell viability can be easily determined using the LIVE/DEAD Viability/Cytotoxicity Assay Kit. The LIVE/DEAD Viability/Cytotoxicity Assay provides a two-color fluorescence cell viability assay that is based on the simultaneous differentiation of live and dead cells. The cell membrane permeable calcein AM could be converted to calcein showing strong green fluorescence, which can be well retained within live cells with the intact plasma membrane. Ethidium homodimer enters cells with damaged plasma membranes (taken as dead cells) and binds to the nucleic acids, producing bright red fluorescence while it is excluded by the intact plasma membrane of live cells. Calcein produces an intense green fluorescence in live cells (excitation wavelength/emission wavelength ~495 nm/~515 nm). EthD-1 undergoes a 40-fold enhancement of fluorescence upon binding to nucleic acids, producing a bright red fluorescence in dead (membrane-compromised) cells (excitation wavelength/emission wavelength ~528 nm/~617 nm) [10,15,20,21,50,51].

Materials and Instruments

Mammalian cells and cell culture reagents
Alginate solution
$CaCl_2$ solution
Mannitol
HEPES buffer solution (1 mol/L)
Syringe (or other devices for generating microdroplets)
Fluorescent microscope
LIVE/DEAD Viability/Cytotoxicity Assay Kit
Glass slide/cover glass

Laboratory Procedure

I. *Preparation of Cell Encapsulation.*

1. Prepare the alginate solution: dissolve alginate in a 0.25 mol/L mannitol solution to prepare a 2.25% (w/v) alginate solution and add 1 mol/L HEPES buffer solution (pH ~ 7.2; final HEPES concentration: 10 mmol/L).
2. Preparation of the $CaCl_2$ solution: dissolve $CaCl_2$ in a 0.25 mol/L mannitol solution to prepare a 150 mmol/L $CaCl_2$ solution and add 1 mol/L HEPES buffer solution (pH ~ 7.2; final HEPES concentration: 10 mmol/L).
   Q1: *Why are HEPES and mannitol used?*
3. Filter both solutions (prevent light exposure).

II. *Cell Encapsulation.*

1. Collect the mammalian cells (detach the adherent cells) and centrifuge the cells (1000 rpm for 3 min) and remove the supernatant (be very careful not to aspirate off the cell pellet).
2. Calculate the volume of Dulbecco phosphate-buffered saline (DPBS, **no** calcium) needed to suspend the cells (e.g., to reach an alginate concentration of 2% (w/v) and cell density of 1×10^6 cells/mL).
3. Resuspend the cells in DPBS: Do NOT use alginate to suspend the cells. Gently swirl the tube after adding DPBS to suspend the cells (gently pipette the cells).
4. Add alginate and gently invert the tube to mix and avoid pipetting.
5. Feed the alginate/cell mixture into a sterile syringe through its tip using a mechanical pipette (do NOT directly draw the mixture into the syringe).
6. Put the syringe needle on.
7. Introduce the cell/alginate suspension into the 150 mmol/L $CaCl_2$ solution dropwise (or use other setups for generating microdroplets).
8. Collect the encapsulated cells (hydrogel beads) by gently and quickly removing the $CaCl_2$ solution and rinsing the hydrogel beads with the complete cell culture medium.
9. Add the complete medium and transfer the encapsulated cells into a culture vessel (optional).

III. *Determination of Encapsulated Cell Viability.*

1. Transfer a small amount of encapsulated cells into a small tube.
2. Add calcein AM and EthD-1 (final concentration of 5 μmol/L of both solutions).
3. Incubate for 5 min.
4. Drop a few hydrogel beads (encapsulated) onto a glass slide.
5. Add cover glass and gently press to deform the beads (for easier visualization).
6. Observe the slide under an inverted fluorescent microscope and take images.

Review and practice questions

1. What is cell encapsulation?
2. What is the major disadvantage of cell macroencapsulation compared with cell microencapsulation?
3. Estimate the surface area/volume ratio of the C_{60} fullerene by simplifying the molecule as a hollow sphere. The atomic radius of carbon is around 77 pm and the diameter of the C_{60} fullerene is about 700 pm.
4. Explain the electrospray mechanism for microsphere/capsule production.
5. Explain the mechanism of microsphere/capsule production using a microfluidic device.
6. Provide an example of cell encapsulation in therapy.

References

[1] Mazzitelli S, Nastruzzi C. Cell encapsulation and delivery. In: Narayan R, editor. Encyclopedia of biomedical engineering. Elsevier; 2019. p. 308–15.
[2] Paez-Mayorga J, et al. Emerging strategies for beta cell transplantation to treat diabetes. Trends Pharmacol Sci 2022;43(3):221–33.
[3] Liu W, et al. Macroencapsulation devices for cell therapy. Engineering 2022;13:53–70.
[4] Zhang W. Encapsulation of transgenic cells for gene therapy. In: Hashad D, editor. Gene therapy. IntechOpen; 2015. p. 191–208.
[5] Majewski RL, et al. Bioencapsulation technologies in tissue engineering. J Appl Biomater Funct Mater 2016;14(4):e395–403.
[6] Lopez-Mendez TB, et al. Cell microencapsulation technologies for sustained drug delivery: latest advances in efficacy and biosafety. J Control Release 2021;335:619–36.
[7] Zhang W, He X. Microencapsulating and banking living cells for cell-based medicine. J Healthc Eng 2011;2(4):875406.
[8] Chick WL, Like AA, Lauris V. Beta cell culture on synthetic capillaries: an artificial endocrine pancreas. Science 1975;187(4179):847–9.
[9] Lim F, Sun AM. Microencapsulated islets as bioartificial endocrine pancreas. Science 1980;210(4472):908–10.
[10] Zhang W, He X. Encapsulation of living cells in small (~100 μm) alginate microcapsules by electrostatic spraying: a parametric study. J Biomech Eng 2009;131(7):074515.
[11] Sarveswaran K, et al. Synthetic capillaries to control microscopic blood flow. Sci Rep 2016;6:21885.
[12] Williams DF. There is no such thing as a biocompatible material. Biomaterials 2014;35(38):10009–14.
[13] Syanda AM, et al. Sulfated alginate reduces pericapsular fibrotic overgrowth on encapsulated cGMP-compliant hPSC-hepatocytes in mice. Front Bioeng Biotechnol 2022;9:816542.
[14] Gasperini L, Mano JF, Reis RL. Natural polymers for the microencapsulation of cells. J R Soc Interface 2014;11(100):20140817.
[15] Zhao S, et al. Coaxial electrospray of liquid core–hydrogel shell microcapsules for encapsulation and miniaturized 3D culture of pluripotent stem cells. Integr Biol 2014;6(9):874–84.
[16] Agarwal P, et al. One-step microfluidic generation of pre-hatching embryo-like core-shell microcapsules for miniaturized 3D culture of pluripotent stem cells. Lab Chip 2013;13(23):4525–33.
[17] Hu C, et al. Ions-induced gelation of alginate: mechanisms and applications. Int J Biol Macromol 2021;177:578–88.
[18] Arifin DR, et al. Microcapsules with intrinsic barium radiopacity for immunoprotection and X-ray/CT imaging of pancreatic islet cells. Biomaterials 2012;33(18):4681–9.
[19] Paredes Juárez GA, et al. Immunological and technical considerations in application of alginate-based microencapsulation systems. Front Bioeng Biotechnol 2014;2:26.
[20] Zhang W, Zhao S, He X. Proliferation and differentiation of mesenchymal stem cells encapsulated in miniaturized 3D core of alginate-chitosan alginate (ACA) microcapsules. Arch Stem Cell Res 2015;2(1):1004.
[21] Zhang W, et al. A novel core-shell microcapsule for encapsulation and 3D culture of embryonic stem cells. J Mater Chem B 2013;1(7):1002–9.
[22] Skinner SJ, et al. Encapsulated living choroid plexus cells: potential long-term treatments for central nervous system disease and trauma. J Neural Eng 2009;6(6):065001.
[23] Ren Y, et al. Comparative investigation of the binding characteristics of poly-l-lysine and chitosan on alginate hydrogel. Int J Biol Macromol 2016;84:135–41.
[24] Kamperman T, et al. Single-cell microgels: technology, challenges, and applications. Trends Biotechnol 2018;36(8):850–65.
[25] Marikar SN, et al. Microencapsulation-based cell therapies. Cell Mol Life Sci 2022;79(7):351.
[26] Ling SD, et al. Enhanced single-cell encapsulation in microfluidic devices: from droplet generation to single-cell analysis. Biomicrofluidics 2020;14(6):061508.
[27] Lopez-Mendez TB, et al. Cell microencapsulation technologies for sustained drug delivery: clinical trials and companies. Drug Discov Today 2021;26(3):852–61.

[28] Neurotech Pharmaceuticals, Inc. Delivery system. Available from: https://www.neurotechpharmaceuticals.com/delivery.
[29] Living Cell Technologies. NTCELL. Available from: https://lctglobal.com/research/ntcell.
[30] Snow B, et al. A phase IIb, randomised, double-blind, placebo-controlled, dose-ranging investigation of the safety and efficacy of NTCELL® [immunoprotected (alginate-encapsulated) porcine choroid plexus cells for xenotransplantation] in patients with Parkinson's disease. Parkinsonism Relat Disord 2019;61:88–93.
[31] PharmaCyte Biotech, Inc. Profile. Available from: https://ir.pharmacyte.com/profile.
[32] Zavala G, et al. Semipermeable cellulose beads allow selective and continuous release of small extracellular vesicles (sEV) from encapsulated cells. Front Pharmacol 2020;11:679.
[33] Sigilon Therapeutics. Science. Available from: https://sigilon.com/science/.
[34] Bashor CJ, et al. Engineering the next generation of cell-based therapeutics. Nat Rev Drug Discov 2022;21(9):655–75.
[35] Farina M, et al. Cell encapsulation: overcoming barriers in cell transplantation in diabetes and beyond. Adv Drug Deliv Rev 2019;139:92–115.
[36] Opara A, et al. Islet cell encapsulation - application in diabetes treatment. Exp Biol Med 2021;246(24):2570–8.
[37] Espona-Noguera A, et al. Review of advanced hydrogel-based cell encapsulation systems for insulin delivery in type 1 diabetes mellitus. Pharmaceutics 2019;11(11):597.
[38] Dolgin E. Diabetes cell therapies take evasive action. Nat Biotechnol 2022;40(3):291–5.
[39] Elliott RB, et al. Live encapsulated porcine islets from a type 1 diabetic patient 9.5 yr after xenotransplantation. Xenotransplantation 2007; 14(2):157–61.
[40] Hillberg AL, et al. Improving alginate-poly-L-ornithine-alginate capsule biocompatibility through genipin crosslinking. J Biomed Mater Res B Appl Biomater 2013;101(2):258–68.
[41] Matsumoto S, et al. Clinical benefit of islet xenotransplantation for the treatment of type 1 diabetes. eBioMedicine 2016;12:255–62.
[42] Bochenek MA, et al. Alginate encapsulation as long-term immune protection of allogeneic pancreatic islet cells transplanted into the omental bursa of macaques. Nat Biomed Eng 2018;2(11):810–21.
[43] Luo Z, et al. A novel insulin delivery system by β cells encapsulated in microcapsules. Front Chem 2023;10:1104979.
[44] Goswami D, et al. Design considerations for macroencapsulation devices for stem cell derived islets for the treatment of type 1 diabetes. Adv Sci 2021;8(16):2100820.
[45] de Klerk E, Hebrok M. Stem cell-based clinical trials for diabetes mellitus. Front Endocrinol 2021;12:631463.
[46] Shapiro AMJ, et al. Insulin expression and C-peptide in type 1 diabetes subjects implanted with stem cell-derived pancreatic endoderm cells in an encapsulation device. Cell Rep Med 2021;2(12):100466.
[47] Ramzy A, et al. Implanted pluripotent stem-cell-derived pancreatic endoderm cells secrete glucose-responsive C-peptide in patients with type 1 diabetes. Cell Stem Cell 2021;28(12):2047–2061.e5.
[48] Ludwig B, et al. Favorable outcome of experimental islet xenotransplantation without immunosuppression in a nonhuman primate model of diabetes. Proc Natl Acad Sci 2017;114(44):11745–50.
[49] Desai T, Shea LD. Advances in islet encapsulation technologies. Nat Rev Drug Discov 2017;16(5):338–50.
[50] Agarwal P, et al. One-step microfluidic generation of pre-hatching embryo-like core–shell microcapsules for miniaturized 3D culture of pluripotent stem cells. Lab Chip 2013;13(23):4525–33.
[51] Thermo Fisher Scientific Inc. LIVE/DEAD Viability/Cytotoxicity Kit *for mammalian cells*. Available from: https://assets.thermofisher.com/TFS-Assets/LSG/manuals/mp03224.pdf.

CHAPTER

8

Diffusion-controlled drug delivery systems

Wujie Zhang

LEARNING OBJECTIVES

- To understand the concept of diffusion and Fick's laws
- To differentiate between the reservoir and matrix systems
- To determine the diffusion coefficient using the Stokes-Einstein equation
- To understand and apply the equations for determining the release profiles of different diffusion-controlled drug delivery systems
- To interpret the lag and burst release effects
- To fit drug release data using different mathematical models
- To discuss the design considerations of diffusion-controlled drug delivery systems
- To design diffusion-controlled drug delivery systems

8.1 Diffusion theory

Two physical phenomena are involved in the transport of molecules: diffusion and convection. Diffusion is the random motion of molecules that arises from the thermal energy transferred by molecular collisions. Convection is a mechanism of transport resulting from the bulk motion of fluids [1]. The focus of this chapter is diffusion because we are examining the drug delivery systems that "release" the drug molecules through diffusion.

To discuss diffusion, we have to start with Fick's laws. Fick's first law relates the diffusion flux (i.e., rate of diffusion through a unit area) to the concentration gradient (steady state):

$$J = -D\frac{dC}{dx},$$

where J is the diffusion flux and D is the diffusion coefficient (diffusivity) (Fig. 8.1). The negative sign arises from the solute molecules moving from a higher concentration region to a lower concentration region. One way to determine the diffusivity (solutes in dilute solutions) is to use the Stokes-Einstein equation:

$$D = \frac{RT}{6\pi\mu\alpha N_A}.$$

https://doi.org/10.1016/B978-0-443-23521-4.00008-4

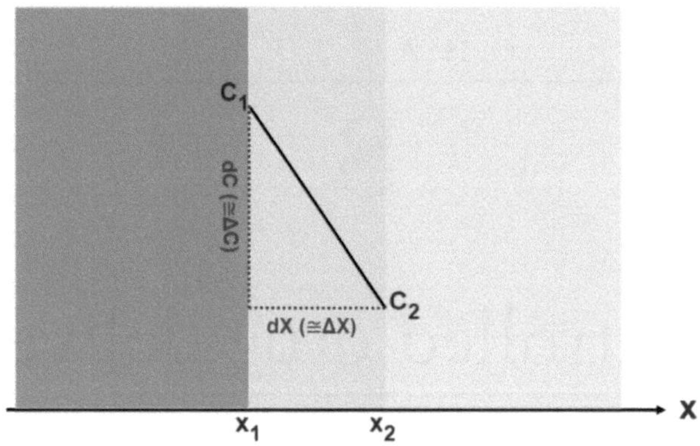

FIGURE 8.1 Steady-state diffusion: The flux is proportional to the concentration gradient, and the rate of diffusion is independent of time.

where R is the ideal gas constant (8.314 J/(mol × K)), T is the temperature in K, μ is the solution viscosity, α is the solute radius, and N_A is the Avogadro constant (6.022 × 10^{23} mol^{-1}). If the solute's molar mass is known, for a spherical molecule with a density of ≈ 1 g/cm^3, the radius can be calculated using

$$\alpha = \left(\frac{3M}{4\pi\rho N_A}\right)^{\frac{1}{3}},$$

where M is the molar mass of the solute molecule, and ρ is the density of the solute molecule [2]. Keep in mind that the Stokes-Einstein equation only applies to the spherical particles in a liquid with a low Reynolds (Re) number [3].

Sample question 8.1

Determine the diffusion coefficient of a spherical therapeutic molecule with a molar mass of 5 × 10^4 g/mol in plasma at 37°C.

Answer: The normal plasma has a viscosity of 1.16 to 1.33 mPa/s at 37°C [4]. Here we use the average value 1.25 mPa/s [= 0.0125 g/(cm × s)]. First, calculate the molecule's radius:

$$\alpha = \left(\frac{3M}{4\pi\rho N_A}\right)^{\frac{1}{3}} = \left(\frac{3 \times 5 \times 10^4 \frac{g}{mol}}{4\pi \times \frac{1g}{cm^3} \times 6.023 \times 10^{23}\frac{1}{mol}}\right)^{\frac{1}{3}} = 2.71 \times 10^{-7}\ cm.$$

then calculate the diffusion coefficient using the Stokes-Einstein equation:

$$D = \frac{RT}{6\pi\mu\alpha N_A} = \frac{8.314\frac{J}{mol \times K} \times \frac{kg \times m^2 \times s^{-2}}{J} \times \frac{1000g}{1kg} \times \frac{10000cm^2}{1m^2} \times (37 + 273)K}{6\pi \times 0.0125\frac{g}{cm \times s} \times 2.71 \times 10^{-7}cm \times 6.023 \times 10^{23}\frac{1}{mol}} = 6.7 \times 10^{-7}\frac{cm^2}{s}$$

Considering the mass balance of a small space element, Fick's second law describes how diffusion causes the concentration to change with time (unsteady state): $\frac{\partial C}{\partial t} = D\frac{\partial^2 c}{\partial x^2}$. In three dimensions, the equation is: $\frac{\partial C}{\partial t} = D\left(\frac{\partial^2 c}{\partial x^2} + \frac{\partial^2 c}{\partial y^2} + \frac{\partial^2 c}{\partial z^2}\right)$.

At steady state:

$$\frac{\partial C}{\partial t} = 0,$$

which gives us

$D\frac{\partial^2 c}{\partial x^2} = 0$. Solving the equation, we get

$\frac{dC}{dx} = constant$ *(back to the first law)*.

Hence, Fick's first law can be considered a specific case of the second law (steady state).

Fick's second law equation can be solved with initial and boundary conditions. The initial conditions concern the initial distribution of the diffusion species in the system, while the boundary conditions deal with the conditions for diffusion at the boundaries of the drug delivery system [5,6] In this chapter, we only discuss the scenarios in which diffusion is the only release-rate limiting factor, with the assumptions that the carrier is not changing with time (not swelling or dissolution/erosion), the diffusion coefficient is constant, and the sink conditions are perfect (the drug concentration in the surrounding bulk fluid is negligible as the drug molecules are quickly removed upon release). Drug diffusion is much slower than release through a medium penetrating into the system and drug dissolution.

8.2 Reservoir systems

Reservoir systems are drugs that are retained within a thin release rate-controlling membrane. These systems can be divided into two groups: nonconstant activity source and constant activity source. For the nonconstant activity source, the drug concentration is below its solubility. Assuming the drug dissolution is much faster compared to its diffusion, the drug release kinetics are first-order:

$$dA = -kAdt,$$

then integrate,

$$\int_0^{\infty} \frac{1}{A} dA = \int_0^{\infty} -kdt$$

$$ln\, A_{\infty} - ln\, A_0 = -k\infty$$

$$\frac{A_{\infty}}{A_0} = e^{-k\infty} = 0$$

$$\int_0^{t} \frac{1}{A} dA = \int_0^{t} -kdt$$

$$ln\, A_t - ln\, A_0 = -kt$$

$$\frac{A_t}{A_0} = e^{-kt}$$

where A_0 is the initial amount of the drug, and A_t is the amount of drug left at time t. To be consistent with the literature, we are switching from A to M for the amount. M_t is used to indicate the amount of the drug released at time t. A_0, the initial drug amount, equals M_{∞} (i.e., given enough time, all the drug molecules are released). Please keep in mind that A_t is not the same as M_t (M_t = -$A_0 - A_t$). Hence, the above equation becomes:

$$\frac{A_t}{A_0} = \frac{A_0 - M_t}{A_0} = \frac{M_{\infty} - M_t}{M_{\infty}} = e^{-kt}$$

$$\frac{M_t}{M_{\infty}} = 1 - e^{-kt}.$$

Here, k is determined by the carrier geometry (e.g., surface area) and drug properties (e.g., diffusion coefficient). Different nonconstant activity source reservoir systems and corresponding mathematical equations for quantifying drug release are shown in Fig. 8.2.

When it comes to the constant-source activity reservoir systems, there is an excess amount of drug (i.e., undissolved plus dissolved drug molecules). The process is simple, for a specific period of time, a specific amount of drug is dissolved and released. This is a typical zero-order process. Recall the general equation for describing the zero-order kinetics:

$$dA = -kdt.$$

Upon integration, we can obtain

$$\int_0^t dA = \int_0^t -kdt$$

$$A_t - A_0 = -kt.$$

$$A_o - A_t = kt$$

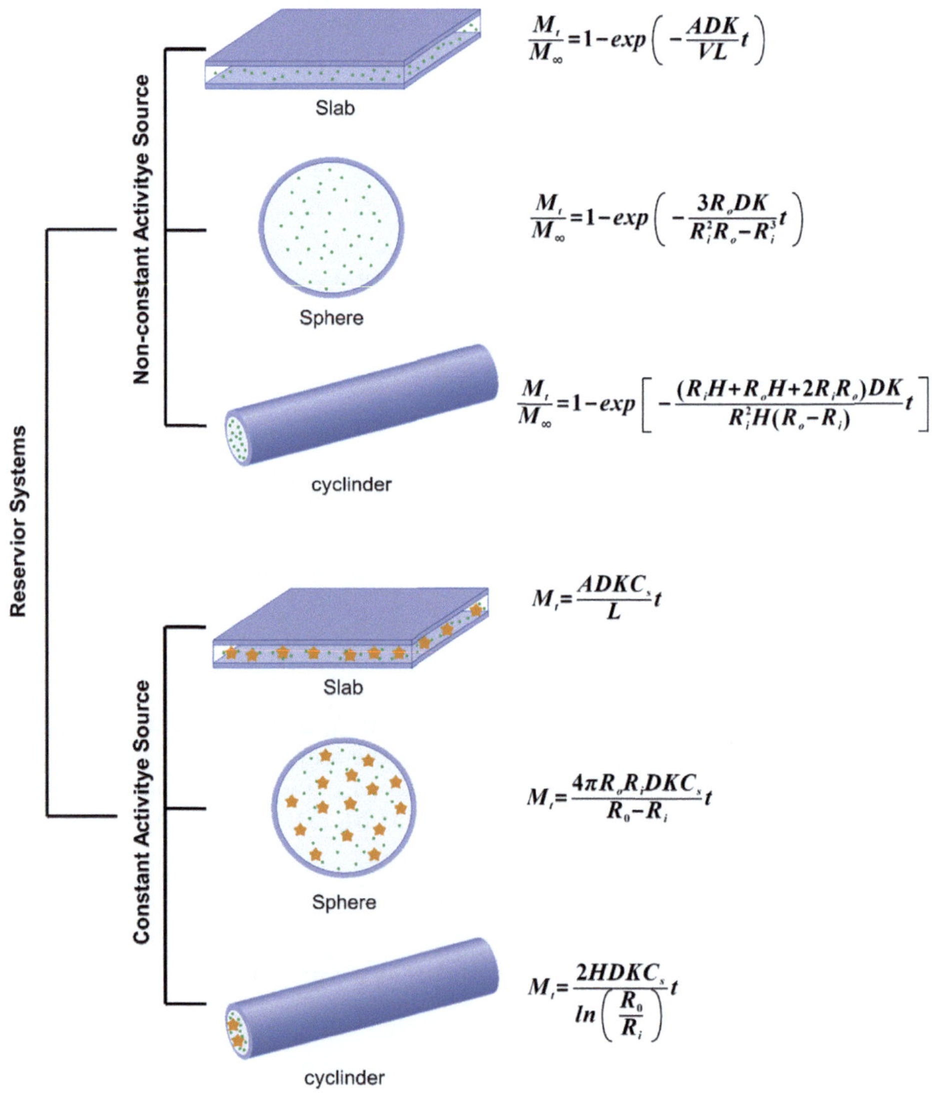

FIGURE 8.2 Different reservoir systems and the corresponding equations for determining the drug release profiles. *A*, Total surface area; *D*, diffusion coefficient; *K*, partition coefficient of the drug between the membrane and reservoir; *L*, thickness of the membrane; *V*, volume of the reservoir; R_o, outer radius; R_i, inner radius; *H*, length of the cylinder; and C_s, solubility of the drug in the core. *Green dots* represent drug molecules, and *orange stars* indicate undissolved drug molecules. Figure information is from Siepmann, J. and F. Siepmann, *Modeling of diffusion controlled drug delivery.* JCR, 2012. **161**(2): p. 351-362.

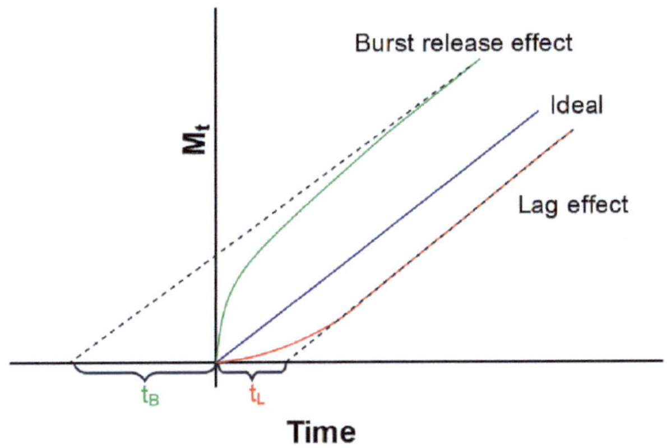

FIGURE 8.3 Graph of the released amount at time t (M_t) over time. The released amount changes with time under different scenarios.

Switching the notation for the amount from A to M, we can obtain $M_t = kt$ ($M_t = A_0 - A_t$; amount released = initial amount − amount remaining). Different constant activity source reservoir systems and corresponding mathematical equations for quantifying drug release are shown in Fig. 8.2. Once the undissolved drug is exhausted, the constant activity source system becomes a nonconstant activity source.

For ideal constant activity source reservoir systems, the accumulated amount of drug released (M_t) is linearly proportional to time (t) (Fig. 8.3). However, if the drug-loaded systems are freshly prepared, drug molecules have to diffuse into the membrane first, which delays the drug release (i.e., lag) (Fig. 8.3). On the contrary, if the systems are stored for a while and drug molecules have saturated the membrane, it will lead to burst release (Fig. 8.3). Burst release is defined as the initial large bolus of a drug being released before the release rate reaches a stable profile. Some of the negative consequences of the burst release effects are local or systemic toxicity, shortened release profile, and requiring more frequent dosing [7]. The extrapolation of the steady-state straight lines can be used to determine either t_B (burst time) or t_L (lag time). For slabs, t_B and t_L are $L^2/3D$ and $L^2/6D$, respectively [5,8].

8.3 Matrix systems

Similar to reservoir systems, matrix systems are divided into monolithic solutions (drug concentration is lower than its solubility) and monolithic dispersions (containing both dissolved and undissolved drug molecules). The term monolithic is used because drug molecules are distributed throughout the matrix rather homogeneously (no local separation between a drug reservoir and a release rate controlling barrier). The drug released is controlled by the diffusion through the matrix. The system's geometry significantly affects the resulting drug release kinetics in matrix systems [6]. Different matrix systems and their corresponding mathematical equations for quantifying drug release are shown in Fig. 8.4. For monolithic solutions, there are early and late time approximations for the equations to avoid the infinite series of exponential functions [5,6].

The equation for the slab geometry of the monolithic solutions is the famous Higuchi equation, which describes a "square root of time" kinetics. Takeru Higuchi published the Higuchi equation in 1961 [9], and the equation has been extended to other geometries. The derivation of the Higuchi equation is shown in Appendix B. Lee [10,11] proposed the following equations for the dispersed drug from a spherical matrix:

$$\frac{M_t}{M_\infty} = \left[1-(1-\delta)^3\right]\left(1-\frac{C_s}{C_0}\right) + 3\delta\frac{C_s}{C_0}\left[\left(\alpha_1+\frac{\alpha_2}{2}+\frac{\alpha_3}{3}\right)-\left(\frac{\alpha_1}{2}+\frac{\alpha_2}{3}+\frac{\alpha_3}{4}\right)\delta\right]$$

$$\frac{Dt}{R^2} = \frac{1}{12}\left[6\frac{C_0}{C_s}-4-\alpha_3\right]-\frac{1}{3}\left(\frac{C_0}{C_s}-1\right)\delta^3$$

FIGURE 8.4 Different matrix systems and the corresponding equations for determining the drug release profiles. *A*, Total surface area exposed to the release medium; *D*, diffusion coefficient; *L*, thickness of the membrane; *R*, radius; *H*, length of the cylinder; C_0, initial drug concentration; C_s, solubility of the drug; *n* and *p*, dummy variables; and q_n, the roots of the Bessel function of the first kind of zero order [$J_0(q_n) = 0$]. *Green dots* represent drug molecules, and *orange stars* indicate undissolved drug molecules. Figure information is from Siepmann, J. and F. Siepmann, *Modeling of diffusion controlled drug delivery.* JCR, 2012. **161**(2): p. 351-362 and Siepmann, J. and F. Siepmann, *Mathematical modeling of drug delivery.* Int. J. Pharm, 2008. **364**(2): p. 328-343.

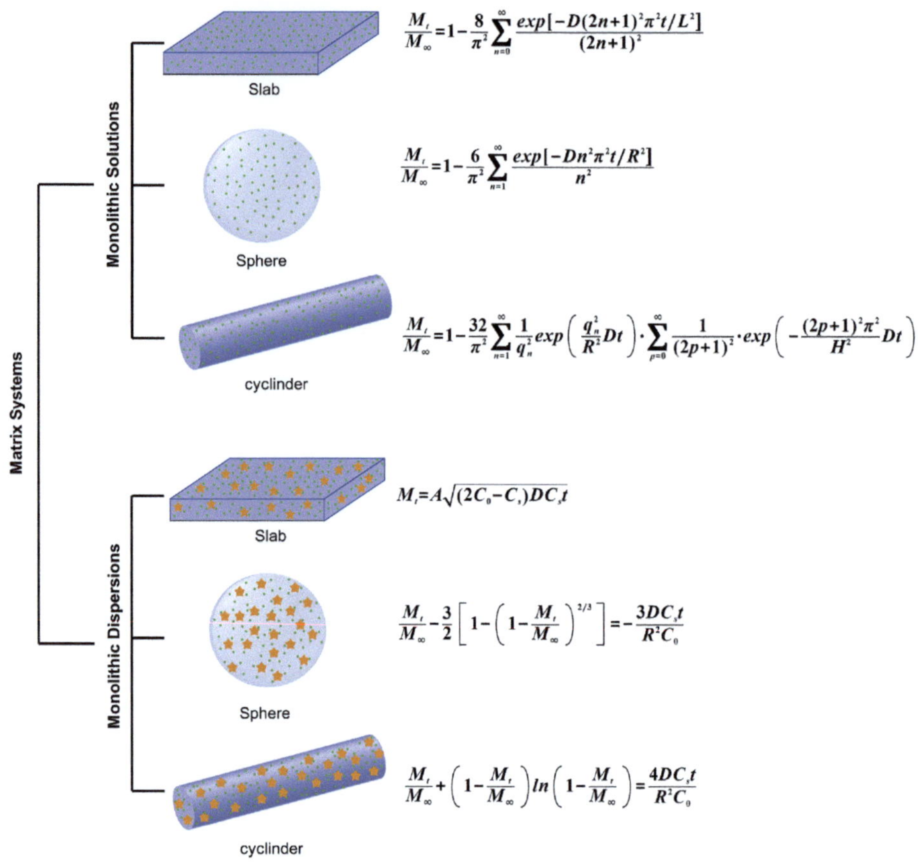

$$\alpha_1 = 1$$

$$\alpha_2 = -\alpha_3 - 1$$

$$\alpha_3 = 1 - \left(1 - \frac{C_0}{C_s}\right)(1-\delta) - \left(\left[1 - \left(1 - \frac{C_0}{C_s}\right)(1-\delta)\right]^2 - 1\right)^{1/2},$$

where δ is the position of the moving diffusion front and R is the radius.

Sample question 8.2

Consider a monolithic dispersion system (slab geometry with a surface area of 3 cm^2 on one side). The loading drug concentration is 0.2 g/cm^3. The drug's solubility and diffusion coefficients are 2.5×10^{-4} g/cm^3 and 1×10^{-7} cm^2/s, respectively. How long will the system take to release 2 mg of the drug if the drug is being released from both sides?

Answer: Use the Higuchi equation:

$$M_t = A\sqrt{D(2C_0 - C_s)C_s t}.$$

Because $C_0 >> C_s$,

$$M_t = A\sqrt{D2C_0C_s t}$$

$$M_t{}^2 = 2A^2DC_0C_s t$$

$$t = \frac{M_t^2}{2A^2DC_0C_s}.$$

Because the drug is released from both sides $A = 2 \times 3\ cm^2 = 6\ cm^2$,

$$t = \frac{(2\ mg)^2 \times \left(\frac{g}{1000\ mg}\right)^2}{2 \times (6\ cm^2)^2 1 \times 10^{-7} \frac{cm^2}{s} \times 0.2 \frac{g}{cm^3} \times 2.5 \times 10^{-4} \frac{g}{cm^3}} = \frac{\left(\frac{2}{1000}\right)^2}{2 \times 6^2 \times 1 \times 10^{-7} \times 0.2 \times 2.5 \times 10^{-4}} s = 1.1 \times 10^4 s$$

Another commonly used model is the Peppas equation (Korsmeyer-Peppas or power law):

$$\frac{M_t}{M_\infty} = kt^n,$$

where k is a constant relating the system's structural and geometric characteristics, and n is the release exponent (also called diffusional or transport exponent) and is dedicated to the mechanism of drug release [10,13]. Transport from swellable systems does not always follow Fickian or Higuchi behavior. Both the zero-order and Higuchi models can be considered as special cases of the Peppas model [14]. The release mechanisms based on n and carrier geometries are summarized in Table 8.1. "Anomalous" transport is an overlapping of different types of phenomena, potentially including drug diffusion and polymer swelling.

The Korsmeyer-Peppas equation is best used to describe the drug release mechanism from a polymeric matrix, but it only applies when $M_0/M_\infty \leq 0.6$ [14]. The Peppas-Sahlin equation is used to describe the relative contributions of Fickian diffusion and macromolecular relaxation [14,15]:

$$\frac{M_t}{M_\infty} = k_1 t^m + k_2 t^{2m},$$

where k_1 and k_2 are the Fickian diffusion kinetic constant and macromolecular relaxation kinetic constant, respectively, and m is the diffusional exponent indicating the release mechanism.

Sample question 8.3

A drug release profile is shown below (data from Zuo, J. et al., *Evaluation of the DDSolver software applications.* Biomed Res. Int, 2014. p. 204925):

Time, min	M_t/M_∞
30	0.3457
60	0.3730
90	0.4456
120	0.5410

(a) Prepare a plot of M_t/M_∞ vs. time.
(b) Determine the mechanism of drug release using the Peppas model.

TABLE 8.1 Release exponent n and drug release mechanism from polymeric controlled drug delivery systems of different geometry.

Exponent, n			
Thin film	**Cylinder**	**Sphere**	**Drug release mechanism**
0.5	0.45	0.43	Fickian diffusion (Case I)
$0.5 < n < 1.0$	$0.45 < n < 0.89$	$0.43 < n < 0.85$	Anomalous transport
1.0	0.89	0.85	Polymer swelling (Case II)

From Siepmann, J. and F. Siepmann, Mathematical modeling of drug delivery. *Int. J. Pharm, 2008.* ***364****(2): p. 328-343, and Morgulchik, N. and N. Kamaly,* Meta-analysis of in vitro drug-release parameters reveals predictable and robust kinetics for redox-responsive drug-conjugated therapeutic nanogels. *ACS Appl. Nano Mater, 2021.* ***4****(5): p. 4256-4268.*

Answer:

(a)

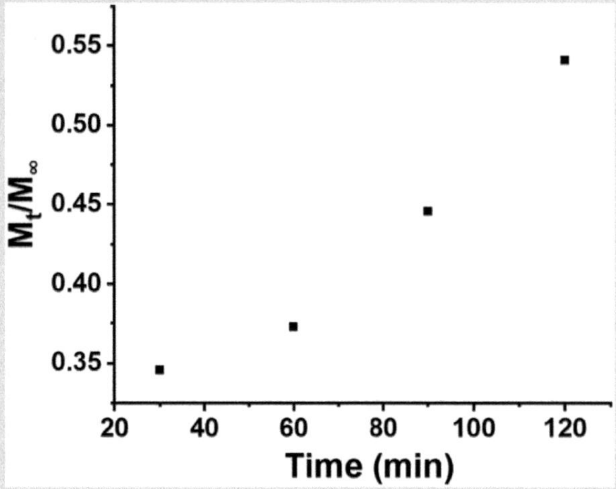

FIGURE 8.5 Plot of M_t/M_∞ vs. time (t).

(b) Change the form of the Peppas model:

$$\frac{M_t}{M_\infty} = kt^n$$

Apply ln on both sides of the equation:

$$ln\left(\frac{M_t}{M_\infty}\right) = ln(kt^n)$$

$$ln\left(\frac{M_t}{M_\infty}\right) = lnk + ln\, t^n = lnk + nlnt$$

Plotting $\ln(M_t/M_\infty)$ vs. lnt should yield a straight line with a slope equal to n.

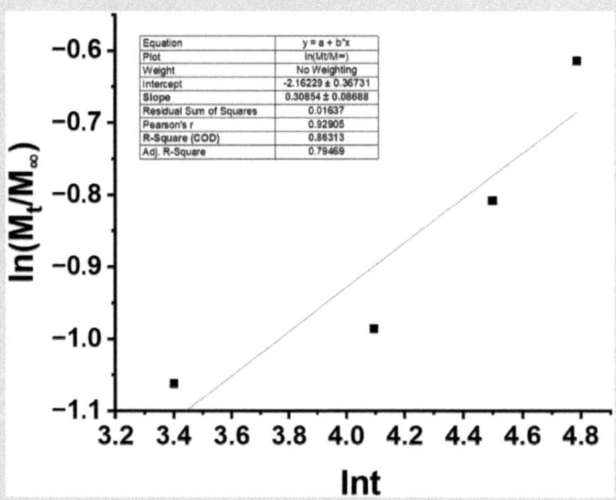

FIGURE 8.6 Plot of $\ln(M_t/M_\infty)$ vs. lnt.

The slope is $0.309 < 0.5$. Hence, the drug release mechanism is Fickian diffusion. Keep in mind that the Peppas model is not universal, and it does not necessarily provide the best fit for this scenario.

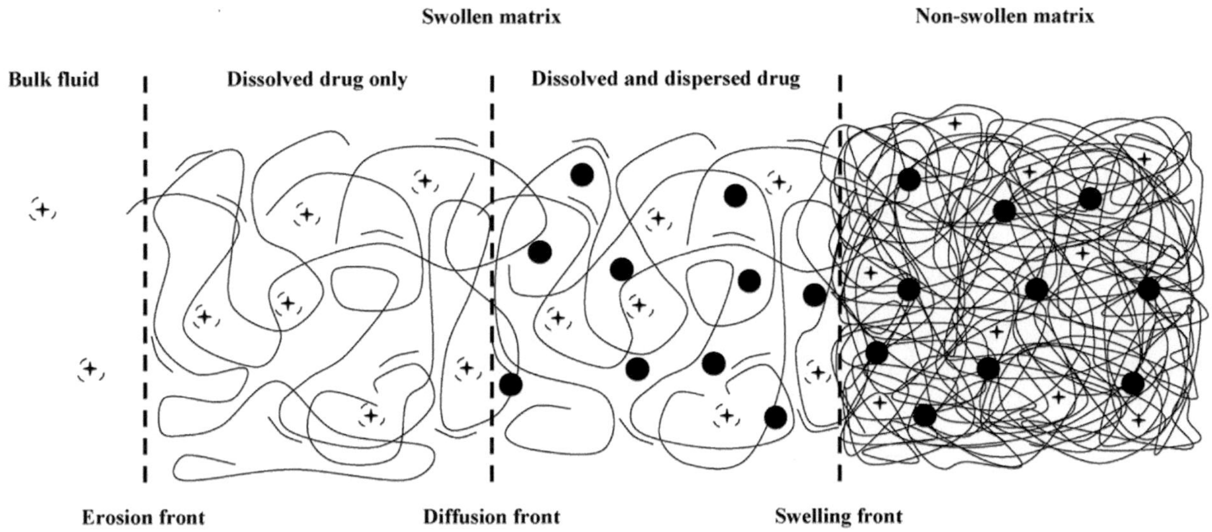

FIGURE 8.7 Schematic of a swelling-controlled drug delivery system containing dissolved *(stars)* and dispersed *(black circles)* drugs exhibiting several moving boundaries: an "erosion front" separating the bulk fluid from the delivery system; a "diffusion front," separating the swollen matrix-containing dissolved drug, and the swollen matrix-containing dissolved and dispersed drug; and a "swelling front," separating the swollen and nonswollen matrix. From Siepmann, J. and F. Siepmann, *Mathematical modeling of drug delivery. Int. J. Pharm*, 2008. **364**(2): p. 328-343, with permission from Elsevier.

Polymer (as a drug carrier) swelling can play a significant role in drug release control: increasing the diffusion pathway (decreasing drug release rates) and increasing the drug molecule's mobility (increasing drug release rates) [6]. Fig. 8.7 shows the mechanisms of controlled drug release from a swellable delivery system. Upon administration, water enters the carrier, and the mobility of the polymer chains increases. Once a certain polymer-specific water concentration is reached, the polymer mobility increases steeply (i.e., polymer chain relaxation or glassy-to-rubbery-phase-transition). For thin slab geometries (eligible edge effects and homogenous distribution of the drug molecules within the matrix), if swelling is the release rate-limiting factor, zero-order kinetics is obtained ($n = 1$; Table 8.1), as the rate of the swelling front does not change.

8.4 Design of diffusion-controlled drug delivery systems

Two advantages of diffusion-controlled drug delivery systems are: zero-order release kinetics can be achieved using the constant activity source reservoir systems and easy modification of the drug release rate is possible by adjusting the physicochemical properties of the drug carriers. One disadvantage is that dangerous dose dumping can occur if the system is damaged [16].

To design diffusion-controlled drug delivery systems, several aspects are to be considered:

a. Controlled pharmacokinetics: If zero-order kinetics is desirable, constant-activity source reservoir systems are preferred.

b. Delivery route: Thin film is preferred for noninvasive transdermal delivery. For an oral drug delivery system, the physiological environment changes greatly along the gastrointestinal tract. Factors that can affect drug diffusion and/or carrier stability, such as pH, should be taken into consideration. For example, the Ca-pectin hydrogel system, in general, is not stable at high pH conditions; hence, modification may be necessary for it to be used as a diffusion-controlled drug delivery system [17]. The size and geometry of the carrier also matter. For intravenous injections, nanoformulations are generally required considering the capillary size.

c. Carrier materials' properties: The materials should be "biocompatible" and relatively stable within the physiological conditions to be used as diffusion-controlled drug carriers. Ideally, the materials exhibit a certain degree of biodegradability and retrieval is not needed after delivering the drugs.

d. Drug properties: Drugs with high solubility are not good candidates for constant-activity source reservoir and monolithic dispersion systems. On the other hand, water penetration into the carrier and drug dissolution should be much faster than drug diffusion, which ensures that the diffusion is rate-limiting. Additionally, the mutual diffusion coefficient and partition coefficients of the drug in the carrier and body fluids (such as blood) should be considered [18].

Review and practice questions

1. What is diffusion?
2. Use the Stokes-Einstein equation to estimate the molar mass of a spherical protein in plasma at 37°C with a diffusion coefficient of 1.25×10^{-6} cm^2/s. **Note:** $\mu = 0.0125$ $g/(cm \times s)$.
3. What is the difference between nonconstant activity and constant activity sources?
4. What is the difference between reservoir and matrix (monolithic) systems?
5. What is the cause of lag?
6. What is burst release? What are the negative effects of burst release?
7. Are the drug release kinetics geometry dependent for the reservoir systems?
8. Are the drug release kinetics geometry dependent for the matrix systems?
9. What are the restrictions of using the Higuchi and Peppas models?
10. A release profile of zidovudine from alginate microspheres is shown below (data are from [19]):

Time, hr	% Drug release
1	3.42
2	4.92
3	25.55
4	38.97
6	56.22
8	87.39
10	96.12

(a) Prepare a plot of M_t/M_∞ vs. time.
(b) Fit the release profile using zero-order, first-order, Higuchi, and Peppas models.

References

[1] Truskey GA. Transport phenomena in biological systems. 2nd ed. Pearson Prentice Hall; 2009.
[2] Fournier RL. Basic transport phenomena in Biomedical Engineering. 4th ed. CRC Press; 2017.
[3] Costigliola L, et al. Revisiting the Stokes-Einstein relation without a hydrodynamic diameter. J Chem Phys 2019;150(2):021101.
[4] Osei-Bimpong A, Burthem J. 6 - Supplementary techniques including blood parasite diagnosis. In: Bain BJ, Bates I, Laffan MA, editors. Dacie and lewis practical haematology. 12th ed. Elsevier; 2017. p. 93–111.
[5] Siepmann J, Siepmann F. Modeling of diffusion controlled drug delivery. J Control Release 2012;161(2):351–62.
[6] Siepmann J, Siepmann F. Mathematical modeling of drug delivery. Int J Pharm 2008;364(2):328–43.
[7] Huang X, Brazel CS. On the importance and mechanisms of burst release in matrix-controlled drug delivery systems. J Control Release 2001; 73(2):121–36.
[8] Kao C-C, Chen S-C, Sheu M-T. Lag time method to delay drug release to various sites in the gastrointestinal tract. J Control Release 1997;44(2): 263–70.
[9] Higuchi T. Rate of release of medicaments from ointment bases containing drugs in suspension. J Pharm Sci 1961;50(10):874–5.
[10] Lee PI. Modeling of drug release from matrix systems involving moving boundaries: approximate analytical solutions. Int J Pharm 2011; 418(1):18–27.
[11] Lee PI. Diffusional release of a solute from a polymeric matrix — approximate analytical solutions. J Membrane Sci 1980;7(3):255–75.
[12] Zuo J, et al. Evaluation of the DDSolver software applications. BioMed Res Int 2014;2014:204925.
[13] Talevi A, Ruiz ME. Korsmeyer-peppas, peppas-sahlin, and brazel-peppas: models of drug release. In: Talevi A, editor. The ADME encyclopedia: a comprehensive guide on biopharmacy and pharmacokinetics. Springer International Publishing; 2022. p. 613–21.
[14] Morgulchik N, Kamaly N. Meta-analysis of in vitro drug-release parameters reveals predictable and robust kinetics for redox-responsive drug-conjugated therapeutic nanogels. ACS Appl Nano Mater 2021;4(5):4256–68.
[15] Peppas NA, Sahlin JJ. A simple equation for the description of solute release. III. Coupling of diffusion and relaxation. Int J Pharm 1989;57(2): 169–72.
[16] Huynh CT, Lee D-S. Controlled release. Encyclopedia of Polymeric Nanomaterials 2014;2014:1–12.
[17] Stealey S, et al. Calcium-oligochitosan-pectin microcarrier for colonic drug delivery. Pharm Dev Technol 2020;25(2):260–5.
[18] Pramanik A, Garg S. Design of diffusion-controlled drug delivery devices for controlled release of Paclitaxel. Chem Biol Drug Design 2019; 94(2):1478–87.
[19] Rao P, Vijayabhaskar K. Formulation and evaluation of zidovudine alginate microspheres. J Drug Deliv Therapeutics 2019;9:57–64.

CHAPTER

9

Erodible drug delivery systems

Wujie Zhang

LEARNING OBJECTIVES

- To understand the difference between surface erosion and bulk erosion
- To discuss different types of chemical erosion
- To discuss different drug release mechanisms of erodible drug delivery systems
- To understand different models for determining the release profiles of different erodible drug delivery systems
- To apply the Hopfenberg model
- To understand and interpret different degradation/erosion mechanisms—hydrolytic, photolytic, and enzymatic
- To discuss the design considerations of erodible delivery systems
- To design the erodible drug delivery systems

9.1 Introduction to erosion

Erodible drug delivery systems are attractive because the removal of the drug carrier is not needed. The systems can be matrix or reservoir, and drugs can be either dissolved, dispersed, or attached to the carrier. Often, degradation and erosion are used interchangeably. However, they are not always the same. Polymer degradation is the chain scission process by which polymer chains are cleaved into oligomers and monomers. Erosion is defined as the process of material loss (in the form of monomer, oligomer, or even parts of the polymer) from the polymer bulk, which can be caused by degradation [1]. Erosion can be either heterogeneous or homogeneous. Heterogenous erosion is also called surface erosion, in which the erosion only occurs at the surface (without losing physical integrity). Homogeneous erosion is bulk erosion. The erosion occurs throughout the matrix, losing physical integrity (Fig. 9.1) [2]. Most biodegradable polymers used for erodible drug delivery systems undergo bulk erosion [3].

There are different types of chemical erosion (Fig. 9.2). Type IA polymer erosion is the cleavage of crosslinks, and type IB is the disintegration of water-soluble polymer backbone. Type II chemical erosion is the conversion of water-insoluble polymers to water-soluble polymers through hydrolysis, ionization, or protonation of the side groups. Type III erosion is the scission of labile bonds of the polymer backbone [2, 4-6].

Fundamentals and Design of Drug Delivery Systems
https://doi.org/10.1016/B978-0-443-23521-4.00009-6

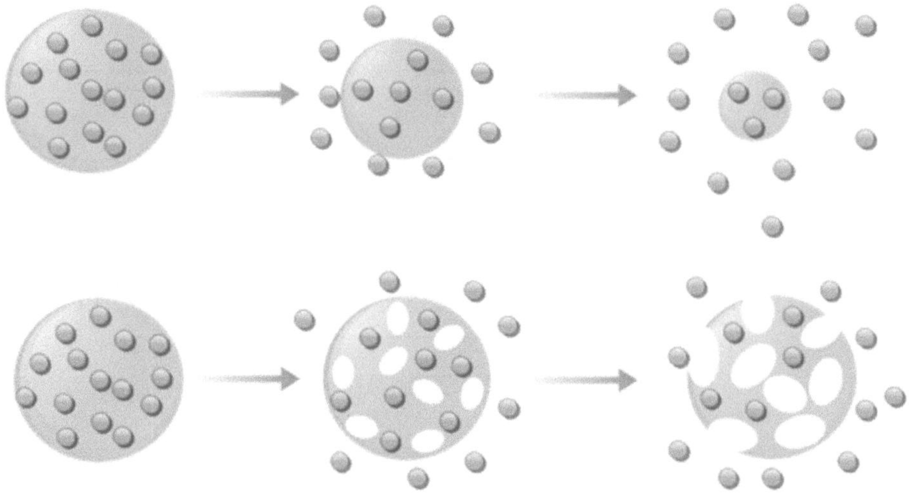

FIGURE. 9.1 Surface erosion *(top)* vs. bulk erosion *(bottom)*. *Green spheres,* drug molecules.

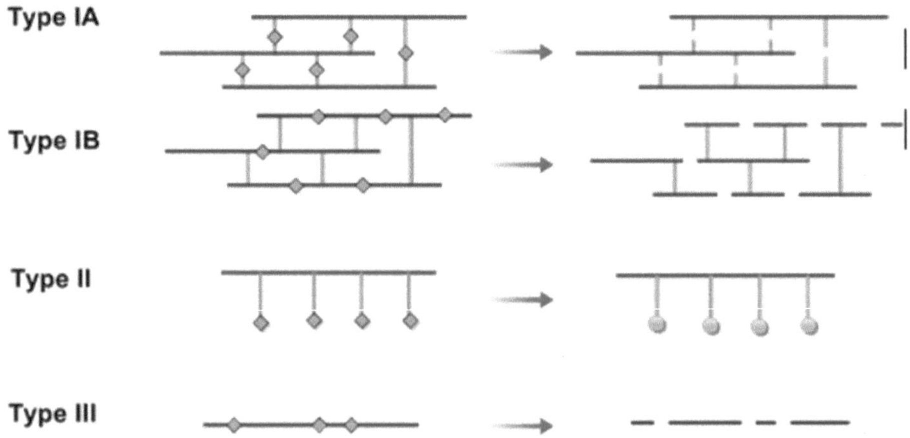

FIGURE. 9.2 Different mechanisms of polymer chemical erosion. *Dark blue,* backbones; *light blue,* crosslinks; *orange diamonds,* bonds involved in erosion; and *green spheres,* drug molecules.

9.2 Drug release from the erodible drug delivery systems

There are different drug release mechanisms of erodible drug delivery systems (Fig. 9.3). Mechanism A (Fig. 9.3A) describes the scenario that drugs are attached to the carrier through labile bonds (such as ester bonds), and the cleavage of these bonds lead to the drug release (pendant chain polymeric systems). Mechanism B (Fig. 9.3B) relates to the reservoir systems where the membrane is erodible. The drug is released through diffusion, and then membrane erosion occurs after the complete drug release. Mechanism C (Fig. 9.3C) shows the erosion of the matrix-induced drug release. Diffusion can also contribute to the drug release [6].

For this chapter, we focus on surface erosion, which is relatively simple to model. Consider a simple slab with surface area A, thickness D (half-thickness R), and initial drug concentration C_0. The amount of drug released at time *t*, can be calculated using the equation:

$$\frac{dM_t}{dt} = AC_0k$$

$$dM_t = AC_0k_edt,$$

where *k* is the surface erosion rate (unit: length/time).

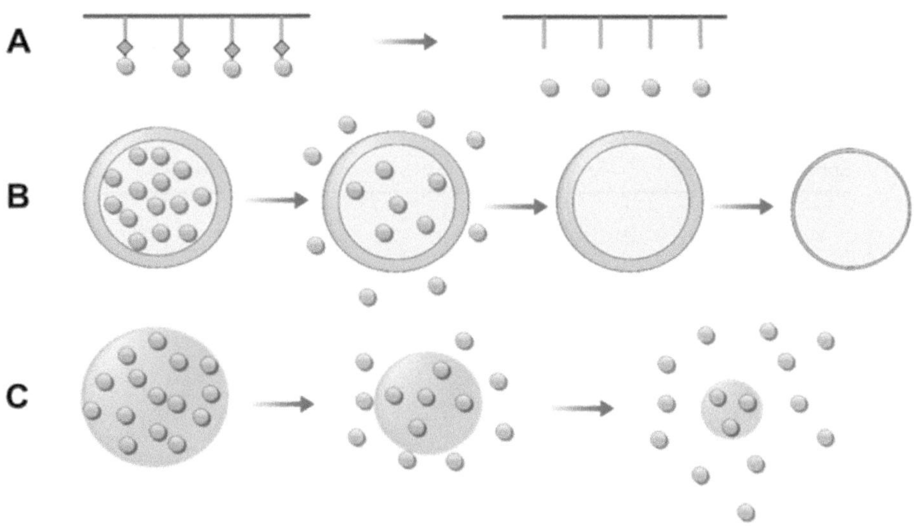

FIGURE. 9.3 Different mechanisms of drug release from erodible drug delivery systems. (A) Cleavage of labile bonds; (B) diffusion followed by membrane erosion; (C) matrix erosion. *Dark blue,* backbones; *light blue,* side chains; *orange diamond,* bonds involved in erosion; and *green spheres,* drug molecules.

Upon integration, we can obtain:

$$\int_0^t dM_t = aC_0k\int_0^t dt$$

$$M_t - M_0 = M_t = AC_0kt$$

$$M_\infty = AC_0D$$

$$\frac{M_t}{M_\infty} = \frac{kt}{D}.$$

Combining k and C_0, we can define a new erosion rate k_e (k_e = ½ × k × C_0; unit: mass/(area × time).

$$\frac{M_t}{M_\infty} = \frac{2k_et}{C_0D} = \frac{k_et}{C_0R} = 1 - \left[1 - \frac{k_e}{C_0R}t\right]^1$$

Now, let's consider the spherical drug delivery system with initial drug concentration C_0, initial radius R, and radius r at time t:

$$\frac{dM_t}{dt} = k_e4\pi r^2,$$

k_e is the erosion rate (unit: mass/(area × time)).
We also have $M_t = \frac{4\pi}{3}C_0(R^3 - r^3)$.
Combining the two equations, we have

$$\frac{d\left[\frac{4\pi}{3}C_0(R^3 - r^3)\right]}{dt} = k_e4\pi r^2.$$

Upon differentiation and simplification, we can get:

$$\frac{dr}{dt} = -\frac{k_e}{C_0}.$$

Then, the relationship between r and t is:

$$r = R - \frac{k_e}{C_0}t$$

TABLE 9.1 Hopfenberg model.

Geometry	n	R
Slab	1	Half-thickness
Cylinder	2	Radius
Sphere	3	Radius

$$\text{and } M_t = \frac{4\pi}{3}C_0\left(R^3 - r^3\right) = \frac{4\pi}{3}C_0\left(R^3 - \left(R - \frac{k_e}{C_0}t\right)^3\right).$$

We also know that $M_\infty = \frac{4\pi}{3}C_0R^3$.

Finally, we can obtain $\frac{M_t}{M_\infty} = \frac{\frac{4\pi}{3}C_0\left[R^3 - \left(R - \frac{k_e}{C_0}t\right)^3\right]}{\frac{4\pi}{3}C_0R^3} = 1 - \left[1 - \frac{k_e}{C_0R}t\right]^3.$

Similarly, we can get the following equation for the cylindrical systems:

$$\frac{M_t}{M_\infty} = 1 - \left[1 - \frac{k_e}{C_0R}t\right]^2.$$

For all the three geometries, the equation can be expressed in the form of $\frac{M_t}{M_\infty} = 1 - \left[1 - \frac{k_e}{C_0R}t\right]^n$. This is the Hopfenberg model [7, 8].

Sometimes, drugs are administered as solid particles. Upon administration, the molecules at the solid-liquid interface are solvated and detached from the solid interface. Then, the solvated molecules diffuse away from the interface to the bulk solution [9]. The process can be described by the Noyes and Whitney equation:

$$\frac{dM}{dt} = A \times \frac{D}{h}\left(C_s - C_b\right),$$

where A is the dissolving surface area, D is the diffusion coefficient, h is the thickness of the diffusion layers, C_s is the solubility, and C_b is the concentration in the bulk solution (Fig. 9.4). The equation looks simple; however, A and h are not constant, and they change with time [9].

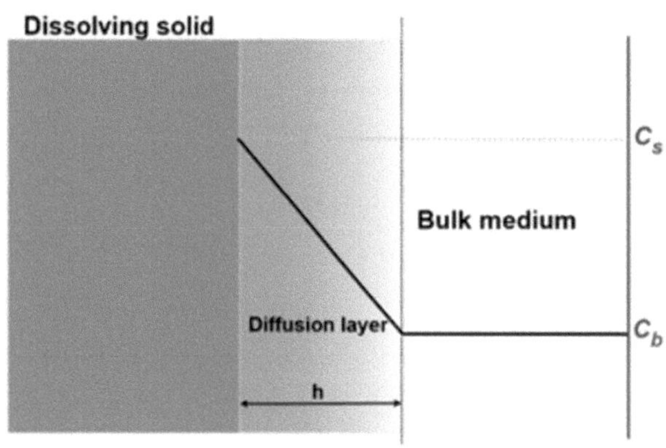

FIGURE. 9.4 Schematic of solid drug particle dissolution.

Sample question 9.1

The release data of a drug from a cylindrical erodible drug delivery system are shown in Table 9.2. Determine the k_e using the Hopfenberg model. R = 0.5 cm and C_0 = 0.1 mg/cm^3.

Answer: Use the Hopfenberg model (n = 2 for cylinder):

$$\frac{M_t}{M_\infty} = 1 - \left[1 - \frac{k_e}{C_0R}t\right]^2$$

TABLE 9.2 Drug release data (M_t/M_∞ [%] vs. time).

Time, hr	M_t/M_∞, %
0	0
1	6
5	22
10	41
15	58
20	71
25	82
30	89
35	95

Transform the equation:

$$\frac{M_t}{M_\infty}=1-\left[1-2\frac{k_e}{C_0R}t+\left(\frac{k_e}{C_0R}t\right)^2\right]=2\frac{k_e}{C_0R}t-\left(\frac{k_e}{C_0R}t\right)^2.$$

The form of the equation is $y = B1x + B2x^2$, where y is M_t/M_∞, x is t, and Bi values are constants. Plot M_t/M_∞ vs. t (Fig. 9.5) and perform regression. The model fits the data very well ($R^2 = 0.99992$).

$$2\frac{k_e}{C_0R}=\frac{4.69}{hr}$$

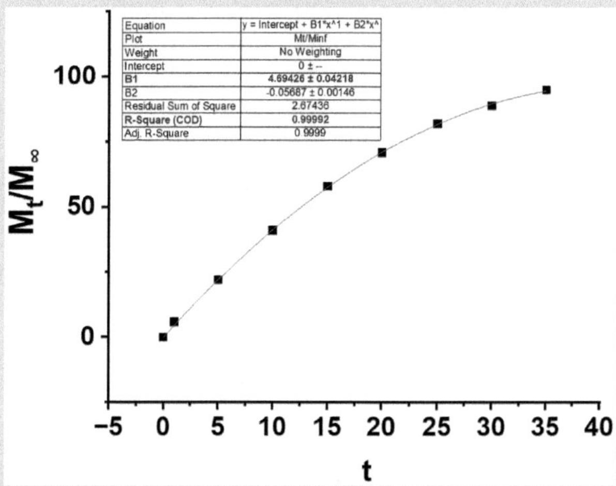

FIGURE. 9.5 Plot of M_t/M_∞ vs. time fitted with the Hopfenberg model.

and $R = 0.5$ cm and $C_0 = 0.1$ mg/cm^3. We can get

$$k_e=\frac{4.69}{2}\times C_0\times R\times\frac{1}{hr}$$

$$k_e=\frac{4.69}{2}\times 0.1\frac{mg}{cm^3}\times 0.5cm\frac{1}{hr}=0.117\frac{mg}{cm^2hr}.$$

Regarding the homogeneous erosion, we will only discuss the slab geometry. For nonerodible slab systems, the Higuchi equation is applicable when C_0 is much higher than C_s (see Chapter 8). We can simply transform the Higuchi equation:

$$M_t=A\sqrt{D2C_0C_st}$$

$$\frac{dM_t}{dt} = \frac{A}{2}\sqrt{\frac{D2C_0C_s}{t}} = \frac{A}{2}\left(\frac{D2C_0C_s}{t}\right)^{\frac{1}{2}} = \frac{A}{2}\left(\frac{2PC_0}{t}\right)^{\frac{1}{2}},$$

where P is the permeability of the slab system. For erodible system, P changes with time. Assuming first-order erosion kinetics, $P = P_0e^{kt}$ (P_0 is the initial permeability and k is the erosion rate constant) [2]. Hence, for the erodible system, the equation becomes:

$$\frac{dM_t}{dt} = \frac{A}{2}\left(\frac{2P_0e^{kt}C_0}{t}\right)^{\frac{1}{2}}.$$

9.3 Design of erodible drug delivery systems

Polymers have been widely used in erodible drug delivery systems. Polyanhydrides, such as poly(sebacic anhydride) (PSA) and poly[bis(*p*-carboxyphenoxy)propane anhydride] (PCCP), are surface-eroding polymers. They have a hydrophobic backbone and water-labile linkages, which allow heterogeneous degradation (the degradation of the polymer bonds is faster than the diffusion of water) [10-12]. Poly(lactic acid) (PLA) and poly(lactic-*co*-glycolic acid) (PLGA), structures shown in Fig. 9.6, are commonly used bulk erosion polymers. However, the degradable polymers can undergo surface erosion and bulk erosion depending on the erosion conditions and the geometry [11].

Some widely used labile bonds are ester, amide, carbonate, and carbamate. There hydrolysis reactions are shown in Fig. 9.7. Photolabile linkers are also being developed, such as *o*-nitrobenzyloxy linkers, *o*-nitrobenzylamino linkers, and α-substituted *o*-nitrobenzyl linkers. Nitrobenzyl-based linkers are the most commonly used photodegradable linkers [12, 13]. Their cleavage mechanism is identified as a Norrish type II reaction—an incident photon (300 to 350 nm) breaks the N=O π-group of the nitro-group (Fig. 9.8) [12]. Enzymatic erosion polymers have also been developed, such as aromatic-aliphatic polycarbonates based on natural phenols, tyrosol, and homovanillyl alcohol (surface erosion by lipase) [14]. Interestingly, some natural polymers can also be used for designing erodible drug delivery systems. Pectin is a good example. There is a large microflora population present within the colon allowing for enzymatic digestion of polysaccharides including pectin [15, 16]. Pectinolytic microorganisms belonging to the phyla Firmicutes and Bacteroidetes use extracellular and cell-bound enzymes for the degradation of the pectin backbone [17]. Pectinases are mixed enzymes that hydrolyze pectic substances, mostly present in microorganisms and higher plants [18]. Fig. 9.9 shows the erosion of Ca-oligochitosan-pectin microspheres in a pectinase solution.

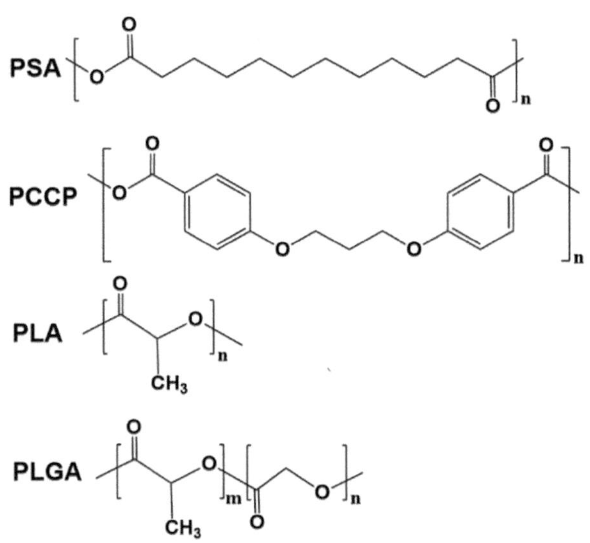

FIGURE. 9.6 Structures of some commonly used degradable polymers in drug delivery.

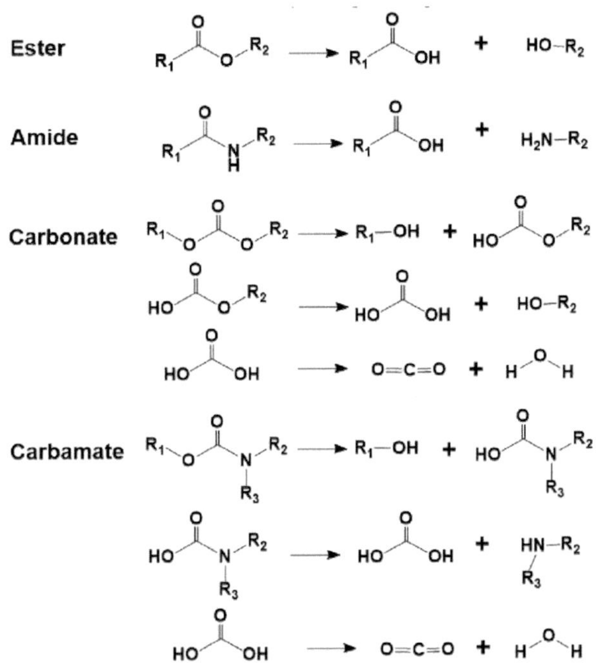

FIGURE. 9.7 Hydrolysis reactions of various labile bonds.

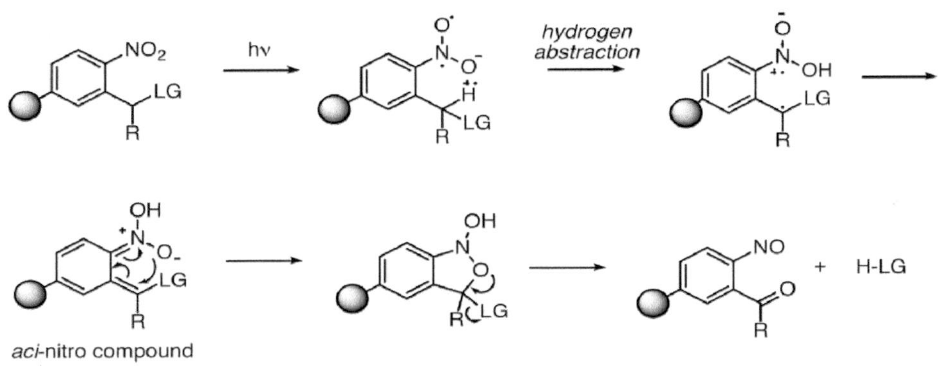

FIGURE. 9.8 Type II mechanism for the photo cleavage of a 2-nitrobenzyl-based linker. *LG*, Leaving group. From Mikkelsen, R.J.T., et al., *Photolabile linkers for solid-phase synthesis.* ACS Comb. Sci, 2018. **20**(7): p. 377-399. Copyright (2018) American Chemical Society.

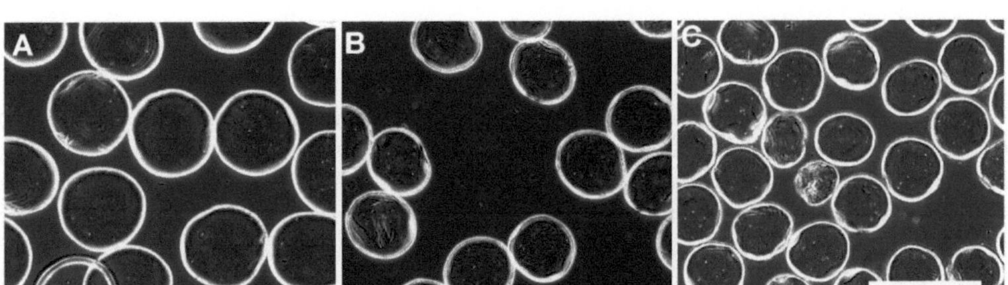

FIGURE. 9.9 Microscopic images of Ca-oligochitosan-pectin microspheres in pectinase solution at 0 (A), 30 (B), and 120 (C) min. The average diameter of microspheres decreased from 288.7 μm (0 min) to 188.2 m (120 μm). Scale bar: 400 μm. From Zhang, W., et al., *Novel pectin-based carriers for colonic drug delivery.* Pharm Dev Technol, 2016. **21**(1): p. 127-130, by permission of the publisher (Taylor & Francis Group).

To design erodible drug delivery systems, there are various factors that should be taken into account besides the general considerations for drug delivery systems design, such as drug properties and delivery route. First, if erosion is the only limiting factor for drug release, the polymer degradation rate should meet the desired drug release rate. Polymer degradation/erosion rate is highly dependent on environmental factors (determined by the delivery route and site), such as pH and enzymes present. On the other hand, if erosion is expected to occur after the drug release, premature erosion may lead to drug dumping (i.e., unintended, rapid release of the entire amount or a significant fraction of the drug over a short period of time [19]). The combination of various erosion/degradation mechanisms for erodible drug delivery systems has also been promising. When it comes to the pendant chain polymeric systems, they can be used for targeted drug delivery by carefully designing degradation conditions of the drug-polymer bonds [3]. It is also worth noting that degradation may produce substances that may modify the system's behavior, such as compatibility and erosion/degradation rate. For example, hydrolysis of PLGA leads to lactic and glycolic acid production. These accumulated acids further catalyze the PLGA hydrolysis (autocatalysis) [20].

Lab Activity VII: Drug release profile determination

Drug release behavior study is critical as it relates to drug stability and therapeutic effects. Clinically, drug release assessment is needed to ensure the product label claims and optimize the *in vitro-in vivo* correlation [21]. The objectives of this experiment are to:

(1) Design the protocol for determining the drug release profile (menthol).
(2) Perform the drug release study and fit the experimental data using different mathematical models.

Background
Cough drops are used to relieve coughs due to minor throat and bronchial irritation from a cold or inhaled irritants and occasional minor sore throat pain. Menthol (Fig. LVII.1) is the active ingredient (about 5 mg/cough drop) [22]. Menthol is a cyclic alcohol obtained from the volatile oils of various species of Mentha. It is also used to relieve symptoms of asthma and rhinitis [23].

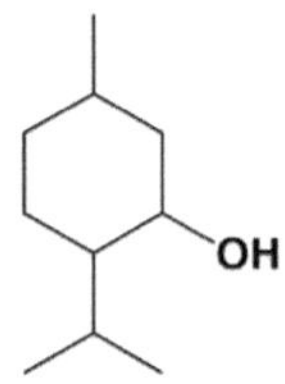

FIG. LVII.1 Structure of menthol.

Materials and Instruments
Cough drops
DI water
Cough drop solution (1 cough drop/100 mL DI water)
UV spectrophotometer

Laboratory Procedure
I. *Design the Procedure for Studying the Release Profile of Menthol*

Materials and Instruments are allowed: cough drops, ingredients of the cough drops, DI water, cough drop solution (1 cough drop/100 mL water), UV spectrophotometer and cuvettes, hot plate with stir bar, and glassware.

Hints: Do not try to measure the absorbance of menthol directly. Study the ingredients list and pay attention to the color of the solution. Assume menthol is homogeneously distributed within the cough drop. A standard curve is needed. Stir speed: ~ 300 rpm. Cover the glassware used for the release study with Parafilm.

II. *Prepare the Standard Curve of Menthol (using Halls cherry flavor cough drops)*

1. Prepare a serial dilution of the cough drop solution (1 cough drop/100 mL DI water: 0.058 mg menthol/1 mL).

2. Measure the absorbance based on FD&C Red 40 using DI water as the blank ($\lambda_{max} \approx$ 504 nm; or use the scanning mode of the UV spectrophotometer to determine the λ_{max} of FD&C Red 40).
3. Graph *Absorbance vs. Menthol Concentration* and perform linear regression (set intercept to 0).

III. *Perform the Menthol Release Study*

1. Place one piece of cough drop in 100 mL DI water and cover the glassware (flask preferred) using Parafilm (stir at 300 rpm).
2. Every 5 min, take 1 mL of sample and quickly measure the absorbance. After measuring, return the sample to the glassware.
3. Determine the menthol concentrations (C_t) using the standard curve.
4. Determine the amount of drug released at time t (M_t): $M_t = C_t \times 100$ mL.
5. Graph M_t vs. time.
6. Compare the curve to the model [24]:

$$M_t = M_\infty \left[1 - e^{\left(\frac{-A_0 C_S k \alpha}{M_0} t\right)}\right] = M_\infty \left[1 - e^{(\beta t)}\right],$$

where M_∞ is the initial drug amount, A_0 is the initial surface area (cm^2), C_s is the solubility of the matrix, *k* is the mass transfer coefficient (cm/s), and α is the mass fraction of drug, menthol. To determine β, the above equation can be simply transformed:

$$M_t - M_\infty = -M_\infty e^{(\beta t)}$$

$$M_\infty - M_t = M_\infty e^{(\beta t)}$$

$$\frac{M_\infty - M_t}{M_\infty} = e^{(\beta t)}$$

$$ln\left(\frac{M_\infty - M_t}{M_\infty}\right) = ln\left(e^{(\beta t)}\right) = \beta t$$

$$ln\left(\frac{M_r}{M_\infty}\right) = \beta t.$$

M_r is the remaining amount of drug. To determine β, plot of $\ln(M_r/M_\infty)$ vs. t should be generated. Then perform the linear regression, the slope is β.

Review and practice questions

1. What is degradation?
2. What is erosion?
3. What are the differences between surface (heterogeneous) and bulk erosion (homogeneous)?
4. What are the different types of chemical erosion mechanisms?
5. What are the drug release mechanisms from erodible drug delivery systems?
6. Derive the equation for the surface erosion of a cylindrical drug delivery system. Initial drug concentration: C_0, radius: R, length: L, and erosion rate: k_e (unit: mass/(area $\times$ time)).

$$\frac{M_t}{M_\infty} = 1 - \left[1 - \frac{k_e}{C_0 R} t\right]^2$$

7. *Assuming heterogeneous degradation, design a device that will yield an increasing release rate.
8. *The data given in the table are for fraction erosion of spheres made of an erodible polyanhydride, poly(CPP=SA) 20:80. This fraction could be derived, similarly from equation $\frac{M_t}{M_\infty} = 1 - \left[1 - \frac{k_e}{C_0 R} t\right]^3$ to yield $\frac{P_t}{P_\infty} = 1 - \left[1 - \frac{k_0}{\rho R} t\right]^3$, where k_0 is defined as the erosion constant, and ρ is the density of the sphere. (a) Plot the expected cumulative fraction of polymer eroded (P_t/P_∞) for spheres with initial diameters of 1000, 660, 475, and 250 μm from t = 0 to t = 100 hr. Use a value of $k_0/p = 2.5$ μm/hr. (b) Compare the experimental data with your results. Comment on the deviation of the experimental results from your theoretical results.

Fraction polymer eroded — P_t/P_∞ (experimental).

Time, hr	1000 μm	660 μm	475 μm	250 μm
0.00	0.000	0.000	0.000	0.000
0.13	0.000	0.000	0.007	0.000
0.25	0.000	0.011	0.013	0.011
0.38	0.001	0.017	0.013	0.011
0.50	0.002	0.020	0.016	0.027
0.63	0.003	0.021	0.016	0.029
0.75	0.003	0.024	0.017	0.032
1.00	0.003	0.025	0.017	0.033
1.25	0.004	0.041	0.019	0.035
1.50	0.004	0.042	0.210	0.036
2.00	0.004	0.042	0.023	0.039
2.50	0.006	0.044	0.034	0.039
3.00	0.008	0.044	0.043	0.045
4.00	0.010	0.050	0.049	0.050
5.00	0.045	0.058	0.055	0.058
6.00	0.067	0.069	0.062	0.069
7.00	0.074	0.075	0.073	0.082
8.50	0.091	0.092	0.101	0.118
14.20	0.216	0.227	0.295	0.381
23.80	0.404	0.455	0.573	0.655
28.00	0.463	0.526	0.634	0.703
32.50	0.517	0.585	0.680	0.738
48.00	0.662	0.719	0.771	0.818
73.50	0.792	0.833	0.860	0.893
96.00	0.854	0.897	0.918	0.932
120.00	0.910	0.936	0.941	0.949
144.00	0.942	0.950	0.951	0.956
193.00	0.960	0.964	0.965	0.970
263.00	0.975	0.975	0.978	0.980
358.00	0.985	0.985	0.986	0.988
477.00	0.993	0.993	0.993	0.995
597.00	0.996	0.997	0.997	0.998
766.00	1.000	1.000	1.000	1.000

9. *Calculate and graph the cumulative release of drug from 100 mg of 10%-loaded spheres (r = 50 μm) after 1, 2, 10, 30, and 60 days if the release persists more than 100 days (heterogeneous erosion). **Hint:** $\frac{k_e}{C_0 R} = \frac{1}{t_\infty}$ and use 100 days for t_∞.
10. Provide an example of a polymer used for erodible drug delivery systems. And describe the degradation/erosion mechanism of the polymer.
11. What is the type of the most commonly used photodegradable linkers? What is the cleavage mechanism?
12. What are the considerations for designing erodible drug delivery systems?

* *Adapted from Kydonieus AF. Treatise on Controlled Drug Delivery: Fundamentals-optimization-applications 1992: CRC Press by permission of Taylor and Francis Group, LLC, a division of Informa plc.*

References

[1] Siepmann J, Siepmann F. Mathematical modeling of drug delivery. Int J Pharm 2008;364(2):328–43.

[2] Kydonieus AF. Treatise on controlled Drug Delivery: fundamentals-optimization-applications. CRC Press; 1992.

[3] Geraili A, Xing M, Mequanint K. Design and fabrication of drug-delivery systems toward adjustable release profiles for personalized treatment. VIEW 2021;2(5):20200126.

[4] Heller J. Controlled release of biologically active compounds from bioerodible polymers. Biomater 1980;1(1):51–7.

[5] Heller J. Biodegradable polymers in controlled drug delivery. Crit Rev Ther Drug Carrier Syst 1984;1(1):39–90.

[6] Robinson J, Lee VHL, editors. Controlled drug delivery: fundamentals and applications. 2nd ed. CRC Press; 1987.

[7] Hopfenberg HB. Controlled release from erodible slabs, cylinders, and spheres. Controlled release polymeric formulations. Paul DR, Harris FW, editors. . ACS symposium series. American Chemical Society; 1976. p. 26–32.

[8] Katzhendler I, et al. Modeling of drug release from erodible tablets. J Pharm Sci 1997;86(1):110–5.

[9] Li X, Jasti BR, editors. Design of controlled release drug delivery systems. McGraw Hill; 2005.

[10] Niaounakis M. 7-Medical, dental, and pharmaceutical applications. In: Niaounakis M, editor. Biopolymers: applications and trends. William Andrew Publishing; 2015. p. 291–405.

[11] von Burkersroda F, Schedl L, Göpferich A. Why degradable polymers undergo surface erosion or bulk erosion. Biomater 2002;23(21):4221–31.

[12] Mikkelsen RJT, et al. Photolabile linkers for solid-phase synthesis. ACS Comb Sci 2018;20(7):377–99.

[13] LeValley PJ, et al. Photolabile linkers: exploiting labile bond chemistry to control mode and rate of hydrogel degradation and protein release. J Am Chem Soc 2020;142(10):4671–9.

[14] Sommerfeld SD, et al. Enzymatic surface erosion of high tensile strength polycarbonates based on natural phenols. Biomacromolecules 2014; 15(3):830–6.

[15] Stealey S, et al. Calcium-oligochitosan-pectin microcarrier for colonic drug delivery. Pharm Dev Technol 2020;25(2):260–5.

[16] Zhang W, et al. Novel pectin-based carriers for colonic drug delivery. Pharmaceutical Development and Technology 2016;21(1):127–30.

[17] Elshahed MS, et al. Pectin in diet: interactions with the human microbiome, role in gut homeostasis, and nutrient-drug interactions. Carbohydrate Polymers 2021;255:117388.

[18] Haile S, Ayele A. Pectinase from microorganisms and its industrial applications. Sci World J 2022;2022:1881305.

[19] Dasgupta A. Chapter 3-Opioid abuse and opioid epidemic. In: Dasgupta A, editor. Fighting the opioid epidemic. Elsevier; 2020. p. 43–60.

[20] Lim YW, et al. Challenges and complications of poly(lactic-co-glycolic acid)-based long-acting drug product development. Pharmaceutics 2022;14(3):614.

[21] Gupta V, Trivedi P. Chapter 15-In vitro and in vivo characterization of pharmaceutical topical nanocarriers containing anticancer drugs for skin cancer treatment. In: Grumezescu AM, editor. Lipid nanocarriers for Drug targeting. William Andrew Publishing; 2018. p. 563–627.

[22] Label: Nice Menthol Cough Drops- menthol lozenge. Available from: https://dailymed.nlm.nih.gov/dailymed/drugInfo.cfm?setid=96d77897-475c-482c-e053-2995a90a2da4.

[23] Mronson JK, editor. Meyler's side effects of drugs. 16th ed. Elsevier; 2016. p. 831–2.

[24] Farrell S, Hesketh RP. An introduction to drug delivery for chemical engineers. Chem Eng Sci 2002;36(3):198–203.

CHAPTER

10

Osmotic-controlled drug delivery systems

Wujie Zhang

LEARNING OBJECTIVES

- To understand osmosis
- To discuss and calculate the osmotic pressure of a solution
- To understand the function(s) of an osmogen
- To determine the orifice size by applying the boundary conditions (A_{min} and A_{max})
- To interpret the working mechanisms of different osmotic-controlled drug delivery systems
- To explain the advantages and disadvantages of osmotic-controlled drug delivery systems
- To discuss the design considerations of osmotic-controlled drug delivery systems
- To design the osmotic-controlled drug delivery systems

10.1 Osmosis

Osmosis is the net movement of water (solvent) across a selectively permeable membrane due to pressure. The pressure applied to the higher-solute-concentration side to resist solvent flow is called the osmotic pressure. Osmotic pressure is a colligative property of a solution in which a nonvolatile solute is dissolved in a volatile solvent [1,2]. For a dilute nonelectrolyte solution that obeys Raoult's law (the vapor pressure of the volatile solvent is proportionally reduced by the number of solute molecules present):

$$n = \frac{\Pi V}{RT},$$

where Π is the osmotic pressure, n is the molar amount of the solute, V is the volume of the solvent, R is the ideal gas constant, and T is the absolute temperature [1]. This relationship was derived by J.H. van't Hoff. Another form of the equation is:

$$\Pi = MRT,$$

Fundamentals and Design of Drug Delivery Systems
https://doi.org/10.1016/B978-0-443-23521-4.00010-2

where M is the solute concentration in molarity. A factor i was introduced to account for the behavior of ionic solutions [3]. For the electrolyte solutions, the equation becomes:

$\Pi = iMRT$. This factor equals to the total number of ions present in one formula unit of the substance.

Sample question 10.1

Five grams of NaCl (Mw = 58.44 g/mol) is dissolved in 1 L of water at 37°C. What is the osmotic pressure of this solution?

Answer:

$$\Pi = iMRT = i\frac{n}{V}RT$$

i = 2 for NaCl
n = 5 g/(58.44 g/mol) = 0.086 mol
R = 0.082 L × atm/(K × mol)
T = (37 + 273.15) K = 310.15 K

Thus,

$$\Pi = i\frac{n}{V}RT = 2 \times \frac{0.086\ mol}{1\ L} \times 0.082\frac{L \times atm}{K \times mol} \times 310.15K$$

$$\Pi = 4.37\ atm.$$

S. Rose and J.F. Nelson were the first to report the osmotic-controlled drug delivery systems. Their work was published in 1955 [4]; the design is shown in Fig. 10.1. This implantable pump was designed for delivering drugs to the gut of animals. The osmotic pressure was generated by a saturated aqueous solution of Congo Red against water with a semipermeable cellophane membrane. The expansion of the latex bag with Congo Red pushes the drug out of the glass ampoule through the "nipple."

The substances used to generate the osmotic pressure are called osmotic agents or osmogens. Commonly used osmogens include lactose, fructose, sorbitol, dextrose, sodium chloride, mannitol, and sodium carboxymethyl cellulose (Table 10.1). It is common that a mixture of osmogens is used, such as lactose-fructose. A drug itself can also act

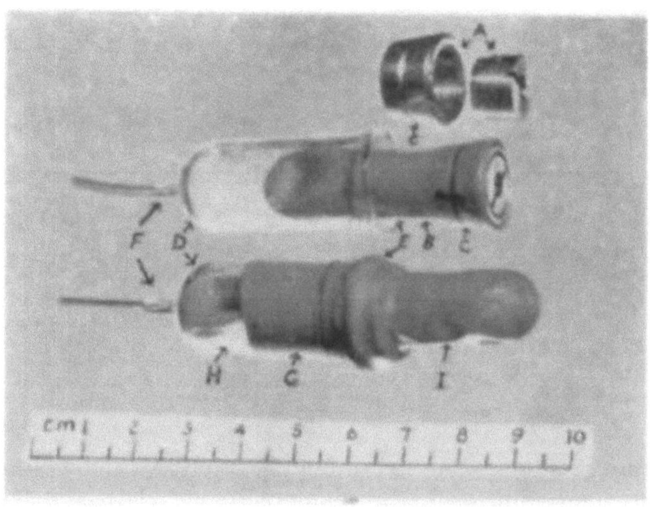

FIGURE 10.1 Component parts and assembled microinjector. (A) Two-piece screw clamp to hold the semipermeable cellophane membrane. (B) Latex bag partially filled with Congo Red. (C) Groove on the outside of the clamp for latex to be pulled in creating a watertight seal. (D) Glass ampoule with a splayed edge (E) and a nipple (F, delivery orifice). (G) Excess latex (turned back over the splayed edge of the glass ampoule and tied with thread). (H) Drug compartment (between B and D). (I) Second latex bag tied over the splayed edge of the glass ampoule (water compartment). *From Rose, S. and J. Nelson,* A continuous long-term injector. *Aust. J. Exp. Biol. Med. Sci, 1955.* **33***(4): p. 415-420, with permission from John Wiley* & Sons, Inc.

TABLE 10.1 Osmotic pressures of saturated solution of commonly used osmogens.

Compound/mixture	Osmotic pressure (atm)
Lactose-fructose	500
Dextrose-fructose	450
Sucrose-fructose	430
Mannitol-fructose	415
Sodium chloride	356
Fructose	335
Lactose-sucrose	250
Potassium chloride	245
Lactose-dextrose	225
Mannitol-dextrose	225
Dextrose-sucrose	190
Mannitol-sucrose	170
Sucrose	150
Mannitol-lactose	130
Dextrose	82
Potassium sulfate	39
Mannitol	38
Sodium phosphate tribasic: 12 H_2O	36
Sodium phosphate dibasic: 7 H_2O	31
Sodium phosphate dibasic: 12 H_2O	31
Sodium phosphate monobasic: H_2O	28
Sodium phosphate dibasic: anhydrous	21

From Gupta, B.P. et al., Osmotically controlled drug delivery system with associated drugs. *J. Pharm. Pharm. Sci., 2010.* ***13****(4): p. 571-588.*

as an osmogen. Water solubility and osmotic activity are the two main factors when choosing a osmogen (or osmogens) [2]. Semipermeable membranes, in general, are polymeric. Cellulose acetate is most commonly used. Other polymers have been applied in designing osmotic-controlled drug delivery systems, including cellulose esters, ethyl cellulose, and polyvinyl chloride [2,5]. Other agents, such as pore-forming agents, may also be needed.

10.2 Elementary osmotic-controlled drug delivery systems

The elementary osmotic pump was first described by Theeuwes and Higuchi in 1970s [7] (more information is given in Case Study V). For an elementary osmotic pump, it consists of a core of drug and osmotic agent(s) surrounded by a rigid semipermeable membrane, with an orifice for releasing drug (Fig. 10.2). This system is good for delivering intermediate water-soluble drugs. For high water-soluble drugs, they would be delivered after a short time upon administration.

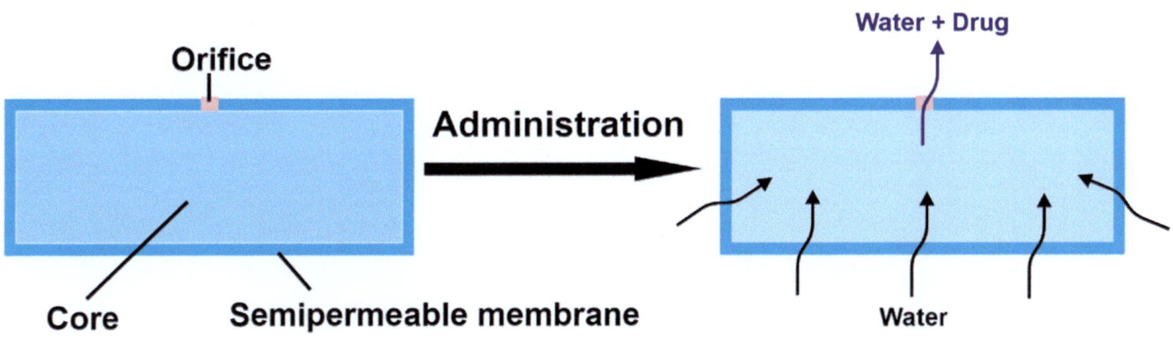

FIGURE 10.2 Schematic of an elementary osmotic pump.

The membrane of an elementary osmotic pump is rigid and does not change (swell, shrink, or degrade). Thus, the system delivers a volume of saturated solution equal to the volume of solvent uptake. Excessive undissolved drug presence can lead to zero-order release kinetics [3]. The volumetric flow rate can be described as:

$$\frac{dV}{dt} = \frac{A}{h} L_p (\sigma \Delta\Pi - \Delta P),$$

where $\Delta\Pi$ is the osmotic pressure difference across the membrane, ΔP is the hydrostatic pressure difference across the membrane, L_p is the mechanical permeability, σ is the reflection coefficient (accounts for the leakage of solute through the membrane), A is the surface area of the membrane, and h is the thickness of the membrane. Also, we have

$$\frac{dm}{dt} = \frac{dV}{dt} C,$$

where C is the drug concentration in the release fluid. Hence,

$$\frac{dm}{dt} = \frac{A}{h} L_p (\sigma \Delta\Pi - \Delta P) C.$$

$\Delta\Pi$ can be changed to Π (pressure of the formulation) because the environmental osmotic pressure is small and ΔP is negligible if the orifice size is big enough and the membrane materials have sufficient low modulus. The simplified equation is

$$\frac{dm}{dt} = \frac{A}{h} L_p \sigma \Pi C.$$

To achieve zero-order release kinetics, Π should be constant, which can be simply done by maintaining a saturated solution of osmotic agent(s). Finally, before all the solids dissolve and the solute concentration begins to fall below saturation, we have

$$\frac{dm}{dt} = \frac{A}{h} k \Pi_s S,$$

where k is $L_p \times \sigma$, Π_s is the osmotic pressure of the saturated system, and S is the solubility (or saturation concentration) [1,3,8].

Sample question 10.2 [1]

Calculate the zero-order delivery rate for drug X with S of 300 mg/mL from an oral osmotic pump with $k\Pi_s$ of 1×10^{-3} cm^2/h, A of 2.5 cm^2, and h of 0.03 cm.

Answer:

$$\frac{dm}{dt} = \frac{A}{h} k\Pi_s S$$

$$k\Pi_s = 1 \times 10^{-3}\ \mathrm{cm^2/h} \quad S = 300\ \mathrm{mg/cm^3}$$

$$A = 2.5\ \mathrm{cm^2} \quad h = 0.03\ \mathrm{cm}$$

$$\frac{dm}{dt} = \frac{2.5\ \mathrm{cm^2}}{0.03\ \mathrm{cm}} \times 0.001 \frac{\mathrm{cm^2}}{\mathrm{h}} \times 300 \frac{\mathrm{mg}}{\mathrm{cm^3}}$$

$$\frac{dm}{dt} = 25.0 \frac{\mathrm{mg}}{\mathrm{h}}.$$

Sample question 10.3 [1]

Using the following information, calculate the permeability coefficient (k) for a semipermeable membrane required to give a delivery rate of 15 mg/hr.

$A = 2.0\ cm^2$ $\quad \Pi_s = 60$ atm
$S = 500\ mg/cm^3$ $\quad h = 0.02$ cm

Answer:

$$\frac{dm}{dt} = \frac{A}{h} k \Pi_s S$$

$$k = \frac{\frac{dm}{dt}}{\frac{A}{h}\Pi_s S} = \frac{\frac{dm}{dt}h}{A\Pi_s S} = \frac{15\frac{mg}{h} \times 0.02\ cm}{2.0\ cm^2 \times 60\ atm \times 500\frac{mg}{cm^3}} = 5 \times 10^{-6} \frac{cm^2}{h \times atm}$$

The size of the orifice is critical. It should be small enough to minimize the drug delivery by diffusion through the orifice but big enough to avoid the hydrostatic pressure buildup damaging the system [5]. The minimum and maximum sizes (areas) can be estimated using the following equations, respectively:

$$A_{min} = 5\left[\left(\frac{L}{\Delta P_{max}}\right)\mu\left(\frac{dV}{dt}\right)\right]^{1/2}$$

and

$$A_{max} = \frac{1}{F}\left(\frac{dm}{dt}\right)\frac{L}{DS},$$

where L is the length of the orifice, μ is the viscosity of the dispersed solution, ΔP_{max} is the maximum hydrostatic pressure across the device, F is the ratio of total delivery rate to diffusive rate, D is the diffusion coefficient of the drug in the permeating solvent, and S is the solubility (or saturation) concentration of the drug [1,3,5].

Sample question 10.4 [1]

Given the following information, calculate the boundary conditions, A_{max} and A_{min}, for an elementary osmotic pump.

$dV/dt = 2.78 \times 10^{-5}\ cm^3/s$ $\quad L = 0.025$ cm
$\mu = 1\ cp = 10^{-3}\ Ns/m^2$ $\quad F = 40$
$dm/dt = 0.0069\ mg/s$ $\quad \Delta P_{max} = 1$ atm
$S = 300\ mg/cm^3$ $\quad D = 2 \times 10^{-5}\ cm^2/s$

Answer:

$$\Delta P_{max} = 1\ atm = 101325\ N/m^2$$

$$A_{min} = 5\left[\left(\frac{L}{\Delta P_{max}}\right)\mu\left(\frac{dV}{dt}\right)\right]^{1/2} = 5\left[\left(\frac{0.025\ cm}{101325\frac{N}{m^2}}\right) \times 10^{-3}\frac{Ns}{m^2} \times 2.78 \times 10^{-5}\frac{cm^3}{s}\right]^{1/2} = 4.141 \times 10^{-7} cm^2$$

$$A_{max} = \frac{1}{F}\left(\frac{dm}{dt}\right)\frac{L}{DS} = \frac{1}{40} \times 0.0069\frac{mg}{s} \times \frac{0.025\ cm}{2 \times 10^{-5}\frac{cm^2}{s} \times 300\frac{mg}{cm^3}} = 7.188 \times 10^{-4} cm^2$$

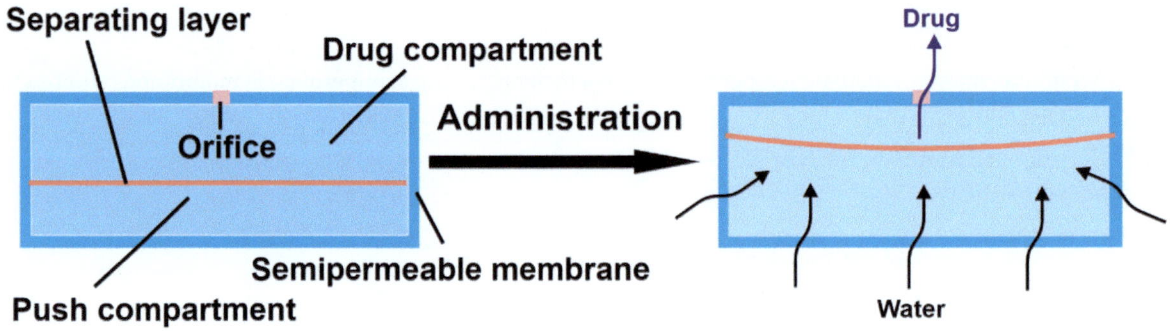

FIGURE 10.3 Schematic of a push-pull system.

10.3 Push-pull systems

A push-pull system has an osmotic core made of two compartments, a drug compartment and a push compartment (Fig. 10.3). While the two compartments are separated by an elastic membrane, the core is covered by a rigid semipermeable membrane. Upon contact with aqueous surroundings, the push compartment containing osmogen(s) draws water and expands. The drug compartment, as a result, has to shrink, releasing drug since the total volume of the two compartments does not change. These systems are useful for the delivery of poor water-soluble drugs [1–3].

The mass delivery rate can be written as:

$$\frac{dm}{dt} = \frac{dV}{dt}C_s,$$

where C_s is the drug concentration in the dispensed liquid or suspension. The osmotic volumetric flow into the push compartment (Q) is $Q = \left(\frac{dV}{dt}\right)_P$, and the volumetric flow into the drug compartment (F) is $F = \left(\frac{dV}{dt}\right)_D$. The concentration of drug released from the formulation can be written as: $C_s = F_D C_0$, where F_D is the fraction of the drug in the drug compartment and C_0 is the concentration of solids dispensed from the system. The assumption is that F_D in the drug compartment is the same in the dispensed formulation. Thus, $\frac{dm}{dt} = (Q+F)F_D C_0$. Q and F can be expressed as

$$Q = \frac{k}{h}A_P \Pi_P$$

$$F = \frac{k}{h}(A - A_P)\Pi_D,$$

where k is the membrane permeability coefficient, h is the membrane thickness, A_P is the surface area of the push compartment, A is the total surface area of the dosage form, Π_P is the imbibition pressure in the push and drug compartment, and Π_D is the imbibition pressure in the push and drug compartment [1,3].

10.4 Design of osmotic-controlled drug delivery systems

Osmotic-controlled drug delivery systems offer multiple advantages: zero-order drug release rate can be achieved, the system is easily formulated, prolonged or sustained drug release is possible, and the release rate is not drug, physiological, or hydrodynamic factor dependent. The disadvantages include dose dumping, system integrity maintenance, and difficulty in achieving the system consistency [2,6].

We have discussed the Rose-Nelson pump, elementary osmotic pump (EOP), and push-pull osmotic pump (PPOP). Their differences are summarized in Table 10.2. There are also other types of osmotic-controlled drug delivery systems, such as liquid oral osmotic systems for liquid forms of drug delivery. The osmotic-controlled drug delivery systems can be classified into implantable pumps (e.g., Rose-Nelson pump) and oral pumps (e.g., EOP).

TABLE 10.2 Comparison of different osmotic delivery systems.

Osmotic system	Differences/drawbacks
Rose-Nelson	The pump is stored empty and in air-tight containers and must be loaded with water before use.
Elementary	It consists of only one compartment and the drug is only released in solution form. Suitable only for water-soluble drugs. Drug release follows zero-order kinetics.
Push-pull	A push-pull system can release drugs both in suspension and solution form. This system is preferred for releasing highly soluble drugs such as oxybutynin hydrochloride and for poorly soluble drugs such as glipizide. A complicated drilling technique is involved in drilling the orifice in the pump.

From Almoshari, Y., Osmotic pump drug delivery systems: a comprehensive review. *Pharmaceuticals, 2022.* ***15****(11): p. 1430.*

To design osmotic-controlled drug delivery systems, these are some of the key factors to consider [2,9]:

Drug solubility. Highly water-soluble drugs generally are not good candidates for the osmotic-controlled drug delivery systems. Excipients can be used to modify the drug solubility. For example, wicking agents can be used for poorly water-soluble drugs. Wicking agents are substances with the ability to absorb water into the porous network of a delivery system. They enhance the contact surface area of drug with the incoming aqueous fluids [2,8]. The fraction of a drug release (F_Z) with zero-order kinetics is given by

$$F_Z = 1 - \frac{S}{P},$$

where S is the drug solubility, and P is the density of the core tablet [1].

Osmotic pressure. Osmotic pressure should be within the desired range as it is proportional to the drug release rate. Osmogen(s) should be used if the osmotic pressure of the drug itself is not adequate. Again, it is possible to maintain a constant osmotic pressure by maintaining a saturated solution of osmotic agent(s).

Orifice size. As discussed in 10.2, the orifice size should be carefully controlled. In general, the optimum size range for a delivery orifice is 600 μm to 1 mm [2]. The orifice can be generated using drilling, such as mechanical and laser drilling (Fig. 10.4), with high precision and reproducibility. Interestingly, there is a report on orifice generation using a modified tablet punch to create an indentation without drilling (Fig. 10.5) [10].

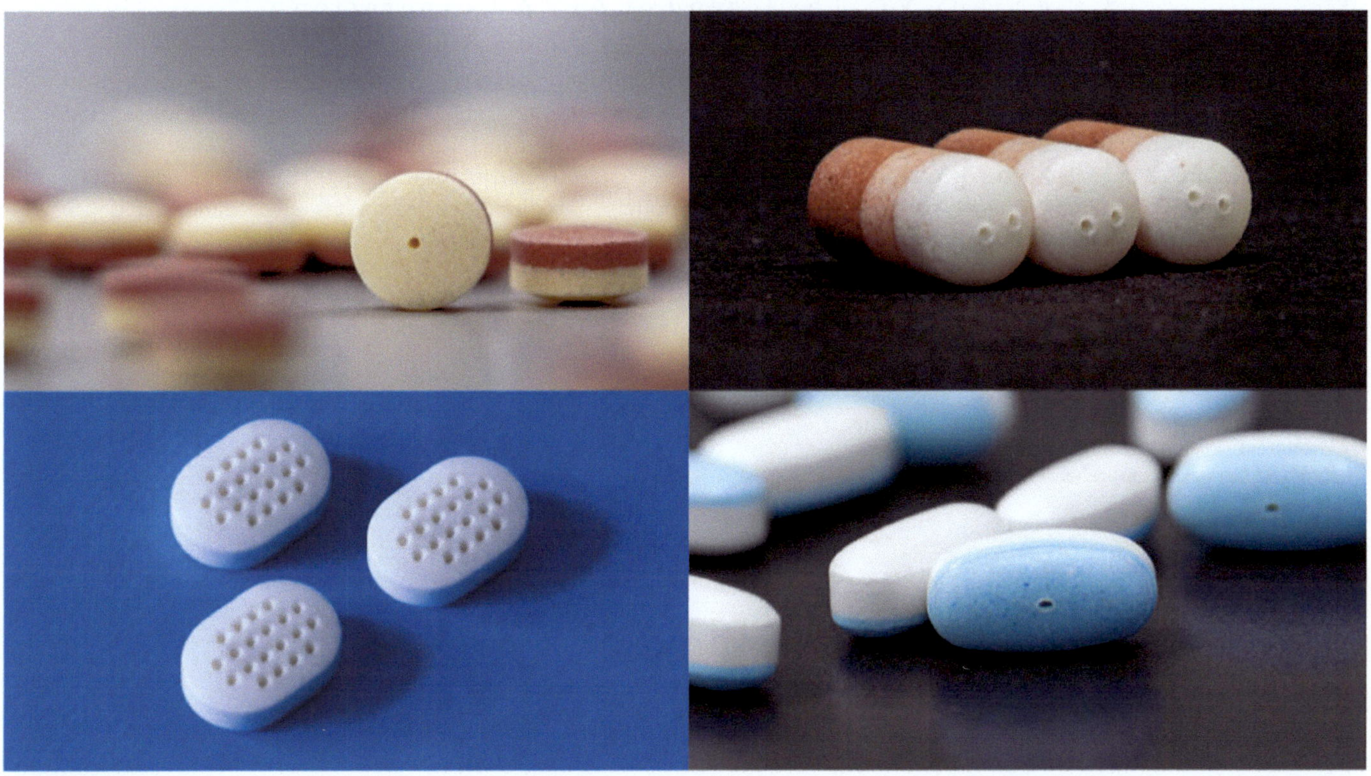

FIGURE 10.4 Single and multiple holes (orifices) in tablets are generated using a commercial laser drilling system. *From Control Micro Systems (CMS Laser). Our Technology. Available from: https://cmslaser.com/products/specialized-laser-systems/pharmaceutical-laser-systems/laser-systems-for-tablet-research-development/, with permission from Control Micro Systems (CMS Laser).*

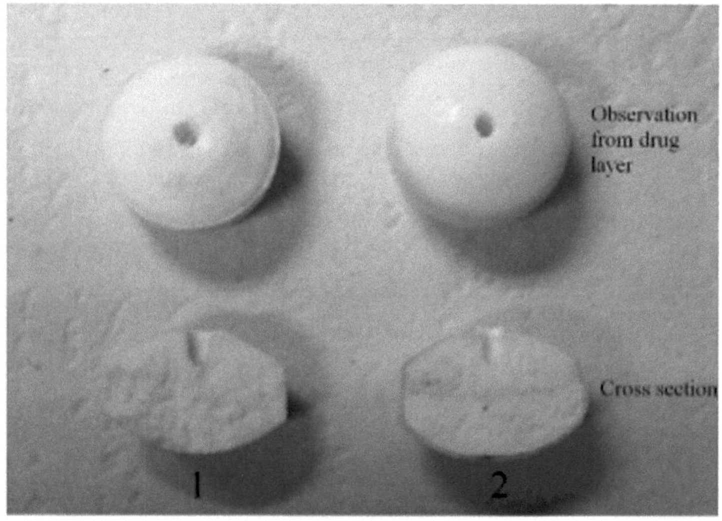

FIGURE 10.5 Bilayer (push and drug compartments) core tablet before (1) and after (2) coating. Nifedipine was the model drug, NaCl was the osmotic agent, and the semipermeable membrane was ethyl cellulose based. *From Liu, L. and X. Xu,* Preparation of bilayer-core osmotic pump tablet by coating the indented core tablet. *Int. J. Pharm, 2008.* ***352****(1): p. 225-230, with permission from Elsevier.*

Semipermeable membrane selection. The membrane should have selective permeability—permeable to water but impermeable to solutes (drugs, osmogen(s), and other substances). Cellulose acetate is the most widely used polymer in osmotic controlled drug delivery systems. Besides biocompatibility, the mechanical strength of the membrane is critical. A damaged membrane may lead to dose dumping. For example, a thick microporous layer can be applied to provide the strength to withstand the internal pressure in addition to the relatively thick semipermeable membrane [8].

Case Study V: The legend of ALZA Corporation

ALZA Corporation, one of the world's leading producers of drug delivery technologies, was founded by Dr. **Al**ejandro **Za**ffaroni. The company merged with Johnson & Johnson in 2001 [12]. ALZA owns the patents on multiple osmotic-controlled drug delivery systems.

Professor Takeru Higuchi set a very fruitful collaboration with the ALZA corporation, leading to the development of several osmotic systems, such as the Higuchi-Leeper pump (Fig. CS 10.1) [13–16]. ALZET Osmotic Pumps were developed during the 1970s by ALZA Corporation with a publication describing the osmotic pump technology in 1976 (Fig. CS 10.2) [17,18]. ALZET Osmotic Pumps entered the marketplace in 1977, and the product line was acquired by DURECT Corporation in 2000 [17]. There are various models with different release rates and durations (Fig. CS. 10.3). ALZET pumps are intended for use in experimental animals only.

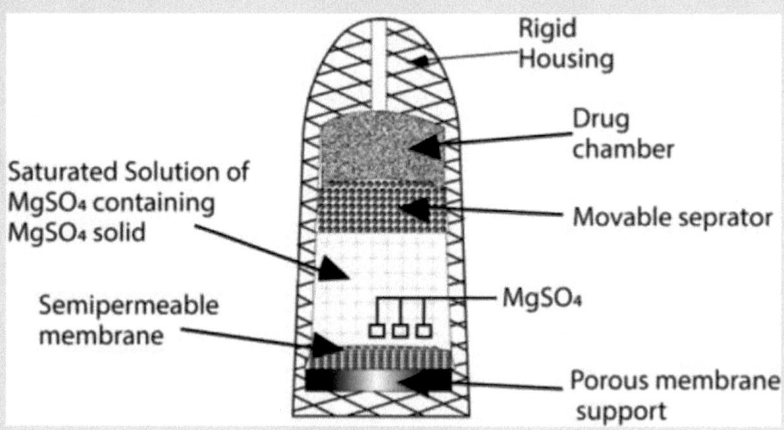

FIGURE CS 10.1 The Higuchi-Leeper pump: a simplified version of the Rose-Nelson pump. The water required for device activation is drawn from the environment. *From Almoshari, Y.,* Osmotic pump drug delivery systems: a comprehensive review. *Pharmaceuticals, 2022.* ***15****(11): p. 1430.*

Case Study V: The legend of ALZA Corporation *(cont'd)*

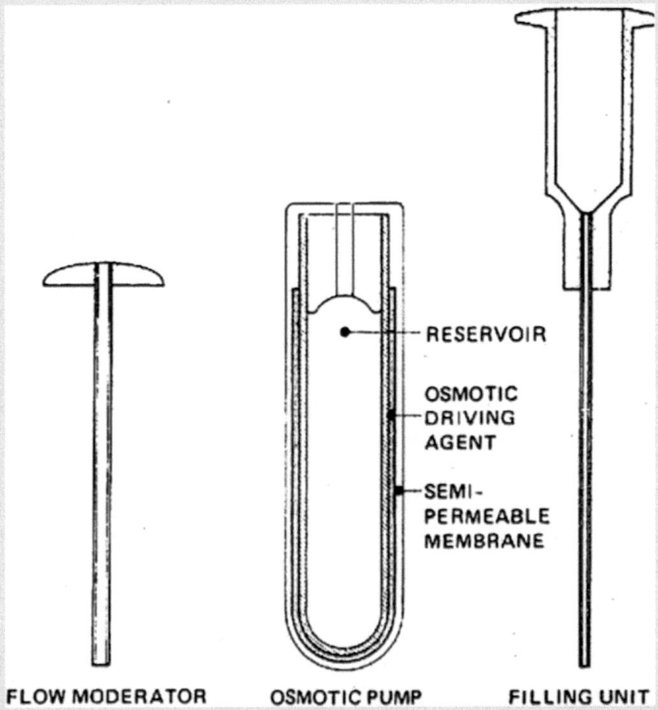

FIGURE CS 10.2 Osmotic pump and components. The osmotic pump is cylindrical in shape and consists of a collapsible reservoir surrounded by a sealed layer of osmotic driving agent, which is contained by a semipermeable membrane. The osmotic pump is filled by using the filling unit and a syringe. A flow moderator is inserted into osmotic pump upon filling. *From Theeuwes, F. and S.I. Yum,* Principles of the design and operation of generic osmotic pumps for the delivery of semisolid or liquid drug formulations. *Ann. Biomed. Eng, 1976. 4(4): p. 343-353, with permission from Springer Nature.*

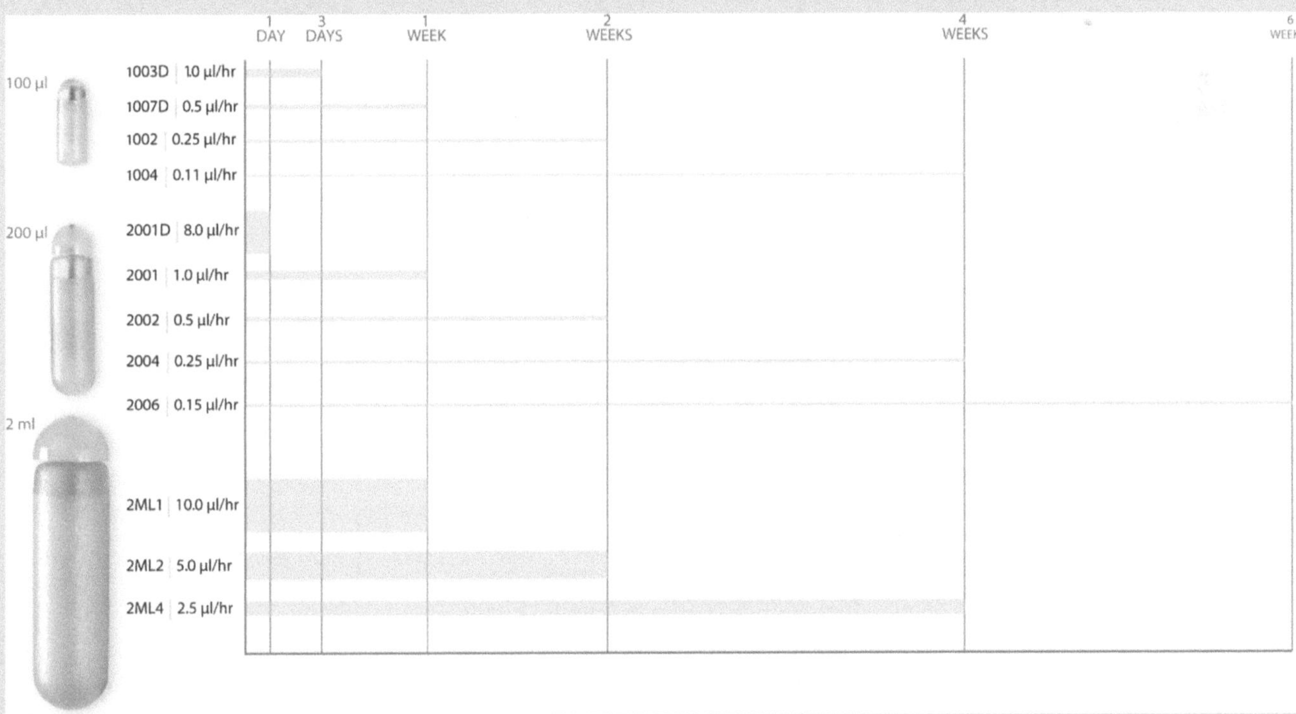

FIGURE CS 10.3 Release rates and durations for all ALZET pumps. Individual lots of pumps will vary from this target within limits. The specific data for each lot of pumps should be used for dose calculations. *From DURECT Corporation. Specifications. Available from: https://www.alzet.com/products/alzet_pumps/specifications/, with permission from the DURECT Corporation.*

Continued

Case Study V: The legend of ALZA Corporation *(cont'd)*

The DUROS implant is an osmotically driven system developed by ALZA Corporation to provide long-term and controlled drug delivery. The first pharmaceutical product used the DUROS technology was Viadur (leuprolide acetate implant). It provides zero-order delivery of leuprolide which is a synthetic nonapeptide gonadotropin-releasing hormone (GnRH) agonist [19]. Unfortunately, the marketing of Viadur was discontinued due to the "limited long-term market viability" [20]. The DUROS implant has also been used for the delivery of other potent biomolecules including those that have a narrow therapeutic window or a short half-life [19]. For example, it has been used for delivering sufentanil for chronic pain management (Chronogesic Sufentanil Pain Therapy System) (Fig. CS 10.4) [21].

Acutrim (withdrawn by FDA), Efidac/24, Efidac 24 Chlorpheniramine, and Volmax (no longer available in the U.S.) are(were) some of the marketed products based on ALZA's EOPs [9,23]. Two main multilayer (multicompartment) osmotically-controlled release oral delivery systems (OROS) have been developed by ALZA Corporation, and are push-pull and push-stick osmotic pumps (PPOP and PSOP) [24]. Procardia XL was one of the first drugs using PPOP for extended release of nifedipine for the treatment of hypertension and angina. In 1992, Procardia XL became the first ALZA-developed product to reach $1 billion in annual sales [25]. PPOP coated with enteric coating without a special onset (OROS-CT) can be used for colon targeting. The OROS-CT system can contain one or multiple push-pull units encapsulated within a hard gelatin capsule. The enteric coating dissolves in the higher pH environment (intestinal region) and allows the drug release [24,26]. COER-24 (controlled onset extended release), mimicking the body's typical 24-hour circadian variations in blood pressure and heart rate, was specially designed to deliver verapamil (Covera HS) [24,27]. PSOP is particularly useful for delivering high doses of water-insoluble drugs. PSOP is longitudinally compressed with one large orifice for the delivery of a high payload. The drug is released as a wet mass that requires subsequent disintegration and dissolution [28]. Concerta uses the PSOP system to deliver methylphenidate HCl for attention deficit hyperactivity disorder treatment in adults and children ages 6 and older. The system comprises an osmotically active trilayer core surrounded by a semipermeable membrane with an immediate-release drug overcoat (Figs. CS 10.5 and 10.6.). The trilayer core is composed of two drug layers and a push layer. Upon administration, the drug overcoat dissolves first and then the drug releases from the core. The release

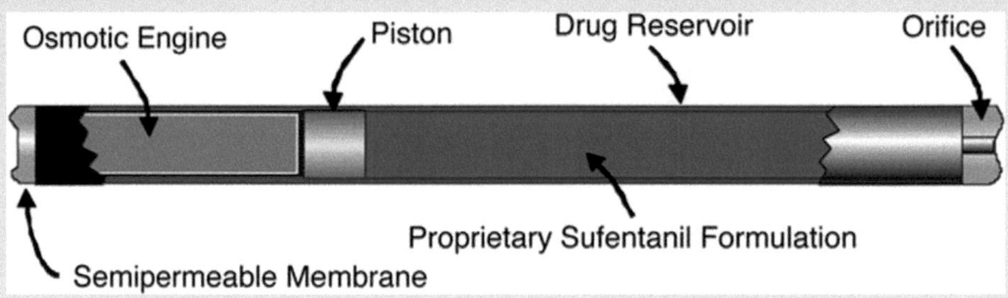

FIGURE CS 10.4 A cross section of the Chronogesic Sufentanil Pain Therapy System. *From Fisher, Dennis M., N. Kellett, and R. Lenhardt,* Pharmacokinetics of an implanted osmotic pump delivering sufentanil for the treatment of chronic pain. *Anesthesiology, 2003.* ***99****(4): p. 929-937, with permission from Wolters Kluwer Health, Inc.*

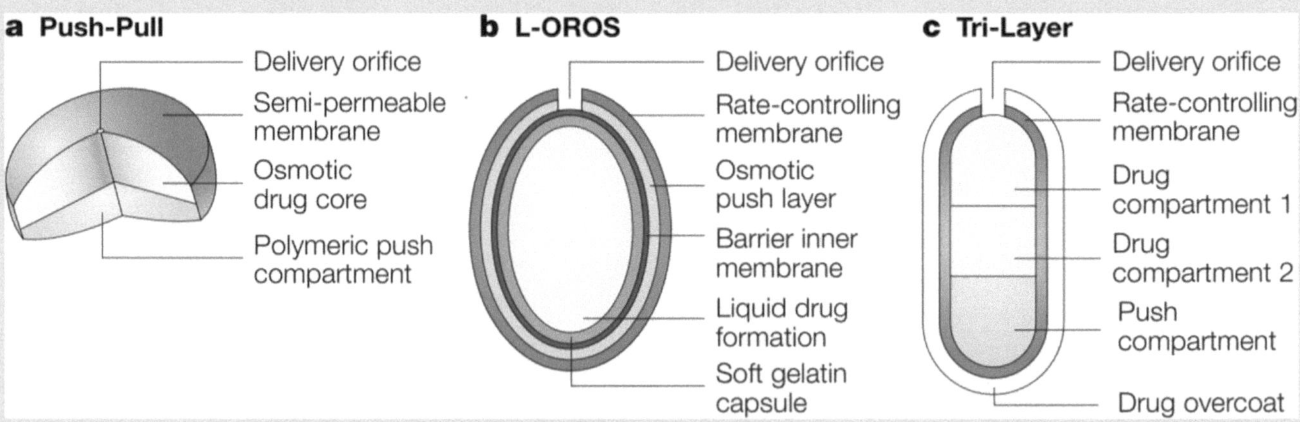

FIGURE CS 10.5 Various controlled-release OROS delivery systems. *From Rosen, H. and T. Abribat,* The rise and rise of drug delivery. *Nat. Rev. Drug Discov, 2005.* ***4****(5): p. 381-385, with permission from Springer Nature.*

Case Study V: The legend of ALZA Corporation *(cont'd)*

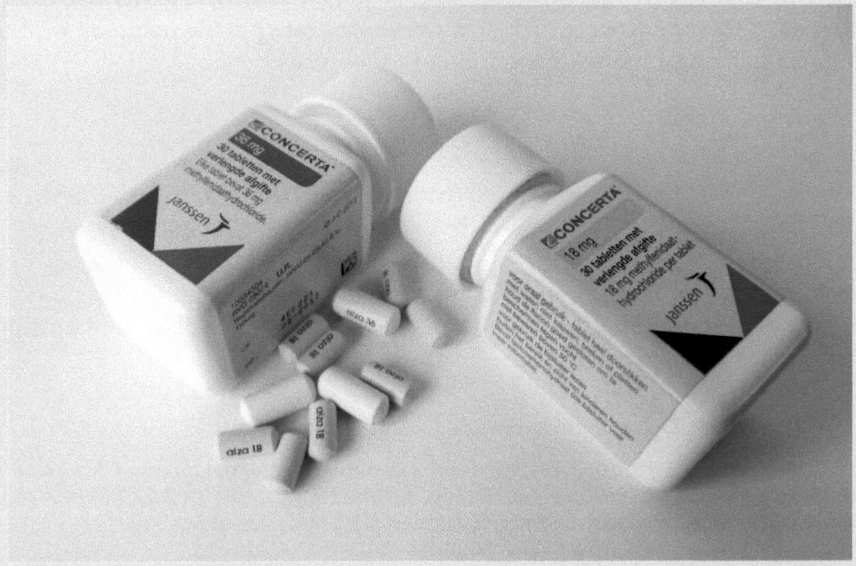

FIGURE CS 10.6 Photo of Concerta 18 and 36-mg tablets. The part "alza" on the tablet indicates ALZA's patented osmotic-controlled release oral delivery system is used, and the number specifies the drug dose. *From Studio. Cobalt/Shutterstock.com.*

rate increases with time due to the drug concentration gradient applied to the two drug layers [29,30]. Recently, there have been concerns over the clinical differences between Concerta and its generics, as well as differences among the generics themselves [31–33].

Regarding capsule-based osmotic systems, Chronset was developed as a pulse-delivery system releasing mucoadhesive particles containing peptides or proteins. Osmet was designed as a miniature osmotic pump to deliver a drug as bolus or over 8 hr in the colon [24]. The liquid osmotic system (L-OROS) was developed by ALZA to overcome drug solubility issues. They are available to provide controlled delivery of liquid, liquid-liquid emulsion, or solid suspension drug formulations (Fig. CS 10.5) [23,24,27].

Review and practice questions

1. What is osmosis? And what is osmotic pressure?
2. Ten grams of mannitol (Mw = 182.17 g/mol) is dissolved in 1 liter of water at 22°C. What is the osmotic pressure of this solution?
3. What is the working mechanism of the osmotic-controlled delivery system designed by Rose and Nelson?
4. Why is there an optimum orifice size range?
5. What is the working mechanism of an elementary osmotic drug delivery system?
6. What is the working mechanism of a push-pull system?
7. *Assume that there is a drug that has an aqueous solubility of 1.2 g/mL and a diffusion coefficient of $5 \times 10^{-6}\ cm^2/s$ in a solution with viscosity of 5 cp. You intend to deliver this drug at a zero-order delivery rate of 24.84 mg/hr by using an elementary osmotic pump which has the following features:

$$dV/dt = 0.1\ mL/h \quad F = 40$$

$$L = 250\ \mu m \quad \Delta P_{max} = 5\ atm$$

* *Adapted from Kydonieus AF, editor. Treatise on Controlled Drug Delivery: Fundamentals-optimization-applications 1992: CRC Press by permission of Taylor and Francis Group, LLC, a division of Informa plc.*

Determine the maximum and minimum boundary conditions for the cross-sectional area (A_0) of the delivery orifice for the pump to be developed.

8. *Assume that there is a drug that has an aqueous solubility of 500 mg/mL and gives an osmotic pressure of 20 atm when it is totally dissolved. You want to deliver it at a zero-order rate profile using an oral osmotic pump that is coated with a semipermeable membrane with the following features:

$$A = 2.0\ \text{cm}^2 \quad h = 400\ \mu\text{m}$$

$$L_p = 10^{-3}\ \text{cm}^2/(\text{h} \times \text{atm})\ \sigma = 0.95$$

Calculate the oral delivery rate for this drug.

9. What are design considerations for osmotic-controlled drug delivery systems?

10. Classify the osmotic pumps discussed in this chapter into two groups: implantable pumps and oral pumps.

References

[1] Kydonieus AF, editor. Treatise on controlled drug delivery: fundamentals-optimization-applications. CRC Press; 1992.

[2] Almoshari Y. Osmotic pump drug delivery systems: a comprehensive review. Pharmaceuticals 2022;15(11):1430.

[3] Li X, Jasti BR, editors. Design of controlled release drug delivery systems. McGraw-Hill; 2005.

[4] Rose S, Nelson J. A continuous long-term injector. Aust J Exp Biol Med Sci 1955;33(4):415–20.

[5] Khavare NB, et al. A review on key parameters and components in designing of osmotic controlled oral drug delivery systems. Indian J Nov Drug Deliv 2010;2:122–31.

[6] Gupta BP, et al. Osmotically controlled drug delivery system with associated drugs. J Pharm Pharm Sci 2010;13(4):571–88.

[7] Theeuwes F, Higuchi T. Osmatic dispensing device for releasing beneficial agent. ALZA CORP; 1972. Available from: https://patents.google.com/patent/US3845770A/en.

[8] Verma RK, Krishna DM, Garg S. Formulation aspects in the development of osmotically controlled oral drug delivery systems. J Control Release 2002;79(1):7–27.

[9] Verma RK, Mishra B, Garg S. Osmotically controlled oral drug delivery. Drug Dev Ind Pharm 2000;26(7):695–708.

[10] Liu L, Xu X. Preparation of bilayer-core osmotic pump tablet by coating the indented core tablet. Int J Pharm 2008;352(1):225–30.

[11] Control Micro Systems (CMS Laser). *Our technology.* Available from: https://cmslaser.com/products/specialized-laser-systems/pharmaceutical-laser-systems/laser-systems-for-tablet-research-development/.

[12] Johnson & Johnson. *Johnson & Johnson announces completion of merger with ALZA corporation.* Available from: https://johnsonandjohnson.gcs-web.com/news-releases/news-release-details/johnson-johnson-announces-completion-merger-alza-corporation.

[13] Barratt G, Puisieux F. Takeru Higuchi, the man and the scientist. Int J Pharm 2011;418(1):3–5.

[14] Higuchi T, Leeper HM. Osmotic dispenser. Alza Corporation; 1973. Available from: https://patents.google.com/patent/US3995632A/en.

[15] Higuchi T, Leeper HM. Osmotic dispenser with means for dispensing active agent responsive to osmotic gradient. Alza Corporation; 1976. Available from: https://patents.google.com/patent/US3995631A/en.

[16] Higuchi T, Leeper HM. Improved osmotic dispenser employing magnesium sulphate and magnesium chloride. 1973. Available from: https://patents.google.com/patent/US3760804A/en.

[17] DURECT Corporation. *Company.* Available from: https://www.alzet.com/company/.

[18] Theeuwes F, Yum SI. Principles of the design and operation of generic osmotic pumps for the delivery of semisolid or liquid drug formulations. Ann Biomed Eng 1976;4(4):343–53.

[19] Wright J, et al. Long-term controlled delivery of therapeutic agents via an implantable osmotically driven system: the DUROS Implant. In: Rathbone M, Hadgraft J, editors. Modified-release drug delivery technology. CRC Press; 2003. p. 657–69.

[20] PharmaTimes. *Bayer discontinues Viadur due to 'diminished market demand'.* Available from: https://www.pharmatimes.com/news/bayer_discontinues_viadur_due_to_diminished_market_demand_991681.

[21] Fisher DM, Kellett N, Lenhardt R. Pharmacokinetics of an implanted osmotic pump delivering sufentanil for the treatment of chronic pain. Anesthesiology 2003;99(4):929–37.

[22] DURECT Corporation. *Specifications.* Available from: https://www.alzet.com/products/alzet_pumps/specifications/.

[23] Keraliya RA, et al. Osmotic drug delivery system as a part of modified release dosage form. ISRN Pharm 2012;2012:528079.

[24] Malaterre V, et al. Oral osmotically driven systems: 30 years of development and clinical use. Eur J Pharm Biopharm 2009;73(3):311–23.

[25] Company-Histories.com. *ALZA Corporation.* Available from: https://www.company-histories.com/ALZA-Corporation-Company-History.html.

[26] Philip AK, Philip B. Colon targeted drug delivery systems: a review on primary and novel approaches. Oman Med J 2010;25(2):79–87.

[27] Baldi A. Recent technological advancements in multiparticulate formulations: the smart drug delivery systems. Asian J Pharm 2015;9(4):481.

[28] Qiu Y, Lee PI. Chapter 19 - Rational design of oral modified-release drug delivery systems. In: Qiu Y, et al., editors. Developing solid oral dosage forms. 2nd ed. Academic Press; 2017. p. 519–54.

[29] Connor DF, Steingard RJ. New formulations of stimulants for attention-deficit hyperactivity disorder. CNS Drugs 2004;18(14):1011–30.

[30] Swanson J, et al. Development of a new once-a-day formulation of methylphenidate for the treatment of attention-deficit/hyperactivity disorder: proof-of-concept and proof-of-product studies. Arch Gen Psychiatry 2003;60(2):204–11.

[31] Fallu A, et al. A randomized, double-blind, cross-over, phase IV trial of oros-methylphenidate (CONCERTA®) and generic novo-methylphenidate ER-C (NOVO-generic). Ther Adv Psychopharmacol 2016;6(4):237–51.

[32] U.S. Food and Drug Administration. *Questions and answers regarding methylphenidate hydrochloride extended release tablets (generic Concerta) made by Mallinckrodt and UCB/Kremers Urban (formerly Kudco)*. Available from: https://www.fda.gov/drugs/drug-safety-and-availability/questions-and-answers-regarding-methylphenidate-hydrochloride-extended-release-tablets-generic.

[33] Lally MD, Kral MC, Boan AD. Not all generic concerta is created equal: comparison of OROS versus non-OROS for the treatment of ADHD. Clin Pediatr 2016;55(13):1197–201.

[34] Rosen H, Abribat T. The rise and rise of drug delivery. Nat Rev Drug Discov 2005;4(5):381–5.

CHAPTER

11

Targeted drug delivery systems

Wujie Zhang

LEARNING OBJECTIVES

- To understand drug targeting
- To discuss the requirements for effective drug targeting
- To discuss different types of drug targets
- To interpret the working mechanisms of physically targeted drug delivery systems
- To interpret the working mechanisms of passive and active targeted drug delivery systems
- To discuss the difference between passive and active targeting
- To design the physically targeted drug delivery systems
- To design the passive and active targeted drug delivery systems

11.1 Requirements for effective drug targeting

The concept of drug targeting can be traced back to the "magic bullet" theory. More than a century ago, Paul Ehrlich, the founder of chemotherapy, postulated the creation of "magic bullets" for selectively targeting a pathogen without harming the host organism [1,2]. Targeted drug delivery systems deliver drug(s) to a specific site rather than the whole body or organ, improving the therapy's effectiveness while reducing the side effects. In general, targeted drug delivery results in increased efficacy, modulated pharmacokinetics, controlled biodistribution, increased specificity of location, decreased toxicity, reduced dose, and improved patient compliance [2]. Additionally, targeted drug delivery systems can be used to improve precision medicines [3].

For a targeted drug delivery system, the following requirements should be met:

1. High loading efficiency: Drug carriers are often involved in targeted drug delivery systems; hence, it is critical to have a high loading efficiency to ensure the required dosage reaches the targeting site.
2. Successful targeting (location): The majority of the drugs should reach the target site following the "expected" targeting approach(es). The premature release of drug(s) should be minimal to avoid systemic drug delivery.
3. Drug release at the targeted site (timing): Upon reaching the targeted site, drug release should start, in particular, triggered by the site-specific environment. Additionally, an insufficient amount of drug(s) released at the site will not lead to the desired therapeutic effects.

Fundamentals and Design of Drug Delivery Systems
https://doi.org/10.1016/B978-0-443-23521-4.00011-4

4. Biocompatible carrier: Again, drug carriers are commonly used to assist targeted drug delivery. The carrier should be biocompatible. Moreover, the "fate" of the carrier should also be considered, especially for those that are not biodegradable.
5. High manufacturability: The manufacturability should be considered for commercialization of the targeted drug delivery systems. Some of the considerations of the manufacturability are complexity, Current Good Manufacturing Practice (cGMP) compliance, and cost-effectiveness.

11.2 Design of targeted drug delivery systems: targets and ligands

Based on the types of targets, drug targeting can be classified into different orders. First-order targeting refers to the restricted distribution to the capillary bed of the targeted organ/tissue. Second-order and third-order targetings indicate targeting specific cells and intracellular sites, respectively. Fourth-order targeting refers to the targeting of macromolecules [2]. To select a disease-specific receptor, there are different factors to consider: receptor expression profile (ratio of targeted receptor expression in diseased versus normal tissues), receptor location (cell-surface receptors are generally preferred over intracellular ones), receptor internalization (whether receptor internalization is desired should be taken into consideration); receptor topography (e.g., allowing for high affinity/specificity binding), and receptor competition (competition with the receptor's natural ligand(s) should be considered) [4].

Various substances, i.e., ligands (targeting moieties), have been used for targeting, including proteins/peptides and aptamers.

Proteins. Antibodies, especially monoclonal antibodies (mAbs), and antibody fragments are commonly used. Among all the mAbs immunoglobulins (Ig) subtypes, IgA, IgD, IgE, IgG, and IgM, IgG is the most relevant for therapies. As shown in Fig. 11.1, IgG contains two separate identical heavy chains (H) and light chains (L). The top part is Fab (fragment, antigen binding) and the base is Fc (fragment, crystalline). Fc region is preferably removed because it triggers antibody-dependent cytotoxicity in the body [5–7]. The antibody's binding region allows selective targeting of certain cells [7]. Drugs can be directly conjugated to antibodies for targeted therapies. Besides antibodies, other proteins, such as transferrin (Tf), have also been used as targeting moieties. The transferrin receptor (TfR) functions in iron uptake through its interaction with Tf (Fig. 11.2) *via* Tf-mediated endocytosis. TfR is upregulated on the surface of many types of cancer cells [8]. Tf has been applied for targeted drug delivery through Tf-drug conjugates and Tf-modified carriers [8]. Moreover, Tf-based delivery systems increase the permeability across a variety of biological

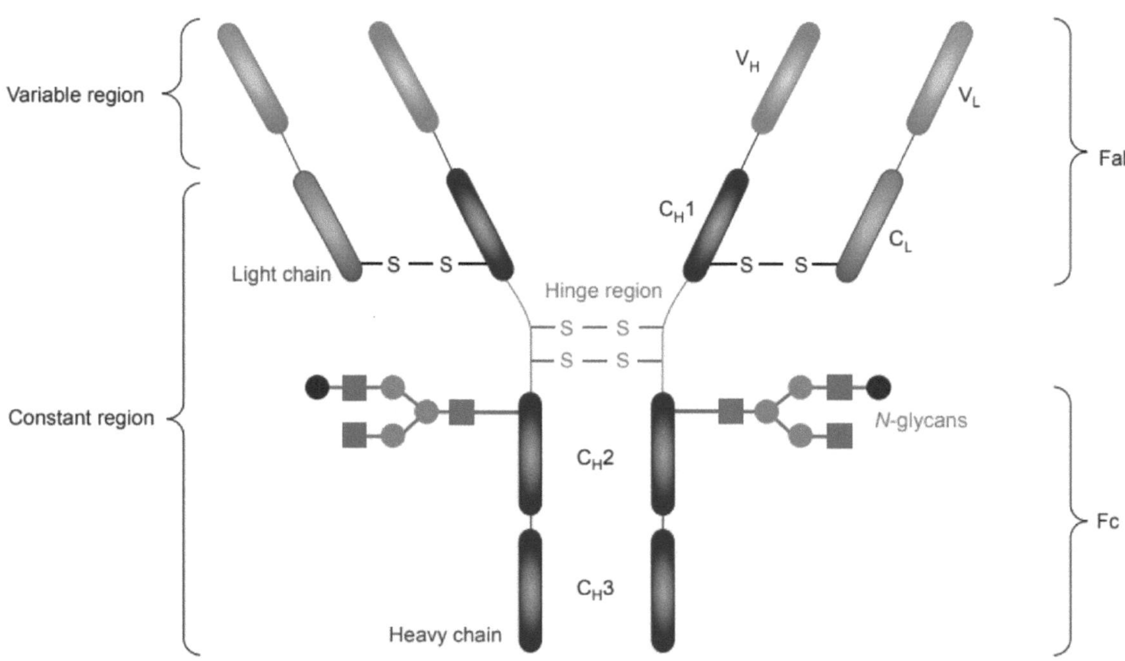

FIGURE 11.1 General structure of IgG1. Fab arms comprise the antigen-binding region and consist of the whole light chain (V_L and C_L) and part of the heavy chain (V_H and C_H^1). Fc consists of identical C_H^2 and C_H^3 fragments. From Chudasama, V., A. Maruani, and S. Caddick, *Recent advances in the construction of antibody–drug conjugates.* Nat. Chem, 2016. **8**(2): p. 114-119, with permission from Springer Nature.

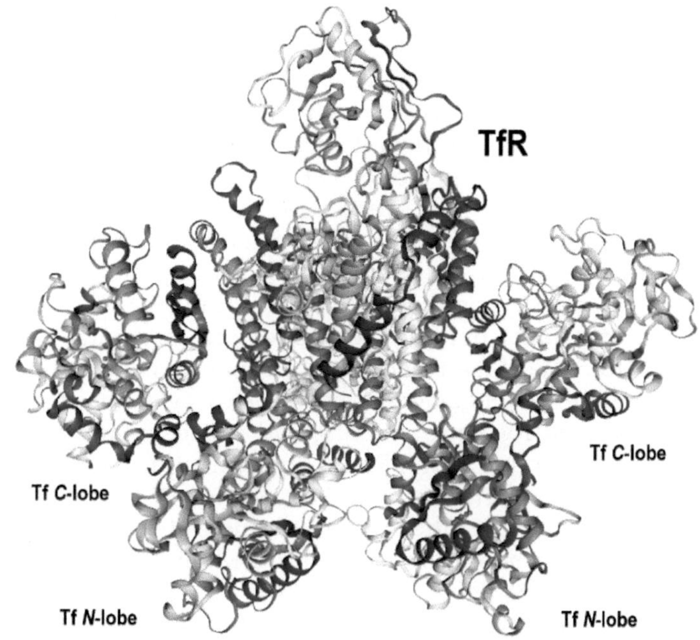

FIGURE 11.2 Structure of human transferrin receptor-transferrin complex: human transferrin receptor (TfR; *center*) bound by two diferric transferrin molecules (Tf). Created with the PDB ID 1SUV and associated publication (From Cheng, Y. et.al., *Structure of the human transferrin receptor-transferrin complex*. Cell, 2004. **116**(4): p. 565-576. Available from: https://doi.org/10.1016/s0092-8674(04)00130-8), NGL Viewer (Rose, A.S. et al., *NGL viewer: web-based molecular graphics for large complexes*. Bioinformatics, 2018. https://doi.org/10.1093/bioinformatics/bty419), and RCSB PDB.

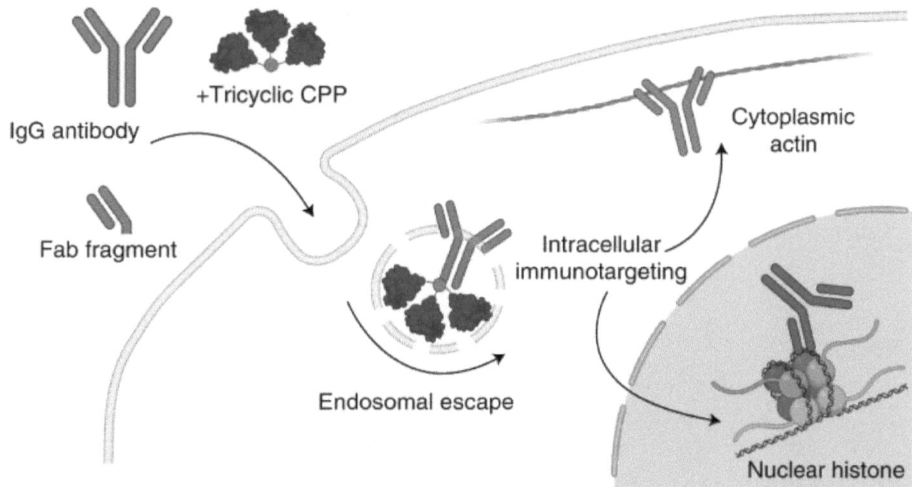

FIGURE 11.3 Mechanism of tricyclic CPPs for intracellular delivery of functional antibodies and Fab fragments. From Tietz, O. et al., *Tricyclic cell-penetrating peptides for efficient delivery of functional antibodies into cancer cells*. Nat. Chem, 2022. **14**(3): p. 284-293, with permission from Springer and Nature.

barriers, such as across the blood-brain barrier through transcytosis. For example, Tf-conjugated nanoparticles can be potentially used for therapy of gliomas [9]. Interestingly, Tf incorporation has been shown to reduce drug resistance and adverse effects of doxorubicin, one of the most commonly used chemotherapeutic drugs [10].

Peptides. Due to their production efficiency and stability in physiological environments, peptides are popular alternatives to antibodies and other proteins for targeting [5,11]. Cell-penetrating peptides (CPPs) are good examples as they are easily internalized across the cell membrane and have excellent transduction efficiency and low cytotoxicity [12]. For example, tricyclic cell—penetrating peptides have been used for efficient delivery of functional antibody Fab fragments into cancer cells (both cytosol and nuclei) at effective concentrations as low as 1 μm (Fig. 11.3) [13].

In general, the higher the specificity, the lower the possibility of having nonspecific reactions and causing side effects [11]. Moreover, positively charged peptides containing arginine (Arg; R) and lysine (Lys; K) residues are preferred for cellular uptake and complexation with nucleic acids. In particular, Arg residues are more advantageous for cellular uptake compared with other positively charged residues, such as Lys [5]. All methods available for targeting peptide selection are based on the screen libraries containing random short amino acid sequences [11]. Angiopep-2, a synthetic peptide with the sequence of TFFYGGSRGKRNNFKTEEY, has been designed to specifically interact with low-density lipoprotein receptor–related protein 1 (LRP1) receptors, which are of great interest for the crossing of the blood-brain barrier and treatment of brain cancer and brain metastases [4,14].

Aptamers. The term "aptamers" is from the Latin word *aptus* (fitting) and the Greek word *meros* (part) [15]. Nucleic acid aptamers are short, chemically synthesized, single-stranded RNA or DNA oligonucleotides that fold into unique three-dimensional structures, binding their target with structural recognition in a manner similar to an antibody-antigen interaction [16]. One of the advantages of aptamers is their short time (within minutes) to be regenerated upon denaturation compared to day(s) for antibodies. However, nuclease activity is a concern for RNA aptamers [17]. Aptamers have been used for both targeting and intracellular drug delivery [18]. Aptamers are selected from a pool of random single-stranded DNA/RNA oligonucleotides through iterative rounds of selection and amplification by the process called Systematic Evolution of Ligands by Exponential Enrichment (SELEX) (Fig. 11.4). SELEX involves three major steps: (1) the binding of single-stranded DNA/RNA to the target, (2) the partitioning of bound DNA/RNA from unbound ones, and (3) the amplification of DNA/RNA with an affinity for the target [19]. Novel methods have been developed to improve the efficiency [20] as well as select aptamers with programmed affinities, such as Pro-SELEX [21]. There are aptamers-based therapies in the market or under clinical trials. Take pegaptanib sodium, for example; it is a PEGylated aptamer that binds to vascular endothelial growth factor (VEGF) with high affinity and selectivity (Fig. 11.5) [22]. Inhibiting neovascularization, pegaptanib sodium has been approved by the Food and Drug Administration for the treatment of neovascular age-related muscular degeneration [23].

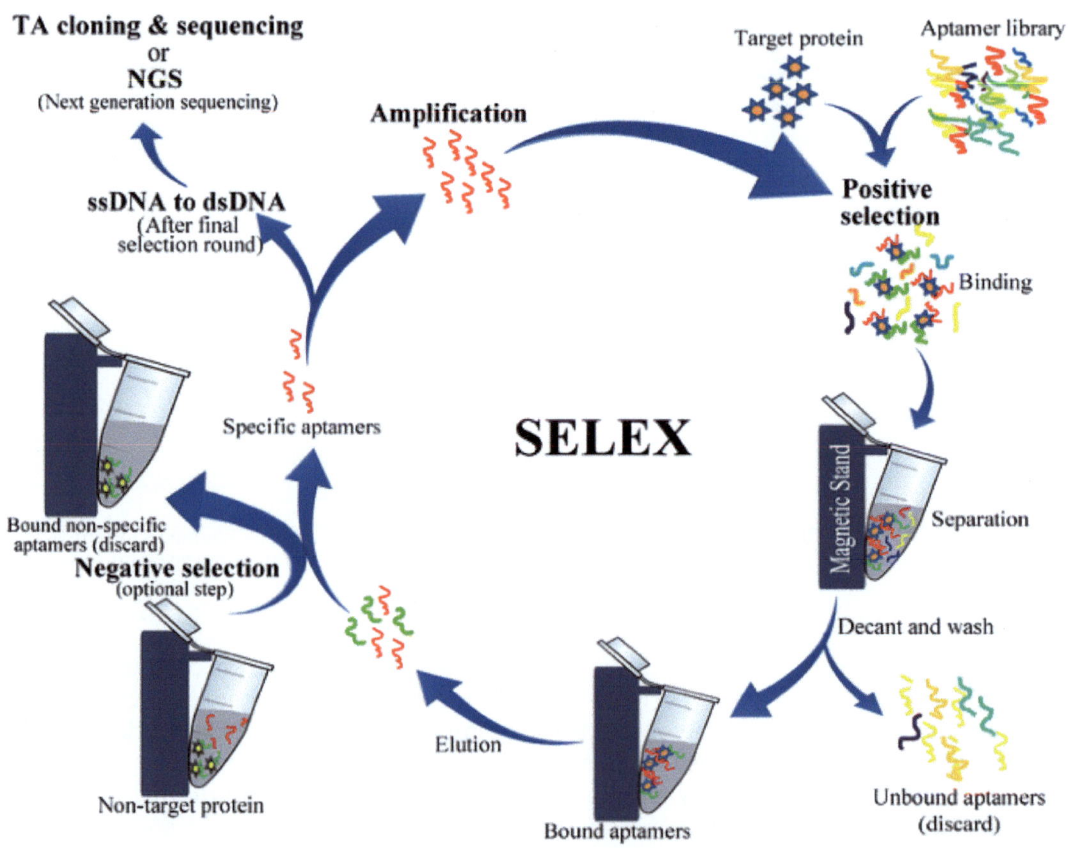

FIGURE 11.4 Schematic of Systematic Evolution of Ligands with Exponential Enrichment (SELEX). From Chandola, C. et al., *Application of aptamers in diagnostics, drug-delivery and imaging*. **J.** Biosci, 2016. **41**(3): p. 535-561, with permission from Springer and Nature.

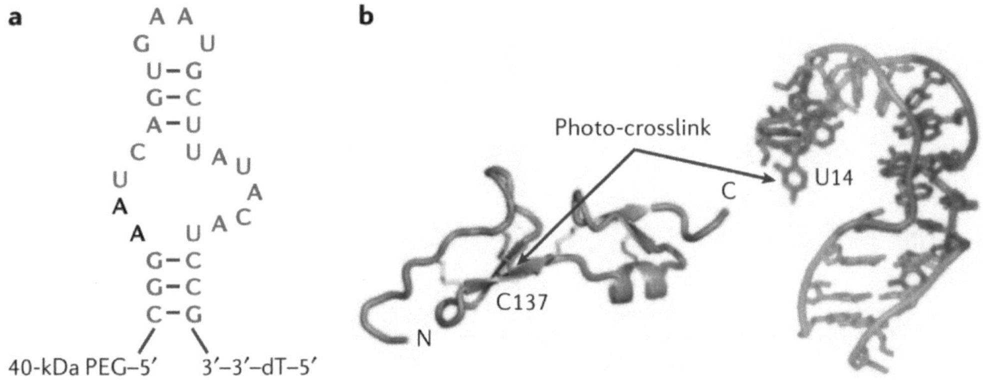

FIGURE 11.5 Pegaptanib structure and target binding. (a) Sequence and predicted secondary structure of pegaptanib. (b) Interaction between the heparin-binding domain of VEGF *(gray)* and pegaptanib *(blue)*. From Ng EWM, et al. Pegaptanib, a targeted anti-VEGF aptamer for ocular vascular disease. Nat Rev Drug Discov 2006;5(2):123–32, with permission from Springer and Nature.

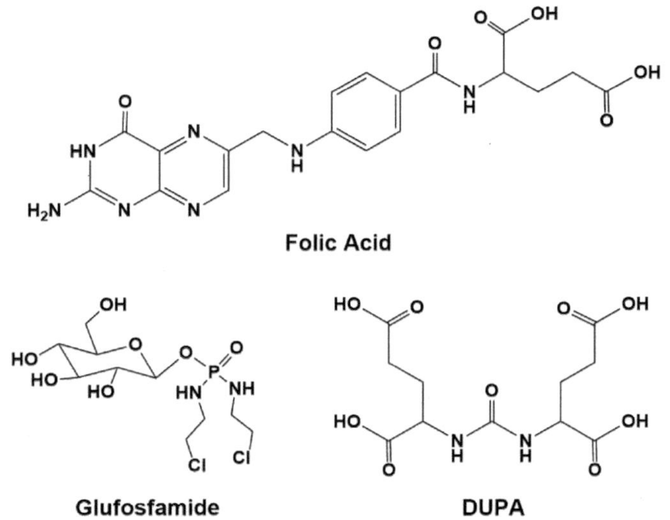

FIGURE 11.6 Chemical structure of some low-molecular-weight ligands.

Low molecular weight molecules. Molecules of low molecular weight have also been explored for targeting. Folic acid (vitamin B9; Fig. 11.6) has been applied for targeting specific cancer cell types (overexpression of folate receptors). Folate receptor–mediated endocytosis can also facilitate intracellular drug delivery [24]. Interestingly, chitosan oligosaccharide has been shown to be able to target the CD44 receptors commonly overexpressed on cancer stem-like cells but not those expressed on normal stem cells [25]. Glufosfamide (Fig. 11.6), a conjugate of glucose and an active alkylating moiety of ifosfamide targets cancer cells that primarily rely on aerobic glycolysis for ATP synthesis [4]. 2-[3-(1,3-Dicarboxypropyl)ureido]pentanedioic acid (DUPA; Fig. 11.6), has been used for targeting the prostate-specific membrane antigen (PSMA) [4,26].

Finally, when selecting a targeting ligand, a few factors should be considered to achieve high affinity and specificity. Ligand size and hydrophobicity may have the largest impact on the pharmacokinetics of a ligand-targeted drug. For example, the apparent tumor permeability of small molecules can be about 10 to 100 times faster than that of an antibody (Fig. 11.7) [4]. On the other hand, the larger ligands may have much longer circulation times. For small ligands, chemical conjugation may affect their affinity for their targets. Hence, ligand conjugation site chemistries should also be taken into account. Last, besides stability and manufacturability, ligand immunogenicity is also critical. Large ligands, such as antibodies, may trigger significant immune responses due to their "foreign" component/nature [4].

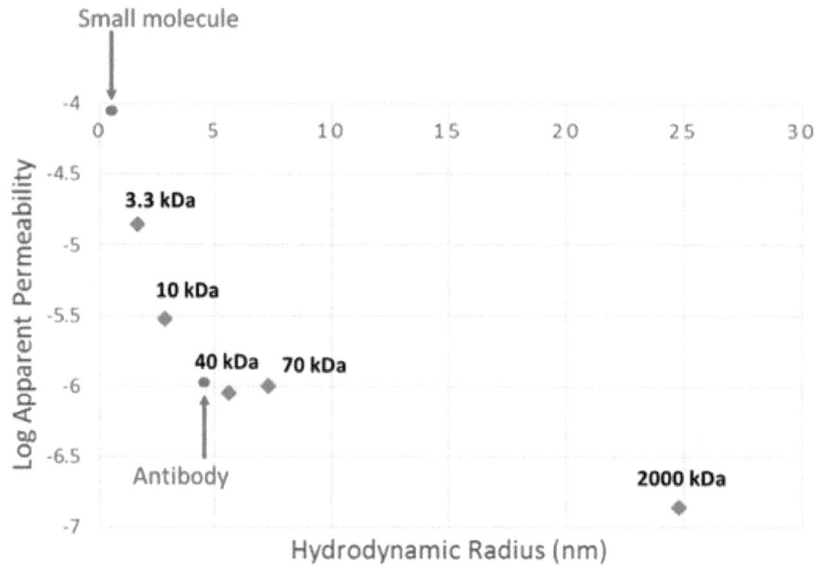

FIGURE 11.7 Effect of molecular size on tumor permeability. From Srinivasarao, M. and P.S. Low, *Ligand-targeted drug delivery*. Chem. Rev, 2017. **117**(19): p. 12133-12164. Copyright (2017), American Chemical Society.

11.3 Design of targeted drug delivery systems: physical targeting

Physical targeting uses various physical forces to accumulate/release therapeutic agents at the desired site(s) [5]. Physical forces include heat/cold, ultrasound, light, and electric and magnetic fields [5,27]. The advantages of physical triggering targeting strategies are minimal invasiveness and the unique capability of spatial targeting and spatiotemporal control [27].

Changing temperature is mostly used to release the drug at targeted sites. For example, thermal-responsive nanocarriers have been widely used for targeted drug release. One good example is Pluronic F-127–based nanocarriers. Pluronic is a copolymer of poly(propylene oxide) and poly(ethylene oxide) (Figs. 6.9 and 14.12). It forms micelles in aqueous solution when reaching the critical micelle concentration [25,28]. Interestingly, both mild hyperthermia (heat) [29] and cryoablation (cold) [30] have been applied to improve the therapeutic outcomes of the Pluronic F-127–based nanocarriers. Another good example is ThermoDox (lyso-thermosensitive liposomal doxorubicin). It is the first heat-activated formulation of a liposomal drug carrier to be utilized in human clinical trials [31]. The working mechanism of ThermoDOX in combination with radiofrequency ablation (RFA) is shown in Fig. 11.8. Unfortunately, the OPTIMA trial, evaluating ThermoDOX in combination with RFA for the treatment of hepatocellular carcinoma, was terminated in 2021. This is not considered as the failure of heat-triggered drug delivery systems, though (see Case Study VI) [32].

As mechanical longitudinal waves, ultrasound (US) has been used as a physical trigger to facilitate therapeutic agents across biological barriers. US can induce cavitations. Propagating US can lead to tissue displacements [27,33]. Cavitation bubbles collapse, releasing a shock wave, and may induce structural changes in the surroundings [34]. Cavitation can enhance stratum corneum (SC) permeability through spherical collapse near the SC surface, the impact of an acoustic micro-jet on the SC surface, and/or micro-jets physically penetrating into the SC (Fig. 11.9) [34,35]. Sonophoresis, the application of US (20 kHz to 1 MHz) has been used for transdermal drug delivery. Sonopermeation (200 kHz to 1 MHz) generally uses acoustically responsive agents, such as microbubbles, for enhancing the acoustic effects locally to the targeted sites [27]. In particular, the combination of US and microbubbles is a promising strategy to enhance vascular permeability, improving drug transport from blood to tissues (Figs. 11.10 and 11.11) [36,37]. Microbubbles can be filled with air or low-solubility gases or simply liquid droplets that change phase at body temperature [38]. Moreover, microbubbles are also commonly used for contrast agents and/or drug carriers [39,40]. To improve their targeting capability, the microbubbles can also be modified with ligands, such as folic acid

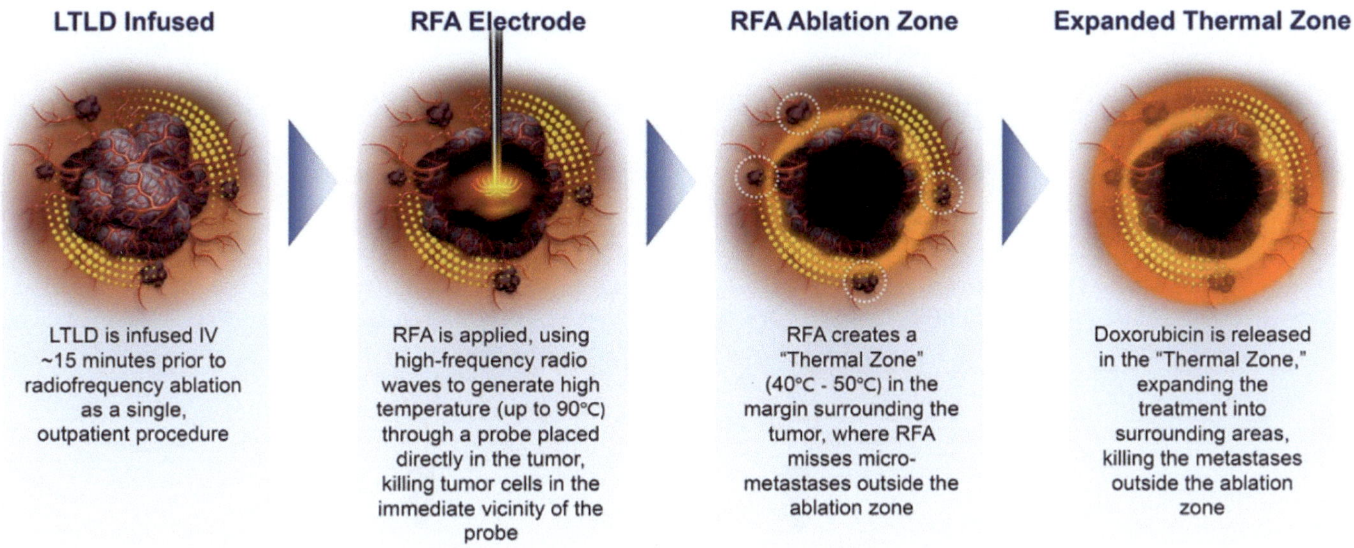

FIGURE 11.8 Working mechanism of ThermoDOX combined with RFA for cancer treatment. *LTLD*, Lyso-thermosensitive liposomal doxorubicin; *RFA*, radiofrequency ablation. From Borys, N. and M.W. Dewhirst, *Drug development of lyso-thermosensitive liposomal doxorubicin: Combining hyperthermia and thermosensitive drug delivery.* Adv. Drug Deliv. Rev, 2021. **178**: p. 113985.

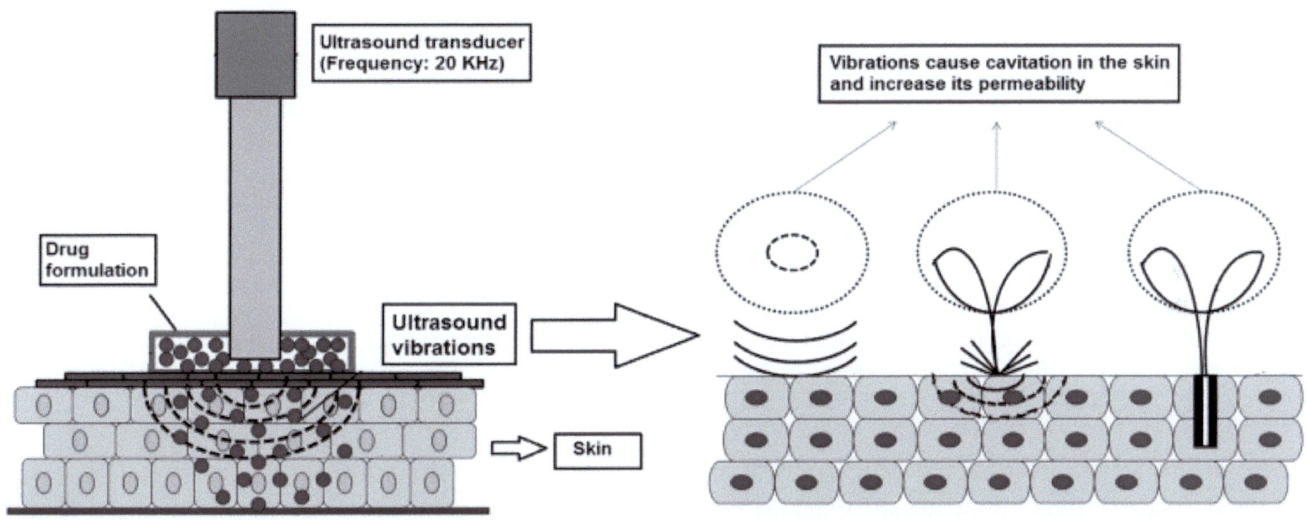

FIGURE 11.9 Possible models for enhanced skin permeability through cavitation. From Manikkath, J. et al., *Chapter 7-Peptide dendrimers in delivery of bioactive molecules to skin.* In: Hamblin MR, Avci P, Prow TW, Editors. *Nanoscience in dermatology.* Boston: Academic Press; 2016. p. 89-97, with permission from Elsevier.

[40]. The major advantages of using US as a physical trigger are high spatiotemporal targeting precision and deep tissue penetration [27].

Light is a form of electromagnetic radiation and can be applied directly for therapeutic intervention or through photosensitive agents for targeted effects [27]. Low-energy infrared exhibits the greatest penetration depth with 750-nm light penetrating about 5 mm below the skin's surface [41]. Light interacts with tissue through transmission, reflection, scattering, and absorption. The depth of penetration depends on absorption and scattering. Light is absorbed by chromophores (e.g., water and melanin). The amount of energy of a laser beam is inversely proportional to the wavelength, and as such the amount of energy available to be scattered [42,43] (Fig. 11.12). Light is mostly used

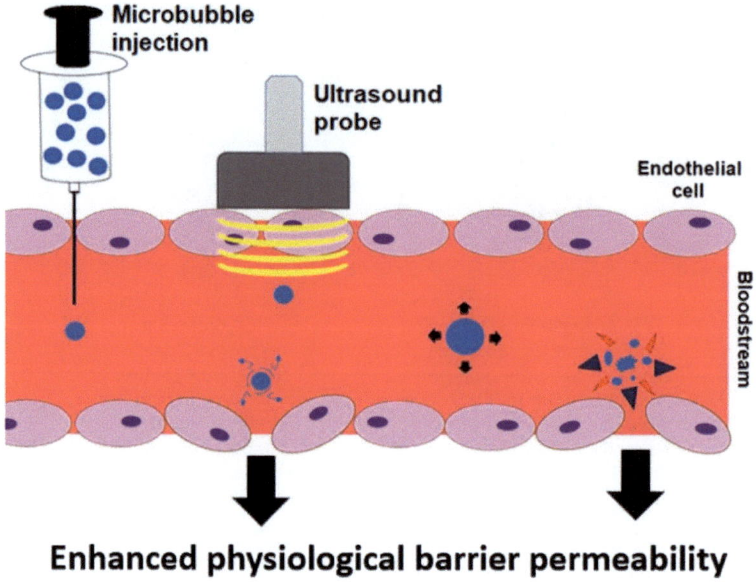

FIGURE 11.10 Impact of ultrasound-induced cavitation through microbubbles on cell membrane permeability: through either microstreaming induced by stable cavitation or microjets and shock waves caused by microbubble bursting. From Al-Jawadi, S. and S.S. Thakur, *Ultrasound-responsive lipid microbubbles for drug delivery: a review of preparation techniques to optimise formulation size, stability and drug loading.* Int. J. Pharm, 2020. **585**: p. 119559, with permission from Elsevier.

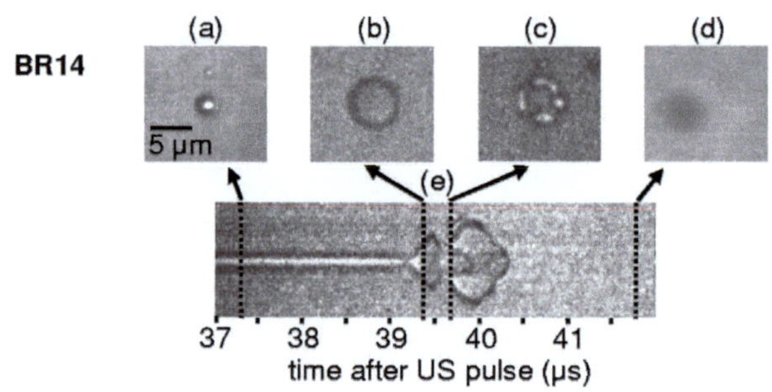

FIGURE 11.11 Destruction of BR 14 (a lipid-shelled US contrast agent filled with perfluorobutane). (a)-(d) Indicate the microbubble before, during, and after exposure to US, and (e) shows the streak image of microbubble width as a function of time. From Bloch, S.H. et al., *Optical observation of lipid- and polymer-shelled ultrasound microbubble contrast agents.* Appl. Phys. Lett, 2004. **84**(4): p. 631-633, with the permission of AIP Publishing.

for targeted release through photosensitive agents *via* photocleavage and photoisomerization. Photocleavage refers to light-induced disassembly or cleavage of molecules/systems [27]. The most common compounds involved are *ortho*-nitrobenzyl, coumarin, and pyrene derivatives. Nitrobenzyl can be cleaved to release a free carboxylic acid and nitrosobenzaldehyde upon UV irradiation (Fig. 11.13). The ester bonds in coumarin and pyrene derivatives can be cleaved into acid and aldehyde upon UV irradiation [27,44]. Photoisomerization is the *cis-trans* isomerization induced by light, and the process is reversible [27]. Photoisomerization changes the properties of a molecule, such as hydrophobicity. For example, azobenzene-containing molecules have been used for designing nanocarriers for specific delivery of cargo into cells [45]. During the *trans-cis* transition, azobenzene transforms from nonpolar to polar (Fig. 11.14). The major advantage of using light as a physical trigger is high spatiotemporal targeting precision. However, shallow tissue penetration and tissue damage can be caused by UV, and short wavelength light remains challenging [27].

Despite the concern over tissue damage and related local adverse events, several electrically based approaches have been developed for enhancing drug delivery across multiple biological barriers in both preclinical and clinical settings. Iontophoresis is the application of low-intensity electrical current around a drug reservoir to force the drug

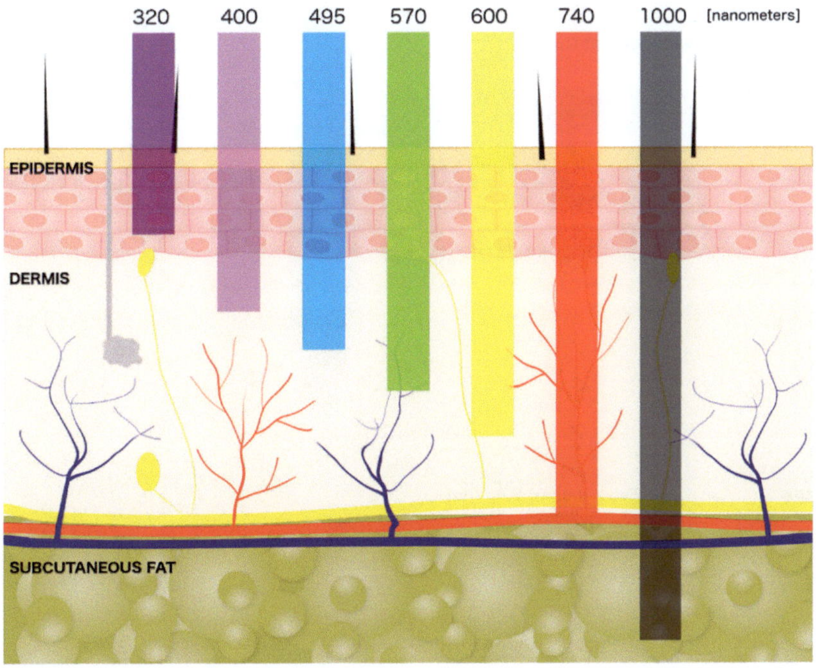

FIGURE 11.12 Dermal penetration by light of different wavelengths. From Cios, A. et al., *Effect of different wavelengths of laser irradiation on the skin cells*. Int. J. Mol. Sci, 2021. **22**(5): p. 2437.

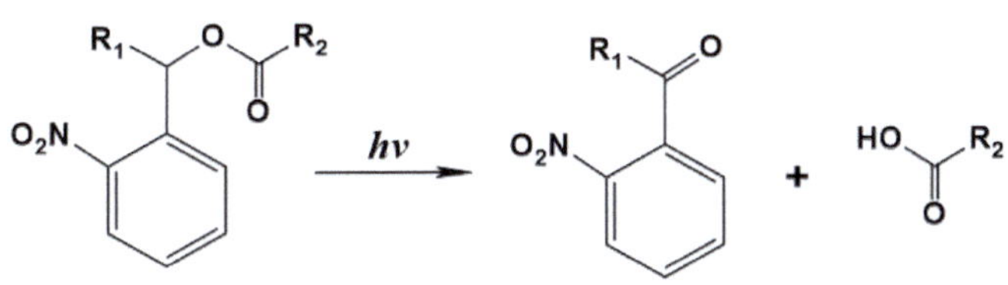

FIGURE 11.13 Photocleavage of the *ortho*-nitrobenzyl ester derivative.

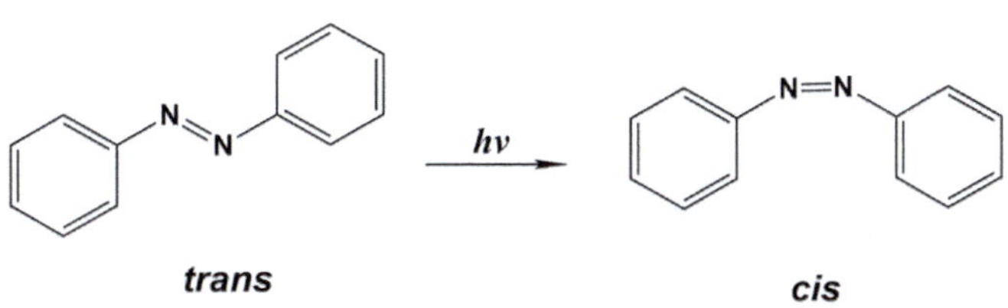

FIGURE 11.14 Photoisomerization of the azobenzene.

to be transported through adjacent biological barriers to the target tissues/organs in a noninvasive way. The system consists of a power supply (self-powered systems are of particular interest), a drug delivery electrode, and a returning electrode (Fig. 11.15) [46,47]. This method has been used for transdermal, ocular, buccal, and other types of drug delivery, especially when combined with microneedles and nanocarriers. Electroporation involving the rearrangement of cellular membranes under an electric pulse has also been used. The advantages of using electroporation for drug delivery include ease of operation and high adaptability to various drug types [27].

Unlike other physical triggers, magnetic approaches can be used to "guide" the delivery system to the targeted site by applying an external magnetic field. The other advantages include high spatiotemporal targeting precision and deep tissue penetration. However, the design of customized magnetic devices can be complicated [27]. The magnetic bioprobes, such as micro/nanoparticles, are commonly involved in magnetic drug delivery. Magnetic bioprobes need to possess high magnetization for efficient magnetic targeting [48]. The magnet systems used for drug targeting can be summarized into two groups: static field magnet systems (the magnetic field remains constant over time) and varying field magnet systems (the magnetic field changes with time) [49]. Drug release can be achieved through various routes, such as magnetic heating of temperature-sensitive drug carriers [50]. Magnetic

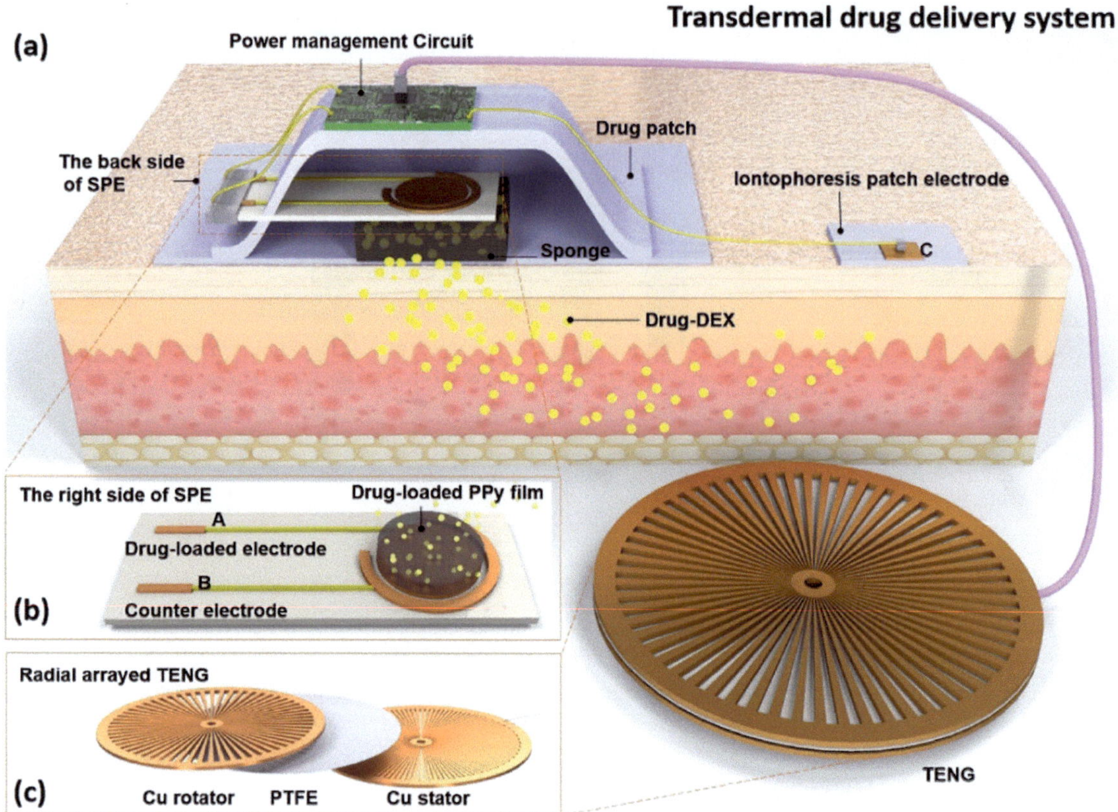

FIGURE 11.15 Schematic illustration of the self-powered, on-demand transdermal drug delivery system. (a) The system consisted of transdermal patches (drug patch and iontophoresis patch electrode), TENG, and power management circuit. (b) Right side of the SPE. (c) Radial-arrayed rotary TENG consists of two copper layers and one PTFE layer. *PTFE,* Polytetrafluoroethylene; *SPE,* screen printed electrode; *TENG,* portable triboelectric nanogenerator. From Ouyang, Q. et al., *Self-powered, on-demand transdermal drug delivery system driven by triboelectric nanogenerator.* Nano Energy, 2019. **62**: p. 610-619, with permission from Elsevier.

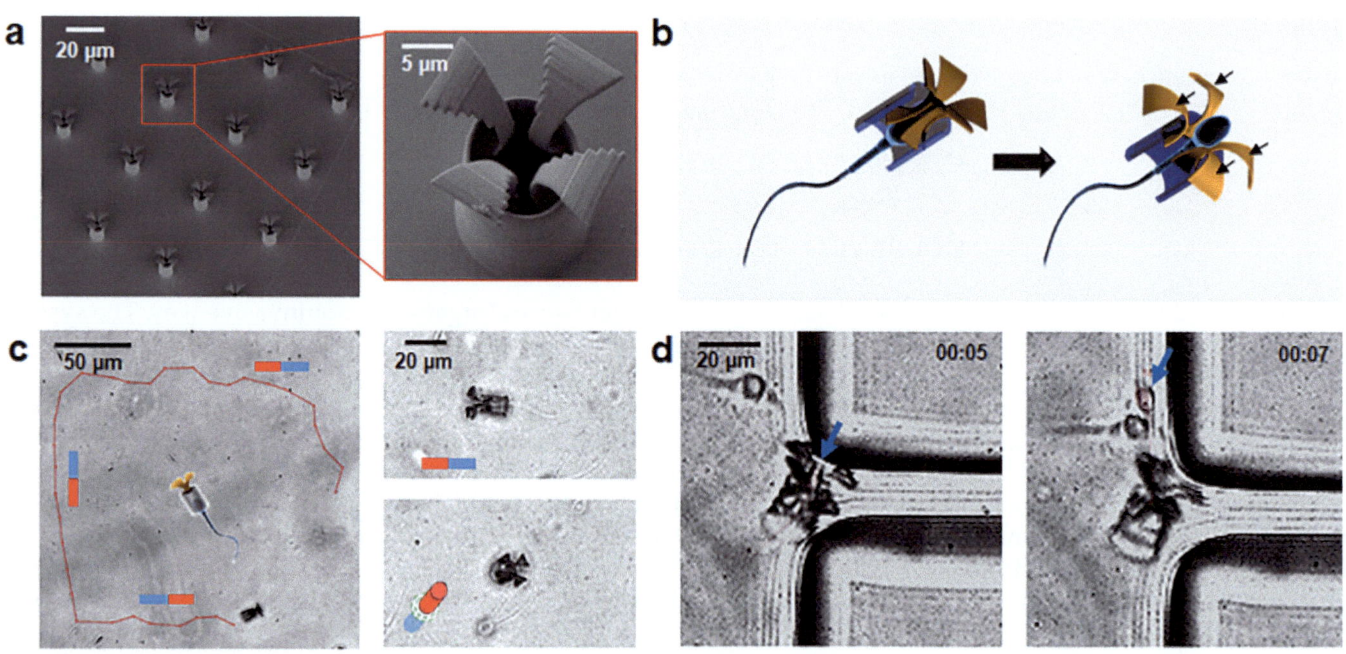

FIGURE 11.16 (a) SEM images of an array of printed tetrapod microstructures. (b) Schematic illustrating the mechanical release mechanism. (c) Track *(red line)* of a sperm-hybrid micromotor under magnetic guidance. (d) Image sequence of a sperm release process when the arms hit the corner of a polydimethilsiloxane wall. *Blue arrows* point at the sperm head. From Xu, H. et al., *Sperm-hybrid micromotor for targeted drug delivery.* ACS Nano, 2018. **12**(1): p. 327-337. Copyright (2018), American Chemical Society.

force has been applied to disrupt endothelial cell-cell junctions for controlled drug delivery [51]. A sperm-driven micromotor, guided magnetically, has been developed for targeted drug delivery (Fig. 11.16) [52]. In the design, sperm cells were utilized as drug carriers for potential treatment of cervical cancer and other gynecologic diseases. Sperm cells were chosen because they are naturally optimized to swim in the female reproductive system (propulsion source). Moreover, they can be used to carry hydrophilic drugs. To guide and release sperms, a magnetic microstructure was used [52].

To design a physically targeted drug delivery system, the target site should be considered first as it is a main consideration for choosing a physical trigger. Feasibility and cost should also be assessed since expensive and complex setups may be involved in activating the physical trigger. Once the physical trigger is determined, approaches to achieve the target ability (i.e., responsiveness to the physical trigger) of the drug delivery system should be considered. These approaches involve the incorporation of the photo-cleavable bond, application of the responsive drug carrier (e.g., microbubbles), and encapsulation/linking magnetic bioprobes. Additionally, it is always necessary to consider the approach of delivering the drug to the target site and accumulating the proper dose of the drug at the target site when designing a physical delivery system because most of the physical triggers are only used to achieve the target release of drug. Hence, it is beneficial to keep the drug delivery efficiency to the target site in mind.

11.4 Design of targeted drug delivery systems: passive and active targeting

Passive targeting is defined as the selective accumulation of a drug in a target site that has unique physiological characteristics relative to other tissues in the body, whereas active targeting involves modifying the surface of a drug carrier with a chemical or biological moiety that specifically binds to receptors or other cellular features highly expressed by cells of a target tissue/organ [5,53]. Fig. 11.17 summarizes passive organ targeting with drug delivery systems. As discussed in Chapter 4 (Section 4.4), the size of drug particles/drug carriers can be specifically controlled (e.g., ~ 3 μm) to achieve drug delivery to the deeper lung *via* inhalation considering the lung physiology/anatomy. The reticuloendothelial system (RES) is the portion of the immune system consisting of phagocytic cells found in reticular connective tissue in the spleen, liver, lungs, bone marrow, and lymph nodes [54]. The system also preferentially captures drug vesicles, such as nanoparticles, which has been used as a strategy of drug accumulation in the liver and spleen for treating tumors metastasized to the liver and spleen and parasitic infestation of the liver [54]. On the other hand, RES is a significant barrier for drug delivery (outside the liver and spleen). PEGylation has been used to reduce the interaction between drug carrier and phagocytes. Novel approaches include the RES-

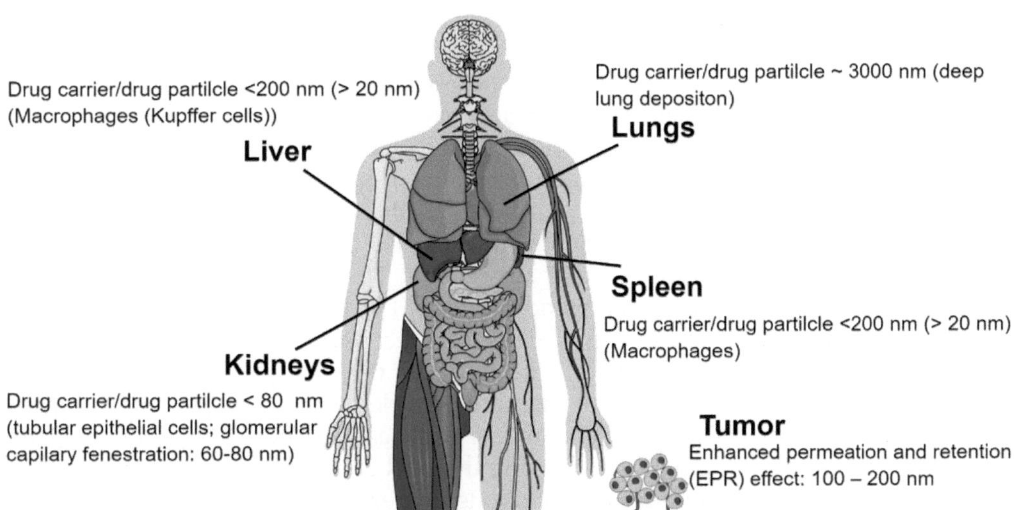

FIGURE 11.17 Passive organ targeting with drug delivery systems.

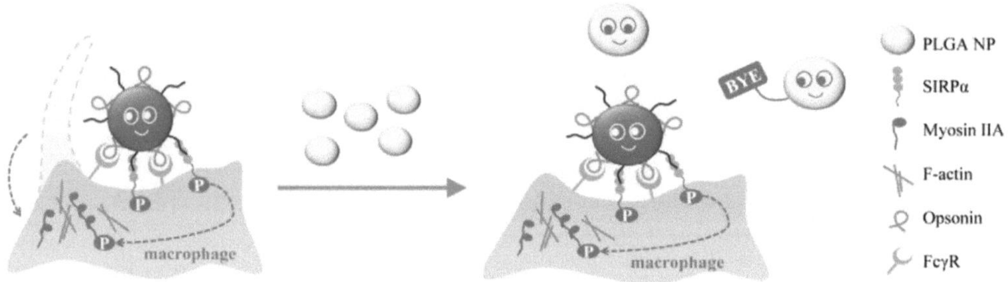

FIGURE 11.18 Schematic depicting PLGA nanoparticle (NP) escape from macrophage uptake after masking the macrophage surface with DSL. *DSL*, D-self-peptide—labeled liposome; *PLGA*, poly(lactic-*co*-glycolic acid). From Tang, Y., et al., *Overcoming the reticuloendothelial system barrier to drug delivery with a "don't-eat-us" strategy.* ACS Nano, 2019. **13**(11): p. 13015-13026. Copyright (2019), American Chemical Society.

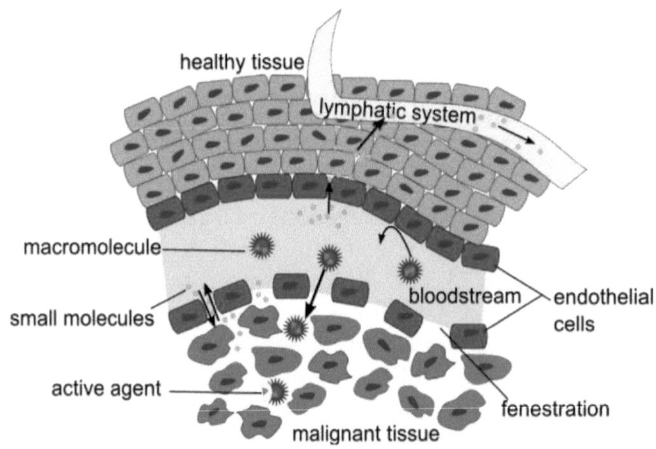

FIGURE 11.19 Enhanced permeability and retention (EPR) effect. From Stockhofe, K. et al., *Radiolabeling of nanoparticles and polymers for PET imaging.* Pharmaceuticals, 2014. **7**(4): p. 392-418.

specific blocking system utilizing a "don't-eat-us" strategy [55]. The strategy used D-self-peptide—labeled liposome to "block" phagocytes by interacting with signal regulatory protein alpha and inhibiting phagocytosis (Fig. 11.18).

The most common passive targeting approach is *via* the enhanced permeability and retention (EPR) effect. EPR effect describes a universal pathophysiological phenomenon and mechanism in which macromolecular compounds such as albumin and other polymer-conjugated drugs beyond certain sizes (> 40 kD) can progressively accumulate in the tumor vascularized area and thus achieve targeting delivery and retention of anticancer compounds into solid tumor tissue [56]. A simpler definition is a transport phenomenon characterized primarily by the presence of fenestrations in tumor vasculature that enables passive accumulation of nanoparticles in tumors [57]. A significantly reduced lymphatic drainage in tumor tissue also contributes to the EPR effect (Fig. 11.19) [58]. The EPR effect was first reported by Matsumura and Maeda in 1986 [59] and has become the "gold standard" in anticancer drug design and anticancer strategies using macromolecular agents [60]. The intervascular spaces in tumors have pores of 100 to 780 nm; such gaps do not exist in normal blood vessels [61]. Unfortunately, targeting therapy *via* the EPR effect in clinical practice is not always successful since the EPR effect varies greatly on the type and location of tumors, the status of blood perfusion in tumors, and the properties of the carrier [56]. Studies have shown the correlation between collagen content in tumor vasculature and nanoparticle permeability, and metalloproteinases may be used as a potential biomarker for EPR (Fig. 11.20) [57]. The size of the carrier should be optimized, and a size range of 100 to 200 nm is generally considered optimal for achieving the EPR effect while escaping the filtration of the liver and spleen [56]. Generally, an increase in the size of a nanoscale carrier prolongs systemic blood circulation and thus an enhanced EPR effect. However, nonspecific tissue uptake could increase proportionally [62]. EPR effects are also modest, providing less than a twofold increase in delivery compared with critical normal organs, which is generally insufficient for achieving therapeutic levels within the tumor [63]. Physical and pharmacological approaches have

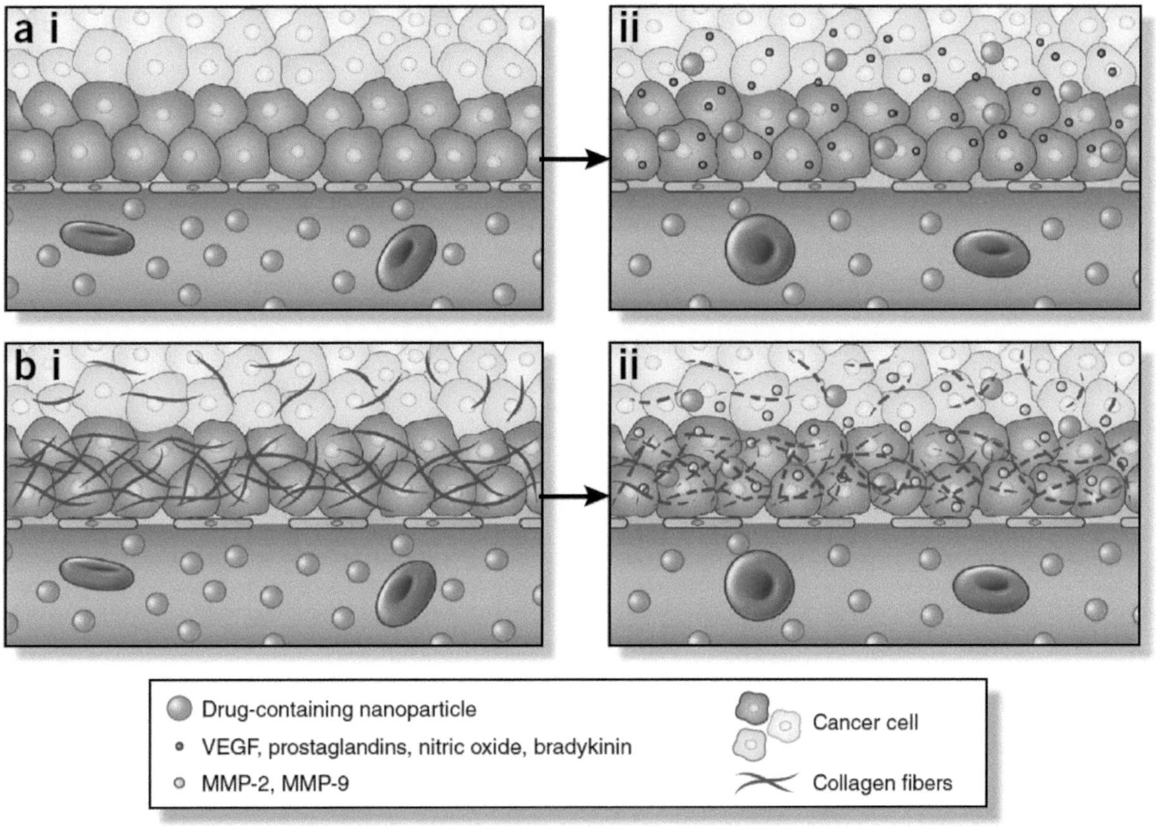

FIGURE 11.20 Determinants of enhanced permeability of nanoparticles into tumor tissues. (a i) Normal vasculature typically possesses tight interendothelial junctions that prevent extravasation of particles into tissues. The imbalance of several factors influences the size of fenestration in tumor vasculature. (a ii) As an example, VEGF and nitric oxide have been shown to increase the size of gaps in the endothelia. (b i) Tumors often possess a dense extracellular matrix that prevents adequate penetration of nanoparticles into the tumor. (b ii) MMP-2 and MMP-9 degrade the dense collagen matrix comprising the basement membrane. These in turn can be exploited pharmacologically to enhance the EPR effect for increased nanoparticle accumulation in tumors. *MMP*, Matrix metalloproteinase; *VEGF*, vascular endothelial growth factor. From Blanco, E., H. Shen, and M. Ferrari, *Principles of nanoparticle design for overcoming biological barriers to drug delivery.* Nat Biotechnol, 2015. **33**(9): p. 941-51, with permission from Springer Nature.

been studied to enhance the EPR effect. Physical approaches use external stimuli, such as radiation, to temporarily increase the permeability in tumor tissues. Pharmacological approaches focus on the tumor microenvironment for improved accumulation [61].

Active targeting generally involves modification of the drug or drug carrier with a ligand (ligands). As discussed in Section 11.2, these ligands can be proteins/peptides, antibodies, aptamers, and small molecules. Under administration, the ligands should be exposed and exhibit correct epitopes. The binding affinity should also be considered and investigated [64]. Low-affinity binding may lead to off-target. Multivalent binding can be used to greatly increase the binding force. Fig. 11.21 shows the ligand-receptor interaction of targeted drug delivery using nanoparticles as an example.

There are different ligand-receptor binding models [65]:

One-step binding/dissociation model: This model is characterized by a one-step association (k_1 or k_{on}) and one-step dissociation (k_2 or k_{off})

$$L + R \underset{k_2}{\overset{k_1}{\rightleftarrows}} L/R$$

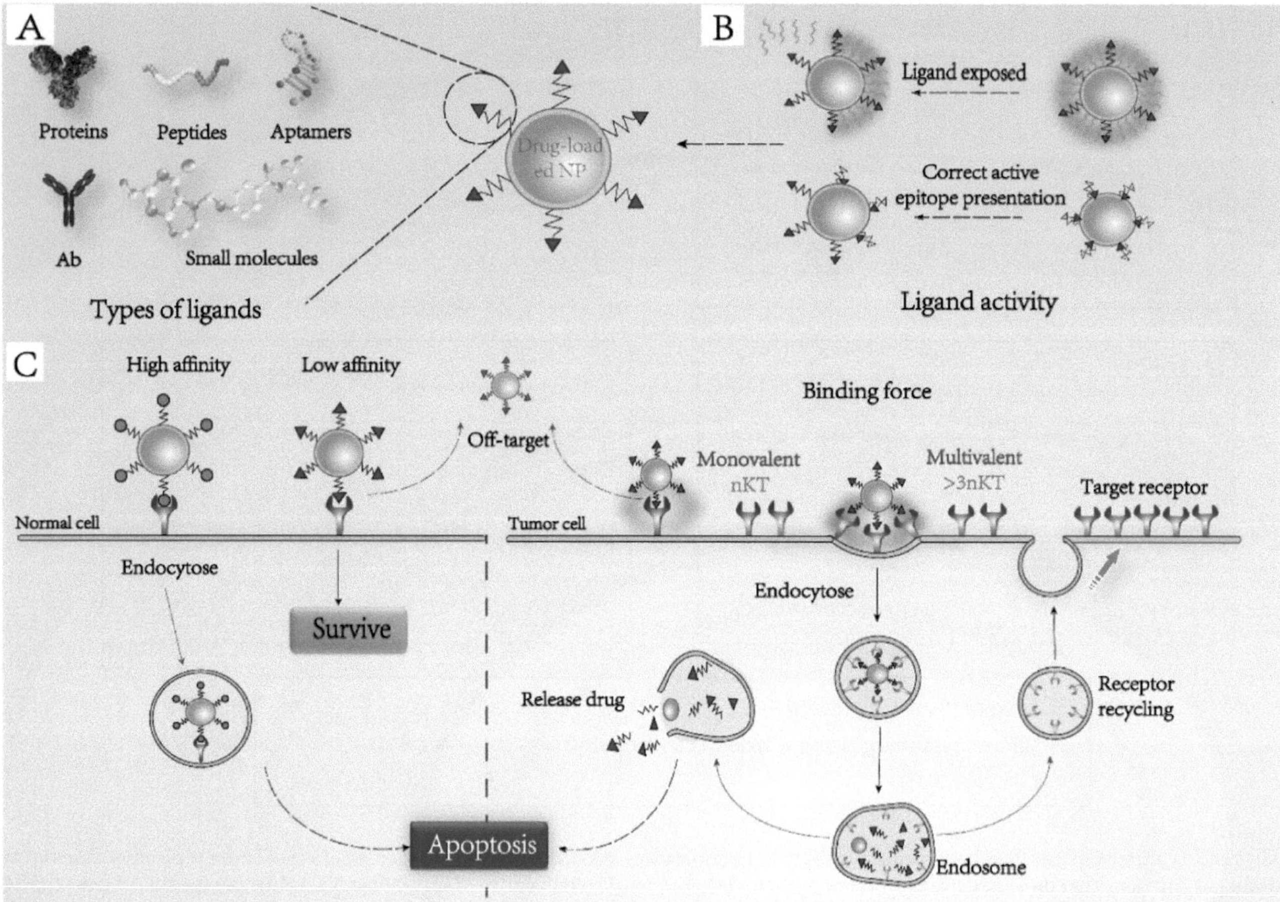

FIGURE 11.21 Schematic of ligand-receptor interaction of targeted drug delivery for cancer treatment. (A) Common types of targeted ligands. (B) The targeting ability is demonstrated only when the ligand modified on the particle surface is exposed and exhibits the correct epitopes. (C) Monovalent binding of the high-affinity ligand mediates endocytosis of drug-loaded particles and induces apoptosis. The multivalent effect, compared with monovalent binding, can significantly increase the binding force between the ligand and receptor. *nKT*, Monovalent binding strength of ligand and receptor. From Yang, T. et al., *"Targeting design" of nanoparticles in tumor therapy.* Pharmaceutics, 2022. **14**(9):1919.

$$K_d = \frac{1}{K_a} = \frac{C_L \times C_R}{C_{L/R}} = \frac{k_2}{k_1}$$

in which R represents the receptor, L is the ligand, L/R is the ligand-receptor complex, C is the concentration, K_d is the equilibrium dissociation constant, and K_a is the equilibrium association constant.

Induced fit model: This model is characterized by an association (k_1) of ligand to a low-affinity state of the receptor, which is followed by a conformation change (k_3) in the receptor, forming a high-affinity ligand-receptor complex (L/R*)

$$L + R \underset{k_2}{\overset{k_1}{\rightleftarrows}} L/R \underset{k_4}{\overset{k_3}{\rightleftarrows}} L/R^*.$$

Conformational selection model: This model is characterized by a conformational change (k_1) in the receptor from a nonselective state (R) to a selective state (R*) and followed by the ligand-receptor complex formation (L/R*)

$$R \underset{k_2}{\overset{k_1}{\rightleftarrows}} R^* \underset{k_4}{\overset{k_3}{\rightleftarrows}} L/R^*.$$

Sample question 11.1

Consider ligand and receptor concentrations of 5×10^{-5} mol/L each. What is the equilibrium concentration of the ligand-receptor complex? K_d is 10^{-4} mol/L.

Answer:

$C_{Ltotal} = C_L + C_{L/R} = 5 \times 10^{-5}$ mol/L
$C_L = C_{Ltotal} - C_{L/R} = 5 \times 10^{-5}$ mol/L $- C_{L/R}$

Similarly, $C_R = C_{Rtotal} - C_{L/R} = 5 \times 10^{-5}$ mol/L $- C_{L/R}$

$$K_d = \frac{C_L \times C_R}{C_{L/R}} = \frac{\left(5\times 10^{-5} - C_{L/R}\right) \times \left(5\times 10^{-5} - C_{L/R}\right)}{C_{L/R}} = 10^{-4}\ M$$

Solving for $C_{L/R}$, the two possible solutions are 1.87×10^{-4} mol/L and 1.34×10^{-5} mol/L. $C_{L/R} = 1.34 \times 10^{-5}$ mol/L, because the maximum value for $C_{L/R}$ is 5×10^{-5} mol/L.

Therapeutic antibodies and related biologics have leveraged multivalency to achieve ultrahigh affinity and selectivity [66]. For multivalent binding, theoretical models are still lacking. One approach is kinetic isothermal titration calorimetry with an invariant subspace projection [67].

To design a targeted drug delivery system, it is beneficial to combine both passive and active targeting approaches. For example, active targeting can be complementary to EPR-mediated tumor targeting to enhance drug delivery, accumulation, and retention in tumors [68]. Even for the active targeting approach alone, different ligands can be used for either sequential (cascade) or synchronized targeting (parallel) [69,70]. In parallel targeting strategy, two (or more) different targeting moieties are used, with each targeting a different receptor. The targeting groups interact simultaneously with one or different types of target cells [70]. One example is to combine peptides against both the epidermal growth factor and transferrin receptors for targeting glioblastomas [71]. During the cascade targeting strategy, the targeting components function in a sequential manner [70]. For example, a core-shell magnetic gold nanostar–based system with both a mitochondrial targeting amphipathic tail-anchoring peptide and a membrane-associated cytokine (tumor necrosis factor–related apoptosis-inducing ligand) was developed. An external magnetic field could facilitate drug delivery and accumulation due to the magnetic core. Tumor necrosis factor–related apoptosis-inducing ligand and amphipathic tail-anchoring peptide could sequentially target and be released toward the plasma membrane and mitochondria (Fig. 11.22) [72].

To summarize, in designing a passive and/or active targeting drug delivery system, drug carriers are commonly involved. Besides modification/functionalization capabilities, the carrier surface properties, shape, and intrinsic properties greatly affect its targeting performance (Fig. 11.23) [64]. Regarding the targeting approach, it is becoming more common to choose more than one strategy. Once reaching/accumulating at the target site, the drug should be released at a desired rate. Hence, drug-releasing mechanism(s) should also considered, e.g., using a physical trigger (Fig. 11.24).

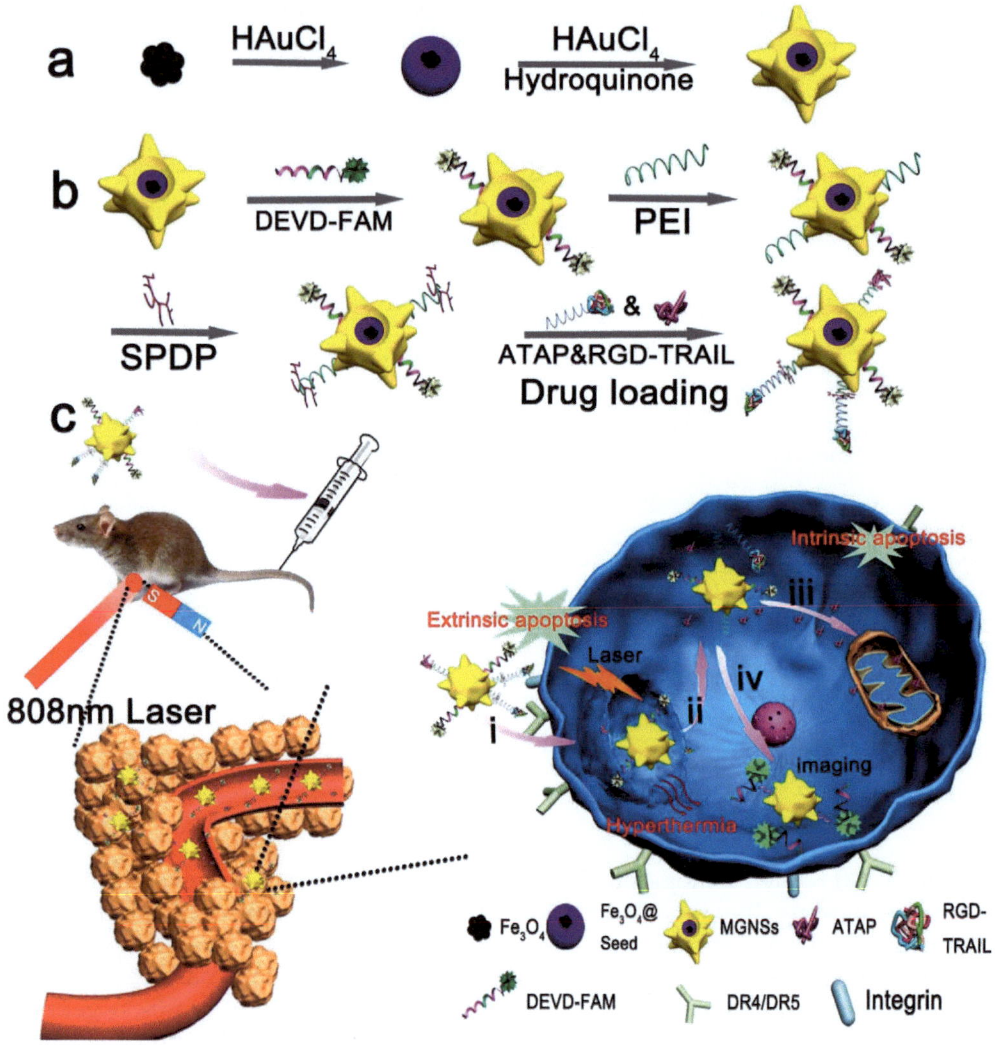

FIGURE 11.22 Schematic illustration of a drug vehicle for triplexed synergistic therapy with real-time monitoring. (a) The synthesis of the magnetic gold nanostars (MGNS). (b) Self-assembly process of MGNSs@ATAP/RGD-TRAIL/FAM-DEVD nanoconstructs. (c) The antitumor mechanism of triplexed synergistic therapy: (i) internalization of vehicle followed by target identification of TRAIL and RGD; (ii) the release of ATAP in the cytoplasm; (iii) the collapse of the mitochondrial structure triggered by ATAP resulting in intrinsic apoptosis; and (iv) imaging triggered by the cleavage of caspase-3. *ATAP,* Amphipathic tail-anchoring peptide; *DEVD*, aspartic-glycine-valine-aspartic acid; *DR,* death receptor; *FAM,* carboxyfluorescein; *PEI,* polyethylenimine; *RGD,* arginine-glycine-aspartic acid; *SPDP, N*-succinimidyl 3-(2-pyridyldithio) propionate; *TRAIL,* tumor necrosis factor–related apoptosis-inducing ligand. From Wu, R. et al., *Sequential delivery and cascade targeting of peptide therapeutics for triplexed synergistic therapy with real-time monitoring shuttled by magnetic gold nanostars.* Analytical Chemistry, 2019. **91**(7): p. 4608-4617. Copyright (2019), American Chemical Society.

Review and practice questions

1. What are targeted drug delivery systems?
2. What are the benefits of using targeted drug delivery systems?
3. What are the considerations for selecting a disease-specific receptor?
4. What is the mechanism for targeting using transferrin?
5. What are the most common amino acid residues in cell-penetrating peptides?
6. What are nucleic acid aptamers? And provide an example of aptamers used for targeting.
7. Provide three examples of low-molecular-weight ligands and their targets.
8. What are the considerations for selecting an effective ligand?
9. Describe the working mechanism of ThermoDOX combined with RFA for cancer treatment.
10. True/False: Temperature can be adjusted for therapeutic purposes, either by increasing or decreasing it.

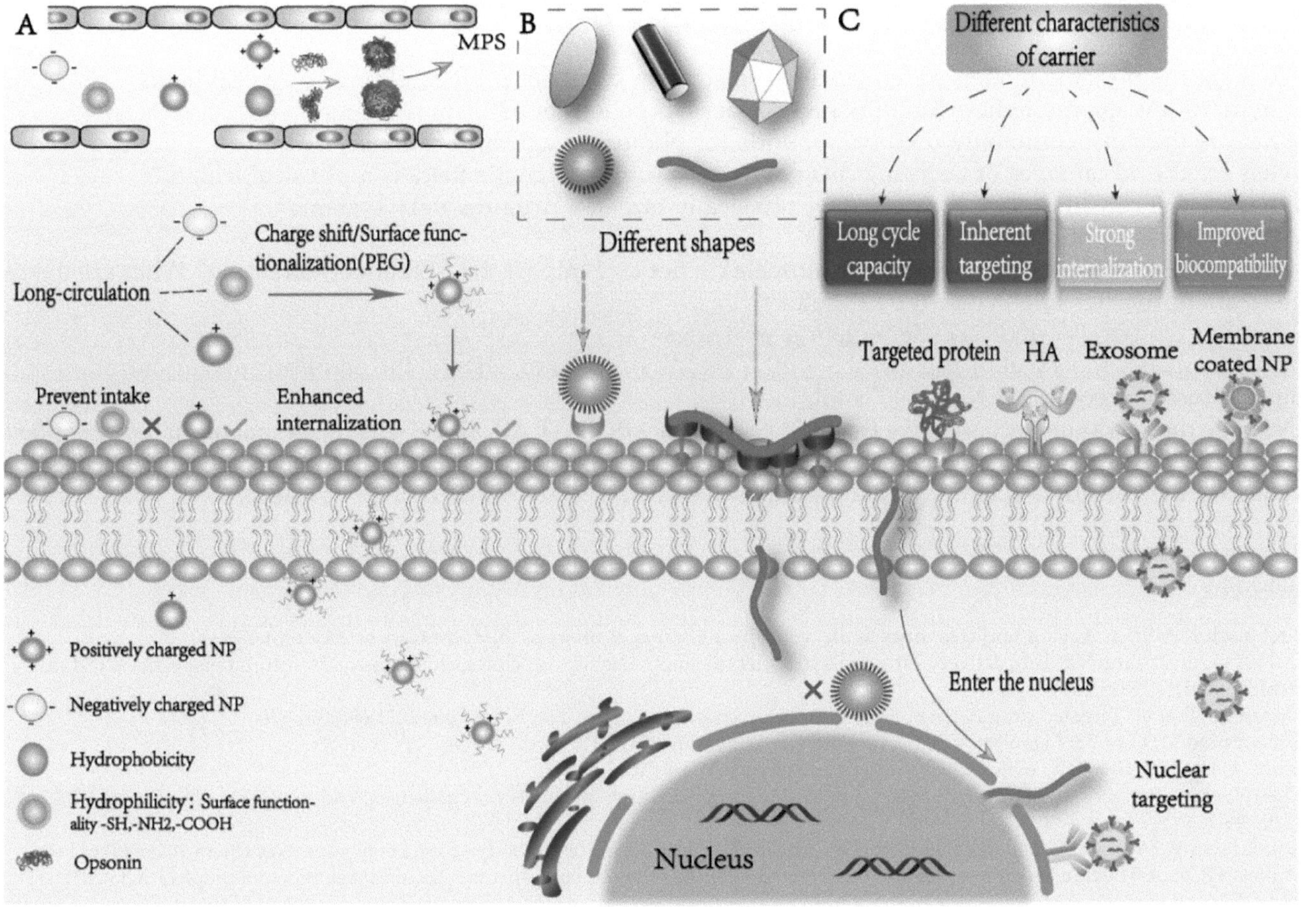

FIGURE 11.23 Effects of surface properties, shape, and intrinsic properties on the targeting of nanoparticles (NPs). (A) Transport of particles with different charge and surface chemical properties *in vivo*. (B) Schematic of cell uptake of NPs with different shapes; vermicular carriers find it easier to enter intracellularly by polyvalent contact with the membrane surface, and they even achieve nuclear targeting. (C) Different intrinsic characteristics of the carrier. *HA*, Hyaluronic acid; *PEG*, polyethylene glycol. From Yang, T. et al., *"Targeting design" of nanoparticles in tumor therapy.* Pharmaceutics, 2022. **14**(9):1919.

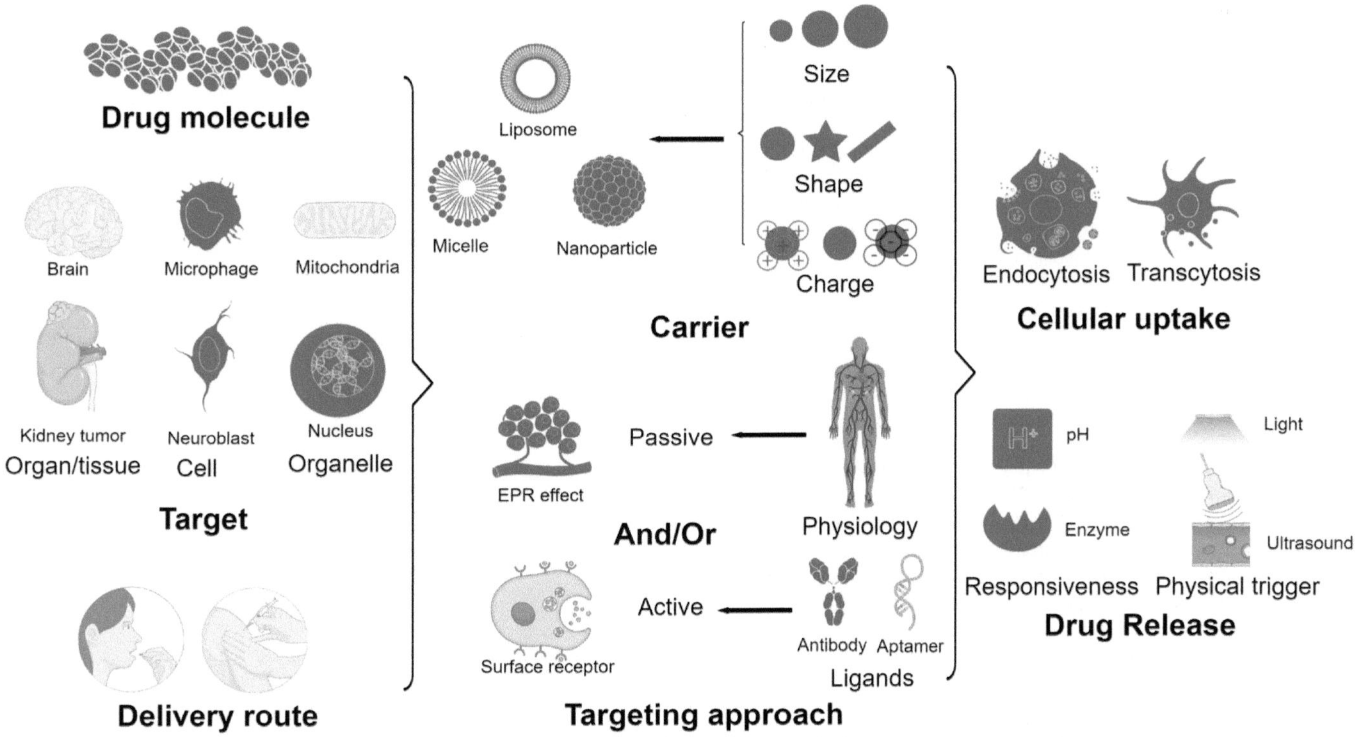

FIGURE 11.24 Design of a passive and/or active targeting drug delivery system.

11. What are the possible models for enhancing the stratum corneum permeability through cavitation?
12. Why does low-energy light exhibit the highest dermal penetration?
13. What are the most commonly used compounds for photocleavage applications?
14. What are the advantages of targeting drug delivery using a magnetic field as a physical trigger?
15. What are the considerations for designing physically targeted drug delivery systems?
16. What are passive and active targeting?
17. What is the EPR effect? How does the nanoscale carrier size impact the EPR effect/targeting? What are the two general approaches to enhance the EPR effect?
18. Compare the parallel and cascade targeting strategies.
19. Consider a 10^{-4} mol/L of ligand and a 5×10^{-5} mol/L of receptor, what is the equilibrium concentration of the ligand/receptor complex? K_d is 10^{-6} mol/L.
20. Describe the working mechanism of the MGNSs@ATAP/RGD-TRAIL/FAM-DEVD nanoconstructs for triplexed synergistic therapy.
21. What are the considerations for designing a passive and/or active drug delivery system?

References

[1] Strebhardt K, Ullrich A. Paul Ehrlich's magic bullet concept: 100 years of progress. Nat Rev Cancer 2008;8(6):473–80.
[2] Tewabe A, et al. Targeted drug delivery - from magic bullet to nanomedicine: principles, challenges, and future perspectives. J Multidiscip Healthc 2021;14:1711–24.
[3] Manzari MT, et al. Targeted drug delivery strategies for precision medicines. Nat Rev Mater 2021;6(4):351–70.
[4] Srinivasarao M, Low PS. Ligand-targeted drug delivery. Chem Rev 2017;117(19):12133–64.
[5] Mitra A, Lee CH, Cheng K, editors. Advanced drug delivery. Wiley; 2013.
[6] Chen Z, et al. Antibody-based drug delivery systems for cancer therapy: mechanisms, challenges, and prospects. Theranostics 2022;12(8): 3719–46.
[7] Chudasama V, Maruani A, Caddick S. Recent advances in the construction of antibody–drug conjugates. Nat Chem 2016;8(2):114–9.
[8] Daniels TR, et al. The transferrin receptor and the targeted delivery of therapeutic agents against cancer. Biochim Biophys Acta 2012;1820(3): 291–317.
[9] Koneru T, et al. Transferrin: biology and use in receptor-targeted nanotherapy of gliomas. ACS Omega 2021;6(13):8727–33.
[10] Wigner P, et al. Doxorubicin–transferrin conjugate alters mitochondrial homeostasis and energy metabolism in human breast cancer cells. Sci Rep 2021;11(1):4544.
[11] Todaro B, et al. Targeting peptides: the new generation of targeted drug delivery systems. Pharmaceutics 2023;15(6):1648.
[12] Kotadiya DD, Patel P, Patel DH. Cell-penetrating peptides: a powerful tool for targeted drug delivery. Curr Drug Deliv 2023;20:1–21.
[13] Tietz O, et al. Tricyclic cell-penetrating peptides for efficient delivery of functional antibodies into cancer cells. Nat Chem 2022;14(3):284–93.
[14] di Polidoro AC, et al. Revealing Angiopep-2/LRP1 molecular interaction for optimal delivery to glioblastoma (GBM). Molecules 2022;27(19): 6696.
[15] Chandola C, et al. Application of aptamers in diagnostics, drug-delivery and imaging. J Biosci 2016;41(3):535–61.
[16] Liebelt BD, Finocchiaro G, Heimberger AB. Chapter 10-Principles of immunotherapy. In: Berger MS, Weller M, editors. Handbook of clinical neurology. Elsevier; 2016. p. 163–81.
[17] Pichon V, Chapuis-Hugon F, Hennion MC. 2.19-Bioaffinity sorbents. In: Pawliszyn J, editor. Comprehensive sampling and sample preparation. Academic Press; 2012. p. 359–88.
[18] Chandola C, Neerathilingam M. Ch. 1 Aptamers for targeted delivery: current challenges and future opportunities. In: Tyagi R, Garg N, Shukla R, Singh Bisen P, et al., editors. Role of novel drug delivery vehicles in nanobiomedicine. IntechOpen; 2019.
[19] Wu D, et al. Directed evolution of aptamer discovery technologies. Acc Chem Res 2022;55(5):685–95.
[20] Cho M, et al. Quantitative selection and parallel characterization of aptamers. PNAS 2013;110(46):18460–5.
[21] Chang D, et al. A high-dimensional microfluidic approach for selection of aptamers with programmable binding affinities. Nat Chem 2023; 15(6):773–80.
[22] Ng EWM, et al. Pegaptanib, a targeted anti-VEGF aptamer for ocular vascular disease. Nat Rev Drug Discov 2006;5(2):123–32.
[23] Stapleton M. Pegaptanib sodium. In: Enna SJ, Bylund DB, editors. xPharm: the comprehensive Pharmacology reference. Elsevier; 2010. p. 1–8.
[24] Carron PM, et al. Targeting the folate receptor: improving efficacy in inorganic medicinal chemistry. Curr Med Chem 2018;25(23):2675–708.
[25] Rao W, et al. Chitosan-decorated doxorubicin-encapsulated nanoparticle targets and eliminates tumor reinitiating cancer stem-like cells. ACS Nano 2015;9(6):5725–40.
[26] Wu J, et al. Functionalized NIR-II semiconducting polymer nanoparticles for single-cell to whole-organ imaging of PSMA-positive prostate cancer. Small 2020;16(19):2001215.
[27] Sun T, et al. Physical triggering strategies for drug delivery. Adv Drug Deliv Rev 2020;158:36–62.
[28] Zhang W, et al. Synthesis and characterization of thermally responsive Pluronic F127–chitosan nanocapsules for controlled release and intracellular delivery of small molecules. ACS Nano 2010;4(11):6747–59.
[29] Rao W, et al. Thermally responsive nanoparticle-encapsulated curcumin and its combination with mild hyperthermia for enhanced cancer cell destruction. Acta Biomater 2014;10(2):831–42.
[30] Rao W, et al. Nanoparticle-encapsulated doxorubicin enhances cryoablation of cancer stem-like cells. Technology 2014;2(1):28–35.

[31] Borys N, Dewhirst MW. Drug development of lyso-thermosensitive liposomal doxorubicin: combining hyperthermia and thermosensitive drug delivery. Adv Drug Deliv Rev 2021;178:113985.
[32] Regenold M, et al. Turning down the heat: the case for mild hyperthermia and thermosensitive liposomes. Nanomedicine 2022;40:102484.
[33] Zhao Z, et al. Ultrasound technology and biomaterials for precise drug therapy. Mater Today 2023;63:210–38.
[34] Manikkath J, et al. Chapter 7-peptide dendrimers in delivery of bioactive molecules to skin. In: Hamblin MR, Avci P, Prow TW, editors. Nanoscience in Dermatology. Academic Press; 2016. p. 89–97.
[35] Park D, et al. Sonophoresis in transdermal drug deliverys. Ultrasonics 2014;54(1):56–65.
[36] Al-Jawadi S, Thakur SS. Ultrasound-responsive lipid microbubbles for drug delivery: a review of preparation techniques to optimise formulation size, stability and drug loading. Int J Pharm 2020;585:119559.
[37] Omata D, et al. Ultrasound and microbubble-mediated drug delivery and immunotherapy. J Med Ultrason 2022.
[38] Bloch SH, et al. Optical observation of lipid- and polymer-shelled ultrasound microbubble contrast agents. Appl Phys Lett 2004;84(4):631–3.
[39] Chen P-Y, et al. Drug-carrying microbubbles as a theranostic tool in convection-enhanced delivery for brain tumor therapy. Oncotarget 2017; 8(26):42359–71.
[40] Patel R, et al. Development of a dual drug-loaded, surfactant-stabilized contrast agent containing oxygen. Polymers 2022;14(8):1568.
[41] Rapp TL, DeForest CA. Targeting drug delivery with light: a highly focused approach. Adv Drug Deliv Rev 2021;171:94–107.
[42] Cios A, et al. Effect of different wavelengths of laser irradiation on the skin cells. Int J Mol Sci 2021;22(5):2437.
[43] Husain Z, Alster TS. The role of lasers and intense pulsed light technology in dermatology. Clin Cosmet Investig Dermatol 2016;9:29–40.
[44] Tao Y, et al. Light: a magical tool for controlled drug delivery. Adv Funct Mater 2020;30(49):2005029.
[45] Mena-Giraldo P, et al. Photosensitive nanocarriers for specific delivery of cargo into cells. Sci Rep 2020;10(1):2110.
[46] Helmy AM. Overview of recent advancements in the iontophoretic drug delivery to various tissues and organs. J Drug Deliv Sci Technol 2021; 61:102332.
[47] Ouyang Q, et al. Self-powered, on-demand transdermal drug delivery system driven by triboelectric nanogenerator. Nano Energy 2019;62: 610–9.
[48] Price PM, et al. Magnetic drug delivery: where the field is going. Front Chem 2018;6:619.
[49] Liu Y-L, et al. A review of magnet systems for targeted drug delivery. J Control Release 2019;302:90–104.
[50] Liu JF, et al. Use of magnetic fields and nanoparticles to trigger drug release and improve tumor targeting. Wiley Interdiscip Rev Nanomed Nanobiotechnol 2019;11(6):e1571.
[51] Qiu Y, et al. Magnetic forces enable controlled drug delivery by disrupting endothelial cell-cell junctions. Nat Commun 2017;8(1):15594.
[52] Xu H, et al. Sperm-hybrid micromotor for targeted drug delivery. ACS Nano 2018;12(1):327–37.
[53] Dilliard SA, Siegwart DJ. Passive, active and endogenous organ-targeted lipid and polymer nanoparticles for delivery of genetic drugs. Nat Rev Mater 2023;8(4):282–300.
[54] Santos E, Pinter J, McCluskey K. Chapter 47 Reticuloendothelial system: vascular, nonvascular, and oncologic. In: Pua BB, Covey AM, Madoff DC, editors. Interventional radiology: fundamentals of clinical practice. Oxford University Press; 2018. p. 626–38.
[55] Tang Y, et al. Overcoming the reticuloendothelial system barrier to drug delivery with a "don't-eat-us" strategy. ACS Nano 2019;13(11): 13015–26.
[56] Wu J. The enhanced permeability and retention (EPR) effect: the significance of the concept and methods to enhance its application. J Pers Med 2021;11(8):771.
[57] Blanco E, Shen H, Ferrari M. Principles of nanoparticle design for overcoming biological barriers to drug delivery. Nat Biotechnol 2015;33(9): 941–51.
[58] Stockhofe K, et al. Radiolabeling of nanoparticles and polymers for PET imaging. Pharmaceuticals 2014;7(4):392–418.
[59] Matsumura Y, Maeda H. A new concept for macromolecular therapeutics in cancer chemotherapy: mechanism of tumoritropic accumulation of proteins and the antitumor agent Smancs1. Cancer Res 1986;46(12_Part_1):6387–92.
[60] Fang J, Nakamura H, Maeda H. The EPR effect: unique features of tumor blood vessels for drug delivery, factors involved, and limitations and augmentation of the effect. Adv Drug Deliv Rev 2011;63(3):136–51.
[61] Ikeda-Imafuku M, et al. Strategies to improve the EPR effect: a mechanistic perspective and clinical translation. J Control Release 2022;345: 512–36.
[62] Kang H, et al. Size-dependent EPR effect of polymeric nanoparticles on tumor targeting. Adv Healthc Mater 2020;9(1):e1901223.
[63] Nakamura Y, et al. Nanodrug delivery: is the enhanced permeability and retention effect sufficient for curing cancer? Bioconjug Chem 2016; 27(10):2225–38.
[64] Yang T, et al. "Targeting design" of nanoparticles in tumor therapy. Pharmaceutics 2022;14(9):1919.
[65] van der Velden WJC, Heitman LH, Rosenkilde MM. Perspective: implications of ligand-receptor binding kinetics for therapeutic targeting of G protein-coupled receptors. ACS Pharmacol Transl Sci 2020;3(2):179–89.
[66] Errington WJ, Bruncsics B, Sarkar CA. Mechanisms of noncanonical binding dynamics in multivalent protein–protein interactions. PNAS 2019;116(51):25659–67.
[67] Erlekam F, et al. *Modeling of* multivalent ligand-receptor binding measu*red by kinITC*. Computation 2019;7(3):46.
[68] Subhan MA, et al. Recent advances in tumor targeting via EPR effect for cancer treatment. J Pers Med 2021;11(6):571.
[69] Shi P, et al. Active targeting schemes for nano-drug delivery systems in osteosarcoma therapeutics. J Nanobiotechnology 2023;21(1):103.
[70] Luo Y, et al. Dual and multi-targeted nanoparticles for site-specific brain drug delivery. J Control Release 2020;317:195–215.
[71] Dixit S, et al. Dual receptor-targeted theranostic nanoparticles for localized delivery and activation of photodynamic therapy drug in glioblastomas. Mol Pharm 2015;12(9):3250–60.
[72] Wu R, et al. Sequential delivery and cascade targeting of peptide therapeutics for triplexed synergistic therapy with real-time monitoring shuttled by magnetic gold nanostars. Anal Chem 2019;91(7):4608–17.

CHAPTER

12

Biomimetic drug delivery systems

Wujie Zhang

LEARNING OBJECTIVES

- To define biomimetics and biomimicry and highlight their differences
- To discuss examples of biomimicry applications
- To discuss various strategies of using cell membranes for drug delivery
- To discuss various approaches for cell membrane modification
- To design biomimetic cell membrane-based drug delivery systems
- To discuss the structure of lipoproteins and various strategies of using lipoproteins for utilizing lipoproteins in drug delivery
- To discuss the mechanisms and benefits of utilizing extracellular vesicles in drug delivery
- To design biomimetic drug delivery systems

12.1 Biomimicry

The term "biomimetics" originates from the Greek words *bios* ("life") and *mimesis* ("to imitate") [1]. Biomimetics is the production of a physical mechanism responsible for a specific functionality exhibited by a biological structure [2]. Schmitt was the first to coin the term "biomimetics" in 1957, and Jack Steele was the first to use the term in an article in 1969 [1]. Biomimicry, one type of bio-inspired design, involves learning nature's design principles in building highly complex and sophisticated engineering models at various length scales and using the wealth of knowledge to solve the critical challenges faced by humanity [3]. "Biomimetics" and "biomimicry" are often used interchangeably. However, biomimicry is focused on reconnection with a new respect for nature, inspiration, ideation, and education, with the greater goal of sustainability. It needs the skills of technical and business specialists to yield commercially viable innovations. Biomimetics focuses on scientific translation, radical technological innovation, and commercialization, with the greater goal of better technologies as well as financial success [4]. Biomimicry has been used, receiving increasing attention, in almost every field (Fig. 12.1). For example, the mosquito proboscis is an optimized "needle" that minimizes the deformation and displacement of surrounding tissue during insertion for accurate guidance to targeted vessels. Mosquito proboscis-inspired insertion has been applied to the biopsy needle to reduce deformation and organ displacement (Fig. 12.2) [5]. Another example is an ingestible self-orienting

Fundamentals and Design of Drug Delivery Systems
https://doi.org/10.1016/B978-0-443-23521-4.00012-6

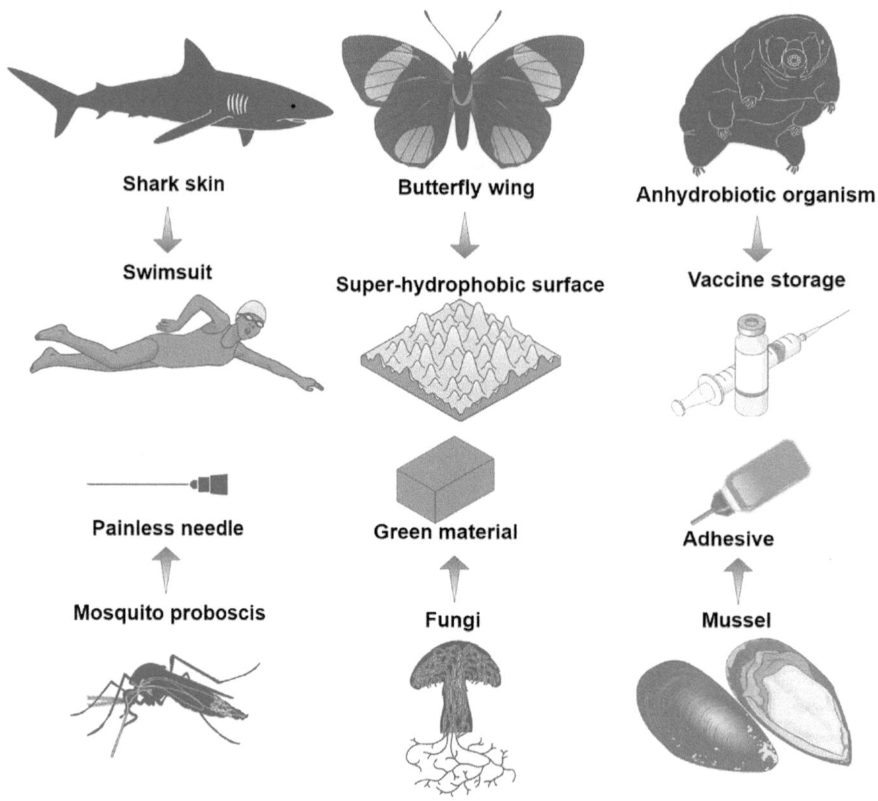

FIGURE 12.1 Examples of biomimicry.

millimeter-scale applicator that autonomously positions itself to engage with gastrointestinal tract tissue, inspired by the self-orienting leopard tortoise (*Stigmochelys pardalis*). The leopard tortoise has a shifted center and a high-curvature upper shell that enables self-orientation to the preferred upright position. The bottom half of the tortoise possesses a low curvature followed by a corner, which helps stabilize the tortoise (Fig. 12.3) [6].

12.2 Cell membrane/lipoprotein-based drug delivery systems

Extensive efforts have been made to imitate natural cells to construct biomimetic drug delivery systems. One simple approach is to use a cell membrane as a coating. The cell membrane can serve as a drug carrier and a valid shield (from the host body's immune system) [7]. During an application, a single type of cell membrane or two (or more) types of cell membranes can be involved [8]. Cell membranes that have been studied include erythrocyte membranes, leukocyte membranes, platelet membranes, stem cell membranes, and cancer cell membranes [7,8].

Red blood cells (RBCs; erythrocytes) are of particular interest. Human RBCs do not have nuclei and many organelles, which is beneficial for drug loading and surface modification [9,10]. Moreover, they have unique longevity in the bloodstream (reduce metabolic clearance), biocompatibility (surface of red blood cells expresses proteins that avoid being engulfed by the immune system), and safe metabolism mechanisms (reduce nonspecific and undesirable off-target effects) [10,11]. Moreover, dark red blood cells are easily heated by near-infrared light and can be used for acousto-optic therapy [10]. Drugs can be either encapsulated or coupled to the surface, when RBCs are used as a carrier directly [11,12]. Fig. 12.4 summarizes the general drug delivery approaches using RBCs as a carrier [12]. Red blood cells were first used to encapsulate enzymes, such as the encapsulation of L-asparaginase for acute lymphoblastic leukemia [10]. A more recent study utilized a photocleavable linker to retain membrane-permeable bioactive agents by attaching cobalamin (vitamin B12) (Fig. 12.5) [13].

Recently, the hybrid cell membrane strategies have been exploited to inherit cell membrane—related moieties, revealing diversified physicochemical properties and cell-specific functions, such as platelet-tumor, neutrophil-macrophage, and red blood cell-tumor hybrid membranes [14—16]. Take the biomimetic neutrophil-macrophage

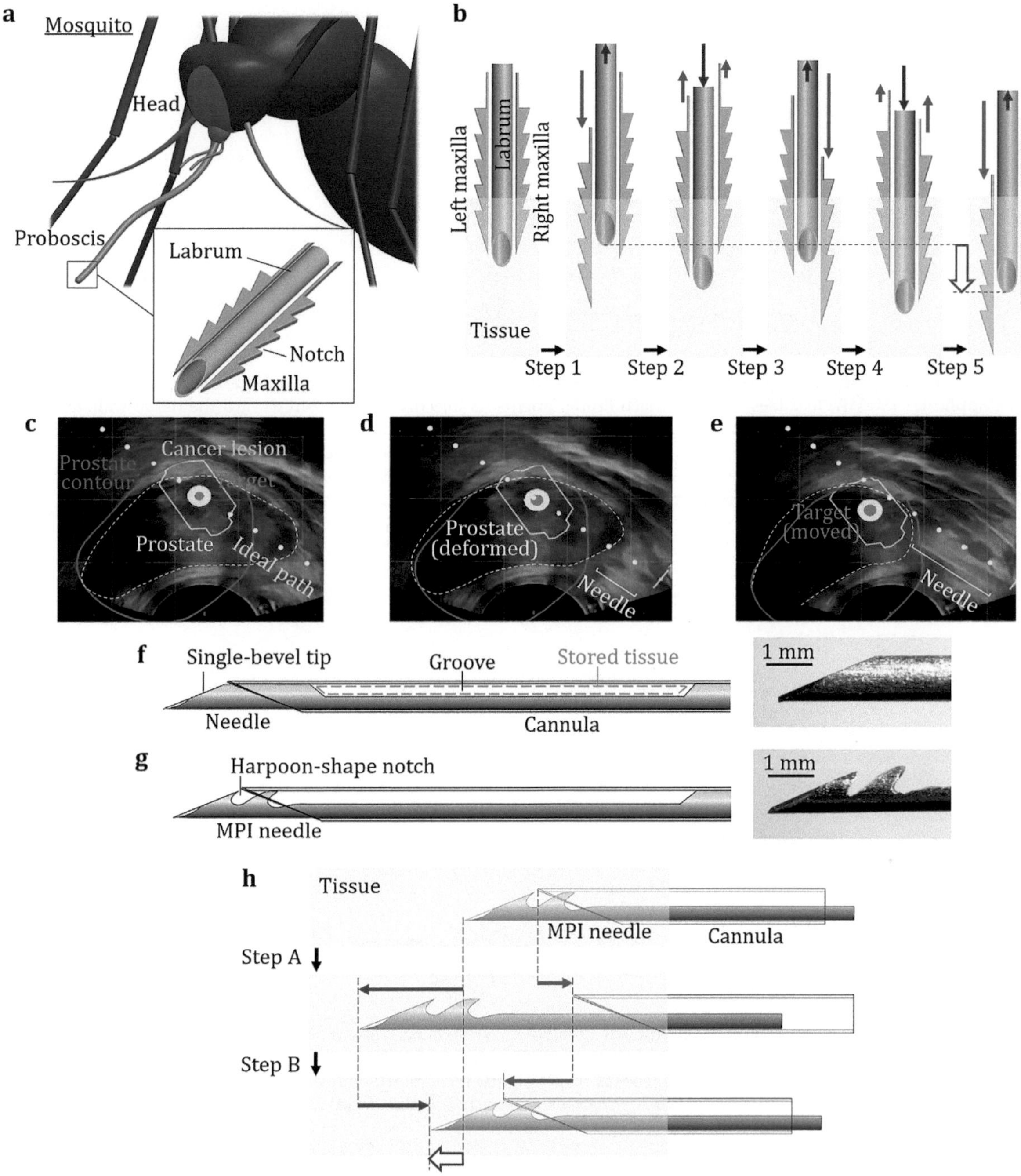

FIGURE 12.2 (a) Mosquito proboscis has a hollow labrum and two harpoon-shaped notched maxillae. (b) The incremental motion during the proboscis insertion reduces insertion force and surrounding tissue deformation. (c) The fused magnetic resonance-ultrasound image with a preidentified cancer lesion allows the targeted sampling of specific lesions in prostate needle biopsy. (d) The currently available needle delivery system deforms and moves the prostate. (e) The deformation and displacement of the prostate and surrounding tissue move the target location away from the predicted path just before biopsy. (f) The current Tru-Cut biopsy needle comprises an outer hollow cannula and an inner solid needle. (g) The mosquito proboscis-inspired needle comprises an outer hollow cannula and a needle with two harpoon-shaped notches at the tip. (h) The needle-cannula incremental motion for vibratory insertion aims to reduce tissue deformation and displacement. From Li, A.D.R. et al., *Mosquito proboscis-inspired needle insertion to reduce tissue deformation and organ displacement.* Sci. Rep, 2020. **10**(1): p. 12248.

dual membrane, for example; it has been used to prepare nanoparticles that are tumor-microenvironment responsive enabling targeted drug delivery. The results showed that the nanoparticles can efficiently transmigrate across the blood brain barrier (BBB), respond to the inflammatory stimuli, and specifically accumulate within the inflammatory (tumor) site (Fig. 12.6) [14].

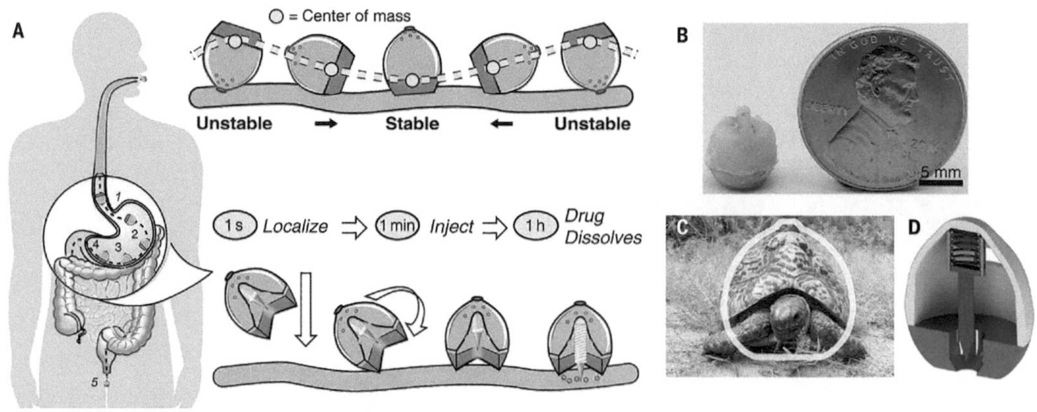

FIGURE 12.3 Mechanical active pharmaceutical ingredient (API) localization and injection for oral gastric delivery. (A) The self-orienting millimeter-scale applicator (SOMA) localizes to the stomach lining, orients its injection mechanism toward the tissue wall, and injects a drug payload through the mucosa. (B) A fabricated SOMA. (C) Shape comparison between the leopard tortoise and SOMA. (D) The SOMA uses a compressed spring fixed in caramelized sucrose *(brown)* to provide a force (hydration-dependent) for drug-loaded millipost *(blue)* insertion. After actuation, the spring remains within the device. From Abramson, A. et al., *An ingestible self-orienting system for oral delivery of macromolecules.* Science, 2019. **363**(6427): p. 611-615, with permission from the American Association for the Advancement of Science.

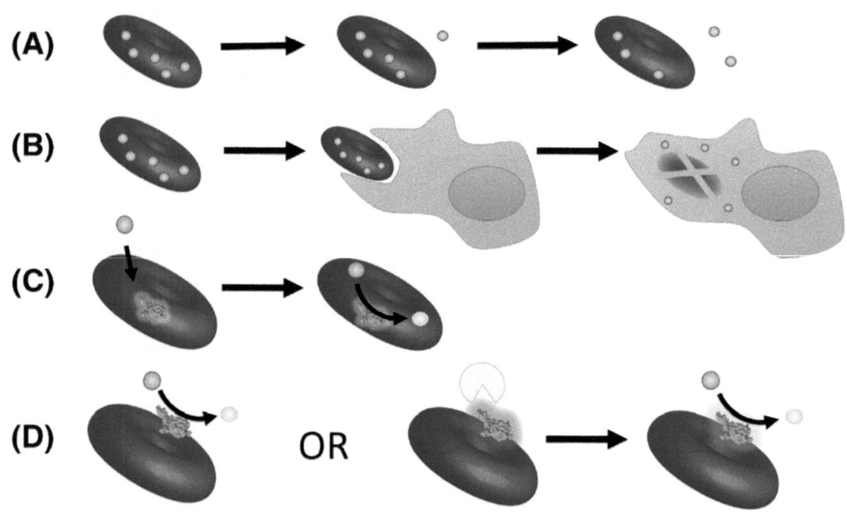

FIGURE 12.4 General approaches to red blood cell (RBC) drug carriers. (A) Sustained release of drugs encapsulated in RBCs. (B) Phagocytosis of drug-loaded RBCs and drug delivery to cells of the reticuloendothelial system. (C) Encapsulated enzymes act on diffusible substrates. (D) Surface-loaded enzymes act on extracellular targets either constitutively or after activation by other substances to an active state *(green). From Villa, C.H. et al., Erythrocytes as carriers for drug delivery in blood transfusion and beyond.* Transfus. Med. Rev, 2017. **31**(1): p. 26-35, with permission from Elsevier.

To design/prepare biomimetic cell membrane–based drug delivery systems, the type or types of cell membranes should be chosen first (Fig. 12.7). Then cell membrane extraction should be performed, such as through freeze-thaw cycles. Membrane modifications are generally beneficial and necessary and can be done through various approaches (Fig. 12.8) [7]. The physical approaches mainly rely on the lipid-lipid interactions. Chemical approaches commonly target the amino, thiol, and hydroxyl residues of the membrane components. Biological approaches, such as genetic engineering, can be used to introduce the desired protein/peptide into the cell membrane [7]. Different cell membranes can be used directly as drug carriers, primarily RBC membrane. The other common approach is to use cell membrane as a coating material. Last, drugs can be encapsulated or attached (physically or chemically) to the surface of the cell membrane–based drug delivery systems.

Lipoprotein assemblies and lipoprotein-based biomimetics represent a flexible nanoparticle platform that can be precisely tailored for various medical applications, including drug delivery. Lipoproteins are a heterogeneous class of biogenic, intrinsically stable, and nonimmunogenic nanoparticles produced by the liver and intestines [17]. They

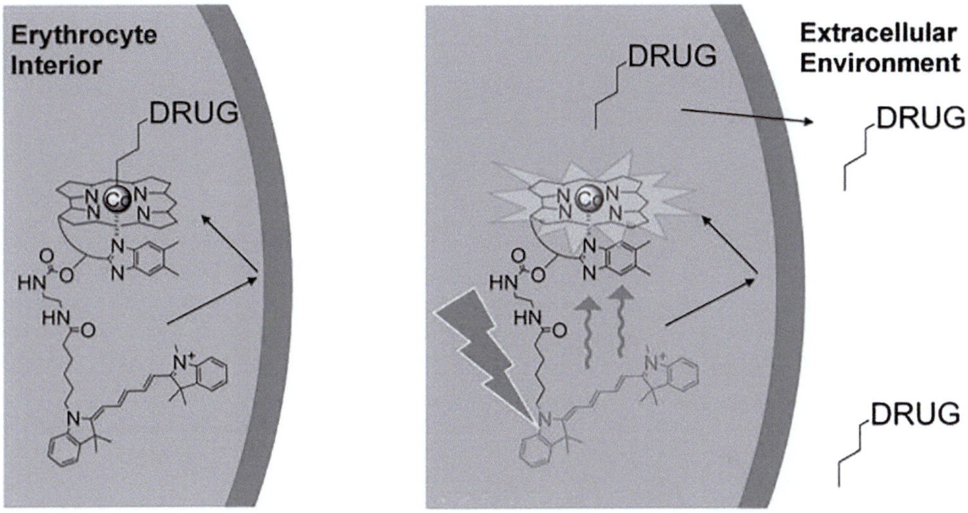

FIGURE 12.5 Photo-triggered release of encapsulated light-responsive compounds. Membrane impermeable cobalamin-bioagents are retained inside red blood cells. Photolysis produces membrane-permeable bioagents that can escape the cell. From Hughes, R.M. et al., *Photo-triggered secretion of membrane compartmentalized bioactive agents.* Angew Chem Int Ed Engl, 2016. **55**(52): p. 16080-16083, with permission from John Wiley & Sons, Inc.

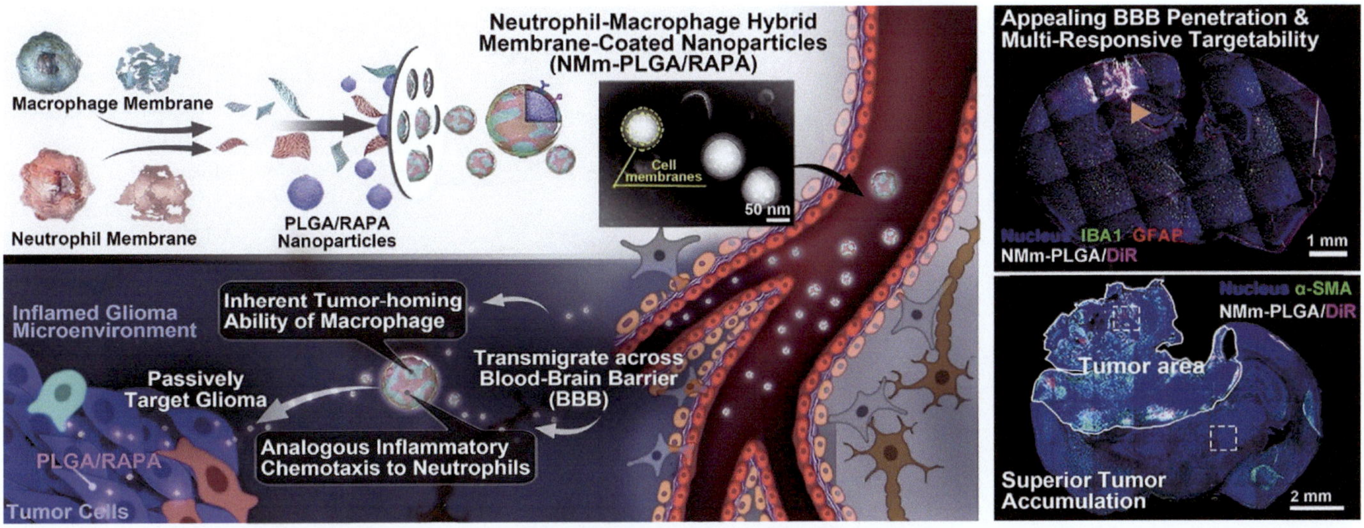

FIGURE 12.6 Schematic showing the preparation of a neutrophil-macrophage hybrid membrane (NMm)-coated PLGA/RAPA nanoparticles. By combining the inflammatory chemotaxis of neutrophil membranes and the tumor-homing ability of macrophage membranes, the nanoparticles are endowed with BBB-crossing and tumor-targeting capabilities and exhibit improved antiglioma therapeutic effects. *BBB*, Blood-brain barrier; *DiR*, 1,1′-dioctadecyl-3,3,3′,3′-tetramethylindotricarbocyanine iodide (a fluorescent dye); *GFAP*, glial fibrillary acidic protein (a marker of astrocytes); *IBA1*, allograft inflammatory factor 1 (a marker of activated microglia associated with glioma progression); *PLGA*, poly(lactic-*co*-glycolic acid); *RAPA*, rapamycin; *SMA*, smooth muscle actin (microvasculature marker in glioma). From Yin, Y. et al., *Biomimetic neutrophil and macrophage dual membrane-coated nanoplatform with orchestrated tumor-microenvironment responsive capability promotes therapeutic efficacy against glioma*. Chem. Eng. J, 2022. **433**: p. 133848, with permission from Elsevier.

are formed from lipid and protein molecule complexes with the primary function of transporting and delivering fatty acids, triacylglycerol, and cholesterol to and from target cells in many organs. The general structure of lipoproteins is a core composed of cholesterol ester and triacylglycerol molecules and a shell primarily made of phospholipids and cholesterol (Fig. 12.9). They can be classified based on their density, such as high-density lipoproteins (HDLs) and low-density lipoproteins (LDLs) [18]. Both isolated and synthesized lipoproteins have been used for drug delivery. They are biocompatible and biodegradable and can be directly used to deliver a range of payloads,

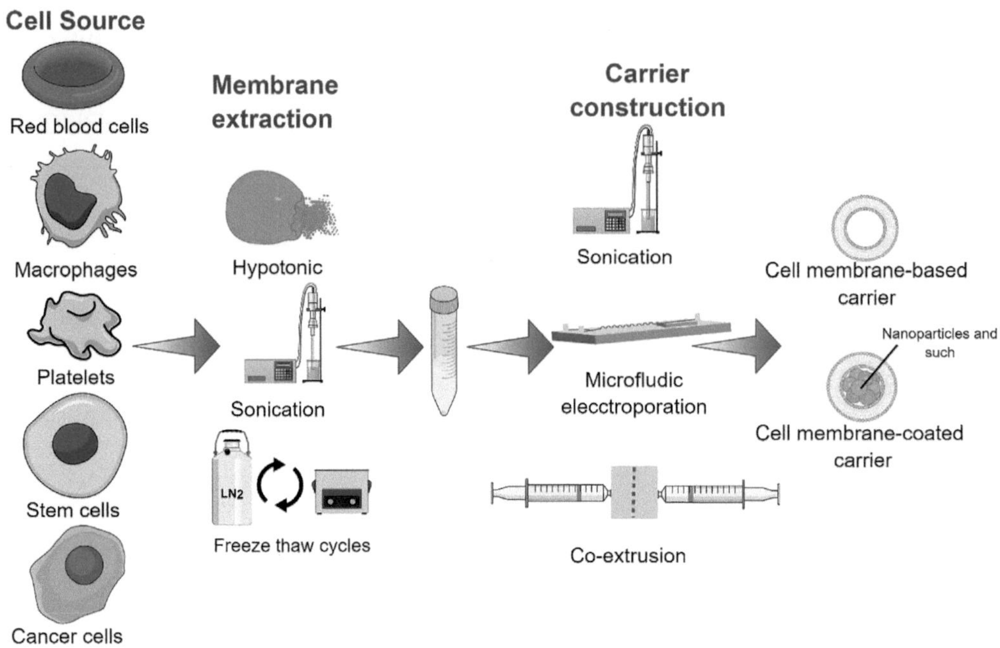

FIGURE 12.7 Schematic showing the process of design/preparation of the biomimetic cell-membrane—based drug delivery systems.

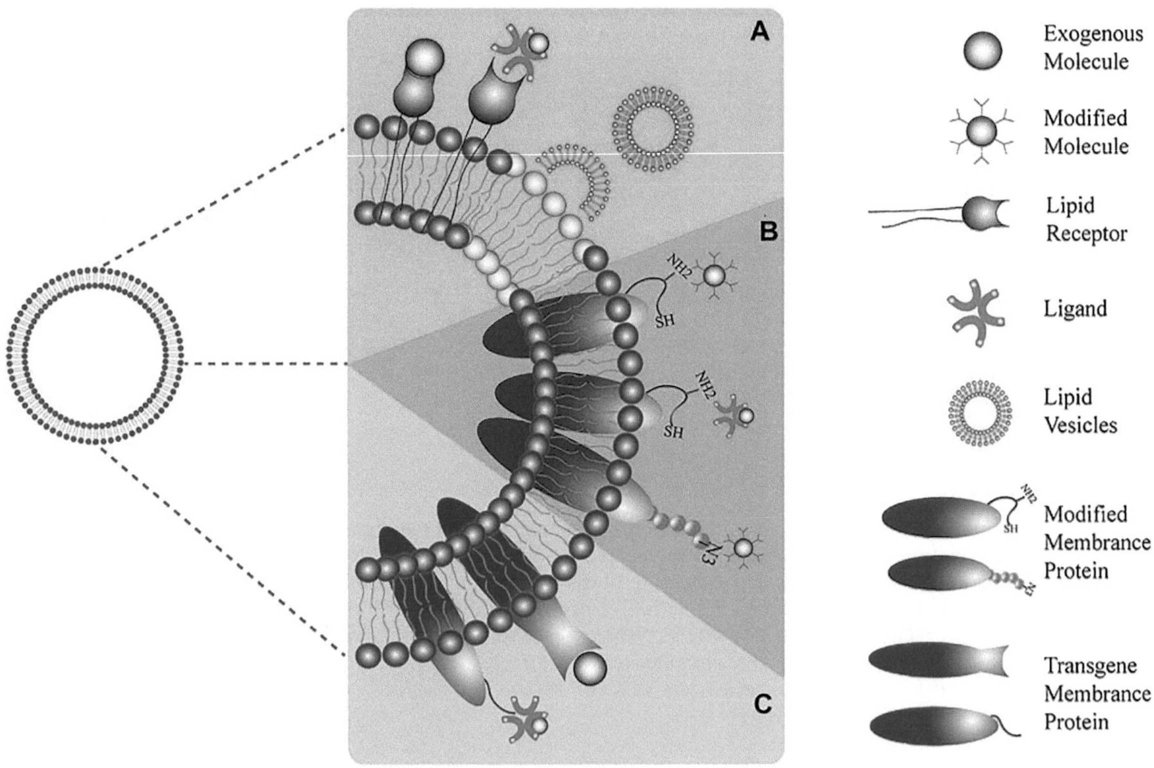

FIGURE 12.8 Cell membrane modification strategies: physical (A), chemical (B), and biological (C). From Guo, M. et al., *Research progress on cell membrane-coated biomimetic delivery systems.* Front Bioeng Biotechnol, 2021. **9**: p. 772522.

can accumulate at several important targets (such as macrophages), and can be rerouted to other targets [18,19]. Drugs can be loaded into lipoproteins through various approaches such as passive loading and chemical conjugation [17]. For example, lipoprotein-biomimetic nanostructure (Fig. 12.10) has been constructed for targeted delivery of siRNA to *Ras*-activated glioblastoma cells *via* micropinocytosis [20].

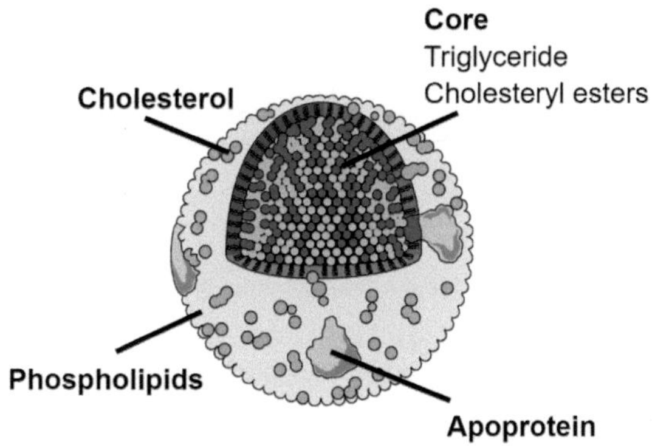

FIGURE 12.9 Structure of lipoproteins.

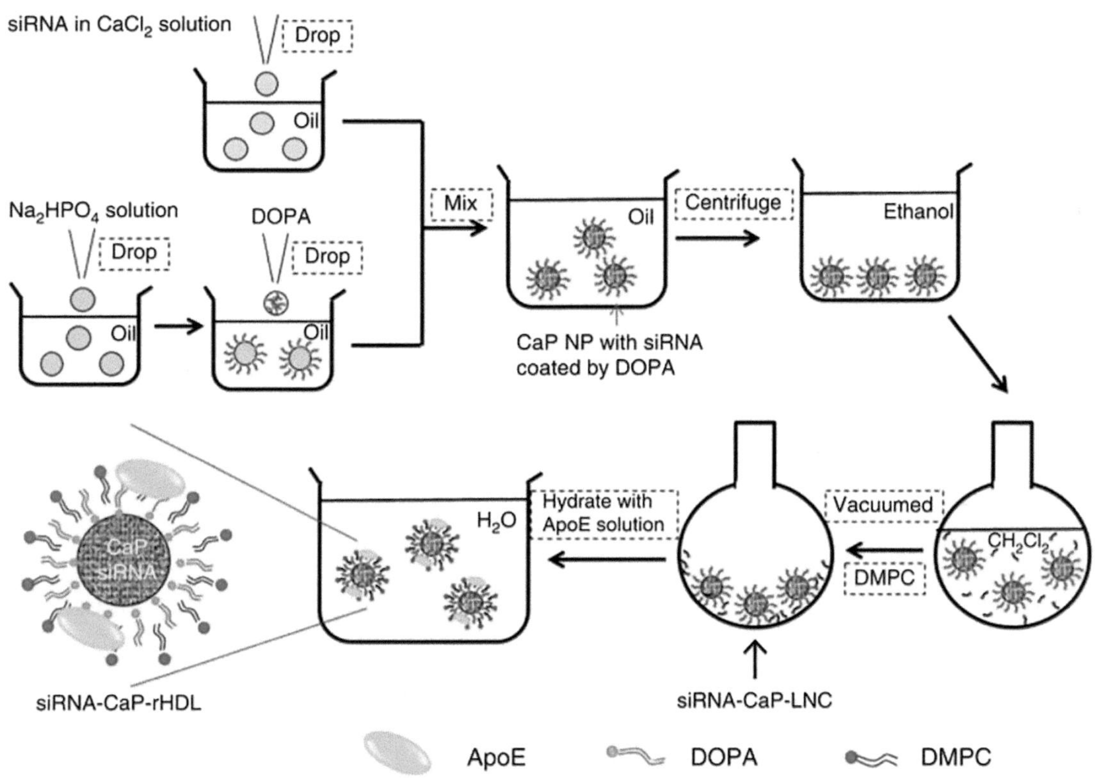

FIGURE 12.10 The outline for the preparation of siRNA-CaP-rHDL. *rHDL*, Reconstituted high-density lipoprotein; *siRNA*, small interfering RNA. From Huang, J.-L. et al., *Lipoprotein-biomimetic nanostructure enables efficient targeting delivery of siRNA to Ras-activated glioblastoma cells via macropinocytosis.* Nat. Commun, 2017. **8**(1): p. 15144.

12.3 Extracellular vesicles—based drug delivery systems

Extracellular vehicles (EVs) are lipid-based structures naturally produced by cells and secreted in the extracellular space through exocytosis [21]. EVs are involved in cell-mediated immune response and chemotaxis and regulating apoptosis, cytokine production, and proliferation [22]. Based on their biogenesis patterns, EVs can be divided into two major groups: EVs that bud outward from the membrane of donor cells (e.g., microvesicles and oncosomes) and exosomes that are generated within the endosomes inside the original cells (Fig. 12.11) [23]. The International Society for Extracellular Vesicles (ISEV) endorses EV as the generic term for particles naturally released from the cell that are determined by a lipid bilayer and cannot replicate (i.e., do not contain a nucleus). It is urged to consider using the operational terms for EV subtypes that refer to (1) physical characteristics of EVs, such as size; (2)

TABLE 12.1 Clinical trial examples of drug-loaded cell membrane/lipoprotein-based drug delivery systems.

ClinicalTrials.gov ID	Project	Carrier	Drug	Conditions	Phase
NCT03674242	Study of eryaspase in combination with chemotherapy versus chemotherapy alone for the treatment of TNBC (TRYbeCA-2)	RBC	L-asparaginase	Triple-negative breast cancer	2/3
NCT04741984	Monocyte antigen carrier cells for newly diagnosed glioblastoma (GBM)	Monocyte	GMV pp65-LAMP mRNA	Glioblastoma and malignant glioma	1
NCT01530698	Single-step antigen loading and TLR activation of dendritic cells in melanoma patients	Dendritic cell	mRNA encoding gp100 and tyrosinase, TLR4 and CD70	Melanoma	1/2
NCT04660929	CAR-macrophages for the treatment of HER2-overexpressing solid tumors	Macrophage	Anti-HER2 CAR M	HER2-positive solid tumors	1
NCT01172964	A pilot feasibility study of oral 5-flurocytosine and genetically-modified neural stem cells expressing *E. coli* cytosine deaminase for treatment of recurrent high grade gliomas	Stem cell	5-FU	Adult anaplastic astrocytoma, etc.	1
NCT06051760	NV-001 in the treatment of advanced solid tumors	Tumor and adjuvant membrane		Malignant neoplasm	1
NCT04616872	Treatment of patients with atherosclerotic disease with methotrexate-associated to LDL-like nanoparticles	LDL-like nanoparticle	Methotrexate	Atherosclerosis, etc.	2/3
NCT04148833	Treatment of patients with atherosclerotic disease with paclitaxel-associated to LDL-like nanoparticles (PAC-MAN)	LDL-like nanoparticle	Paclitaxel	Coronary artery disease, etc.	2/3

Note: this is by no means an exhaustive list and is subject to updates and additions. Data were collected from ClinicalTrials.gov (Nov 2024).

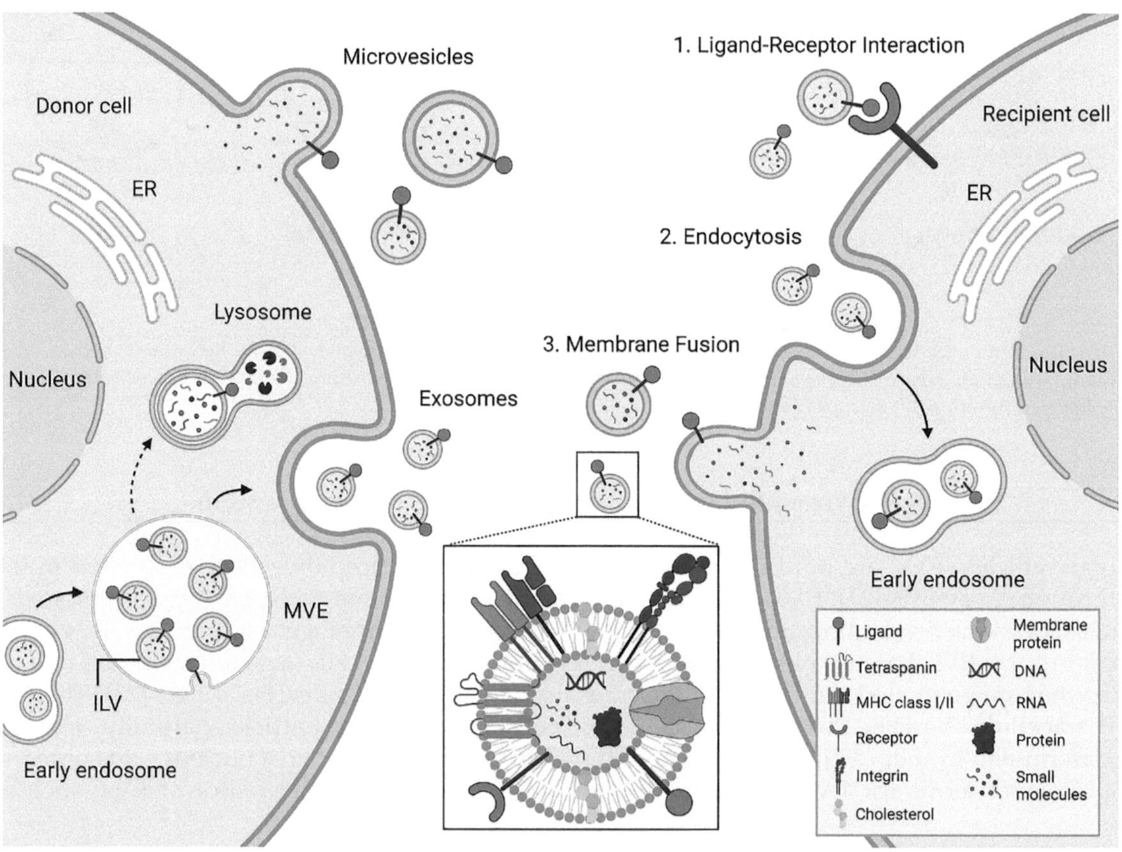

FIGURE 12.11 Extracellular vesicle biogenesis and intracellular communication patterns. *ER*, Endoplasmic reticulum; *ILV*, intraluminal vesicle; *MVE*, multivesicular endosome. From Song, X., L. Xu, and W. Zhang, *Biomimetic synthesis and optimization of extracellular vesicles for bone regeneration.* J Control Release, 2023. **355**: p. 18-41, with permission from Elsevier.

biochemical composition, such as $CD63^{+}/CD81^{+}$ EVs; or (3) descriptions of conditions or cell of origin, such as apoptotic bodies [24]. EV-mediated communication can be unidirectional or reciprocal. EV uptake by target cells involves receptor-mediated endocytosis, lipid raft interactions, phagocytosis, and direct fusion (Fig. 12.11) [21,25].

The idea of exploring EVs for targeted drug delivery was introduced in 2011 [21]. As shown in Fig. 12.12, the advantages of using EV biomimetics include natural tropism, inherent targeting ability, deceased immune clearance, ability to cross biological barriers, and biological stability [21,22,25]. On the other hand, some of the challenges for clinical translation of EV biomimetics include safety concerns (especially for nonautologous EVs) and the inherent complexity and heterogeneity of EVs [21,25]. To develop EV biomimetics, a novel strategy is to mimic the natural EVs in terms of lipid composition with a consideration of the protein signature (rather than focusing on the surface protein profile or nucleic acids). In reality, lipids are essential and actively involved in the biological function of EVs. As shown in Fig. 12.13, the starting point is the lipidomic studies of well-known cells/cell lines and their EVs showing the desired tropism/homing capabilities. Simplifications, such as grouping phospholipids of similar lipidic component characteristics, can be beneficial. To improve drug delivery efficiency, key molecules identified through the study of tropism and internalization mechanisms of EVs can be incorporated into EV biomimetics [21].

EVs/biomimetic EVs have been applied for various diseases treatment, such as drug-resistant infections, diabetes, SARS-CoV-2 pneumonia, and cancer (Table 12.2) [25]. For example, grapefruit-derived EVs decorated with doxorubicin-loaded heparin-based nanoparticles (biomimetic EV-DNs), were designed for glioma therapy (Fig. 12.14). Grapefruit EVs have large amounts of phosphatidylethanolamine and cell membrane proteins and can provide reactive amino groups to react with the carboxyl groups of heparin-based nanoparticles. Moreover, grapefruit-derived EVs also showed higher efficiency in cell recognition compared with synthetic lysolipid liposomes. cRGD (cyclic Arg-Gly-Asp) peptide was used since it can specifically bind with integrin $\alpha_v\beta_3$ (highly expressed on activated endothelial cells and some cancer cells) and pH-sensitive adipic acid dihydrazide was used to provide the pH-responsiveness of the nanoparticle assisting its endosomal escape [26].

When it comes to the scale-up and manufacturing of drug-loaded EVs/EV mimetics, the process/unit operations include cell culture for EV production (or components for constructing EV biomimetics), isolation, purification, drug loading, and formulation (Fig. 12.15) [25]. At present, differential ultracentrifugation is considered the standard method for EV extraction. Cells and large cell fragments can be removed at low-speed centrifugation (e.g., 300*g*) while removing larger vesicles at a higher speed centrifugation (e.g.,10,000*g*). Then, a high-speed centrifugation

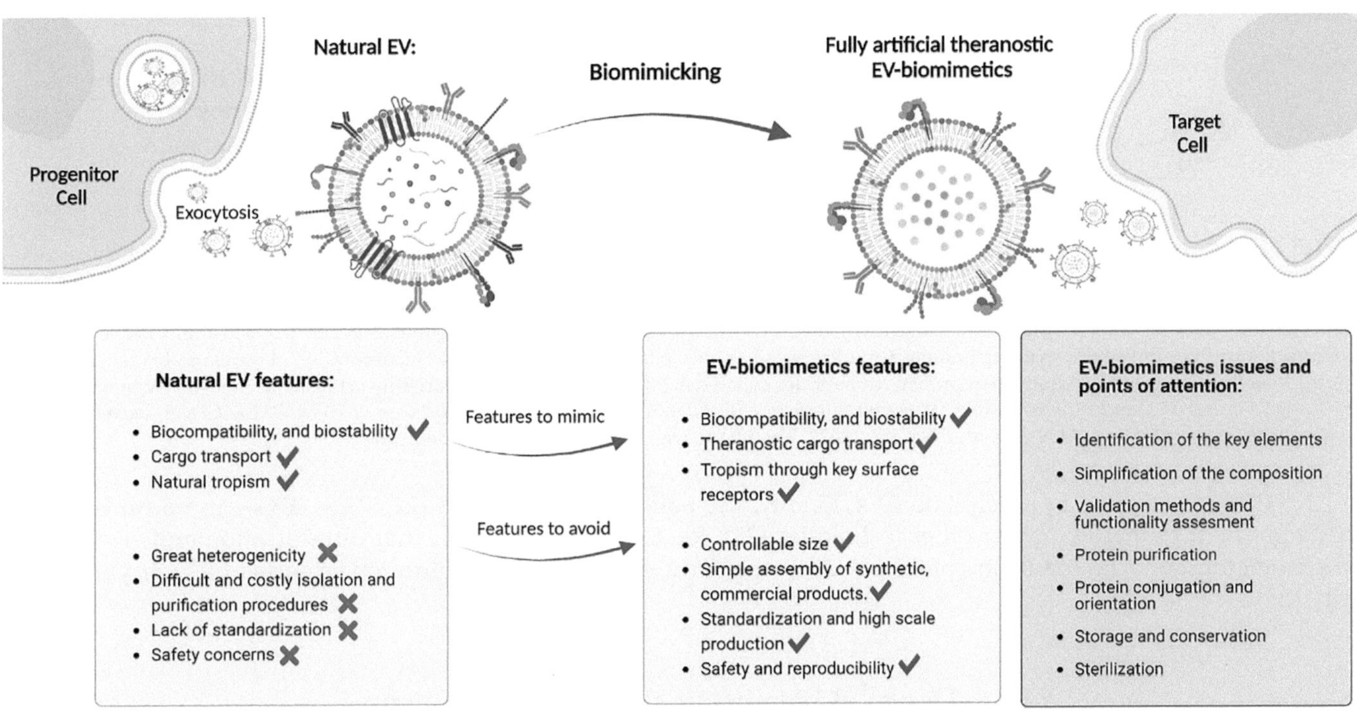

FIGURE 12.12 Schematic of the advantages and issues of extracellular vesicle (EV) biomimetics obtained through the bottom-up approach. From Rosso, G. and V. Cauda, *Biomimicking extracellular vesicles with fully artificial ones: a rational design of EV-BIOMIMETICS toward effective theranostic tools in nanomedicine.* ACS Biomater. Sci. Eng, 2022. The image was created with BioRender.com.

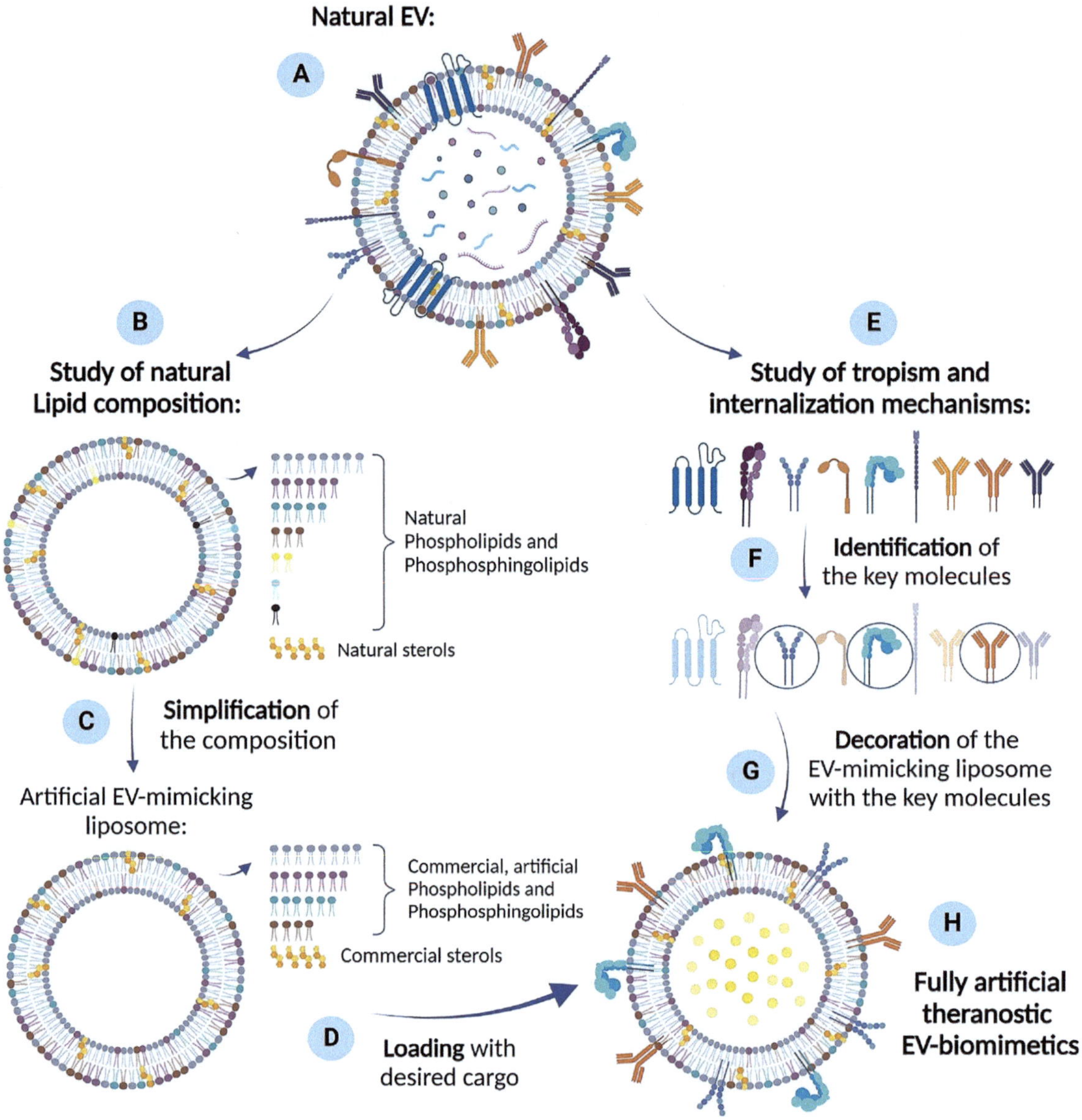

FIGURE 12.13 Schematic of a novel, practical approach to develop extracellular vesicle (EV) biomimetics. The choice of (A) a natural EV population with the desired characteristics and homing capabilities is the starting point. (B) Lipidomic studies of natural EVs provide a reference composition, from which simplifications (C) can be introduced. (C) Through the simplification of the composition, artificial EV-mimicking liposomes can be produced and (D) loaded with a cargo. (E) The study of the biological mechanisms behind a specific tropism ability can lead to the (F) identification of key molecules enabling homing attitude toward a specific target cell receptor. (G) The decoration of the cargo-loaded, artificial EV-mimicking liposome with the designated proteins or peptides concludes the process to produce (H) fully artificial theranostic EV biomimetics. From Rosso, G. and V. Cauda, *Biomimicking extracellular vesicles with fully artificial ones: a rational design of EV-BIOMIMETICS toward effective theranostic tools in nanomedicine*. ACS Biomater. Sci. Eng, 2022. The image was created with BioRender.com.

(e.g., 100,000*g*) is applied to precipitate EVs. Finally, the pellet is resuspended [22,27,28]. EVs can be purified by density gradient centrifugation or other techniques [22]. Recent studies indicate that ultrafiltration and size exclusion chromatography (alone or in combination) outperform differential ultrafiltration in terms of both yield and purity [25].

12.4 Design of biomimetic drug delivery systems

Problem-driven biological-inspired design (BID) is one approach to biomimetic design. A unified problem-driven process model is shown in Fig. 12.16. It consists of eight steps. The first phase (steps 1-4) focuses on a technology-to-

TABLE 12.2 Clinical trials with drug-loaded EVs/biomimetic EVs.

ClinicalTrials.gov ID	Project	Vesicle	Drug	Conditions	Phase
NCT04879810	Plant exosomes +/− curcumin to abrogate symptoms of inflammatory bowel disease	Ginger exosome	Curcumin	Irritable bowel disease	NA
NCT03608631	iExosomes in treating participants with metastatic pancreas cancer with KrasG12D mutation	Mesenchymal stromal cell derived exosome	KrasG12D siRNA	KRAS NP_004976.2: p.G12D, etc.	1
NCT01294072	Study investigating the ability of plant exosomes to deliver curcumin to normal and colon cancer tissue	Plant exosome	Curcumin	Colon cancer	1
NCT04664738	PEP on a skin graft donor site wound	Platelet derived extracellular vesicle	Anti-inflammatory and angiogenic growth factors	Skin graft	1
NCT05043181	Exosome-based nanoplatform for LDLR mRNA delivery in FH (ENDFH)	Bone marrow MSCs—derived exosome	LDLR mRNA	Familial hypercholesterolemia	1
NCT05375604	A study of exoASO-STAT6(CDK-004) in patients with advanced hepatocellular carcinoma (HCC) and patients with liver metastases from either primary gastric cancer or colorectal cancer (CRC)	Cell-derived exosome	Synthetic lipid-tagged oligonucleotide	Advanced hepatocellular carcinoma, etc.	1
NCT03384433	Allogenic mesenchymal stem cell—derived exosome in patients with acute ischemic stroke	Mesenchymal stem cells—derived exosome	MiR-124	Cerebrovascular disorders	1/2
NCT05947747	Safety and efficacy of EXO-CD24 in preventing clinical deterioration in patients with mild-moderate ARDS	Exosome	CD24	Mild-moderate ARDS	2
NCT04969172	A phase II randomized, double-blind, placebo-controlled study to evaluate the safety and efficacy of exosomes overexpressing CD24 to prevent clinical deterioration in patients with moderate or severe COVID-19 infection	Human embryonic kidney T-REx-293 cell derived exosome	CD24	COVID-19	2
NCT04902183	Safety and efficacy of exosomes overexpressing CD24 in two doses for patients with moderate or severe COVID-19	Exosome	CD24	COVID-19	2
NCT01159288	Trial of a vaccination with tumor antigen-loaded dendritic cell—derived exosomes (CSET 1437)	Dendritic cell derived exosome	Tumor antigen	Non small cell lung cancer	2

Note: this is by no means an exhaustive list and is subject to updates and additions. Data were collected from ClinicalTrials.gov (Nov 2024).

biology transition, while the second phase (steps 5–8) tackles its way back from biology to technology. The required contributions are indicated with the light (biological) and dark (technological) arrows. The initial step is the problem analysis followed by the abstraction of the problem leading to a functional model. The problem can be then transposed to biology with the envisaged function. Biological models can be set up through literature search and/or gathering existing knowledge. Once a biological model is selected and abstracted, the transposition of the biological strategy to technology follows. The whole process is iterative. For example, after step 4, with a better understanding of the initial problem, a new cycle of steps 1 to 3 may be necessary [29]. Abstraction (identification and concentration on specific properties/functions) is done at least twice during the problem-driven BID process as shown in Fig. 12.16. First, the technical problem is abstracted from the initial analysis of the design problem. Second, key biological principles/strategies are abstracted from the understanding of a biological phenomenon and brought into a form useful for design work [30].

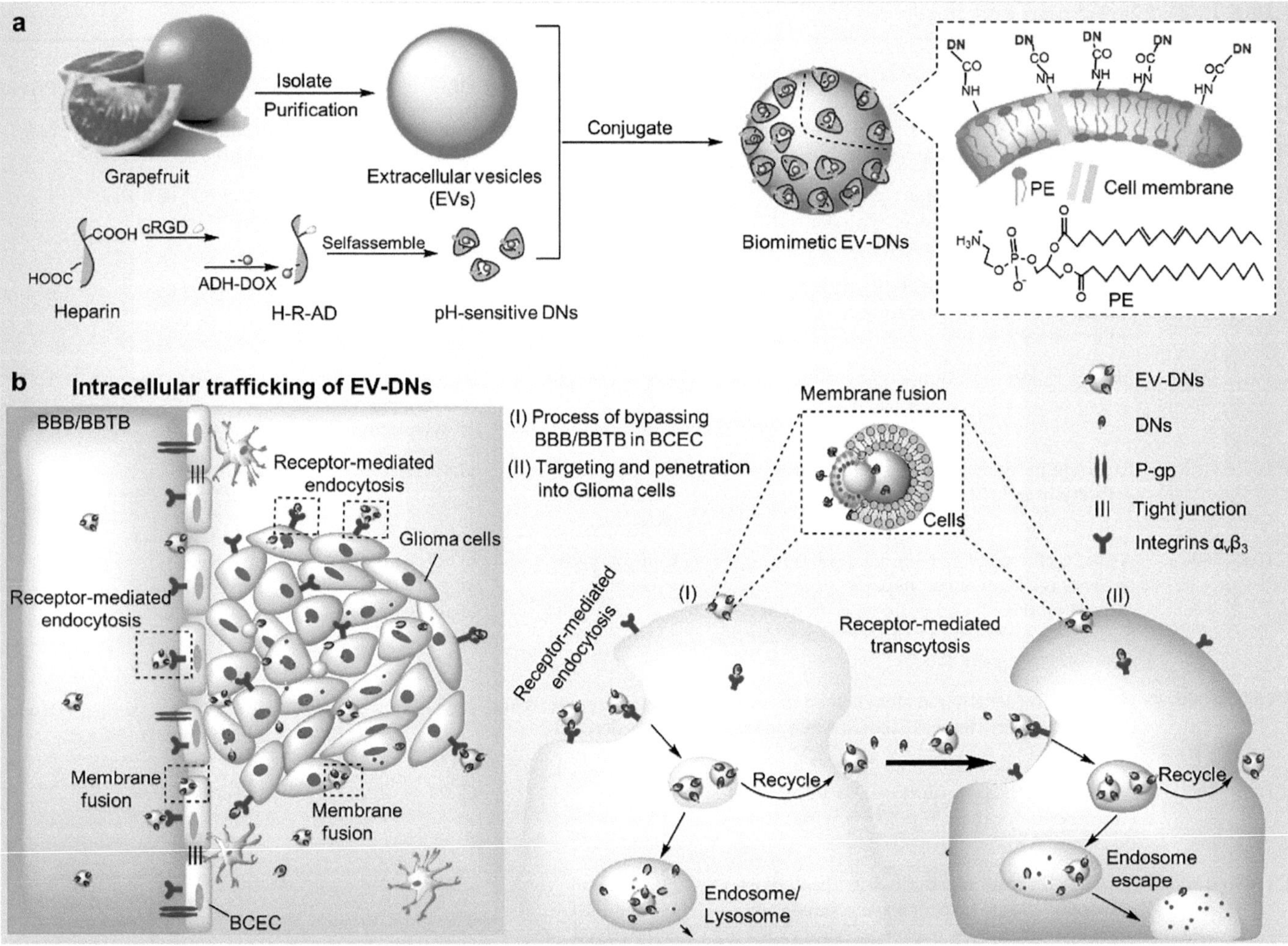

FIGURE 12.14 Schematic of the preparation (a) of biomimetic delivery system of EV-DNs and the mechanism (b) of EV-DNs bypassing BBB/BBTB and penetrating glioma. The pH-sensitive DNs using natural biomacromolecule heparin as a carrier were devised to incorporate onto the surface of grapefruit EVs for the treatment of glioma. Uptake of EV-DNs could occur by BCEC *via* receptor-mediated endocytosis and membrane fusion, and then parts of EV-DNs and DNs could be recycled to the outside BCEC and enter into glioma cells. After uptake by glioma cells *via* receptor-mediated endocytosis and membrane fusion, DOX could be further released from pH-sensitive EV-DNs or DNs in the acidic tumor microenvironment and penetrate into the nucleus by triggering endosomal escape. *ADH*, Adipic acid dihydrazide; *BBB/BBTB*, blood-brain barrier/blood-brain tumor barrier; *BCEC*, brain capillary endothelial cells; *cRGD*, cyclic Arg-Gly-Asp; *DN*, doxorubicin (DOX)-loaded heparin-based nanoparticle; *PE*, phosphatidylethanolamine; *P-gp*, P-glycoprotein. From Niu, W. et al., *A biomimetic drug delivery system by integrating grapefruit extracellular vesicles and doxorubicin-loaded heparin-based nanoparticles for glioma therapy.* Nano Lett, 2021. **21**(3): p. 1484-1492. Copyright (2021), American Chemical Society.

Another approach for biomimetic design is solution-driven BID. This approach is often initiated by biologists with deep insights into biological functionalities [31]. One good example is the self-cleaning property of lotus leaves inspired the development of superhydrophobic surfaces. The eight steps of an approach to implement solution-driven BID are summarized in Fig. 12.17 [31,32]. The most challenging part of the solution-driven BID is the identification of technical applications that will benefit from the "solutions" presented by the biological world [31].

Finally, we can examine some examples of both approaches. First, the problem-driven approach, starting with the problem of low residence time of encapsulated drugs resulting in suboptimal therapeutic efficacies and even toxic effects. It is beneficial to improve the "adhesiveness" of the drug carrier. Examining the biological world, geckos exhibit exceptional ability to stick to various surfaces. A gecko's foot has nearly 500,000 keratinous setae, and each seta contains hundreds of projections terminating in 0.2- to 0.5-μm spatula-shaped structures (Fig. 12.18). This topographic design increases the surface contact area, leading to extraordinary adhesive properties [33–36]. Hence, engineering the drug carrier surface with this unique topographic design can be a potential approach to increase the residence time [37]. When it comes to the solution-driven approach, we must keep reminding ourselves to

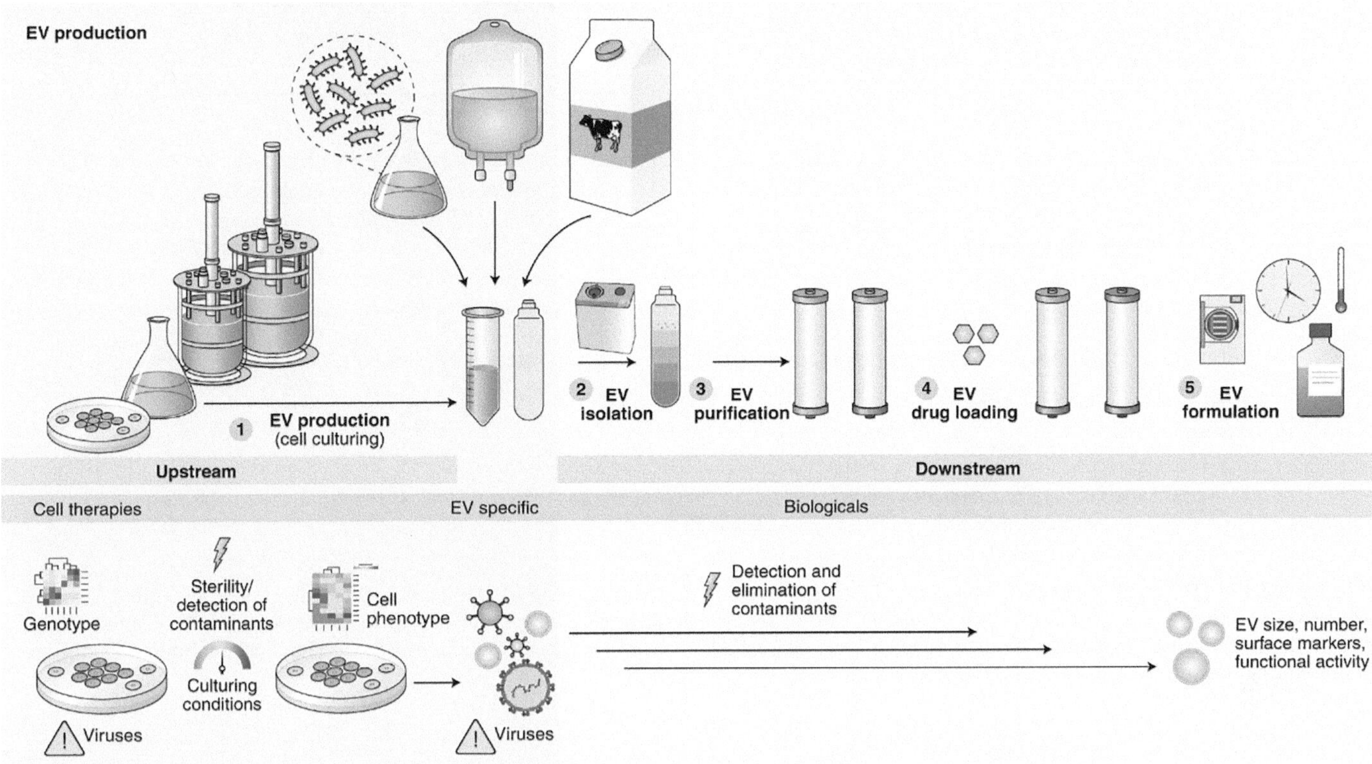

FIGURE 12.15 Process steps and key unit operations in the production process of drug-loaded extracellular vesicles (EVs). Upstream processing can adapt safety and quality concepts used in the production of cells for cell therapies, while downstream processing can partially adapt the concepts used in the production of biologicals. From Herrmann, I.K., M.J.A. Wood, and G. Fuhrmann, *Extracellular vesicles as a next-generation drug delivery platform.* Nat. Nanotechnol, 2021. **16**(7): p. 748-759, with permission from Springer Nature.

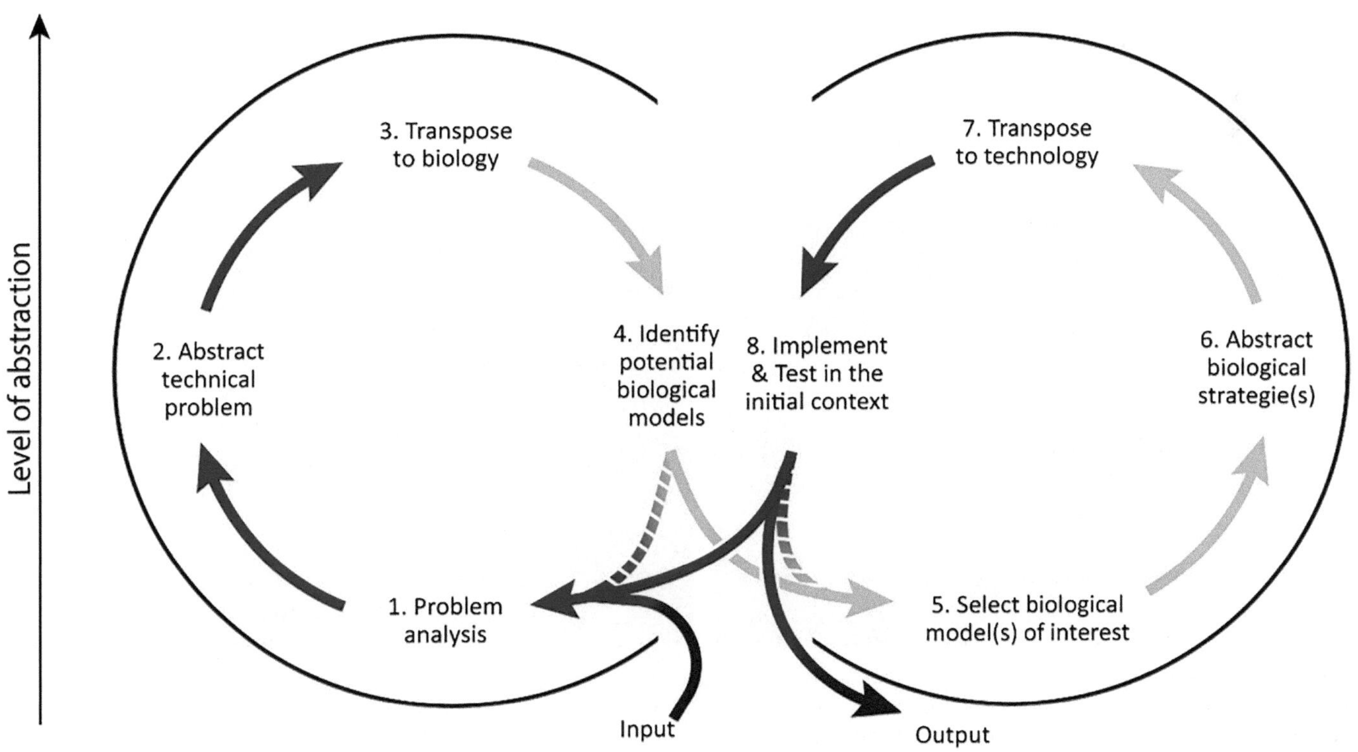

FIGURE 12.16 The unified problem-driven process of biomimetics. From Fayemi, P.E. et al., *Biomimetics: process, tools and practice.* Bioinspir Biomim, 2017. **12**(1): p. 011002, with permission from IOP Publishing Ltd.

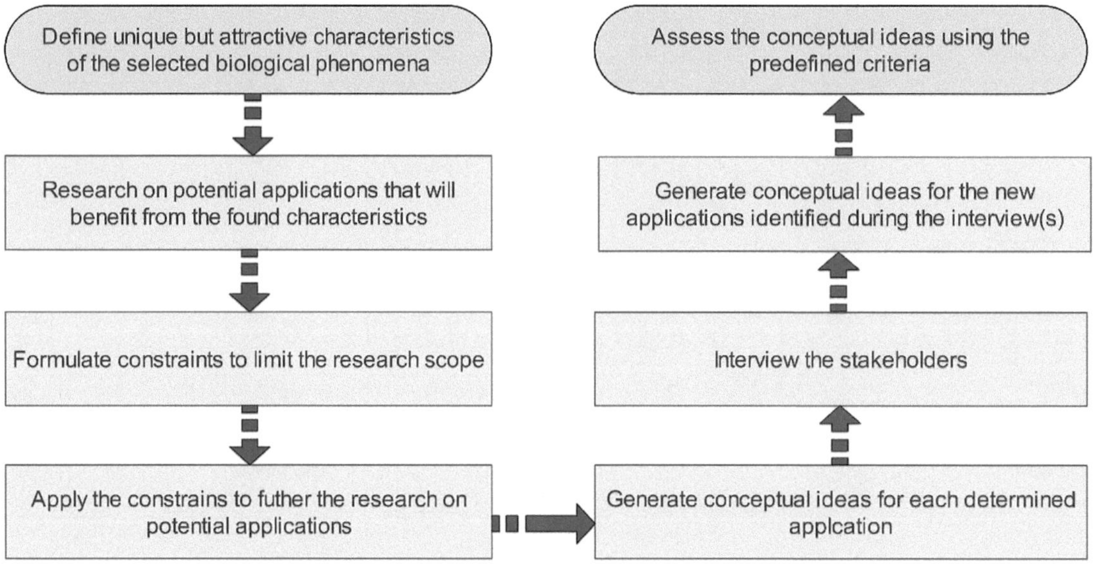

FIGURE 12.17 The eight steps of solution-driven biological-inspired design (searching for applications). The diagram is generated based on Lenau TA, Lakhtakia A, *Solution-driven biologically inspired design.* In: *Biologically inspired design: a primer.* Springer International Publishing: Cham; 2021. p. 61-76; Lenau TA, *Application Search in Solution-Driven Biologically Inspired Design.* Proceedings of the Design Society: International Conference on Engineering Design, 2019. 1(1) p. 269-278.

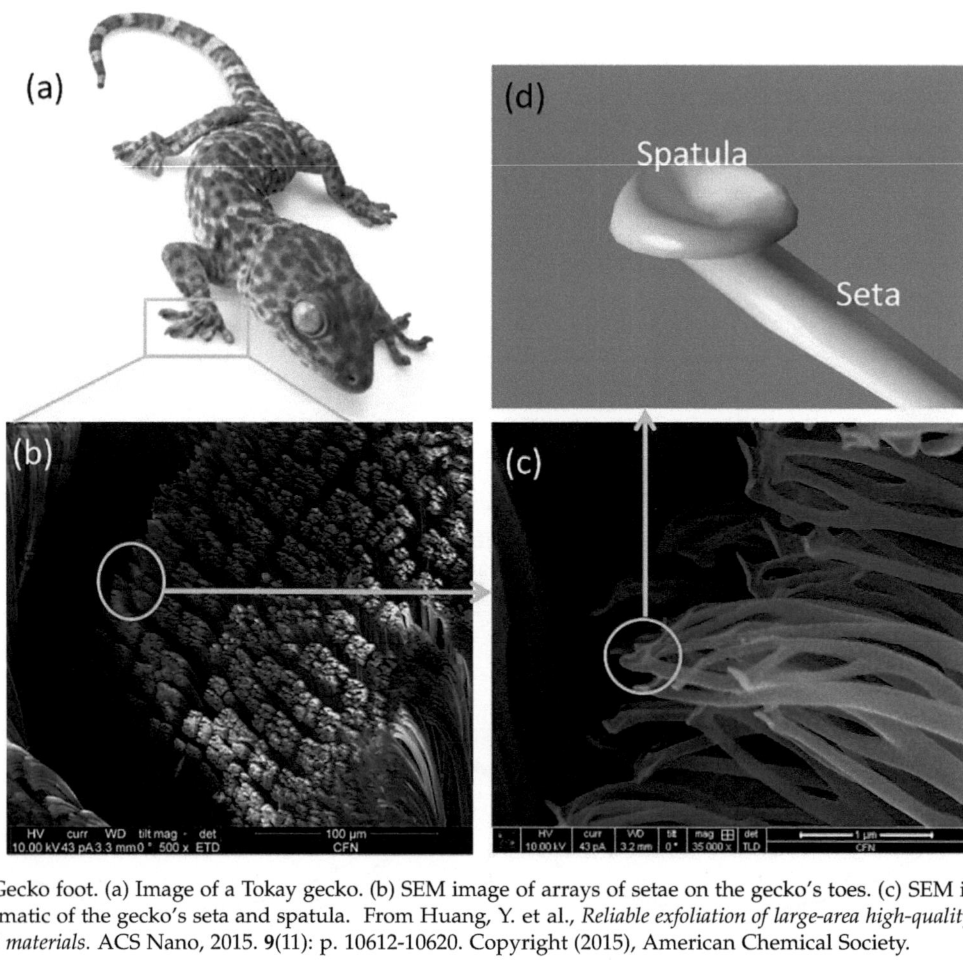

FIGURE 12.18 Gecko foot. (a) Image of a Tokay gecko. (b) SEM image of arrays of setae on the gecko's toes. (c) SEM image of spatulae and setae in (b). (d) Schematic of the gecko's seta and spatula. From Huang, Y. et al., *Reliable exfoliation of large-area high-quality flakes of graphene and other two-dimensional materials.* ACS Nano, 2015. **9**(11): p. 10612-10620. Copyright (2015), American Chemical Society.

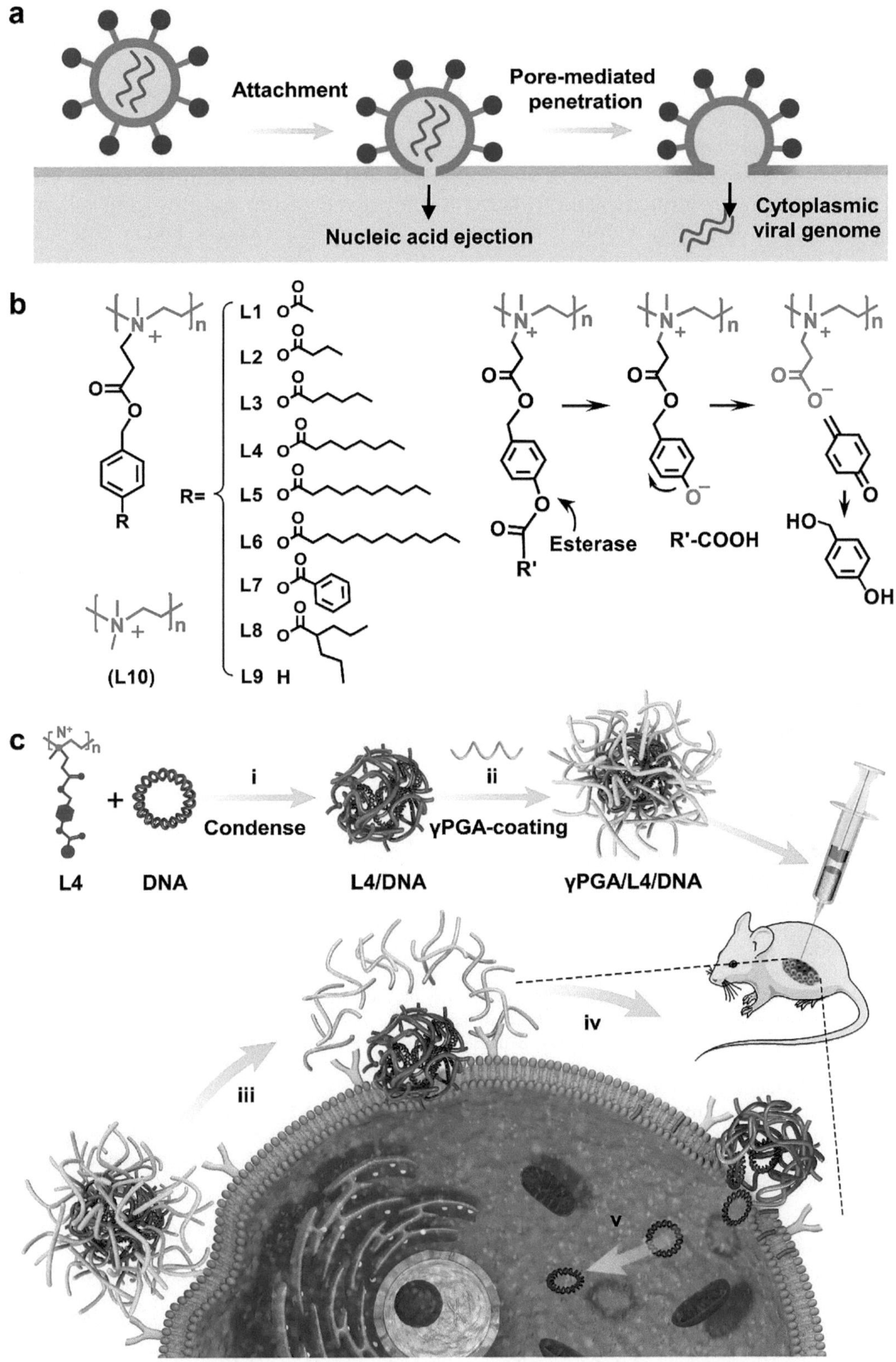

FIGURE 12.19 Scheme of DNA-ejecting vector for gene delivery. (a) Illustration of a virus delivering its genome *via* DNA ejection. (b) Structures of quaternized linear PEI with esterase-responsive moieties (L1-L8) or esterase-irresponsive controls, L9 and L10; and the esterase-catalyzed hydrolysis-triggered elimination reaction. (c) Scheme of fabrication and gene delivery of γPGA/L4/DNA. DNA is condensed by L4 to form L4/DNA polyplex (i) and then coated with γPGA (ii). Once contacting a cell, γPGA can strip off and expose L4/DNA, then the L4 long acyl chains inserts into the lipid bilayer and anchor the L4/DNA on the cell membrane (iii); Some of the L4 exposed to the cytoplasm are hydrolyzed by cytosolic esterase, thereby turning neutral to liberalize the DNA (iv); finally, the liberalized DNA are squeezed into the cytoplasm by its electrostatic repulsion (v) for effective gene transfection. *γPGA*, Poly(γ-glutamic acid). From Wang, G. et al., *Virus-mimetic DNA-ejecting polyplexes for efficient intracellular cancer gene delivery.* Nano Today, 2021. **39**: p. 101215, with permission from Elsevier.

learn from nature, the best teacher. For example, viruses use their protruding coat proteins (spikes) to induce multivalent interactions with cell membranes to initiate cellular binding and uptake and also utilize nanoscale "needles" to inject genetic materials directly into the target cells [33]. One potential application is to design drug carriers with virus-inspired DNA/RNA-ejecting vectors to improve cellular uptake through direct membrane penetration [33,38]. For example, a virus-mimicking vector capable of sticking to the cell membrane and ejecting DNA into cytosol without entering the cells has been developed. The vector utilizes the esterase-catalyzed charge-reversal polymer with long acyl chains, *N*-[*p*-octanoyloxybenzyloxycarbonyl]-*N*-methyl ammonium of linear polyethyleneimine (L4). And it is coated with poly(γ-glutamic acid) (γPGA) for improved serum stability [39]. γPGA is nonimmunogenic and biodegradable and has been widely used for drug delivery. The cationic L4 can interact with DNA and form nanocomplex. It contains a large number of free carboxyl groups which can be used to enhance the solubility of the drug delivery systems and control the drug release [40]. As shown in Fig. 12.19, γPGA comes off upon contacting the cells, and L4's long acyl chains insert into the cell membrane. The part of the L4 exposed to the cytosolic esterase becomes neutral and releases DNA [39].

Review and practice questions

1. What is biomimetics? What is biomimicry? What is the major difference between the two terms?
2. Provide an example of biomimetic drug delivery systems which are not discussed in this chapter.
3. What are the advantages of using red blood cell-based systems for drug delivery?
4. What are the benefits of utilizing biomimetic hybrid-membrane systems for drug delivery?
5. What are the three general approaches for cell membrane modification?
6. What is the typical structure of lipoproteins?
7. What are extracellular vesicles (EVs)? What are the advantages of using EVs/EV biomimetics for drug delivery?
8. What are the process steps and key unit operations in the production process of drug-loaded EVs?
9. Describe the general process of the problem-driven biomimetic design.
10. Describe the general process of the solution-driven biomimetic design.

References

[1] Hwang J, et al. Biomimetics: forecasting the future of science, engineering, and medicine. Int J Nanomedicine 2015;10:5701–13.
[2] Lenau TA, Lakhtakia A. Chapter 1 Definitions. In: Biologically inspired design: a primer. Springer International Publishing; 2021. p. 1–4.
[3] Introduction: Bioinspired and biomimetic materials. Chem Rev 2017;117(20):12581–3.
[4] Bio-Inspired Buzzwords: Biomimicry and Biomimetics. Available from: http://businessinspiredbynature.com/bio-inspired-buzzwords-biomimicry-biomimetics/.
[5] Li ADR, et al. Mosquito proboscis-inspired needle insertion to reduce tissue deformation and organ displacement. Sci Rep 2020;10(1):12248.
[6] Abramson A, et al. An ingestible self-orienting system for oral delivery of macromolecules. Science 2019;363(6427):611–5.
[7] Guo M, et al. Research progress on cell membrane-coated biomimetic delivery systems. Front Bioeng Biotechnol 2021;9:772522.
[8] Li J, et al. Cell-membrane-coated nanoparticles for targeted drug delivery to the brain for the treatment of neurological diseases. Pharmaceutics 2023;15(2):621.
[9] Yan J, et al. Red blood cells for drug delivery. Small Methods 2017;1(12):1700270.
[10] Chen M, et al. Red blood cells: a potential delivery system. J Nanobiotechnology 2023;21(1):288.
[11] Muzykantov VR. Drug delivery by red blood cells: vascular carriers designed by mother nature. Expert Opin Drug Deliv 2010;7(4):403–27.
[12] Villa CH, et al. Erythrocytes as carriers for drug delivery in blood transfusion and beyond. Transfus Med Rev 2017;31(1):26–35.
[13] Hughes RM, et al. Phototriggered secretion of membrane compartmentalized bioactive agents. Angew Chem Int Ed Engl 2016;55(52):16080–3.
[14] Yin Y, et al. Biomimetic neutrophil and macrophage dual membrane-coated nanoplatform with orchestrated tumor-microenvironment responsive capability promotes therapeutic efficacy against glioma. Chem Eng J 2022;433:133848.
[15] Wu L, et al. Platelet-tumor cell hybrid membrane-camouflaged nanoparticles for enhancing therapy efficacy in glioma. Int J Nanomedicine 2021;16(null):8433–46.
[16] Shi W, et al. Hybrid membrane-derived nanoparticles for isoliquiritin enhanced glioma therapy. Pharmaceuticals 2022;15(9):1059.
[17] Busatto S, et al. Lipoprotein-based drug delivery. Adv Drug Deliv Rev 2020;159:377–90.
[18] Moini J. Chapter 5 - Epidemiology of diet and diabetes mellitus. In: Moini J, editor. Epidemiology of diabetes. Elsevier; 2019. p. 57–73.
[19] Ma X, Song Q, Gao X. Reconstituted high-density lipoproteins: novel biomimetic nanocarriers for drug delivery. Acta Pharm Sin B 2018;8(1):51–63.
[20] Huang J-L, et al. Lipoprotein-biomimetic nanostructure enables efficient targeting delivery of siRNA to Ras-activated glioblastoma cells via macropinocytosis. Nat Commun 2017;8(1):15144.
[21] Rosso G, Cauda V. Biomimicking extracellular vesicles with fully artificial ones: a rational design of EV-BIOMIMETICS toward effective theranostic tools in nanomedicine. ACS Biomater Sci Eng 2022.

[22] Shi R, et al. Biomimetic extracellular vesicles for the tumor targeted treatment. Eng Regen 2023;4(4):427–37.
[23] Song X, Xu L, Zhang W. Biomimetic synthesis and optimization of extracellular vesicles for bone regeneration. J Control Release 2023;355: 18–41.
[24] Théry C, et al. Minimal information for studies of extracellular vesicles 2018 (MISEV2018) a position statement of the International Society for Extracellular Vesicles and update of the MISEV2014 guidelines. J Extracell Vesicles 2018;7(1):1535750.
[25] Herrmann IK, Wood MJA, Fuhrmann G. Extracellular vesicles as a next-generation drug delivery platform. Nat Nanotechnol 2021;16(7): 748–59.
[26] Niu W, et al. A biomimetic drug delivery system by integrating grapefruit extracellular vesicles and doxorubicin-loaded heparin-based nanoparticles for glioma therapy. Nano Lett 2021;21(3):1484–92.
[27] Doyle LM, Wang MZ. Overview of extracellular vesicles, their origin, composition, purpose, and methods for exosome isolation and analysis. Cells 2019;8(7):727.
[28] Momen-Heravi F, et al. Current methods for the isolation of extracellular vesicles. Biol Chem 2013;394(10):1253–62.
[29] Fayemi PE, et al. Biomimetics: process, tools and practice. Bioinspir Biomim 2017;12(1):011002.
[30] Lenau TA, Lakhtakia A. Chapter 5 Problem-driven biologically inspired design. In: Biologically inspired design: a primer. Springer International Publishing; 2021. p. 47–60.
[31] Lenau TA, Lakhtakia A. Chapter 6 Solution-driven biologically inspired design. In: Biologically inspired design: a primer. Springer International Publishing; 2021. p. 61–76.
[32] Lenau TA. Application search in solution-driven biologically inspired design. Proceedings of the Design Society: International Conference on Engineering Design 2019;1(1):269–78.
[33] Finbloom JA, et al. Bioinspired nanotopographical design of drug delivery systems. Nat Rev Bioeng 2023;1(2):139–52.
[34] Autumn K, et al. Adhesive force of a single gecko foot-hair. Nature 2000;405(6787):681–5.
[35] Autumn K, et al. Effective elastic modulus of isolated gecko setal arrays. J Exp Biol 2006;209(18):3558–68.
[36] Huang Y, et al. Reliable exfoliation of large-area high-quality flakes of graphene and other two-dimensional materials. ACS Nano 2015;9(11): 10612–20.
[37] Mahdavi A, et al. A biodegradable and biocompatible gecko-inspired tissue adhesive. PNAS 2008;105(7):2307–12.
[38] Liao Z, et al. Virus-inspired nanosystems for drug delivery. Nanoscale 2021;13(45):18912–24.
[39] Wang G, et al. Virus-mimetic DNA-ejecting polyplexes for efficient intracellular cancer gene delivery. Nano Today 2021;39:101215.
[40] Khalil IR, et al. Poly-gamma-glutamic acid (γ-PGA)-based encapsulation of adenovirus to evade neutralizing antibodies. Molecules 2018; 23(10):2565.

CHAPTER

13

Site-specific drug delivery

Wujie Zhang

LEARNING OBJECTIVES

- To understand the physiology of the blood-brain barrier and the major challenges for brain drug delivery
- To discuss the three major approaches for brain drug delivery
- To understand the physiology of the colon
- To interpret the major design principle of oral colonic drug delivery systems
- To discuss the challenges of drug delivery for cancer therapy
- To interpret the general working mechanism of responsive and multifunctional drug delivery systems for cancer therapy
- To discuss the significance of circulating tumor cells and cancer stem cells in cancer therapy
- To design site-specific drug delivery systems

13.1 Drug delivery to the brain

Brain diseases, from stroke and Alzheimer disease to multiple sclerosis, epilepsy, traumatic brain injury, and more, affect millions worldwide [1]. The adult brain has five principal interfaces that protect the central nervous system (CNS): the blood-brain barrier (BBB), the arachnoid barrier, the blood—cerebrospinal fluid (CSF) barrier, the circumventricular organs, and the ependyma. Among them, the BBB is the most selective physical barrier [2]. The existence of the BBB was first found by Paul Ehrlich and proved by Edwin Goldmann [3], although some believe that the credit goes to Humphrey Ridley, who noticed the difference in the permeability of beeswax and mercury in brain tissues from other tissues [4,5]. As shown in Fig. 13.1, the BBB is composed of endothelial cells, astroglia (astrocytes), pericytes, and junctional complexes. Endothelial cells are the BBB's core anatomical structure for lining the cerebral blood vessels and interacting with different types of cells in the CNS [3]. Pericytes are perivascular cells embedded in the basement membrane and are located abluminal to the endothelial cells. Pericytes regulate vesicular transport across the BBB and modulate capillary diameter. The endfeet plasma membrane (astrocytes) of the neurovascular unit is responsible for maintaining water homeostasis, ionic concentration, and a functionally mature

Fundamentals and Design of Drug Delivery Systems
https://doi.org/10.1016/B978-0-443-23521-4.00013-8

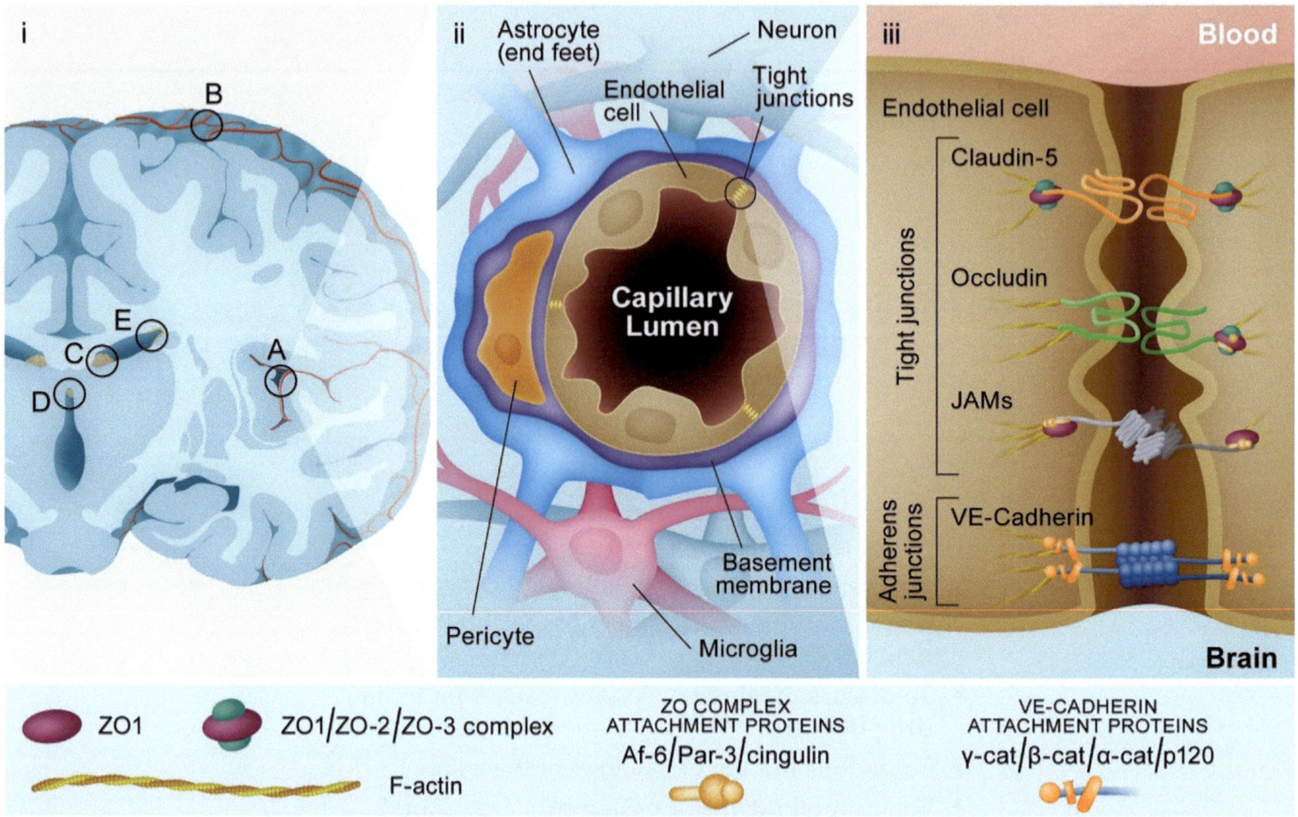

FIGURE 13.1 Barriers in the adult human brain. (i) The adult human brain has five barrier interfaces that regulate the molecular traffic into the brain parenchyma. (A) The blood-brain barrier (BBB), (B) the arachnoid barrier, (C) the blood-CSF barrier, (D) the circumventricular organs, and (E) the ependyma. (ii) The properties of the BBB are primarily dictated by the endothelial cells. The BBB also comprises the acellular basement membrane, pericytes, and astrocytes, with further contributions from neurons and glial cells. (iii) Junctions between the endothelial cells are responsible for regulating paracellular permeability through the complex molecular architecture of junction and scaffolding proteins and their interactions with the cytoskeleton. *From Pandit, R., L. Chen, and J. Götz,* The blood-brain barrier: physiology and strategies for drug delivery. *Adv. Drug Deliv. Rev., 2020.* ***165-166****: p. 1-14, with permission from Elsevier.*

BBB [4]. The BBB excludes more than 98% of small-molecule drugs and all macromolecular therapeutics from crossing into the brain. The tight gap only allows passive diffusion of small (~ 500 Da) lipid-soluble drugs [3]. The first indication that the BBB would be a problem in brain drug delivery occurred in 1994: neurosyphilis, the most serious effect of syphilis, could not be treated by neosalvarsan due to the lack of transport of this drug across the BBB [5]. With the development of novel drug delivery approaches/systems, the transport of drug molecules across the BBB has also been achieved *via* other pathways such as receptor-mediated transcytosis (Fig. 13.2) [3].

Regarding the transvascular approaches, specific peptides/proteins can enter the brain by binding to receptors on endothelial cells *via* receptor-mediated transcytosis. These receptors include transferrin receptor (TfR), insulin receptor (IR), insulin-like growth factor (IGF), leptin receptor (LEP-R), vasopressinergic receptor (V1), low-density lipoprotein receptors (LDLR), and receptors for advanced glycation end products (RAGE). Cationization enhances cellular uptake through absorptive-mediated endocytosis (*via* the interaction with the negatively charged endothelial membrane and proteoglycans in the basement membrane). The BBB carrier-mediated transporters are members of the solute carrier (SLC) gene superfamily. Some of the carriers/transporters are glucose transporter 1 (GLUT1), L-type amino acid transport 1(LAT1), B vitamin carriers, thyroid hormone carriers, and organic cation carriers. However, for drug molecules that are ligands for efflux pumps, such as P-glycoprotein (P-gp), inhibition of these transporters should be taken into consideration [2,5].

Various natural/biomimetic and synthetic drug carriers have also been used for brain drug delivery. As shown in Table 13.1, natural/biomimetic carriers include the red blood cell membrane, brain tumor cell membrane, exosomes, and viruses (e.g., adeno-associated virus [AAV]). Synthetic ones are mostly nanoparticle and liposome based [3,6].

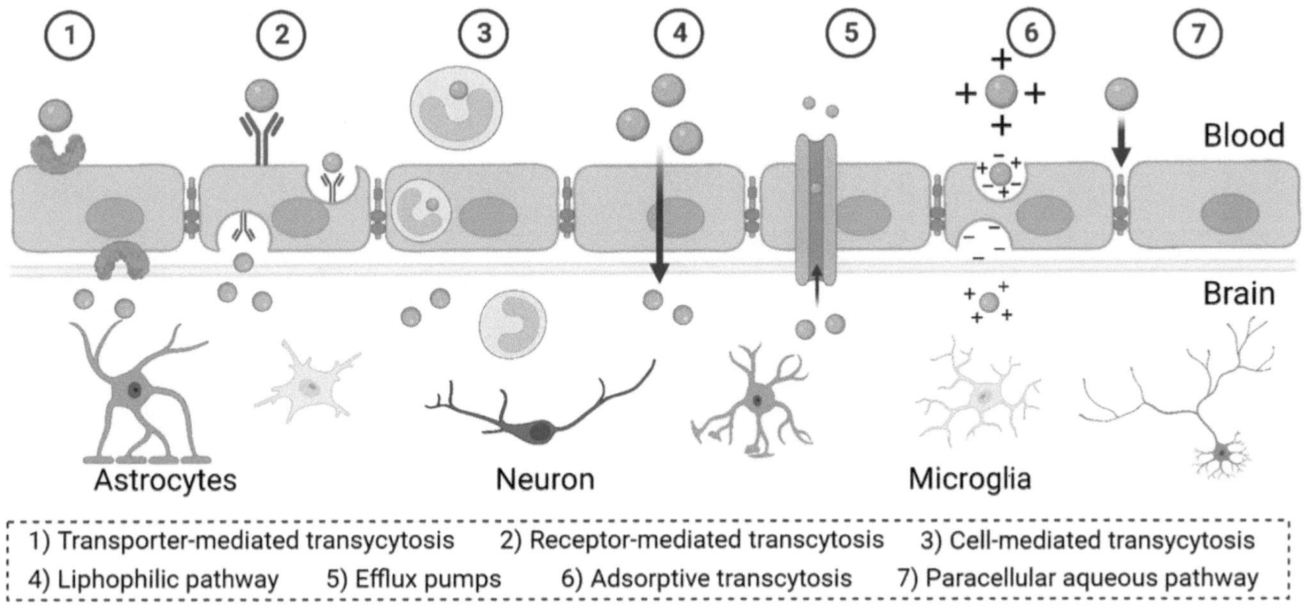

FIGURE 13.2 Schematic of different mechanisms for crossing the BBB (transvascular). *From* Wu, D. et al., The blood–brain barrier: structure, regulation, and drug delivery. *Signal Transduct Target Ther, 2023. 8(1): p. 217.*

TABLE 13.1 Transvascular brain drug delivery approaches.

Approach	Examples
Receptor-mediated transcytosis	Transferrin receptor (TfR); insulin receptor (IR); leptin receptor (LEP-R); low-density lipoprotein receptors (LDLR)
Carrier/transporter-mediated transcytosis	Glucose transporter (GLUT1); cationic L-amino acid transporter (CAT1); fatty acid transporters (FATP-1); vitamin carriers
Absorptive-mediated transcytosis	Cationization
Efflux pump inhibition	P-glycoprotein (P-gp); multidrug resistance–associated proteins (MRPs)
Drug carrier	
Natural biomimetic	Red blood cell membrane; brain tumor cell membrane; macrophage membrane; exosomes; viruses (e.g., adeno-associated virus [AAV])
Synthetic	Targeted nanoparticles; dendrimers

Viruses have developed various approaches to cross the BBB: direct transcytosis, *via* immune cell migration, and retrograde transport (Fig. 13.3) [7]. A recent study engineered AAV capsid variants that selectively target neurons after intravenous injection in mice and marmosets with CNS enrichment and decreased targeting of the liver (Fig. 13.4) [8,9]. When it comes to synthetic drug carriers, nanoparticles, dual and multitargeted ones, in particular, are of great interest [10]. For example, a dopamine-loaded nanoparticle system was developed to circumvent the BBB restoring motor function for Parkinson's disease [11]. Another example to cross BBB *via* caveolin-1–dependent transcytosis is to use P-selectin targeting [12]. As shown in Fig. 13.5, the nanoparticles, FiVis, are incorporated with the polysaccharide fucoidan for P-selectin targeting and loaded with the Smoothened inhibitor vismodegib. P-selectin includes transendothelial transport across the BBB *via* caveolin-1–dependent transcytosis and irradiation enhances the P-selectin expression. However, nanoparticles administered intravenously encounter multiple barriers besides the BBB, such as protein opsonization and macrophage uptake (Fig. 13.6) [13]. These should be carefully considered when designing a nanoparticulate system for brain drug delivery.

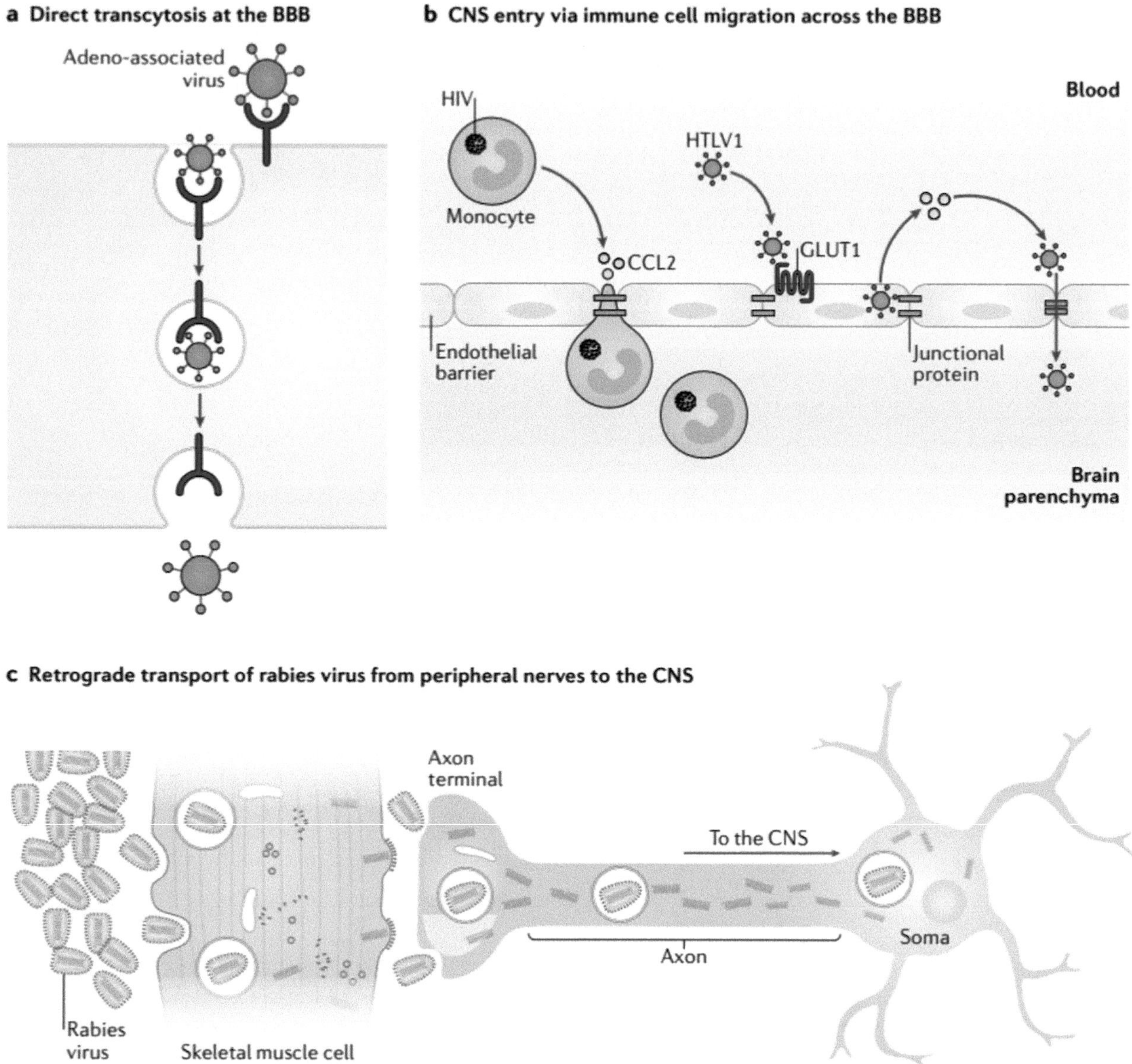

FIGURE 13.3 Viral entry into the central nervous system (CNS). (a) Viruses such as adeno-associated viruses (AAV) enter the brain parenchyma by binding to a surface protein on neurovascular endothelial cells, triggering receptor-mediated transcytosis. (b) Viruses such as HIV infect monocytes, which they use as Trojan horses to cross the BBB. Infected monocytes either pass through the BBB during normal turnover of perivascular macrophages or compromise the barrier by producing proinflammatory cytokines such as CC-motif ligand 2 (CCL2). Other viruses, such as human T- cell lymphotropic virus type 1 (HTLV-1), are able to infect the BBB to gain entry into the brain. For example, glucose transporter 1 (GLUT1) has been described as a receptor for HTLV-1. (c) Sensory and motor neurons that extend beyond the BBB are another entry point for viruses such as the rabies virus, which can bind to neurons at the neuromuscular junction. After entry, the viruses use the axonal transport system for retrograde transport. *From Testappen, G. et al.,* Strategies for delivering therapeutics across the BBB. *Nat. Rev. Drug Discov, 2021.* ***20****: p. 362-383, with permission from Springer Nature.*

Noninvasive nose-to-brain drug delivery approaches have also been becoming increasingly attractive (Fig. 13.7). A few hydrophilic, high-molecular-weight peptides/proteins have shown to appear in the brain rapidly after intranasal administration with higher levels compared to intravenous administration. Some advantages of the nose-to-brain drug delivery include self-administration capability, rapid onset of action, and minimized systemic exposure. Upon intranasal administration, a portion of the drug molecules may reach the innermost olfactory region, where they can be transported to the brain through intracellular, and/or transcellular pathways. At the same time, the respiratory pathway may also lead to the drug delivery to the brain [14–16]. Nanoparticles and micelles have been

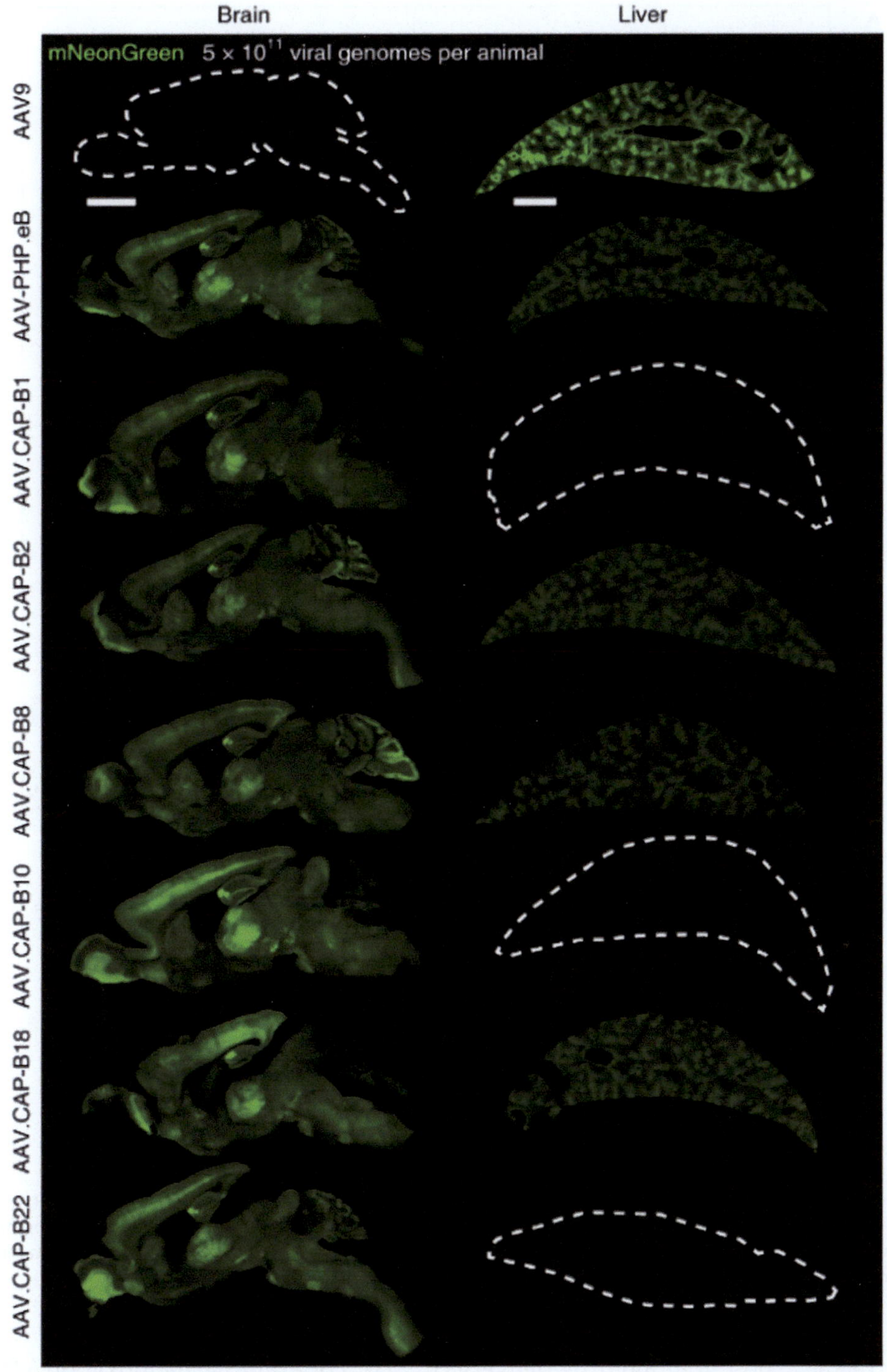

FIGURE 13.4 mNeonGreen was packaged in each AAV capsid variant under the control of the ubiquitous CAG promoter and intravenously administered to mice at a dose of 5×10^{11} viral genomes per animal. Transgene expression was assayed by mNeonGreen fluorescence throughout the brain and liver after 2 weeks. Direct comparison of the expression profiles in the brain and liver of the top-performing variants shows a correlation between validated tropisms and those predicted by the NGS data. Scale bars, 2 mm. *AAV,* Adeno-associated virus; *NGS,* next-generation sequencing. *From Goertsen, D. et al.,* AAV capsid variants with brain-wide transgene expression and decreased liver targeting after intravenous delivery in mouse and marmoset. *Nat. Neurosci, 2022.* ***25****(1): p. 106-115, with permission from Springer Nature.*

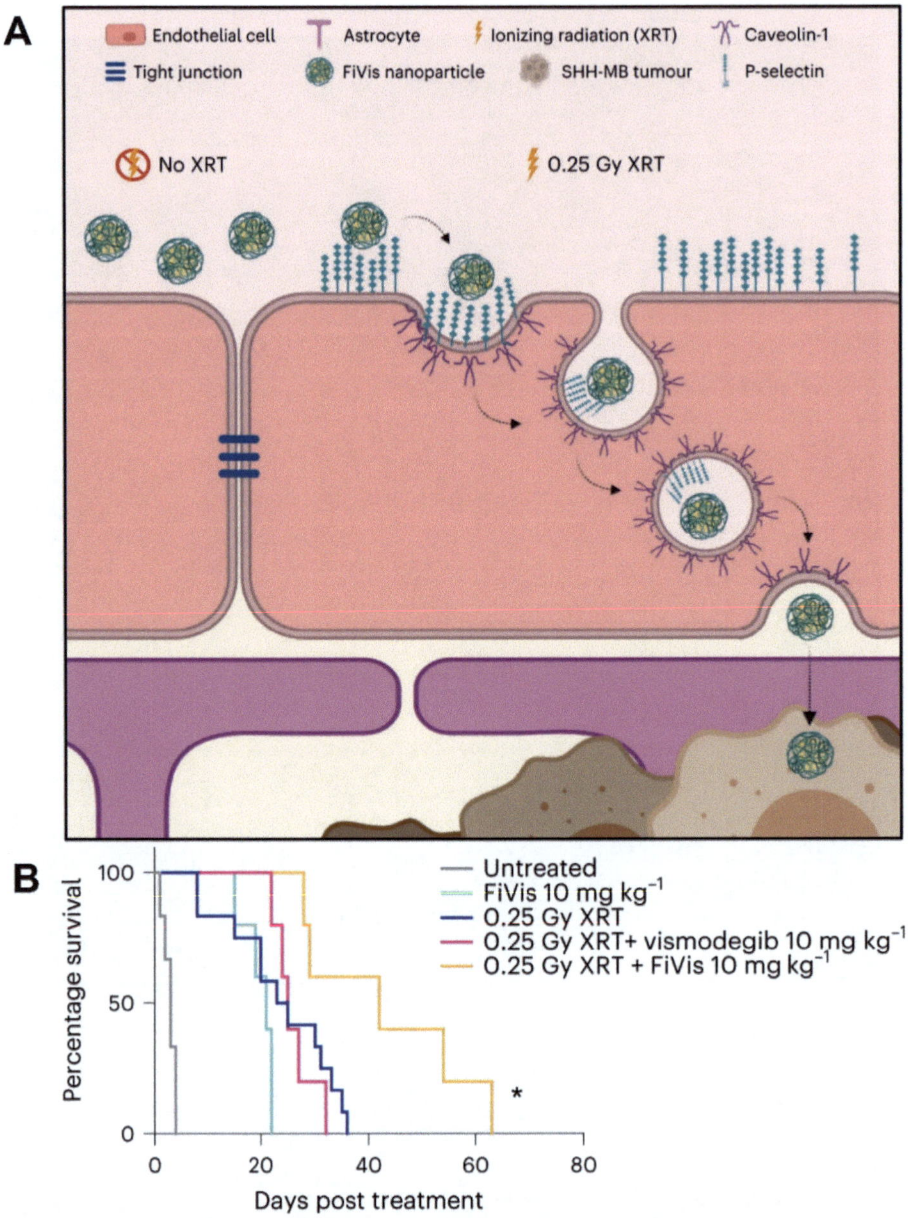

FIGURE 13.5 P-selectin–targeted nanocarriers induce active crossing of the blood-brain barrier (BBB). (A) Schematic of the proposed mechanism for FiV is nanoparticle across the BBB. (B) Kaplan-Meier survival analysis of advanced-stage Sonic hedgehog medulloblastoma (SHH-MB) mice under different conditions. *XRT*, X-ray irradiation. *Figure from Tylawsky, D.E. et al.*, P-selectin-targeted nanocarriers induce active crossing of the blood–brain barrier via caveolin-1-dependent transcytosis. *Nat. Mater, 2023.* **22***(3): p. 391-399.*

studied as carriers to achieve nose-to-brain drug delivery [15–21]. For example, methoxypoly(ethylene glycol)-poly(D,L-lactide) (mPEG-PDLLA) micelles (PMs) and HIV-1 transactivator of transcription (TAT) peptide functionalized PMs (TAT-PMs) have been investigated for nose-to-brain drug delivery. The studies indicated that the trigeminal nerve is the main transportation pathway for nose-to-brain delivery of the intact micelles. The TAT modification improved the cellular uptake of the intact micelles and was critical for the penetration of micelles into the olfactory bulb (Fig. 13.8) [20]. When it comes to commercialization, companies such as Zeteo Biomedical LLC have developed platforms for nose-to-brain drug delivery (Fig. 13.9) [22].

Over the past 40 years, invasive brain drug delivery and BBB disruption brain drug delivery have emerged (Fig. 13.10). During invasive brain drug delivery, the BBB is circumvented such as by transcranial direct injection into

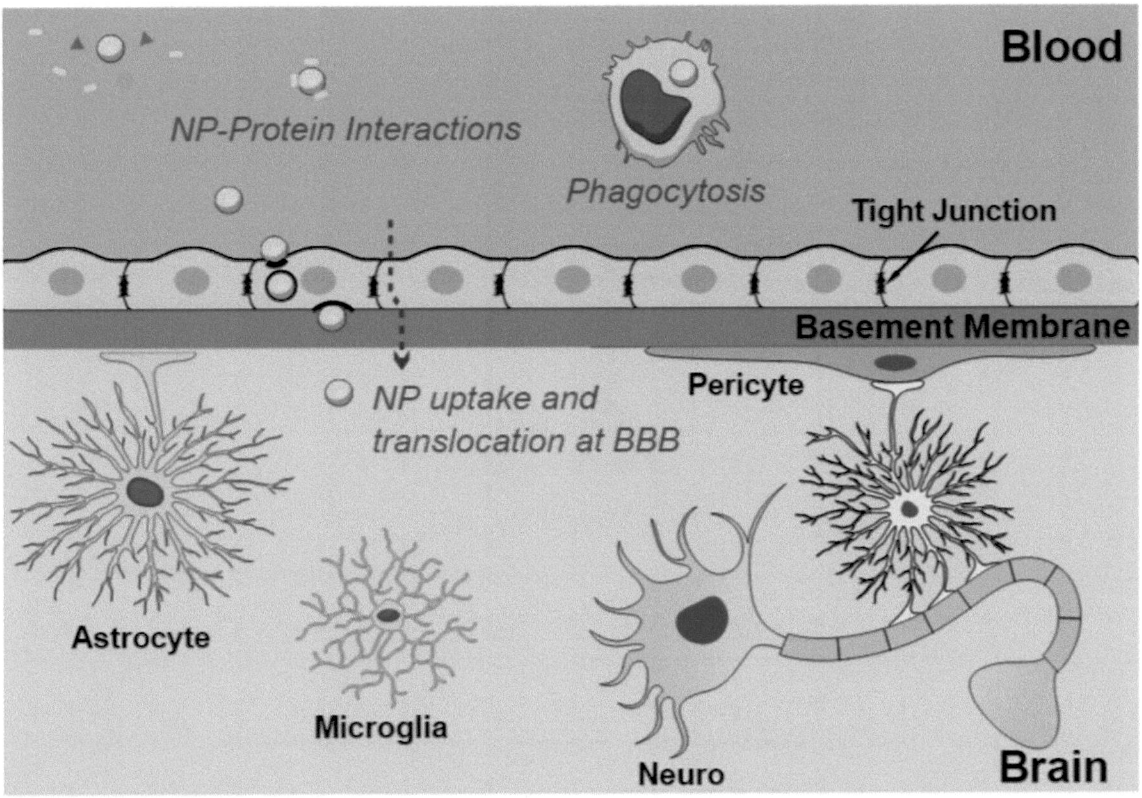

FIGURE 13.6 During the journey of nanoparticles (NPs) toward the brain parenchyma, they encounter different types of cells (e.g., macrophage) and interact with biological barriers (e.g., the BBB) as well as plasma proteins. *Figure adapted from Rabanel, J.-M. et al.,* Nanoparticle shell structural cues drive in vitro transport properties, tissue distribution and brain accessibility in zebrafish. *Biomaterials, 2021.* ***277****: p. 121085.*

brain tissue through convection-enhanced delivery (CED) [5]. CED generates a pressure gradient at the tip of an infusion microcatheter to deliver therapeutics directly through the interstitial spaces of the CNS (Fig. 13.11). This technique allows drug delivery throughout large volumes of brain tissue while minimizing the side effects [23,24]. However, high flow rates may damage the tissue near the site of infusion and induce backflow along the insertion tract [25]. Implants, miniaturized ones, in particular, have been developed for localized and controllable drug delivery to the brain. Implants with integrated micro-fluidic pumps or wireless control allow convenient adjustment of drug delivery profiles for long-term application compared with those with external pumps [26]. For example, Jongha Lee *et al.* developed a flexible and biodegradable wireless device for drug delivery to brain tumors (Fig. 13.12) [27].

Cerebrospinal fluid (CSF) is a clear, proteinaceous fluid that exists in the surrounding spaces of mammalian CNS. There is about 150 mL CSF circulating at any given moment in the average adult human [28]. It is produced at the choroid plexus that lines the four cerebral ventricles and is absorbed into the peripheral blood, primarily across the arachnoid villi into the superior sagittal sinus of the venous system. Both lumbar and ventricular CSF have been used for drug delivery. For example, nusinersen (marketed as Spinraza) is used for spinal muscular atrophy treatment through lumbar injection. However, the intrathecal injection generally results in drug distribution to the brain surface rather than brain parenchyma [5].

When it comes to the BBB disruption, different approaches have been developed through both physical and biochemical methods (Fig. 13.10) [5,29]. Various physical methods, including focused ultrasound and pulsed electrical field, have been employed for transient BBB disruption. In particular, ultrasound, in combination with microbubbles, shows great potential for brain drug delivery. In a recent study, cisplatin-loaded microbubbles in combination with ultrasound were investigated for glioblastoma therapy (Fig. 13.13) [30].

Osmotic agents have been extensively studied for BBB disruption. Mostly, inert sugars, such as mannitol (Fig. 13.14), are used to prepare hypertonic solutions for short-term carotid artery infusion. The underlying

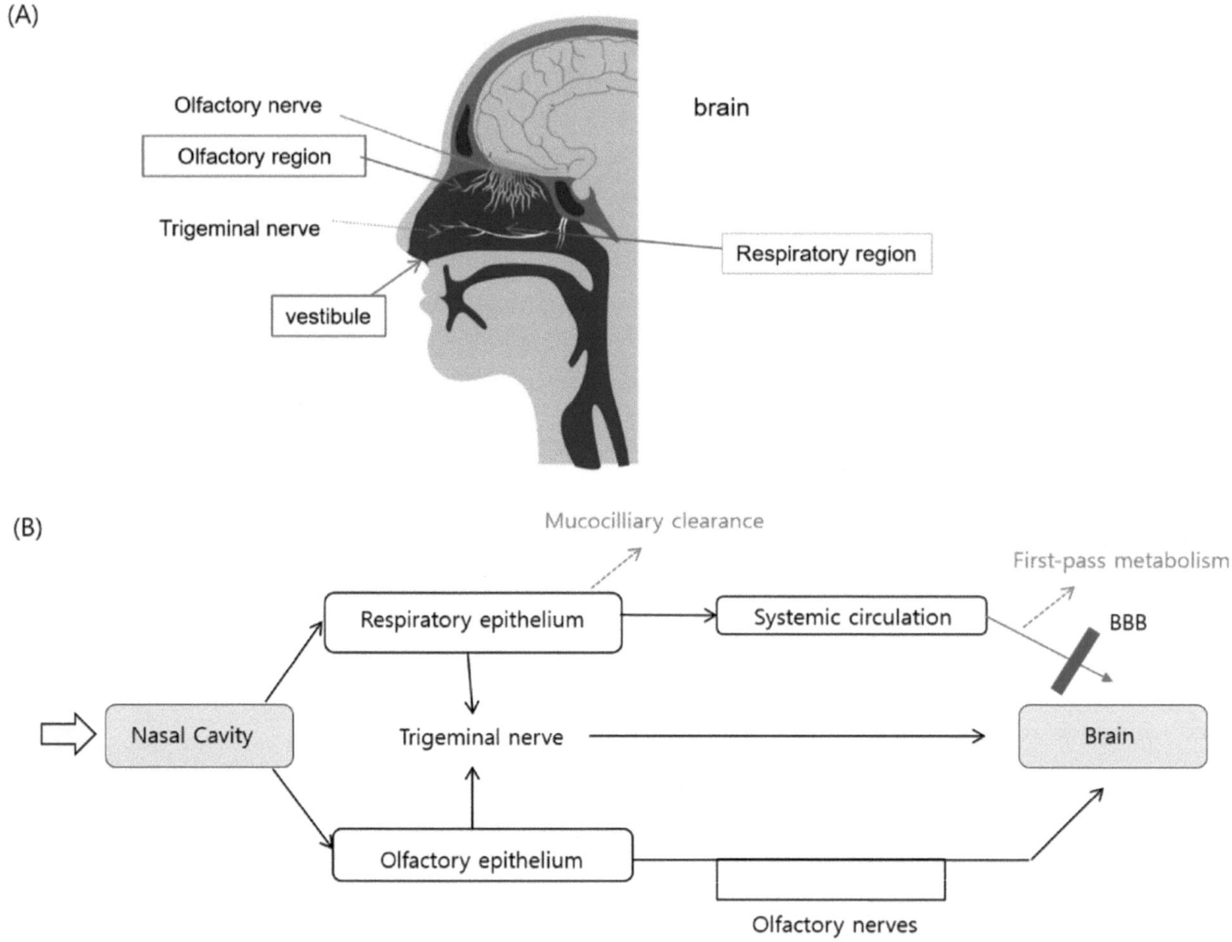

FIGURE 13.7 Nose-to-brain delivery. (A) Intranasal structure involved in the possible drug transport. (B) Potential drug transport routes leading to brain uptake following intranasal administration. *From Hong, S.-S. et al.,* Liposomal formulations for nose-to-brain delivery: recent advances and future perspectives. *Pharmaceutics, 2019.* ***11****(10): p. 540.*

mechanisms for increasing the BBB permeability are thought to be the alteration of endothelial cells and tight junction (TJ) integrity, and expansion of the blood volume [21,31]. The increase of BBB permeability has been reported to be rapid, 30 seconds to 2 minutes, in response to hyperosmolar mannitol. And the barrier properties re-establishment is also fast—within 20 min after infusion [21]. However, a recent study showed that the intracarotid artery hyperosmotic mannitol infusion can lead to a transient sterile neuroinflammatory response (marked by increased production of cytokines, chemokines, and trophic factors) and innate immune response [31]. Other molecules, such as bradykinin and histamine (Fig. 13.14), have also been used for biochemical BBB disruption [21]. Bradykinin acts on bradykinin receptors to release nitric oxide and trigger a wide range of biological effects including increasing vascular permeability [32]. Other possible mechanisms include TJ loosening and transcytosis [33]. Histamine, derived from amino acid histidine, increases BBB permeability by opening the tight junctions of interendothelial cells [33].

13.2 Drug delivery to the colon

Colon-targeted drug delivery systems have been mainly used for the treatment of local diseases such as ulcerative colitis, Crohn's disease, irritable bowel syndrome, and colon cancer. There has been an increasing need for colonic-targeted delivery systems. For example, inflammatory bowel disease has become a global disease with accelerating incidence in newly industrialized countries [34]. Moreover, colon cancer is the second leading cause of cancer-related deaths worldwide [35]. We will focus on the oral drug delivery systems in this section. The rationales are

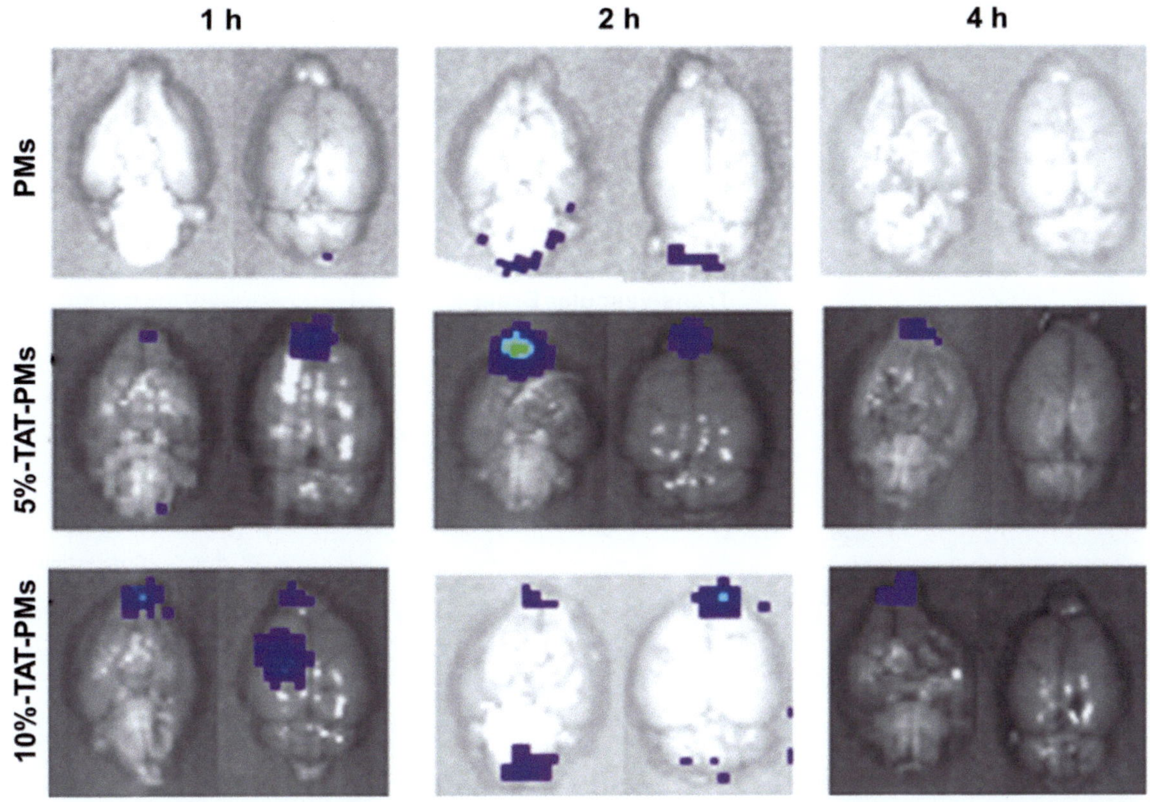

FIGURE 13.8 *Ex vivo* imaging of P2 (an aggregation-caused quenching (ACQ) probe) signals in dorsal *(right)* and ventral *(left)* sides of the brains of rats treated with PMs, 5%-TAT-PMs, and 10%-TAT-PMs at 1, 2, and 4 hr post-administration. *PM*, mPEG-PDLLA, methoxypoly(ethylene glycol)-poly(D,L-lactide) micelle; *TAT*, HIV-1 transactivator of transcription. *From Ahm, E. et al.*, TAT modification facilitates nose-to-brain transport of intact mPEG-PDLLA micelles: evidence from aggregation-caused quenching probes. *Appl. Mater. Today, 2020.* ***19****: p. 100556, with permission from Elsevier.*

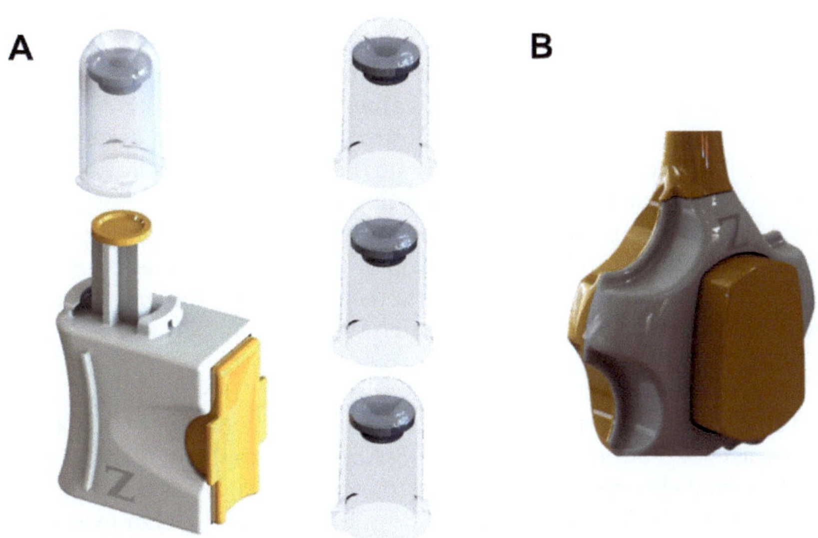

FIGURE 13.9 ZTECH-L OrionMRS mono-dose reloadable nasal liquid delivery system (A) and ZTECH-P CygnusSDX nasal powder delivery system (B). *Courtesy Zeteo Biomedical LLC (Austin, Texas).*

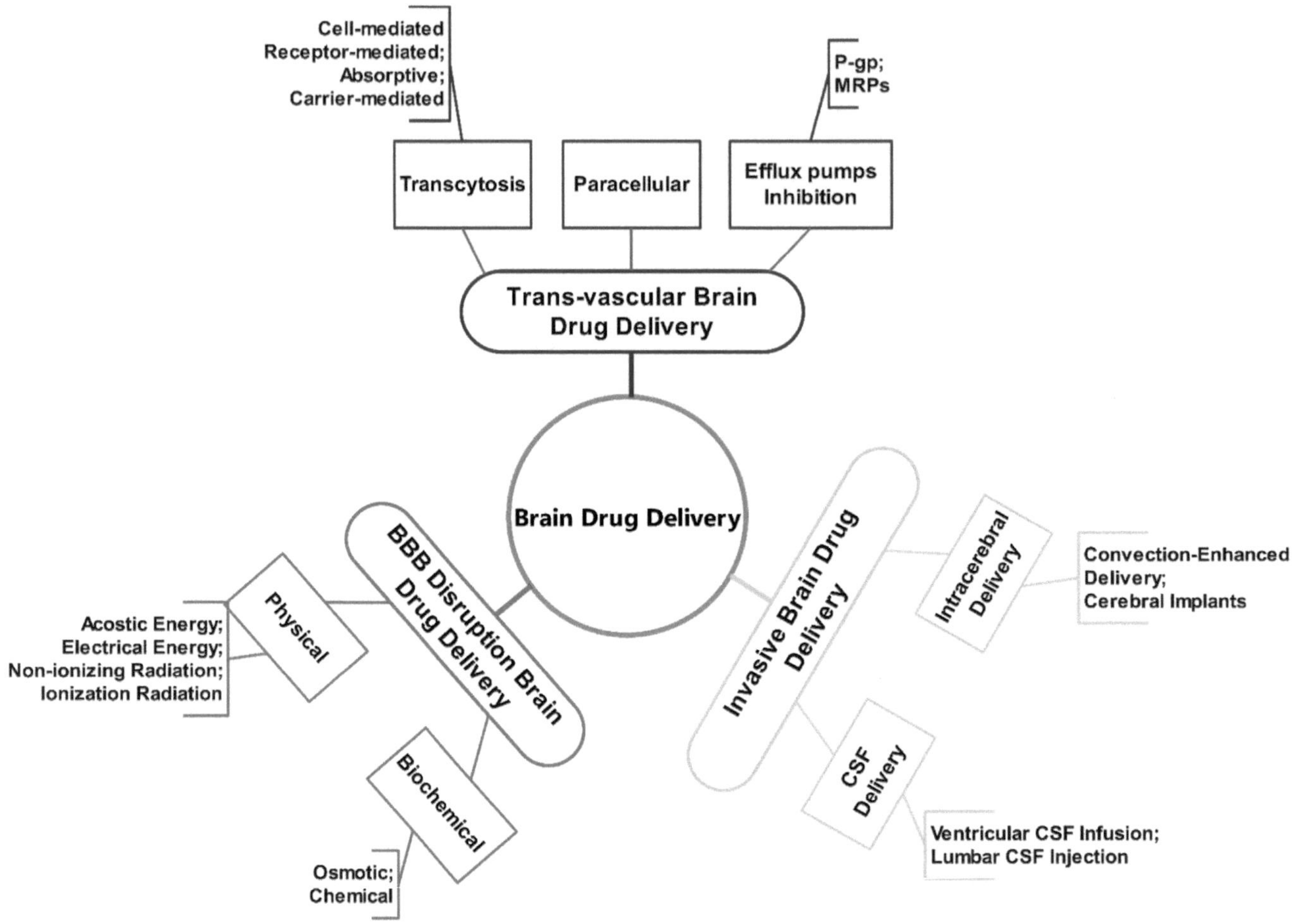

FIGURE 13.10 Overview of brain drug delivery approaches.

that oral systems allow for a greater degree of flexibility in their design, manufacturing, noninvasive and improved patient adherence, while direct rectal delivery of drugs is challenging [36,37]. It is critical for oral drug delivery systems to retain the drug in the stomach and small intestine before reaching the colon. As discussed in Chapter 4, the gastrointestinal tract's physiology is very complex in pH values, fluid volumes, and transit times [36]. The colon is the longest/largest portion of the large intestine and is composed of cecum and ascending colon, transverse colon, and sigmoid colon (Fig. 13.15). The cecum and colon cultivate the most dense and diverse microbial communities of all body habitats. The most common bacterial phyla inhabiting the colon are the Bacteroidetes, Firmicutes, Proteobacteria, and Actinobacteria [38]. These microorganisms are responsible for the breakdown of otherwise "resistant" polysaccharides that are not metabolized in the upper parts of the gstrointestinal tract [39]—which can be utilized for designing colon-targeted drug delivery systems. Bacteria responsible for dietary polysaccharide fermentation are mostly located within the proximal colon [38]. However, microbiome composition differs significantly along distinct colon regions [39].

Common approaches for targeting the colon include prodrugs, pH-dependent systems, microbiota-dependent systems, and integrated systems. Azo-based prodrugs such as sulfasalazine have been studied for colonic drug delivery [40]. Sulfasalazine consists of 5-aminosalicylic acid (5-ASA; or mesalazine) and sulfapyridine (both are pharmacologically active) with minimal absorption in the small intestine (~ 90% reach the colon). The active compounds are released in the colon through the bacterial metabolism (Fig. 13.16) [41,42]. Other examples are metronidazole sulfate (TMZS) and *N*-nicotinoyl-2-{2-(2-methyl-5-nitroimidazol-1-yl)ethyoloxy}-D,L-glycine (NMG), prodrugs of metronidazole (TMZ) (Fig. 13.17). Both chemical modifications greatly decreased the apparent partition coefficient. Microbial nitroreductases may lead to the metabolization of prodrugs to TMZ [43,44].

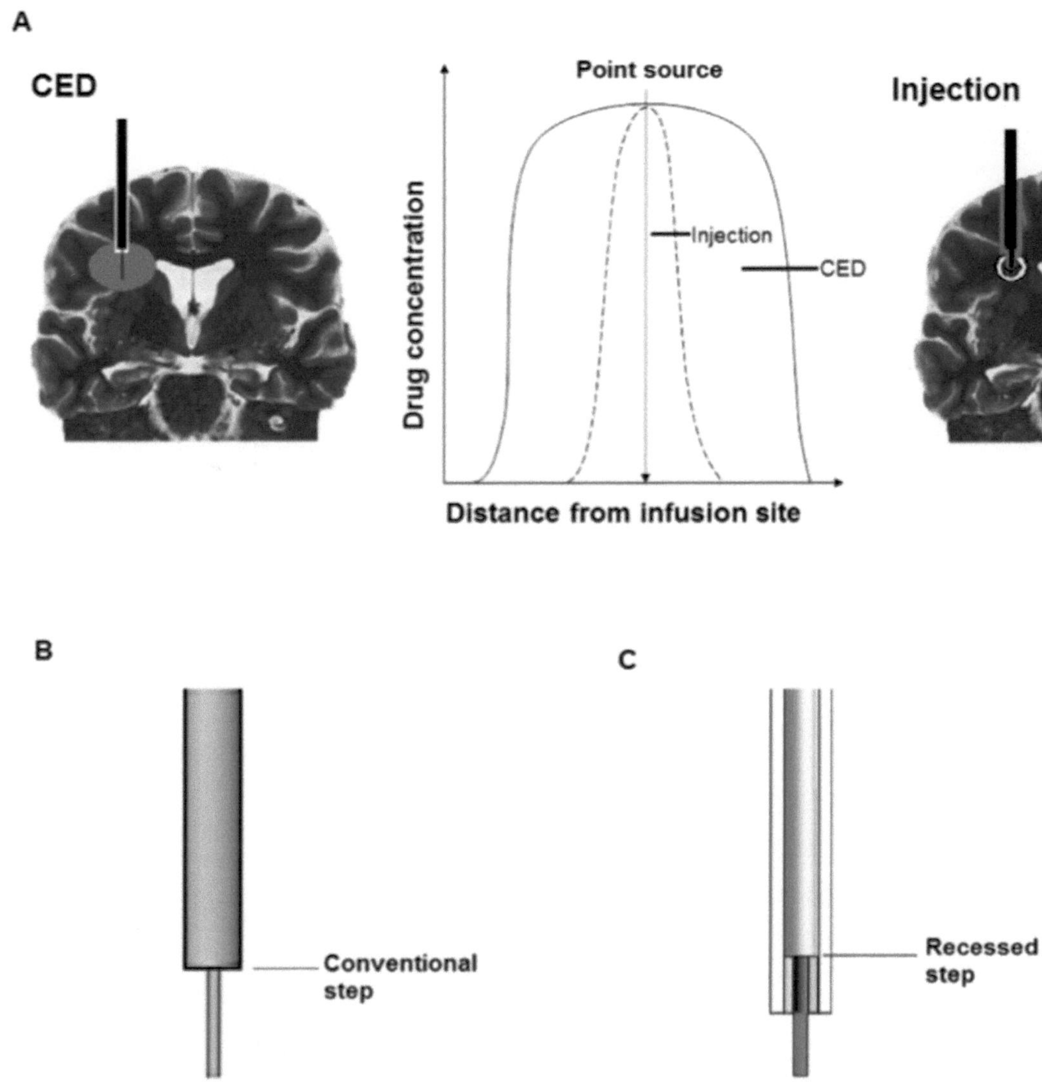

FIGURE 13.11 (A) Convection-enhanced delivery (CED) facilitates homogeneous drug distribution through large, clinically relevant brain volumes. In contrast, local injection methods are associated with significant reflux of drug, tissue trauma, and inhomogeneous drug distribution. (B) Conventional "stepped" catheter designs incorporate an abrupt change in catheter diameter proximal to catheter tip, which acts to reduce reflux. (C) Novel "recessed-step" catheter in which the stepped element is held within an outer guide tube. *From Barua, N.U., S.S. Gill, and S. Love,* Convection-enhanced drug delivery to the brain: therapeutic potential and neuropathological considerations. *Brain Pathol, 2014.* ***24****(2) p. 117-127, with permission from John Wiley & Sons Inc.*

Polymeric coatings and/or polymer-based delivery systems have widely been used for colonic drug delivery, e.g., Eudragit polymers (Evonik Industries AG) for pH-triggered release and hydroxypropyl methylcellulose (HPMC) for time-triggered release [38]. Eudragit polymers, synthesized by radical polymerization, are used for enteric coating, precise temporal release, and targeting the entire gastrointestinal tract [45]. Eudragit S 100, S 12.5, FS 30 D, and FS 100 are for colonic drug delivery, and they are soluble above pH 7.0. Insoluble and pH-independent swelling Eudragit RS (high permeability) and RL (low permeability) polymers are for sustained release (Fig. 13.18) [45–47]. Nanoparticles, dual pH/time-dependent, composed of both Eudragit FS 30 D and RS 100 have been developed for colon-targeted delivery [48]. HPMC is a partly *O*-methylated and *O*-(2-hydroxypropylated) cellulose ether derivative and is commonly used to prepare hydrophilic matrices (viscous gel) to adjust the delivery system degradation and drug release rate [49]. For example, it has been combined with amylose to design enzyme-controlled colonic drug delivery systems. Amylose can be made resistant to pancreatic enzymes (not colonic bacteria) through the

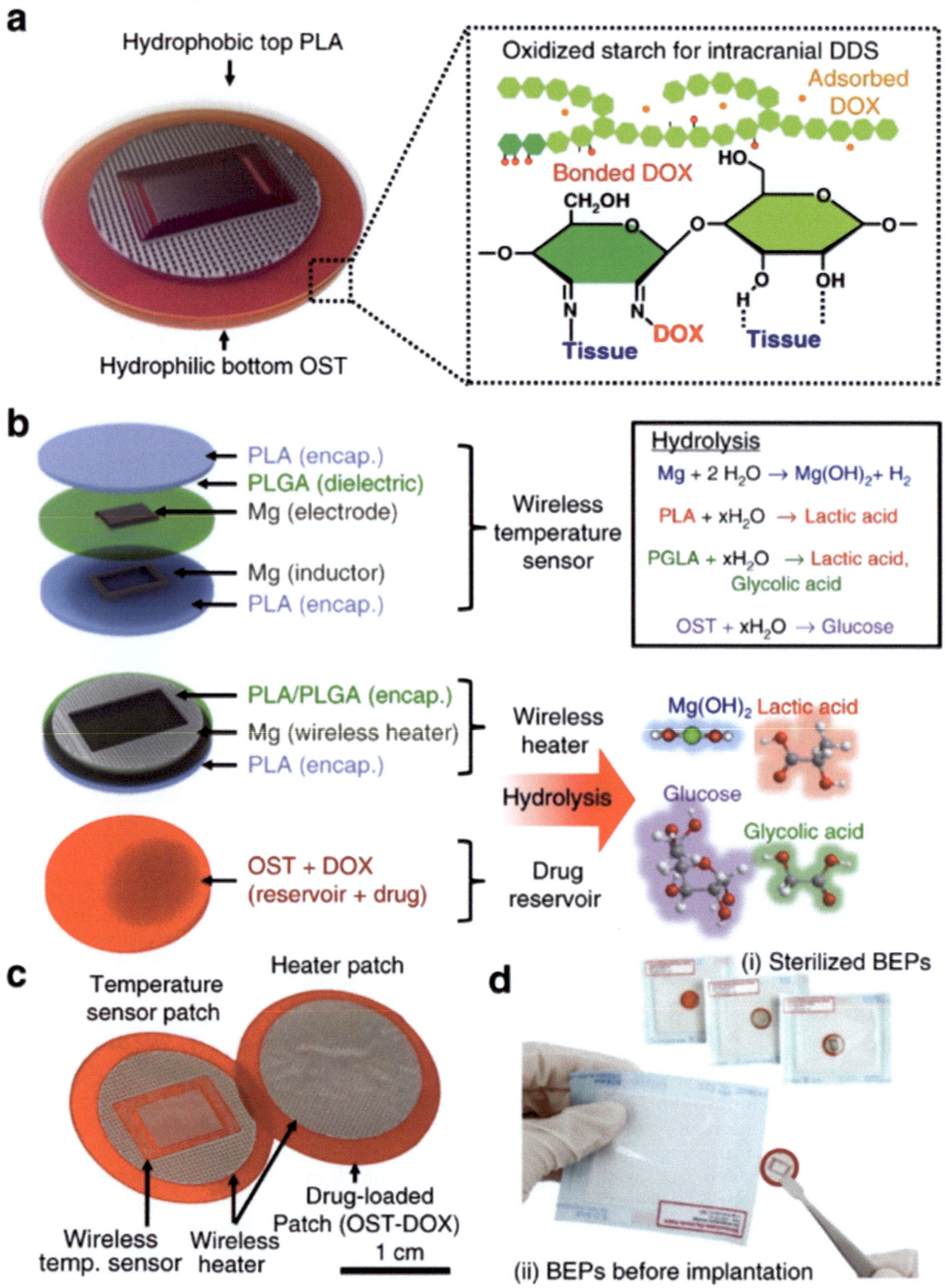

FIGURE 13.12 Materials, device design, and wireless actuation of the bioresorbable electronic patch (BEP). (a) Schematic illustration of the BEP *(left)* and the molecular structure of drug-containing oxidized starch (OST) *(right)*. (b) Schematic illustration of the BEP and its constituent materials *(left)*, and their biodegradation into hydrolyzed products *(right)*. (c) Image of the BEP, which includes a bioresorbable wireless heater and a temperature sensor on an OST patch containing doxorubicin (DOX). (d) Sterilized BEP before implantation. *DDS*, Drug delivery system; *Mg*, magnesium; *PLA*, poly(lactic acid); *PLGA*, poly(lactic-*co*-glycolic acid). *From Lee, J. et al.,* Flexible, sticky, and biodegradable wireless device for drug delivery to brain tumors. *Nat Comm, 2019.* ***10****(1): p. 5205.*

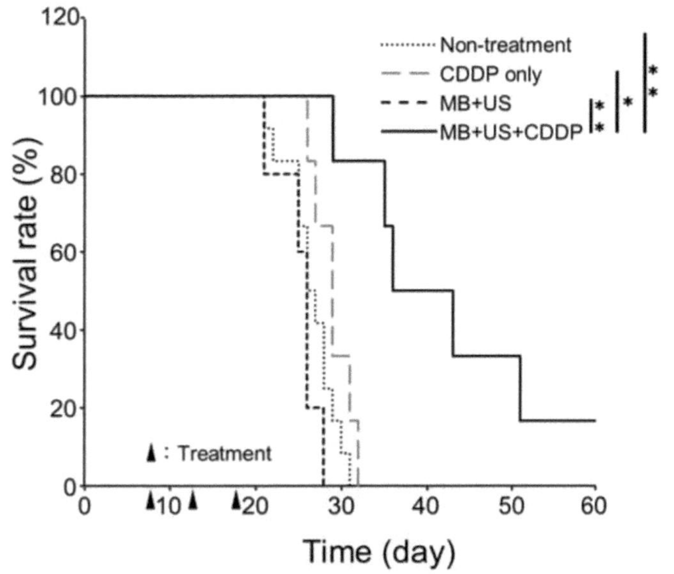

FIGURE 13.13 Comparison of survival in specific treatment groups in a mouse model of glioblastoma. The mice were treated with cisplatin (CDDP) delivered with MBs and ultrasound (MB + US + CDDP), MBs and US alone (MB + US), cisplatin alone (CDDP), or left untreated (non-treatment) 7 days after tumor transplantation. *MBs*, Microbubbles; *US*, ultrasound. *From Hagiwara, F. et al.*, Brain delivery of cisplatin using microbubbles in combination with ultrasound as an effective therapy for glioblastoma. *Pharmaceuticals, 2023.* ***16****(11): p. 1599.*

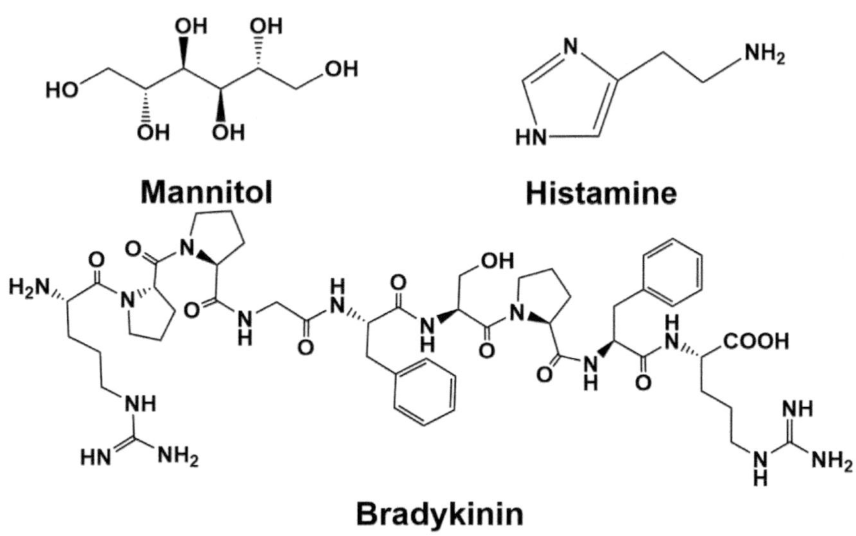

FIGURE 13.14 Chemical structure of mannitol, bradykinin, and histamine.

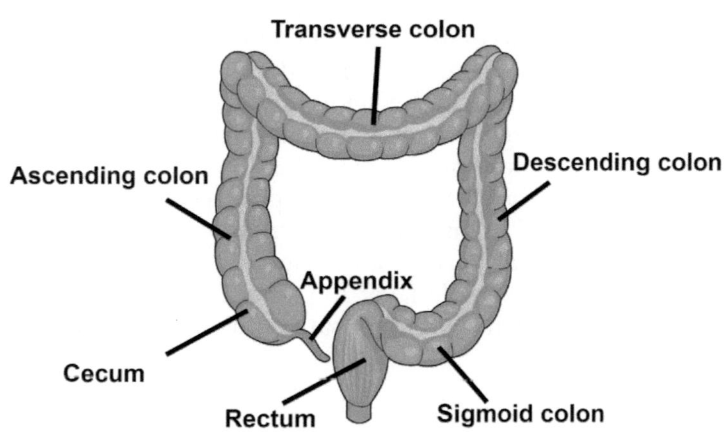

FIGURE 13.15 Anatomical structure of the large intestine.

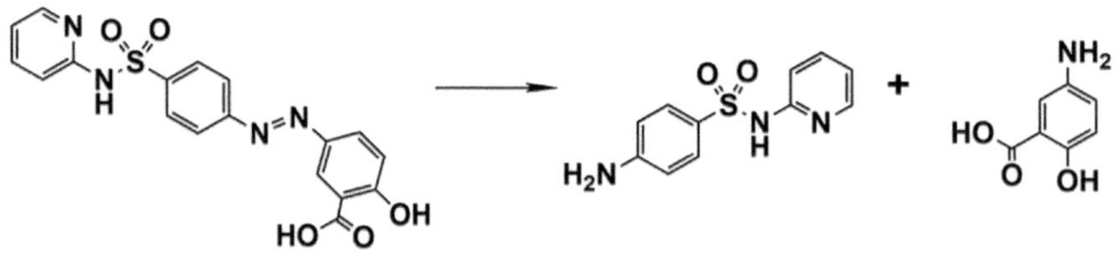

FIGURE 13.16 Chemical structures of sulfasalazine and its metabolites.

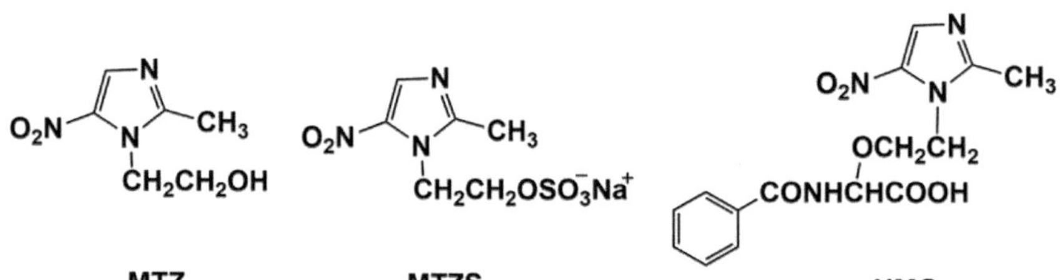

FIGURE 13.17 Chemical structures of metronidazole (MTZ), metronidazole sulfate (MTZS), and *N*-nicotinoyl-2-{2-(2-methyl-5-nitroimidazol-1-yl)ethyloxy}-D,L-glycine (NMG).

formation of an amorphous structure. However, the amylose matrix tends to swell in water. The addition of HPMC and other cellulose derivatives can improve the matrix properties [50,51]. Natural polymers, such as alginate, chitosan, guar gum, hyaluronic acid, and pectin, have also been extensively studied for colonic drug delivery [37,52]. Among them, pectin is of particular interest due to its dual responsiveness to the high pH environment and enzymatic activity of the colon. Pectin is a naturally occurring polysaccharide found in citrus fruits and apple peels. Pectin extracted from citrus fruits is generally a block copolymer of linear (poly-α(1-4)-D-galacturonic acid) and branched (poly-α(1-2)-L-rhamnosyl-α(1-4)-D-galacturonosyl with side branches of either α-L-arabinofuranose or α-D-galactopyranose) (Fig. 13.19) [53]. Pectin is generally characterized by the degree of methyl esterification. In particular, low methyl (LM) pectin has been shown to have excellent capability for developing hydrogel-based drug delivery systems [54,55]. A novel type of pectin-based microcarriers dual crosslinked with a mixture of calcium and oligochitosan (COP) showed great promise for colonic drug delivery. Calcium-pectin (CP) and oligochitosan-pectin (OP) systems have different crosslinking mechanisms—Ca^{2+} forming a macromolecular aggregate "egg-box" structure and oligochitosan forming a polyelectrolyte complex. Neither CP nor OP systems can be used for colonic drug delivery as they are unstable within the small intestine environment [54]. The results showed that the COP showed highly improved stability in simulated small intestine fluid but retained the responsiveness to the simulated colonic fluid (Fig. 13.20) [55]. A recent study used oral OP microspheres for colon-specific controlled release of quercetin for inflammatory bowel disease treatment [56].

When it comes to proprietary technologies, the Phloral system (Intract Pharma) was the first dual-triggered technology (pH-and microbiota-triggered) to be successfully marketed for colonic drug delivery, which is composed of a single-layer coating system of a homogeneous mixture of Eudragit S and biodegradable polysaccharide (high amylose starch resistant to bacterial degradation in the small intestine) [38,57]. OPTICORE (Tillotts Pharma) is a more recent system designed for rapid drug release in the ileocolonic region. The system has two layers—an inner alkaline to accelerate drug release and an outer Phloral coat [38,58].

There are also more sophisticated approaches, i.e., integrated approaches, for colonic drug delivery. Pulsatile systems are good examples and are composed of an insoluble body capsule filled with the drug content. The capsule is sealed at one end with a time-dependent plug to control the lag time and covered with a water-soluble cap. The entire capsule is then coated with an acid-insoluble layer to prevent the drug release in the stomach [37,59]. El-Hady *et al.* developed a nano-mixed micelles (NMMs)/pulsatile system, which showed protective effects against colitis (Fig. 13.21) [59].

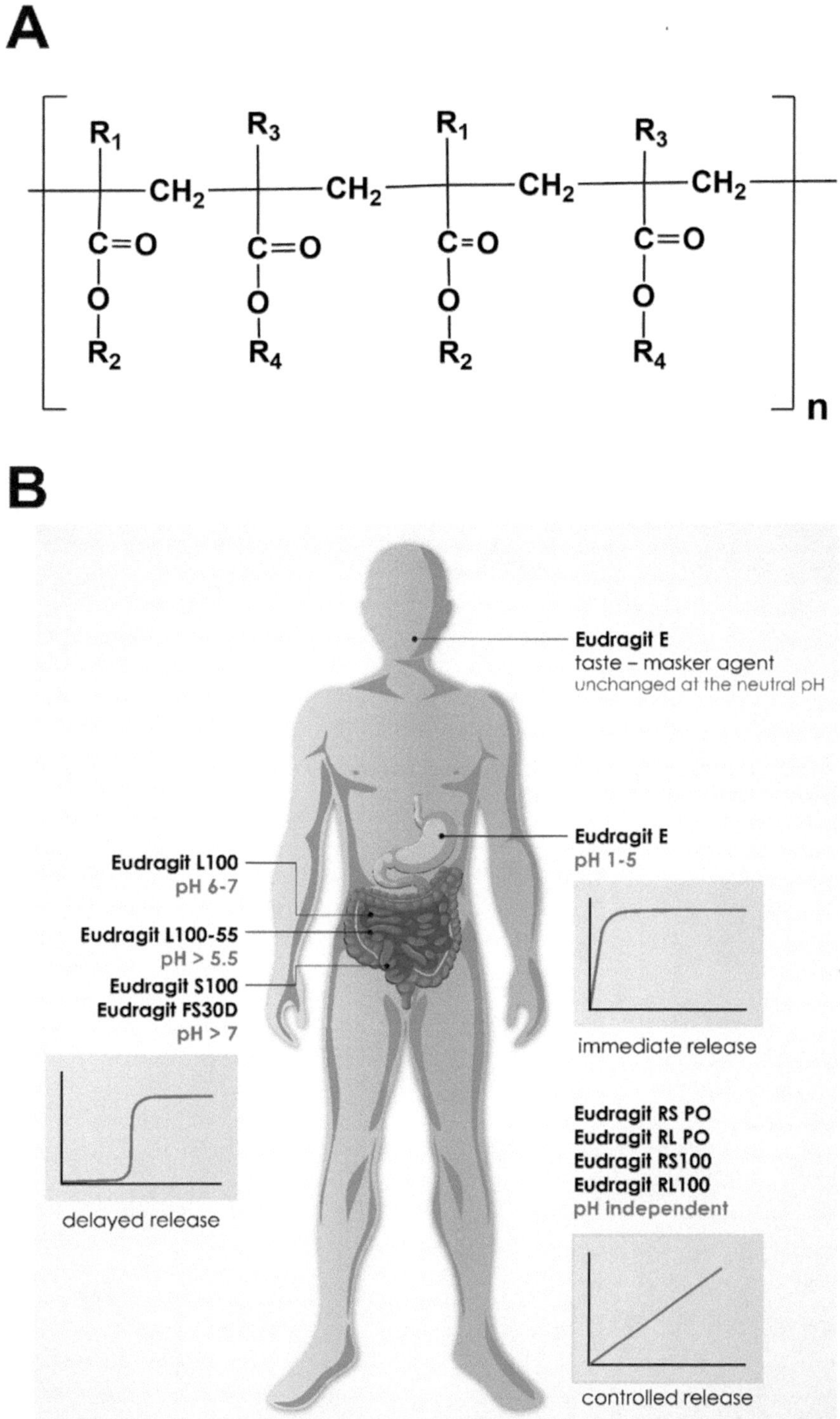

FIGURE 13.18 (A) General structure of Eudragit polymers. (B) Predictable drug release site from dosage forms produced with Eudragit polymers, according to their physicochemical properties. *(B) From dos Santos, J. et al.,* Eudragit: a versatile family of polymers for hot melt extrusion and 3D printing processes in pharmaceutics. *Pharmaceutics, 2021.* ***13****(9): p. 1424.*

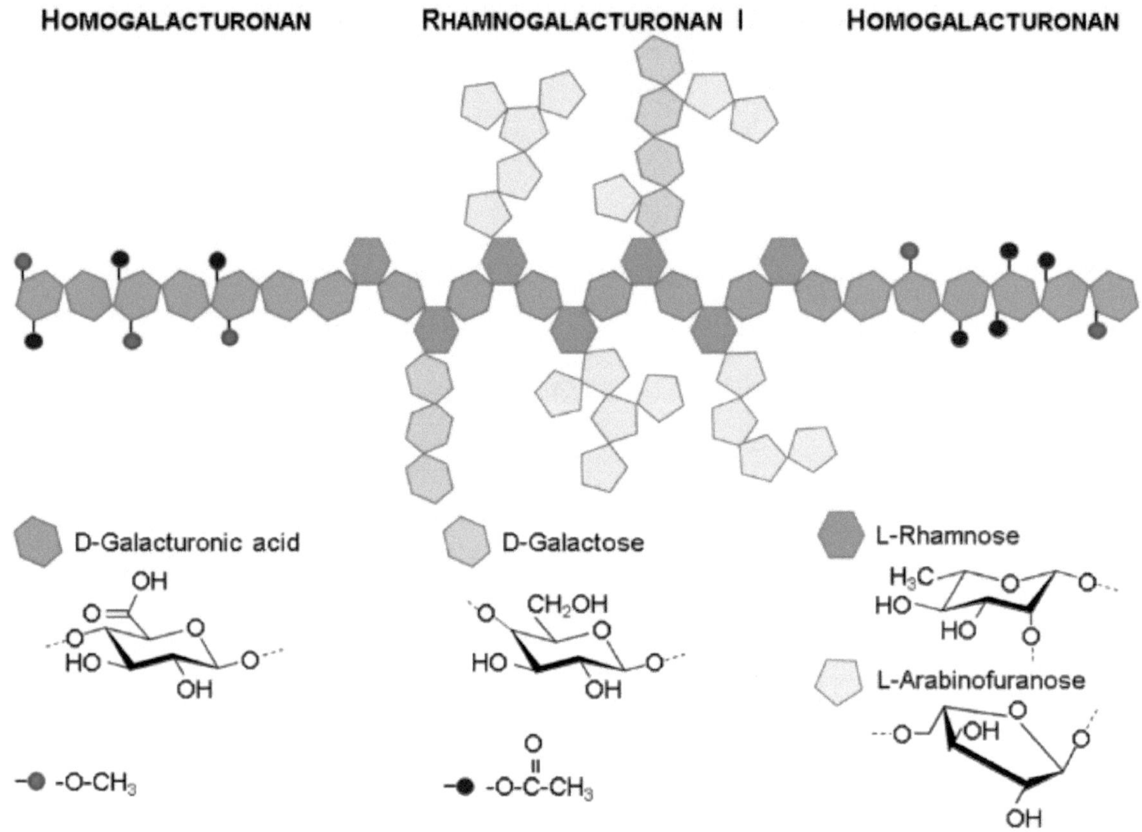

FIGURE 13.19 Schematic model of citrus fruit pectin block copolymer structure. *From Meneguzzo, F. et al.,* Real-scale integral valorization of waste orange peel via hydrodynamic cavitation. *Processes, 2019.* ***7****(9): p. 581.*

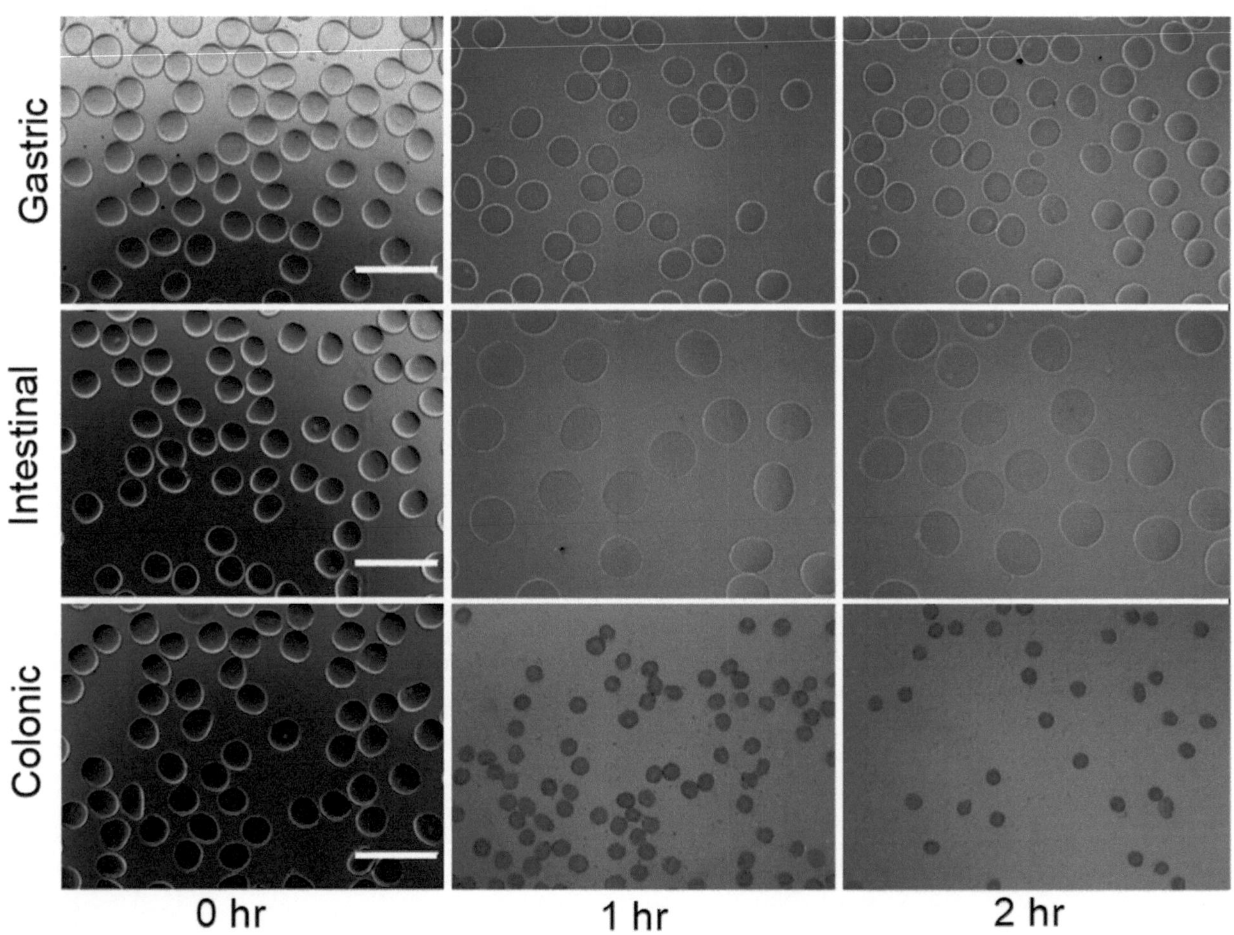

FIGURE 13.20 Responsiveness of calcium-oligochitosan-pectin (COP) microcarriers to simulated gastrointestinal environments. The scale bar represents 1,000 μm. *From Zhang, W. et al.,* Novel pectin-based carriers for colonic drug delivery. *Pharm Dev Technol, 2016.* ***21****(1) p. 127-130, with permission from Taylor & Francis.*

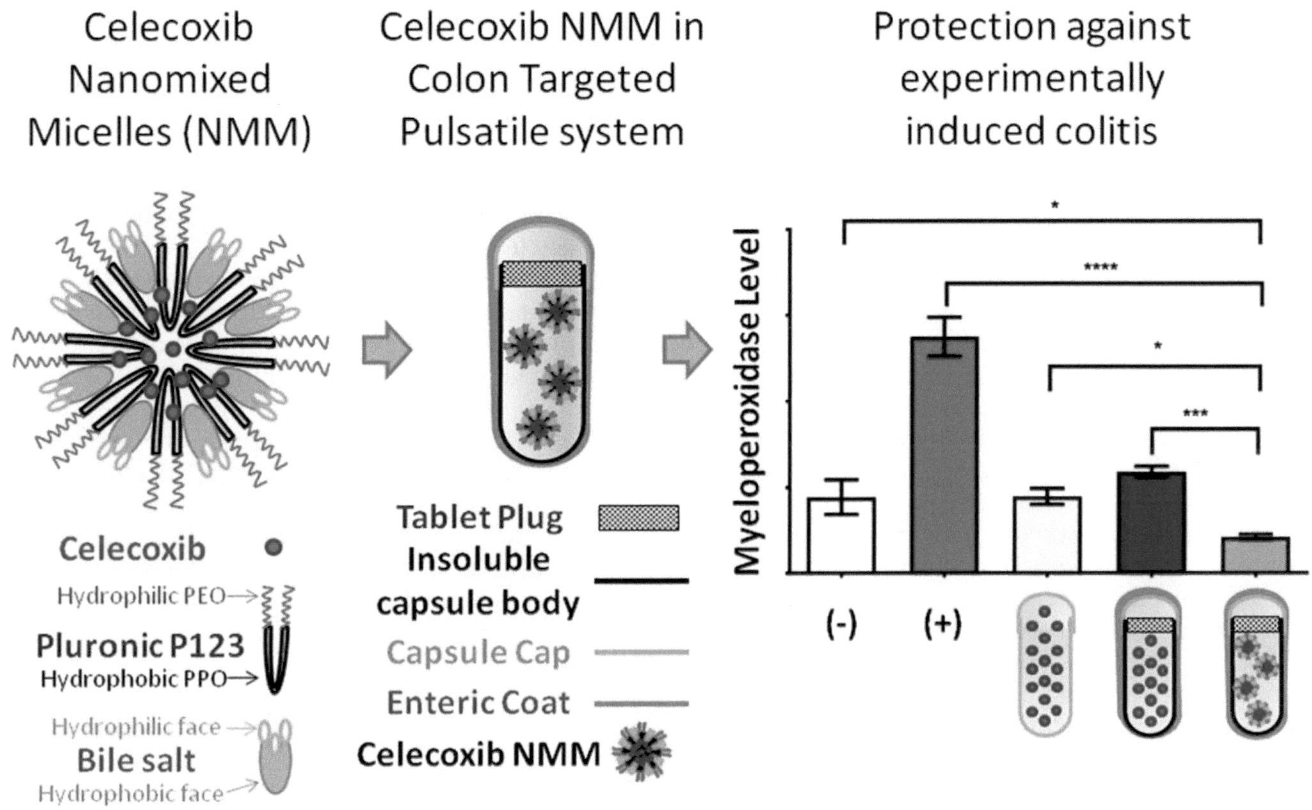

FIGURE 13.21 Pulsatile systems loaded with nano-mixed micelles (NMMs) showed protective effects against ulcerative colitis induced in the mice. Myeloperoxidase (MPO) was used as a biomarker for intestinal inflammation. *From El-Hady, S.M. et al.,* Colon targeting of celecoxib nanomixed micelles using pulsatile drug delivery systems for the prevention of inflammatory bowel disease. *Int. J. Pharm, 2020.* ***576****: p. 118982, with permission from Elsevier.*

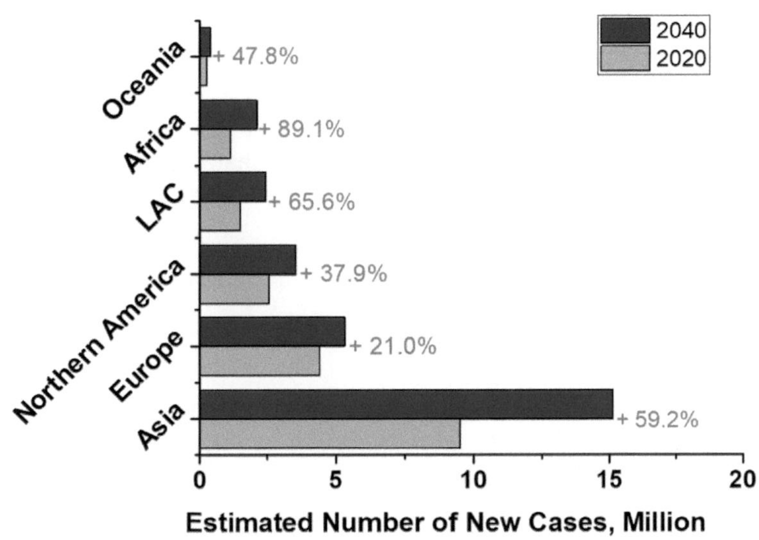

FIGURE 13.22 Estimated number of new cases from 2020 to 2040—all genders. *LAC,* Latin America and the Caribbean. *Data from the International Agency for Research on Cancer of the World Health Organization [62].*

13.3 Drug delivery in cancer therapy

Cancer is a leading cause of death worldwide (Fig. 13.22). Around one-third of deaths from cancer are due to tobacco use, high body mass index, alcohol consumption, low fruit and vegetable intake, and lack of physical activity. The most common cancers (in terms of new cases) are breast, lung, colon and rectum, prostate, skin (non-melanoma), and stomach cancers. And the most common causes of cancer death are lung, colon and rectum, liver, stomach, and breast cancers. However, the most common cancer varies between countries. In general, cancer mortality is reduced when cases are detected (diagnosis and screening) and treated early [60].

The major goal for developing drug delivery systems in cancer therapy is to target cancerous cells with improved therapeutic efficacy but reduced side effects [62,63]. Local delivery is preferred due to improved pharmacological benefits and reduced systemic toxicity. GLIADEL is a good example. It is a polymeric wafer (made of polifeprosan 20; a copolymer of 1,3-bis-(p-carboxyphenoxy)propane and sebacic acid in 20:80 ratio) containing 3.85% carmustine (BCNU) to treat malignant gliomas. They are placed during surgery and provide sustained drug release [64,65]. Unfortunately, systemic delivery through IV has to be used in most cases. Currently, platforms based on nanoparticles, liposomes, polymeric micelles, antibody-drug conjugates, polymer-drug conjugates, and targeted radionuclides have been extensively investigated in clinical trials [66]. Nanoscale drug delivery systems, nanoparticles/capsules, in particular, are of great interest for cancer therapy through systemic delivery. As extensively discussed in Chapter 11, nanoscale systems have great potential for both passive and active targeting. Nanocarriers of 100- to 200-nm size can be used for passive targeting of tumors through the enhanced permeation and retention (EPR) effect. Chemical modification can be used to achieve active targeting [62,64]. Fig. 13.23 summarizes the workflow in the development of actively targeted nanocarriers.

Another major hurdle that limits the therapeutic efficacy of nanocarriers is the premature and nonspecific release of encapsulated therapeutics. Stimuli-responsive nanocarriers that can respond to specific microenvironments releasing the therapeutics "on-demand" [64]. Intrinsic stimuli include pH, redox, and enzymes. Take pH, for example; the proton sponge effect can be considered for releasing carrier/drug uptaken through endocytosis (Chapter 6). Although no consensus has been reached, the effective endosomal escape by the use of proton sponge-based polymers depends on a delicate balance between osmotic pressure, polymer swelling, and

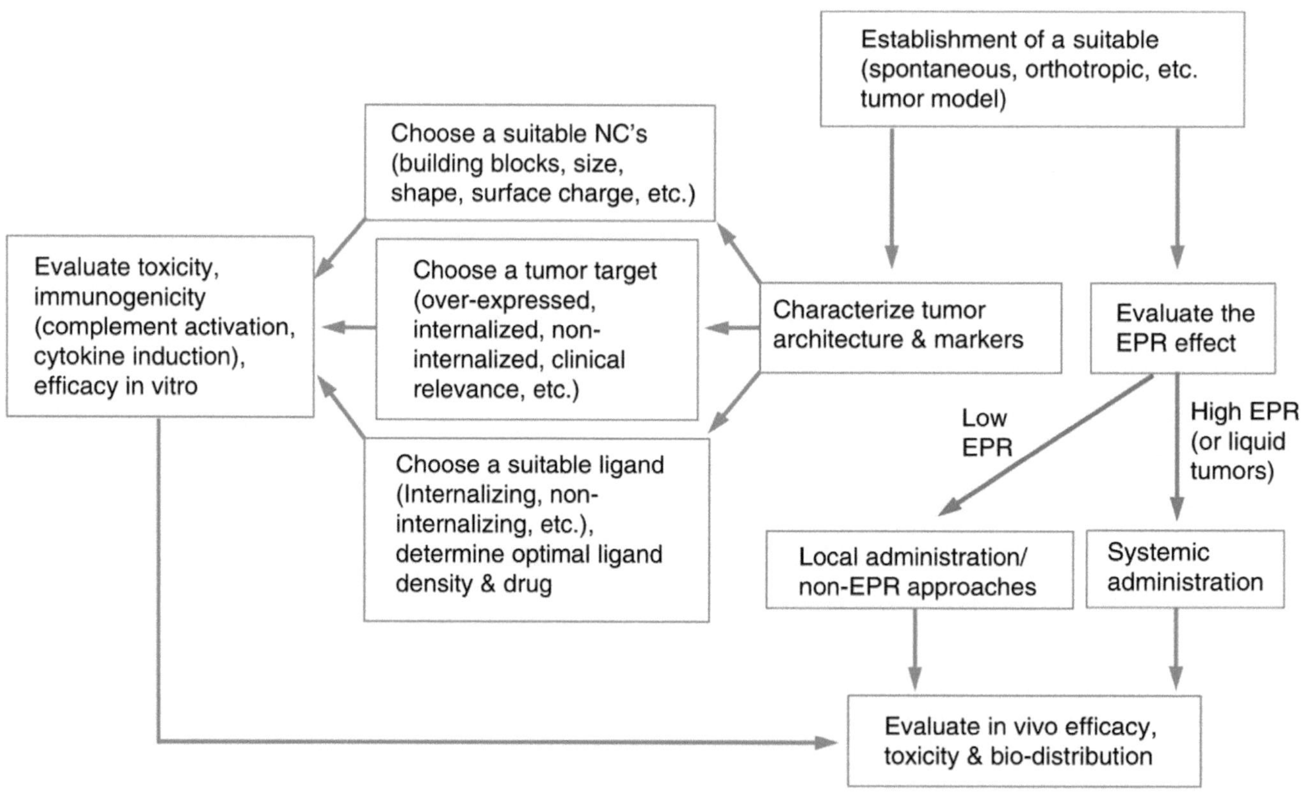

FIGURE 13.23 Schematic illustration of the proposed workflow in the development of actively targeted nanocarriers (NCs). *From Rosenblum, D. et al.,* Progress and challenges towards targeted delivery of cancer therapeutics. *Nat Comm, 2018.* ***9****(1): p. 1410.*

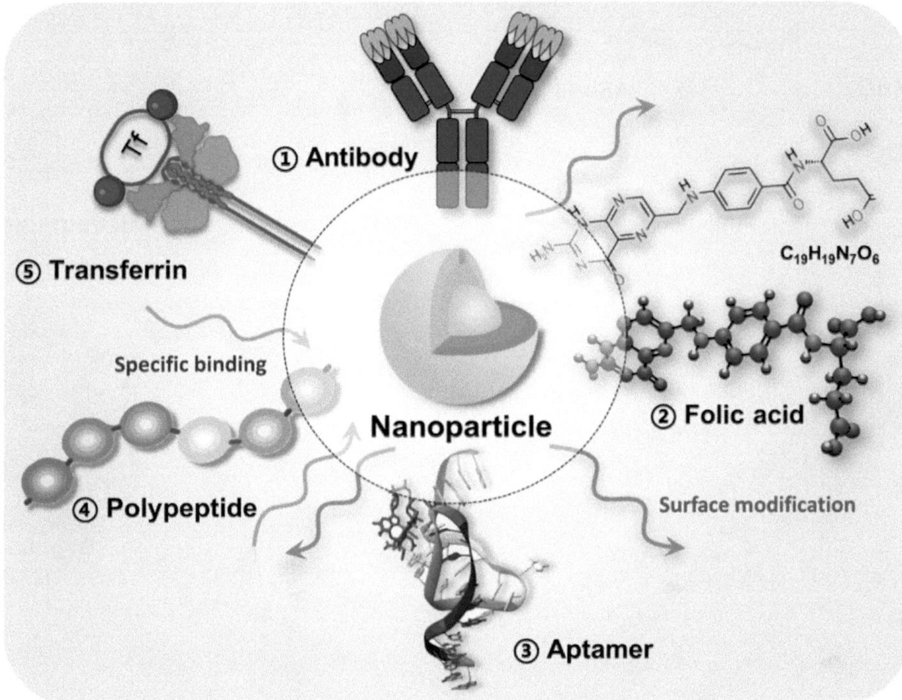

FIGURE 13.24 Tumor-specific target modification of nanoparticles categorized by aptamer, antibody, peptide, folic acid, and transferrin. *From Sun, L. et al.,* Smart nanoparticles for cancer therapy. *Signal Transduct Target. Ther, 2023.* ***8****(1): p. 418.*

destabilizing of the endosomal membrane [67]. External stimuli include temperature, magnetic field, electric field, light, and ultrasound [64]. Chapter 14 discusses the stimuli-responsive drug delivery systems in detail.

The newly developed nanoscale systems are mostly multifunctional: bioimaging, targeted delivery of drugs, and thermo/radiotherapies [68–70]. As discussed in Chapter 11, a targeting moiety can be linked to the drug or drug carrier for active targeting. As shown in Fig. 13.24, these targeting moieties can be peptides/proteins, aptamers, or other molecules such as folic acid (overexpressed on the surface of a variety of cancers such as breast cancers) and transferrin (transferrin receptor is overexpressed on a variety of metastatic and drug-resistant tumors). In cancer therapy, antibodies are commonly used for targeting epidermal growth factor receptor (overexpressed in cancer cells), vascular endothelial growth factor (tumor angiogenesis), human epidermal growth factor receptor (*HER2* is highly expressed in ~ 30% of breast cancers and 20% of ovarian cancers), fibroblast growth factor receptor 3 (*FGR3* is overexpressed in ~ 20% of advanced bladder cancer), p-glycoprotein (overexpressed in tumor drug-resistant cells), prostate-specific membrane antigen (a biomarker for prostate cancer), ephrin type-a receptor 3 (overexpressed in the stoma and vasculature of gliomas), glypican-3 (overexpressed in hepatocellular carcinoma tissues), and epithelial cell adhesion molecule (higher expressed in circulating tumor cells). Peptides have also been widely used for cancer cell targeting, such as C16Y peptide for targeting $\alpha_v\beta_3$ integrin [71]. Excitingly, The Cancer Surfaceome Atlas (TCSA) is now available, which can be used to identify cancer-specific genes encoding cell-surface proteins (GESPs) as actionable targets [72,73]. Moreover, tumor microenvironment–mediated targets should also be considered, such as cancer-associated fibroblasts and angiogenesis [74]. Regarding the multifunctional nanocarrier with targeting capability, a good example is a nanoplatform based on manganese dioxide (MnO_2) coated gold nanoclusters delivering indocyanine green (ICG) (Fig. 13.25) [75]. ICG is a photothermal agent, photosensitizer, and fluorescence imaging probe [75]. Aptamer AS141 is used for targeting, and the system is coupled with turn-on and always-on fluorescence probes for imaging-guided photodynamic/chemodynamic/photothermal therapy [76]. Photodynamic therapy (PDT) incorporates a laser of a specific wavelength to produce photochemical reactions producing reactive oxygen species or singlet oxygen ($^1O_2$) and such. Chemodynamic therapy (CDT) is based on the acidic tumor environment in which the overexpressed H_2O_2 is catalyzed by transition metals (such as Fe and Mn), causing a Fenton or Fenton-like reaction in tumor cells (e.g., generating hydroxyl radical ($\cdot$OH)). Photothermal

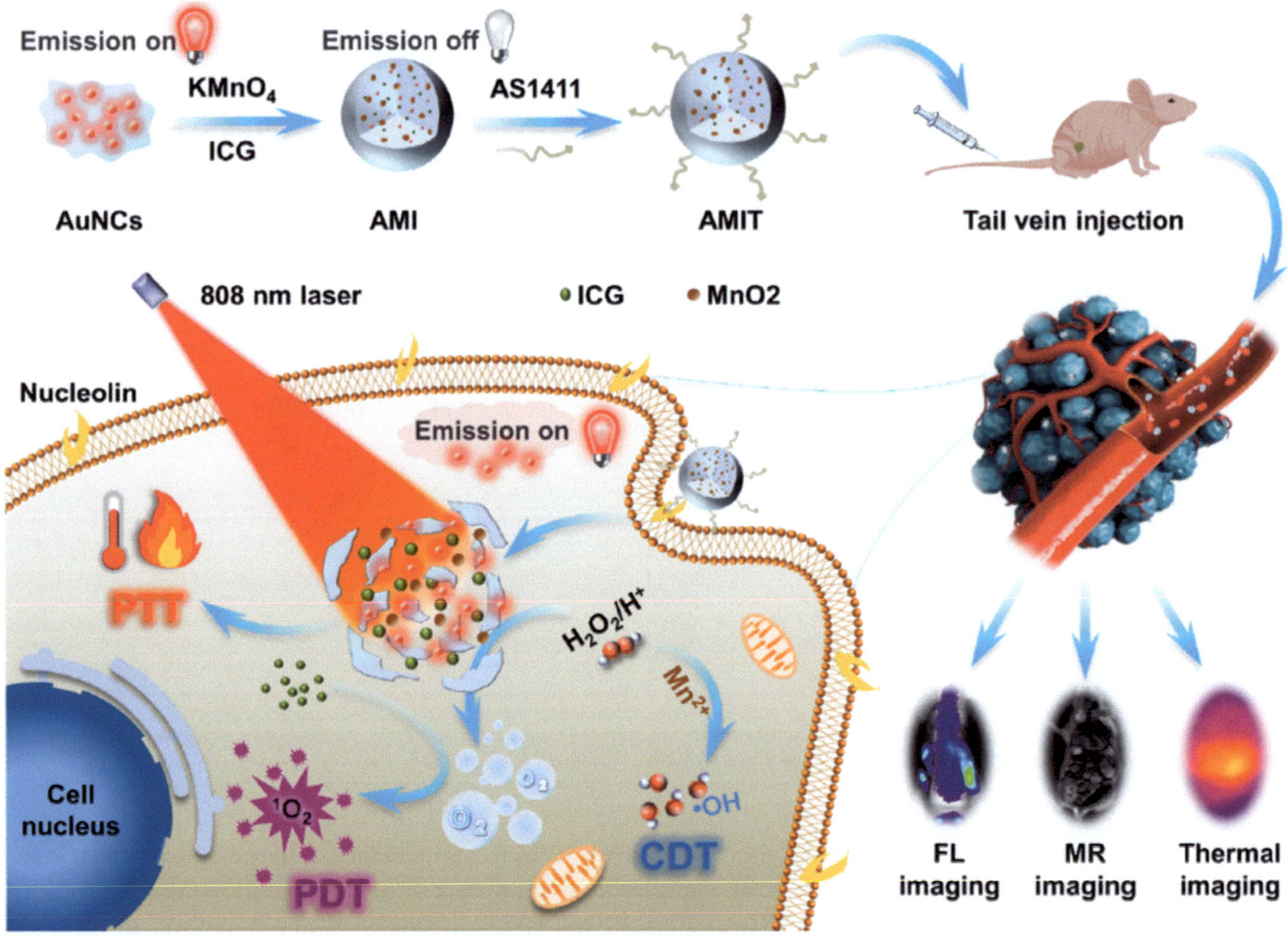

FIGURE 13.25 Schematic diagram of AuNCs@MnO2-ICG@AS1411 (AMIT) nanoparticles as a multifunctional nanoplatform for effective cancer theranostics through intrinsic tumor environment (TME)-activated triple-modal imaging-guided enhanced PDT/CDT/PTT. *AuNCs*, Au nanoclusters; *CDT*, chemodynamic therapy; *ICG*, indocyanine green; *FL*, fluorescence; *MR*, magnetic resonance; *PDT*, photodynamic therapy; *PTT*, photothermal therapy. *From Sun, Y. et al.,* Intelligent tumor microenvironment-activated multifunctional nanoplatform coupled with turn-on and always-on fluorescence probes for imaging-guided cancer treatment. *ACS Appl. Mater. Interfaces, 2021.* **13***(45): p. 53646-53658. Copyright (2021), American Chemical Society.*

therapy (PTT) uses photothermal agents to absorb the energy of near-infrared light and convert it into thermal energy leading to thermal damage to cells/tissues [70]. In this example, the dissociation of MnO_2 generated sufficient O_2 and Mn^{2+} which improved the ICG-guided PDT efficacy (producing singlet oxygen) and resulted in Fenton-like reaction-mediated CDT (producing hydroxyl radical). Simultaneously, the released ICG and gold nanoclusters facilitated PDT and PTT efficacy *via* deep tumor penetration (Fig. 13.25). Additionally, the turn-on fluorescence of gold nanoclusters revealed the real-time MnO_2 degradation process, and the always-on ICG fluorescence enabled the *in situ* monitoring of the payload distribution *in vitro* and *in vivo* [75,76]. Another example is a photo-triggered self-accelerated nanoplatform combining an aggregation-induced emission luminogen (AIEgen) and hypoxia-responsive paclitaxel prodrug for multifunctional image-guided combination cancer immunotherapy. The nanoplatform is based on the co-assembly of AIEgen and prodrug with Pluronic F127 and then coated with M1 macrophage membrane for tumor targeting. The PDT effect induced immunogenic cell death (ICD) and accelerated the activation of the prodrug by decreasing the local oxygen level (Fig. 13.26) [77].

Nanoscale systems can also be developed through the self-assembly of drugs/prodrugs. Drugs or prodrugs serve as both cargo and vehicle materials simultaneously. Chemical drug-based nanoassembly generally exhibits high loading efficiency [78]. For example, Yinxian Yang *et al.* developed the trisulfide bond-mediated doxorubicin dimeric prodrug nanoassemblies using doxorubicin homodimeric prodrugs. The nanoassemblies showed high drug loading

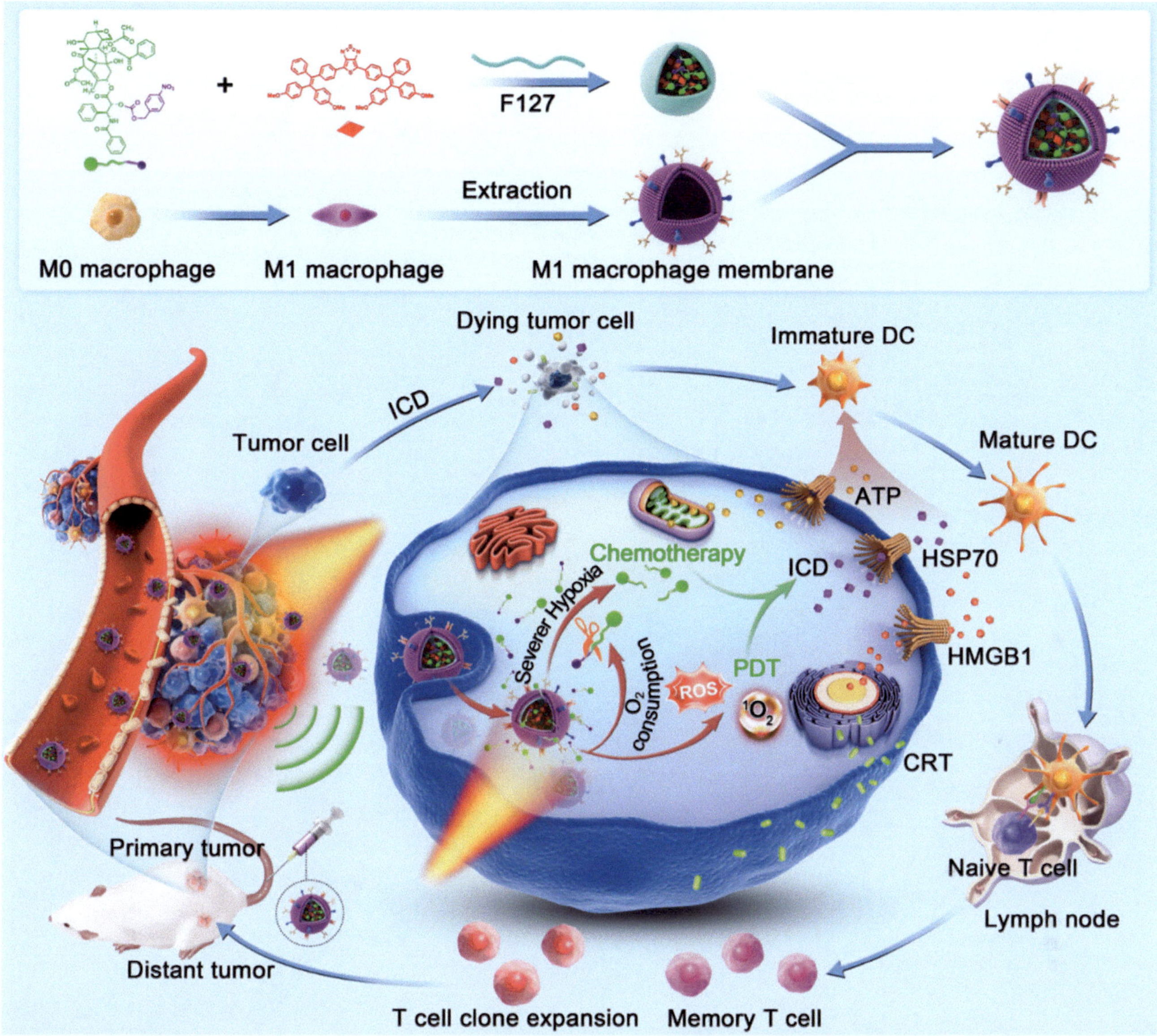

FIGURE 13.26 Schematic illustration of the photo-triggered self-accelerated nanoplatform for fluorescence and photoacoustic imaging-guided combination immunotherapy. *ATP*, Adenosine triphosphate; *CRT*, calreticulin; *DC*, dendritic cells; *HSP70*, heat shock protein 70; *HMGB1*, high mobility group protein B1; *ICD*, immunogenic cell death; *PDT*, photodynamic therapy; *ROS*, reactive oxygen species. *From Kang, X. et al.,* A photo-triggered self-accelerated nanoplatform for multifunctional image-guided combination cancer immunotherapy. *Nat Commun, 2023.* ***14****(1): p. 5216.*

(67.24%, w/w), high stability, and high tumor selectivity. The trisulfide bond also showed higher glutathione (GSH) sensitivity compared to the disulfide bond, enabling efficient tumor-specific drug release as GSH is generally overexpressed in tumor cells (Fig. 13.27) [79].

Last, let us examine the circulating tumor cells (CTCs) and cancer stem-like cells (CSCs). CTCs are tumor cells that have sloughed off the primary tumor and extravasate into the blood, and then circulate in the blood. However, only a small proportion of CTCs can survive and eventually trigger metastases (Fig. 13.28). CTCs have been detected in patients with early-stage cancers and have great potential for early detection of clinically relevant cancer. Moreover, studies focusing on these strongly metastatic CTCs may provide insights into CTCs-related therapeutic targets [80–82]. CSCs, a subpopulation of cancer cells, possess remarkable capability in proliferation, self-renewal, and differentiation, which plays a crucial factor in tumor progression and metastasis. Conventional cancer treatments

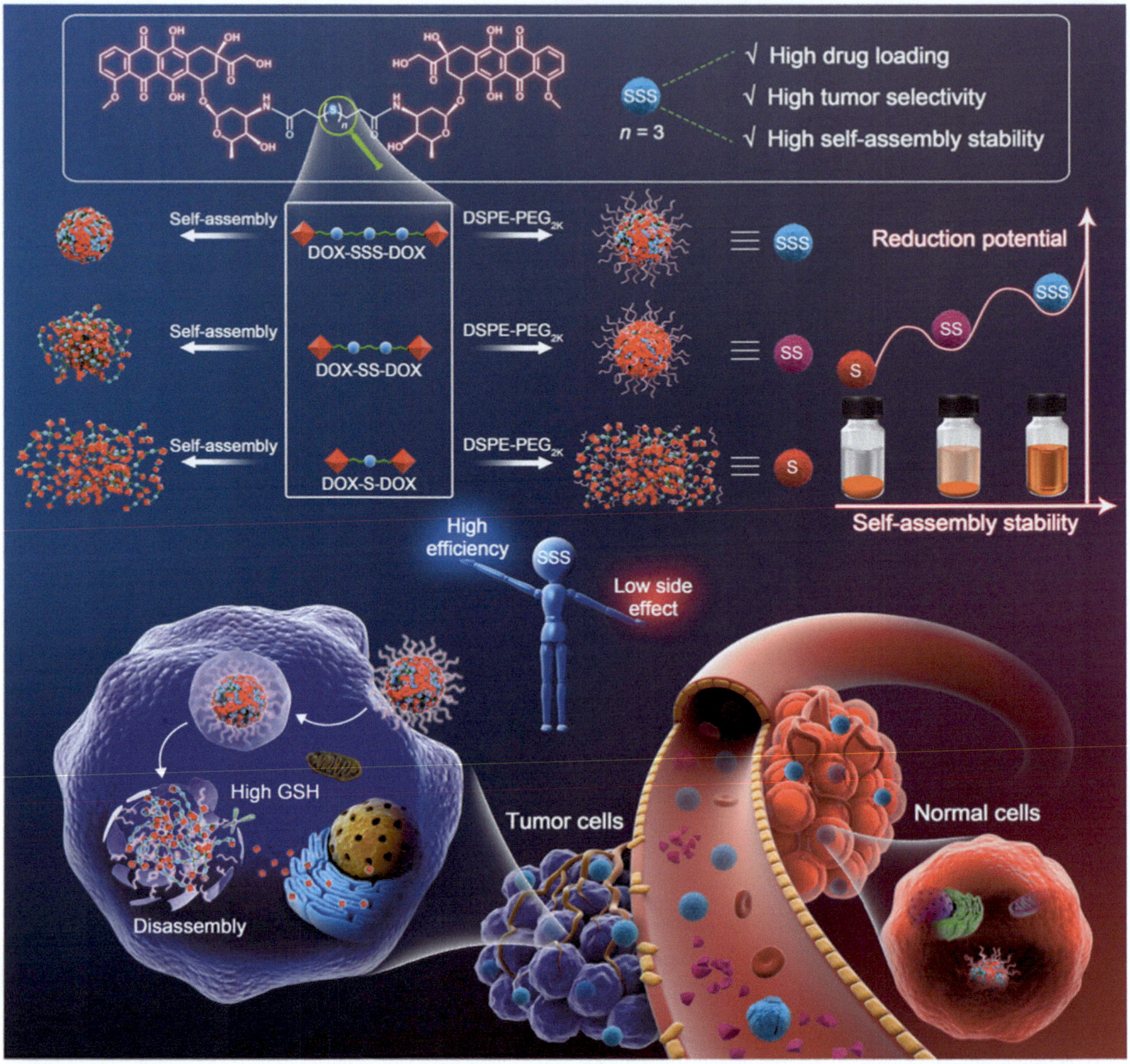

FIGURE 13.27 The trisulfide bond–bridged prodrug nanoassemblies for cancer therapy. *GSH*, Glutathione. *From Yang, Y. et al.*, Trisulfide bond–mediated doxorubicin dimeric prodrug nanoassemblies with high drug loading, high self-assembly stability, and high tumor selectivity. *Science Advances, 2020.* ***6****(45): p. eabc1725, with perimission from The American Association for the Advancement of Science.*

generally only target the bulk of the tumor and fail to target CSCs as they have higher resistance, causing metastasis and tumor recurrence. One hot research topic related to cancer therapy is to target and eradicate CSCs, overcoming CSC-mediated therapy resistance [83–85]. Interestingly, oligochitosan has been shown to be able to target CD44 receptors on CSCs [86]. Yi Hou *et al.* combined the genipin-crosslinked-Pluronic F127 oligochitosan nanoplatform (gnDOX) with cryoablation for the destruction of chemoresistant mammary CSCs (Fig. 13.29). The gnDOX showed both thermal responsiveness and pH sensitivity and the genipin crosslinking improved the hydrophilic anticancer drugs' loading efficiency. The combination of the gnDOX with cancer cryotherapy enhanced the CSC destruction both *in vitro* and *in vivo* [87].

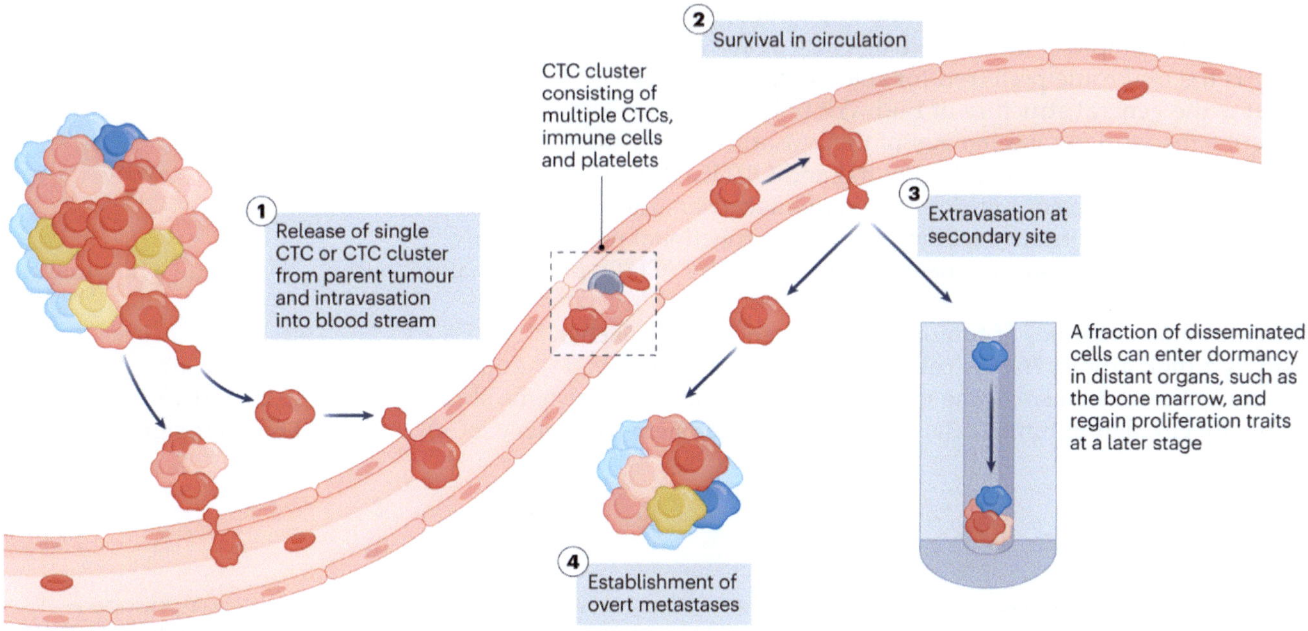

FIGURE 13.28 Key steps in the formation of metastases by circulating tumor cells (CTCs). *From Lawrence, R. et al.,* Circulating tumour cells for early detection of clinically relevant cancer. *Nat. Rev. Clin. Oncol, 2023.* ***20****(7): p. 487-500, with permission from Springer Nature.*

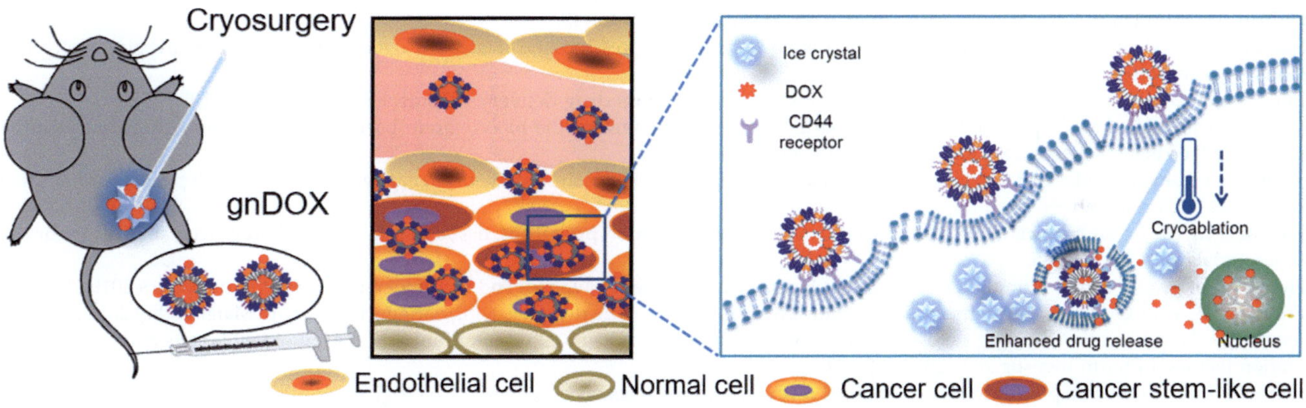

FIGURE 13.29 The genipin-crosslinked Pluronic F127–chitosan nanoparticle encapsulated doxorubicin (DOX) hydrochloride (gnDOX) combined with cryoablation for cancer treatment. *From Hou, Y. et al.,* Cryoablation-activated enhanced nanodoxorubicin release for the therapy of chemoresistant mammary cancer stem-like cells. *J. Mater. Chem. B, 2020.* ***8****(5): p. 908-918, with permission from the Royal Society of Chemistry.*

Review and practice questions

1. Describe the structure of the blood-brain barrier (BBB).
2. What are the different mechanisms for crossing the BBB (transvascular)? And what are some of the receptors involved in the receptor-mediated transcytosis?
3. What are some of the transvascular brain drug delivery approaches?
4. Describe the nose-to-brain drug delivery mechanism.
5. Describe the convection-enhanced drug delivery (CED) mechanism.
6. Regarding BBB disruption brain drug delivery, what are some of the examples of physical approaches?
7. Describe the mechanism of using mannitol for biochemical BBB disruption.
8. Describe the mechanism of using bradykinin for biochemical BBB disruption.
9. Describe the mechanism of using histamine for biochemical BBB disruption.

10. Draw the anatomical structure of the large intestine.
11. Provide an example of using prodrugs for colonic drug delivery.
12. Why is the oral route preferred for colonic drug delivery?
13. What is the general structure of Eudragit polymers?
14. Describe the working mechanism of the pulsatile system shown in Fig. 13.21.
15. Describe the mechanisms of the Phloral and OPTICORE systems.
16. What are the two major hurdles of using nanocarriers for cancer therapy?
17. What are the major functionalities of the multifunctional nanocarriers?
18. Describe the mechanisms of chemodynamic therapy (CDT), photodynamic therapy (PDT), and photothermal therapy (PTT).
19. Provide some examples of tumor-specific targeting approaches.
20. Why is a high affinity for the cell membranes or the membrane receptors not always beneficial?
21. Describe the mechanism of the multifunctional nanocarrier systems shown in Figs. 13.25 and 13.26.
22. What are circulating tumor cells (CTCs) and cancer stem-like cells (CSCs)? And explain their significance in cancer therapy.

References

[1] American Brain Foundation. Brain diseases and disorders. Available from: https://www.americanbrainfoundation.org/diseases/.

[2] Pandit R, Chen L, Götz J. The blood-brain barrier: physiology and strategies for drug delivery. Adv Drug Deliv Rev 2020;165-166:1–14.

[3] Wu D, et al. The blood–brain barrier: structure, regulation, and drug delivery. Signal Transduct Target Ther 2023;8(1):217.

[4] Alahmari A. Blood-brain barrier overview: structural and functional correlation. Neural Plast 2021;2021:6564585.

[5] Pardridge WM. A historical review of brain drug delivery. Pharmaceutics 2022;14(6):1283.

[6] Dong X. Current strategies for brain drug delivery. Theranostics 2018;8(6):1481–93.

[7] Testappen G, et al. Strategies for delivering therapeutics across the BBB. Nat Rev Drug Discov 2021;20:362–83.

[8] Le Bras A. Optimizing AAV delivery to the brain. Lab Anim 2022;51(2). 45–45.

[9] Goertsen D, et al. AAV capsid variants with brain-wide transgene expression and decreased liver targeting after intravenous delivery in mouse and marmoset. Nat Neurosci 2022;25(1):106–15.

[10] Luo Y, et al. Dual and multi-targeted nanoparticles for site-specific brain drug delivery. J Control Release 2020;317:195–215.

[11] Monge-Fuentes V, et al. Dopamine-loaded nanoparticle systems circumvent the blood–brain barrier restoring motor function in mouse model for Parkinson's disease. Sci Rep 2021;11(1):15185.

[12] Tylawsky DE, et al. P-selectin-targeted nanocarriers induce active crossing of the blood–brain barrier via caveolin-1-dependent transcytosis. Nat Mater 2023;22(3):391–9.

[13] Rabanel J-M, et al. Nanoparticle shell structural cues drive in vitro transport properties, tissue distribution and brain accessibility in zebrafish. Biomaterials 2021;277:121085.

[14] Hong S-S, et al. Liposomal formulations for nose-to-brain delivery: recent advances and future perspectives. Pharmaceutics 2019;11(10):540.

[15] Formica ML, et al. On a highway to the brain: a review on nose-to-brain drug delivery using nanoparticles. Appl Mater Today 2022;29:101631.

[16] Jeong S-H, Jang J-H, Lee Y-B. Drug delivery to the brain via the nasal route of administration: exploration of key targets and major consideration factors. J Pharm Investig 2023;53(1):119–52.

[17] Rohrer J, Lupo N, Bernkop-Schnürch A. Advanced formulations for intranasal delivery of biologics. Int J Pharm 2018;553(1–2):8–20.

[18] Bhattamisra SK, et al. Nose to brain delivery of rotigotine loaded chitosan nanoparticles in human SH-SY5Y neuroblastoma cells and animal model of Parkinson's disease. Int J Pharm 2020;579:119148.

[19] Wang F, et al. Facile nose-to-brain delivery of rotigotine-loaded polymer micelles thermosensitive hydrogels: in vitro characterization and in vivo behavior study. Int J Pharm 2020;577:119046.

[20] Ahmad E, et al. TAT modification facilitates nose-to-brain transport of intact mPEG-PDLLA micelles: evidence from aggregation-caused quenching probes. Appl Mater Today 2020;19:100556.

[21] Ndemazie NB, et al. Multi-disciplinary approach for drug and gene delivery systems to the brain. AAPS PharmSciTech 2021;23(1):11.

[22] Zeteo Biomedical LLC. Nose to brain drug delivery devices. Available from: https://zeteobiomed.com/nose-to-brain-drug-delivery/.

[23] Mehta AM, Sonabend AM, Bruce JN. Convection-enhanced delivery. Neurotherapeutics 2017;14(2):358–71.

[24] Barua NU, Gill SS, Love S. Convection-enhanced drug delivery to the brain: therapeutic potential and neuropathological considerations. Brain Pathol 2014;24(2):117–27.

[25] Ramadi KB, et al. Computationally guided intracerebral drug delivery via chronically implanted microdevices. Cell Rep 2020;31(10):107734.

[26] Zhao X, et al. Miniaturized neural implants for localized and controllable drug delivery in the brain. J Mater Chem B 2023;11(27):6249–64.

[27] Lee J, et al. Flexible, sticky, and biodegradable wireless device for drug delivery to brain tumors. Nat Commun 2019;10(1):5205.

[28] Khasawneh AH, Garling RJ, Harris CA. Cerebrospinal fluid circulation: what do we know and how do we know it? Brain Circ 2018;4(1):14–8.

[29] Partridge B, et al. Advancements in drug delivery methods for the treatment of brain disease. Front Vet Sci 2022;9:1039745.

[30] Hagiwara F, et al. Brain delivery of cisplatin using microbubbles in combination with ultrasound as an effective therapy for glioblastoma. Pharmaceuticals 2023;16(11):1599.

[31] Burks SR, et al. Blood–brain barrier opening by intracarotid artery hyperosmolar mannitol induces sterile inflammatory and innate immune responses. PNAS 2021;118(18):e2021915118.

[32] Zhang Q, et al. Increase in blood-brain barrier permeability is modulated by tissue kallikrein via activation of bradykinin B1 and B2 receptor-mediated signaling. J Inflamm Res 2021;14:4283–97.
[33] Luo H, Shusta EV. Blood-brain barrier modulation to improve glioma drug delivery. Pharmaceutics 2020;12(11):1085.
[34] Ng SC, et al. Worldwide incidence and prevalence of inflammatory bowel disease in the 21st century: a systematic review of population-based studies. Lancet 2017;390(10114):2769–78.
[35] World Health Organization. Colorectal cancer. Available from: https://www.who.int/news-room/fact-sheets/detail/colorectal-cancer#:~:text=Colon%20cancer%20is%20the%20second%20leading%20cause%20of,variations%20in%20incidence%20and%20mortality%20rates%20were%20observed.
[36] Amidon S, Brown JE, Dave VS. Colon-targeted oral drug delivery systems: design trends and approaches. AAPS PharmSciTech 2015;16(4): 731–41.
[37] Arévalo-Pérez R, Maderuelo C, Lanao JM. Recent advances in colon drug delivery systems. J Control Release 2020;327:703–24.
[38] McCoubrey LE, et al. Colonic drug delivery: formulating the next generation of colon-targeted therapeutics. J Control Release 2023;353: 1107–26.
[39] Donaldson GP, Lee SM, Mazmanian SK. Gut biogeography of the bacterial microbiota. Nat Rev Microbiol 2016;14(1):20–32.
[40] Belali N, Wathoni N, Muchtaridi M. Advances in orally targeted drug delivery to colon. J Adv Pharm Technol Res 2019;10(3):100–6.
[41] Najjar A, Karaman R. The prodrug approach in the era of drug design. Expert Opin Drug Deliv 2019;16(1):1–5.
[42] Shah K, et al. Prodrugs of NSAIDs: a review. Open Med Chem J 2017;11:146–95.
[43] Kim H, et al. Synthesis and evaluation of sulfate conjugated metronidazole as a colon-specific prodrug of metronidazole. J Drug Target 2012; 20(3):255–63.
[44] Kim D, et al. Synthesis and evaluation of N-nicotinoyl-2-{2-(2-methyl-5-nitroimidazol-1-yl)ethyloxy}-D,L-glycine as a colon-specific prodrug of metronidazole. J Pharm Sci 2009;98(11):4161–9.
[45] Nikam A, et al. A systematic overview of Eudragit® based copolymer for smart healthcare. Pharmaceutics 2023;15(2):587.
[46] Evonik. The global market leader for enteric release coatings. Available from: https://healthcare.evonik.com/en/drugdelivery/oral-drug-delivery/oral-excipients/eudragit-portfolio/delayed-release.
[47] dos Santos J, et al. Eudragit: a versatile family of polymers for hot melt extrusion and 3D printing processes in pharmaceutics. Pharmaceutics 2021;13(9):1424.
[48] Naeem M, et al. Colon-targeted delivery of budesonide using dual pH- and time-dependent polymeric nanoparticles for colitis therapy. Drug Des Devel Ther 2015;9:3789–99.
[49] Brady J, et al. Chapter 7 - Polymer properties and characterization. In: Qiu Y, et al., editors. Developing solid oral dosage forms. 2nd ed. Academic Press; 2017. p. 181–223.
[50] Kshirsagar SJ, et al. Development of enzyme-controlled colonic drug delivery using amylose and hydroxypropyl methylcellulose: optimization by factorial design. Drug Deliv 2011;18(6):385–93.
[51] McConnell E, Basit A. Targeting the colon using COLAL™: a novel bacteria-sensitive drug delivery system. In: Rathbone MJ, Roberts MS, editors. Modified-release drug delivery technology. 2nd ed. Informa Healthcare; 2008. p. 343–8.
[52] Lee SH, et al. Strategic approaches for colon targeted drug delivery: an overview of recent advancements. Pharmaceutics 2020;12(1):68.
[53] Meneguzzo F, et al. Real-scale integral valorization of waste orange peel via hydrodynamic cavitation. Processes 2019;7(9):581.
[54] Zhang W, et al. Novel pectin-based carriers for colonic drug delivery. Pharm Dev Technol 2016;21(1):127–30.
[55] Stealey S, et al. Calcium-oligochitosan-pectin microcarrier for colonic drug delivery. Pharm Dev Technol 2020;25(2):260–5.
[56] Jing S, et al. Oral pectin/oligochitosan microspheres for colon-specific controlled release of quercetin to treat inflammatory bowel disease. Carbohydr Polym 2023;316:121025.
[57] Ibekwe VC, et al. A new concept in colonic drug targeting: a combined pH-responsive and bacterially-triggered drug delivery technology. Aliment Pharmacol Ther 2008;28(7):911–6.
[58] Varum F, et al. OPTICORE™, an innovative and accurate colonic targeting technology. Int J Pharm 2020;583:119372.
[59] El-Hady SM, et al. Colon targeting of celecoxib nanomixed micelles using pulsatile drug delivery systems for the prevention of inflammatory bowel disease. Int J Pharm 2020;576:118982.
[60] World Health Organization. Cancer. Available from: https://www.who.int/news-room/fact-sheets/detail/cancer.
[61] International Agency for Research on Cancer. Cancer tomorrow. Available from: https://gco.iarc.fr/tomorrow/en/dataviz/bars?types=0&sexes=0&mode=population&group_populations=0&multiple_populations=1&multiple_cancers=1&cancers=39&populations=903_904_905_908_909_935&apc=cat_ca20v1.5_ca23v-1.5&group_cancers=1.
[62] Senapati S, et al. Controlled drug delivery vehicles for cancer treatment and their performance. Signal Transduct Target Ther 2018;3(1):7.
[63] Bahrami B, et al. Nanoparticles and targeted drug delivery in cancer therapy. Immunol Lett 2017;190:64–83.
[64] Rosenblum D, et al. Progress and challenges towards targeted delivery of cancer therapeutics. Nat Commun 2018;9(1):1410.
[65] Bota DA, et al. Interstitial chemotherapy with biodegradable BCNU (Gliadel) wafers in the treatment of malignant gliomas. Ther Clin Risk Manag 2007;3(5):707–15.
[66] Lu Z-R, Qiao P. Drug delivery in cancer therapy, quo vadis? Mol Pharm 2018;15(9):3603–16.
[67] Vermeulen LMP, et al. The proton sponge hypothesis: fable or fact? Eur J Pharm Biopharm 2018;129:184–90.
[68] Bao G, Mitragotri S, Tong S. Multifunctional nanoparticles for drug delivery and molecular imaging. Annu Rev Biomed Eng 2013;15(1): 253–82.
[69] Dang Y, Guan J. Nanoparticle-based drug delivery systems for cancer therapy. Smart Mater Med 2020;1:10–9.
[70] Gao Y, et al. Multifunctional nanoparticle for cancer therapy. MedComm 2023;4(1):e187.
[71] Sun L, et al. Smart nanoparticles for cancer therapy. Signal Transduct Target Ther 2023;8(1):418.
[72] Hu Z, et al. The Cancer Surfaceome Atlas integrates genomic, functional and drug response data to identify actionable targets. Nat Cancer 2021;2(12):1406–22.
[73] The Cancer Surfaceome Atlas (TCSA). Available from: http://fcgportal.org/TCSA.
[74] Hahn WC, et al. An expanded universe of cancer targets. Cell 2021;184(5):1142–55.

[75] Shirata C, et al. Near-infrared photothermal/photodynamic therapy with indocyanine green induces apoptosis of hepatocellular carcinoma cells through oxidative stress. Sci Rep 2017;7(1):13958.
[76] Sun Y, et al. Intelligent tumor microenvironment-activated multifunctional nanoplatform coupled with turn-on and always-on fluorescence probes for imaging-guided cancer treatment. ACS Appl Mater Interfaces 2021;13(45):53646–58.
[77] Kang X, et al. A photo-triggered self-accelerated nanoplatform for multifunctional image-guided combination cancer immunotherapy. Nat Commun 2023;14(1):5216.
[78] Wang X, et al. Smart drug delivery systems for precise cancer therapy. Acta Pharm Sin B 2022;12(11):4098–121.
[79] Yang Y, et al. Trisulfide bond–mediated doxorubicin dimeric prodrug nanoassemblies with high drug loading, high self-assembly stability, and high tumor selectivity. Sci Adv 2020;6(45):eabc1725.
[80] Eslami-S Z, et al. Functional analysis of circulating tumour cells: the KEY to understand the biology of the metastatic cascade. Br J Cancer 2022;127(5):800–10.
[81] Lawrence R, et al. Circulating tumour cells for early detection of clinically relevant cancer. Nat Rev Clin Oncol 2023;20(7):487–500.
[82] Lin D, et al. Circulating tumor cells: biology and clinical significance. Signal Transduct Target Ther 2021;6(1):404.
[83] Mai Y, et al. The strategies to cure cancer patients by eradicating cancer stem-like cells. Mol Cancer 2023;22(1):171.
[84] Ayob AZ, Ramasamy TS. Cancer stem cells as key drivers of tumour progression. J Biomed Sci 2018;25(1):20.
[85] Yang L, et al. Targeting cancer stem cell pathways for cancer therapy. Signal Transduct Target Ther 2020;5(1):8.
[86] Rao W, et al. Chitosan-decorated doxorubicin-encapsulated nanoparticle targets and eliminates tumor reinitiating cancer stem-like cells. ACS Nano 2015;9(6):5725–40.
[87] Hou Y, et al. Cryoablation-activated enhanced nanodoxorubicin release for the therapy of chemoresistant mammary cancer stem-like cells. J Mater Chem B 2020;8(5):908–18.

CHAPTER

14

Stimuli-responsive drug delivery systems

Wujie Zhang

LEARNING OBJECTIVES

- To differentiate and discuss internal and external stimuli
- To interpret the working mechanism of pH-responsive drug delivery systems
- To interpret the working mechanism of redox-responsive drug delivery systems
- To interpret the working mechanism of enzyme-responsive drug delivery systems
- To interpret the working mechanisms of external stimuli-responsive drug delivery systems
- To design the stimuli-responsive drug delivery systems

14.1 Internal and external stimuli

Stimuli-responsive drug carriers are a significant part of novel drug delivery systems. Two of the major advantages of using stimuli-responsive drug delivery systems are achieving site-specific release (at desired rates) and avoiding premature drug release [1]. At the same time, targeting aims to deliver the drug to the desired site. For novel drug delivery systems, stimuli-responsive systems are commonly coupled with targetability (Fig. 14.1). In general, stimuli can be categorized into either internal (endogenous) or external (exogenous) (Fig. 14.2). Internal stimuli include pH, enzyme, redox, O_2 (e.g., hypoxia), glucose (hyperglycemia), and ATP (extracellular environment: < 5 μmol/L and intracellular cytosol: $1 \sim 10$ mmol/L) [2–4]. Temperature, light, ultrasound, electric field, and magnetic field are commonly used external stimuli [3].

14.2 pH-responsive drug delivery systems

pH-responsive drug delivery systems have the ability to respond to disease microenvironments triggering the release of drugs [5]. As shown in Fig. 14.3, differential pH environments at different levels, organ, tissue, and cellular, can be exploited for pH-responsive drug delivery systems [6]. At the organ level, the gastrointestinal tract is a good example as it is characterized by a pH gradient (Fig. 4.7). In general, extracellular pH values of normal tissues are in the range of 7.2 to 7.5 compared to 6.4 to 7.0 for tumors. Take lung tissues, for example; the average extracellular pH

Fundamentals and Design of Drug Delivery Systems
https://doi.org/10.1016/B978-0-443-23521-4.00014-X

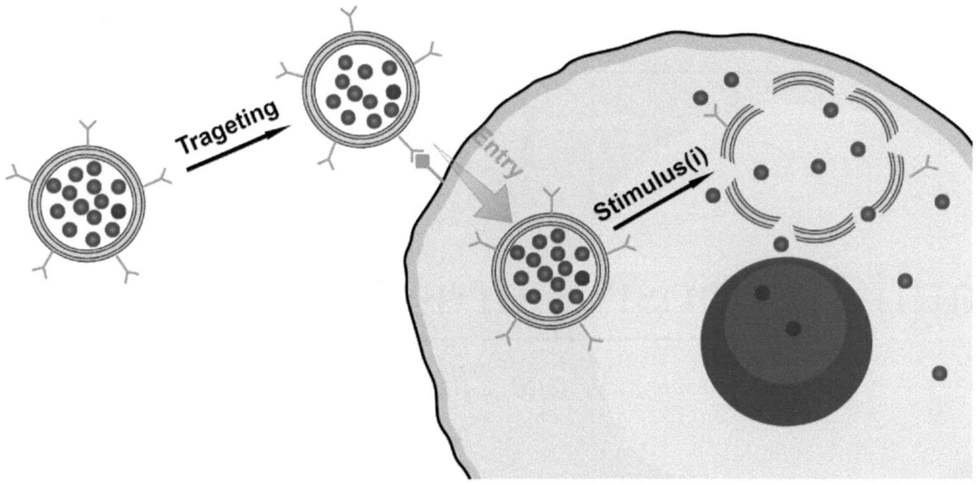

FIGURE 14.1 Targetability (Chapter 11) and stimuli-responsiveness (Chapter 14) of drug delivery systems—a demonstration using a nanoscale carrier.

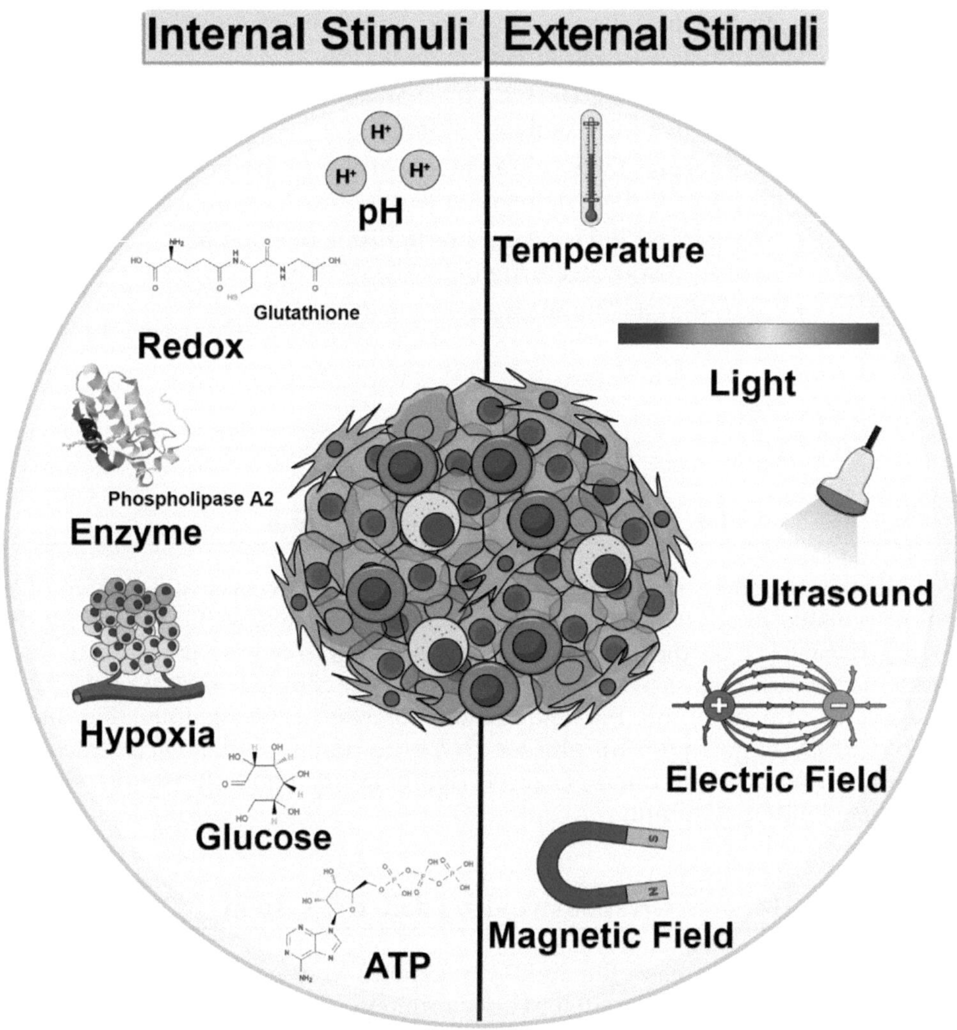

FIGURE 14.2 Internal and external stimuli for designing stimuli-responsive drug delivery systems.

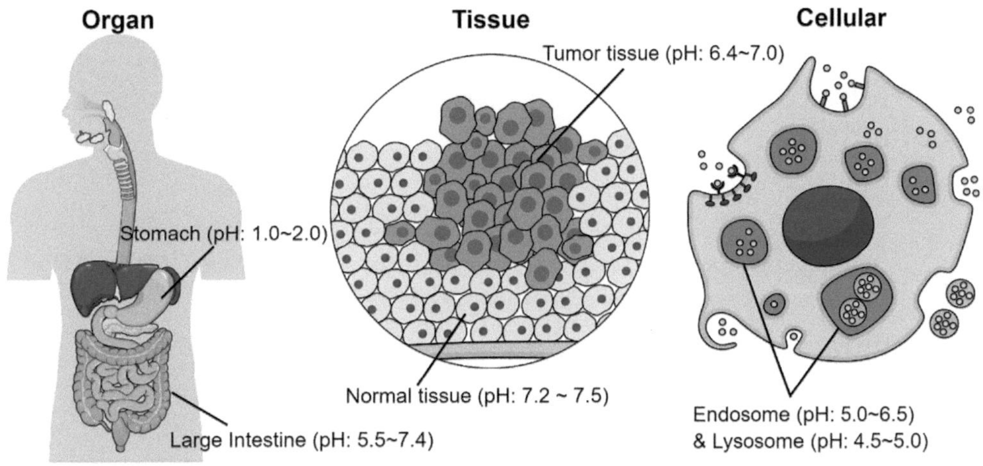

FIGURE 14.3 Differential pH environment at the organ, tissue, and cellular levels that could be used for developing pH-responsive drug delivery systems.

is around 7.3 and 6.5 for normal and tumor tissues, respectively [7]. When it comes to the cellular level, pH-responsiveness is of particular interest as it can assist the endosomal escape of drug carriers/drugs. Particularly, nanoscale drug carriers end up in endo/lysosomes during cellular uptake (endocytosis), and endosomes (pH 5-6.5) and lysosomes (pH 4.5-5) are acidic [3,8].

Drug release can be triggered by the physical and/or chemical dissociation of the carrier or chemical bond-cleavage of the drug from its carrier [5,6]. Commonly used acid-labile chemical bonds are shown in Fig. 14.4 [2,5,9]. Protonation and deprotonation of functional groups (e.g., interrupting ionic interactions and changing hydrophilicity) at different pH values can also trigger drug release. For example, reversible ionization of carboxyl and/or amino groups has been widely used to design pH-responsive drug delivery systems [9]. Some of the pH-responsive polymers include alginate, pectin, chitosan, Eudragit, poly(methacrylic-g-ethylene glycol), poly(γ-glutamic acid), polyacrylic acid, poly(amidoamine), poly[2-dimethylaminoethylmethacrylate], and poly(β-aminoester) [4,9–12].

pH-responsiveness drug delivery systems, liposomes, micelle, dendrimers, and micro/nanospheres have been applied in treating many diseases, including cancer, diabetes, inflammation, bacterial infection, and neurological diseases [4,9,11,12]. For example, Haibin Zhang *et al.* developed a pH-sensitive *O*-carboxymethyl chitosan/sodium alginate nanohydrogel for oral insulin delivery, which could release the drug for more than 12 hours [13]. Huiru Zhu *et al.* designed pH-responsive nanoparticles for paclitaxel delivery to inhibit vascular restenosis. The nanoparticle system is poly(D,L-lactic-*co*-glycolic acid) (PLGA) based and loaded with the drug paclitaxel and $NaHCO_3$. The pH at the site of vascular inflammation is slightly acidic. $NaHCO_3$ reacts with protons, resulting in CO_2 production and drug release (Fig. 14.5) [14]. A pH-responsive delivery system has also been used for ischemic stroke treatment. The succinobucol-loaded pH-sensitive polymeric nanovehicle (PP/SCB) was coated with a 4T1 cell membrane (MPP/SCB). The nanovehicle was based on methoxy poly(ethylene glycol)-*block*-poly(2-diisopropyl methacrylate) (PEG-PDPA; PP) (Fig. 14.6). This biomimetic coating enabled the penetration of the blood-brain barrier targeting the inflammation lesions [15].

14.3 Redox-responsive drug delivery systems

Redox-responsive drug delivery systems are typically designed to be triggered by reactive oxygen species (ROS) such as superoxide dismutase and hydrogen peroxide (H_2O_2). Diselenide bond (-Se-Se-), disulfide bond (-S-S-), thiol (sulfhydryl) group (-SH), thioether bond (-S-), and boronic ester are widely utilized in designing redox-responsive systems [3,16–18]. The reaction (oxidation) scheme is shown in Fig. 14.7 [18,19]. Glutathione (GSH) is also a common "target" for designing redox-responsive systems. GSH is a triple peptide: γ-Glu-Cys-Gly. It is a marker of the redox state in many diseases and plays a critical role in maintaining the redox homeostasis of the cells [20]. For example, GSH concentration is four times higher in tumors than in healthy tissues [3]. Disulfide bonds are the most commonly used GSH-cleavable bonds in drug delivery systems (disulfide bonds are cleaved into sulfhydryl groups) [2,21].

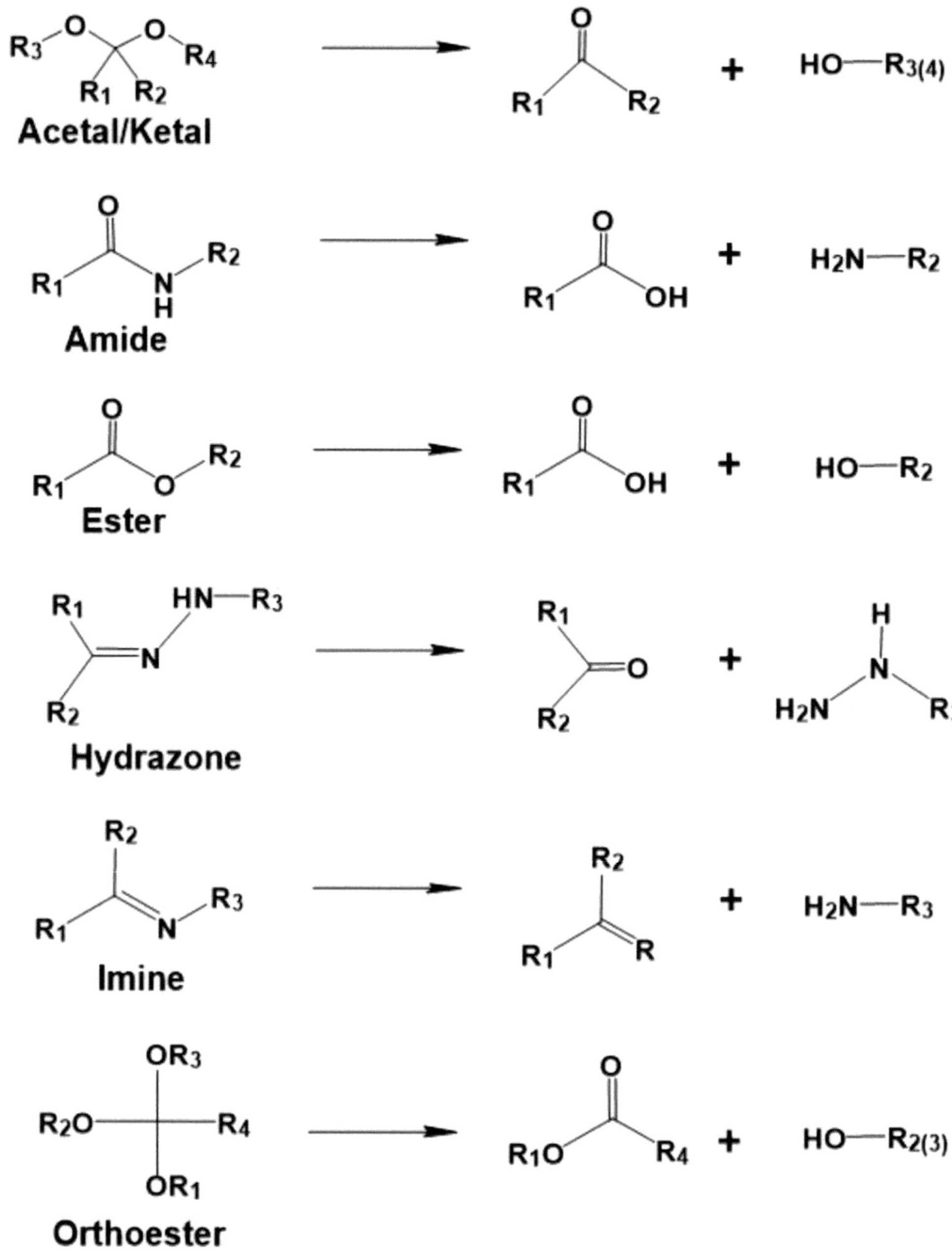

FIGURE 14.4 pH-responsive chemical bonds and their hydrolysates.

Novel redox-responsive systems are mostly in the nanoscale and in the form of liposomes, micelles, particles/capsules, and hydrogel. Both synthetic and natural polymers are used in the design of these systems—poly(ethylene glycol), polycaprolactone, poly(glycolic acid), poly(L-lactic acid), polypropylenimine, poly(*N*-isopropylacrylamide), β-cyclodextrin, hyaluronic acid, chitosan, heparan sulfate, and more [4,16]. Redox-responsive systems have been used in numerous biomedical fields including cancer therapy, anti-inflammation, and vaccination [4]. Here, let's examine examples of redox-responsive drug delivery systems targeting either ROS or GSH. Ziyin Zhao *et al.* developed an H_2O_2-responsive "system (i.e., pro-protein)" for endocytosis-independent and cancer-selective cytosolic protein delivery. Drugs (proteins) are sequentially modified with 4-nitrophenyl,4-(4,4,5,5-tetramethyl-1,3,2-dioxaborolan-2-yl)benzyl carbonate (H_2O_2-responsive domain) and 3,4-dihydroxy-L-phenylalanine (substrate of L-type amino acid transporter 1 (LAT1), which is overexpressed on the cancer cell membrane). After the direct transport into cancer cells by LAT1, the overproduced H_2O_2 in cytosol restores the protein drug activity (Fig. 14.8) [22]. Recently, chitosan-based redox-responsive nanoparticles were developed for treating airway inflammation in

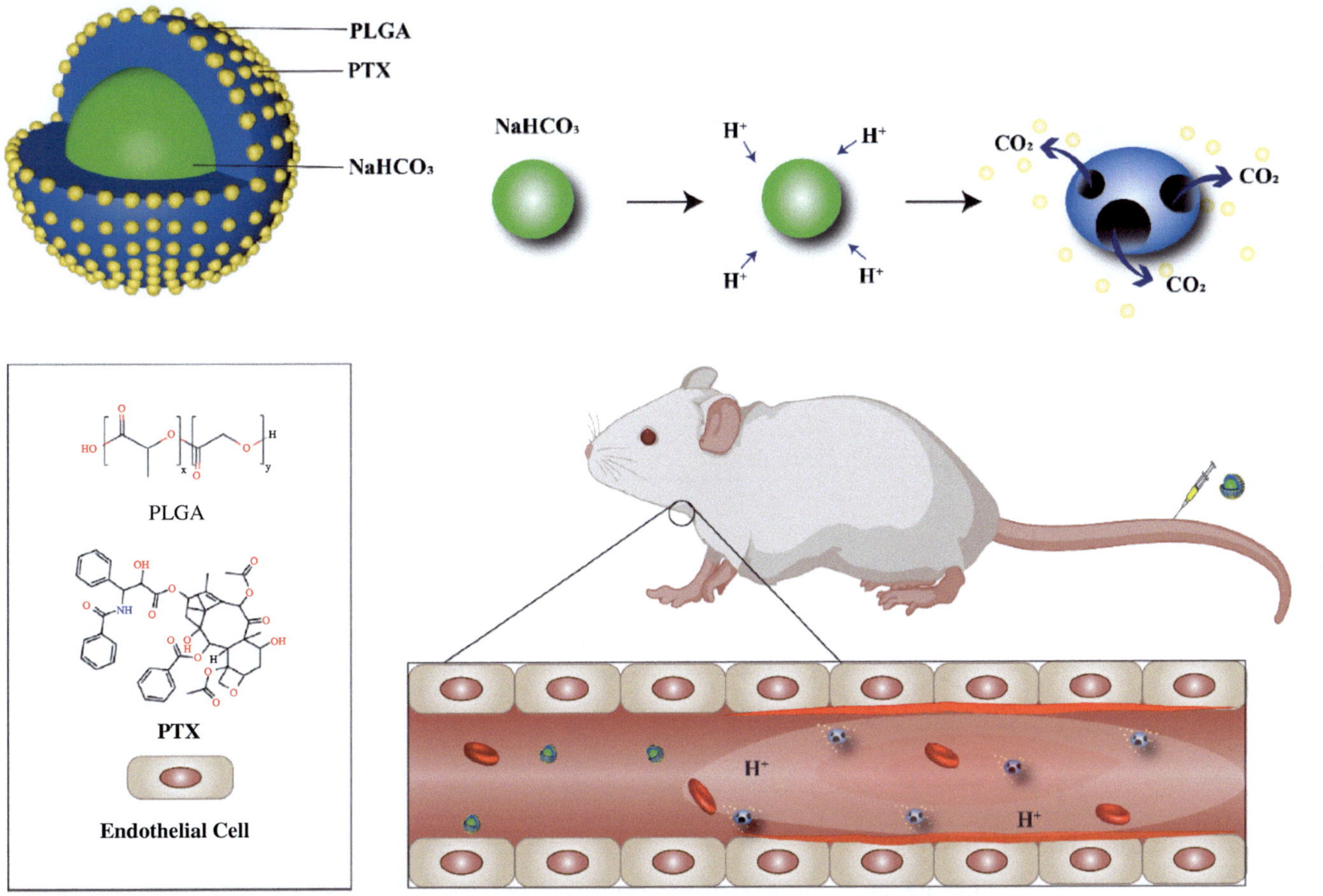

FIGURE 14.5 pH-responsive nanoparticles for the vascular restenosis treatment. *PLGA*, Poly(D,L-lactic-*co*-glycolic acid); *PTX*, paclitaxel. *From Zhu, H., et al.,* pH-responsive nanoparticles for delivery of paclitaxel to the injury site for inhibiting vascular restenosis. *Pharmaceutics, 2022.* ***14****(3): p. 535.*

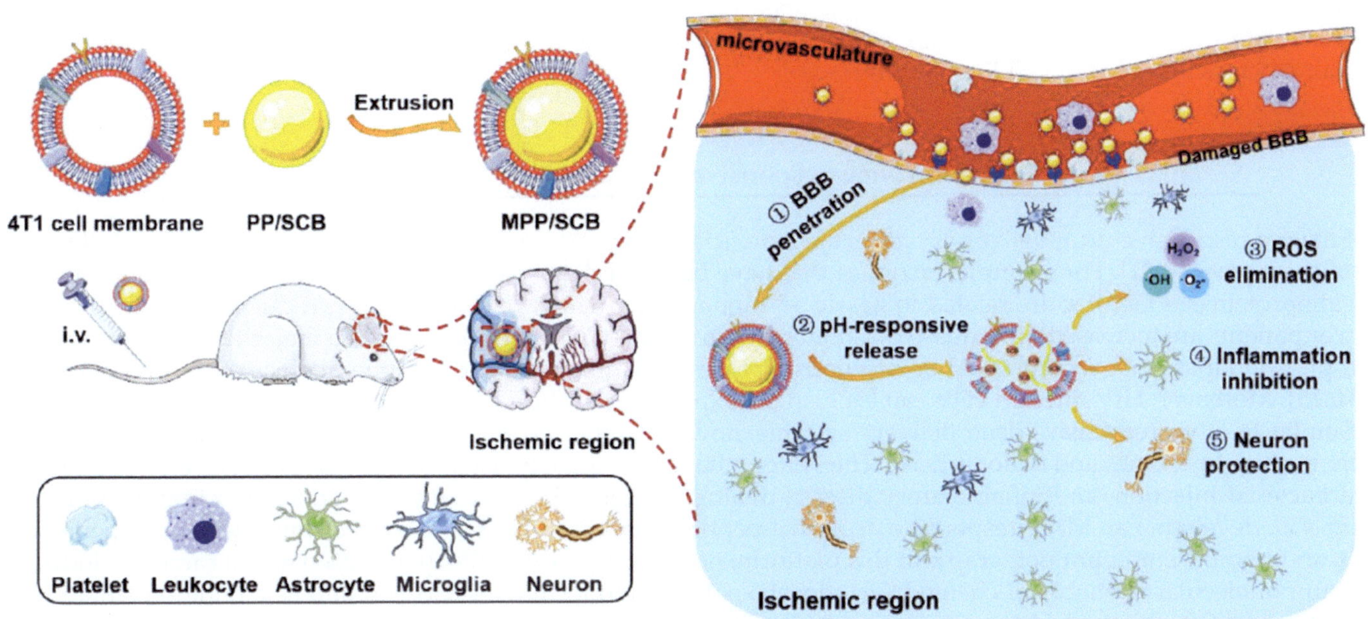

FIGURE 14.6 Schematic illustration of the preparation of the membrane camouflaged nanovehicles of MPP/SCB and their preferential targeting of cerebral ischemic lesions in a biomimetic manner to attenuate the ischemia/reperfusion injury for ischemic stroke treatment. *M*, 4T1 cell membrane; *PP*, methoxy poly(ethylene glycol)-*block*-poly(2-diisopropyl methacrylate); *SCB*, succinobucol. *From He, W., et al.,* Preferential targeting cerebral ischemic lesions with cancer cell-inspired nanovehicle for ischemic stroke treatment. *Nano Lett, 2021.* ***21****(7): p. 3033-3043. Copyright (2021), American Chemical Society.*

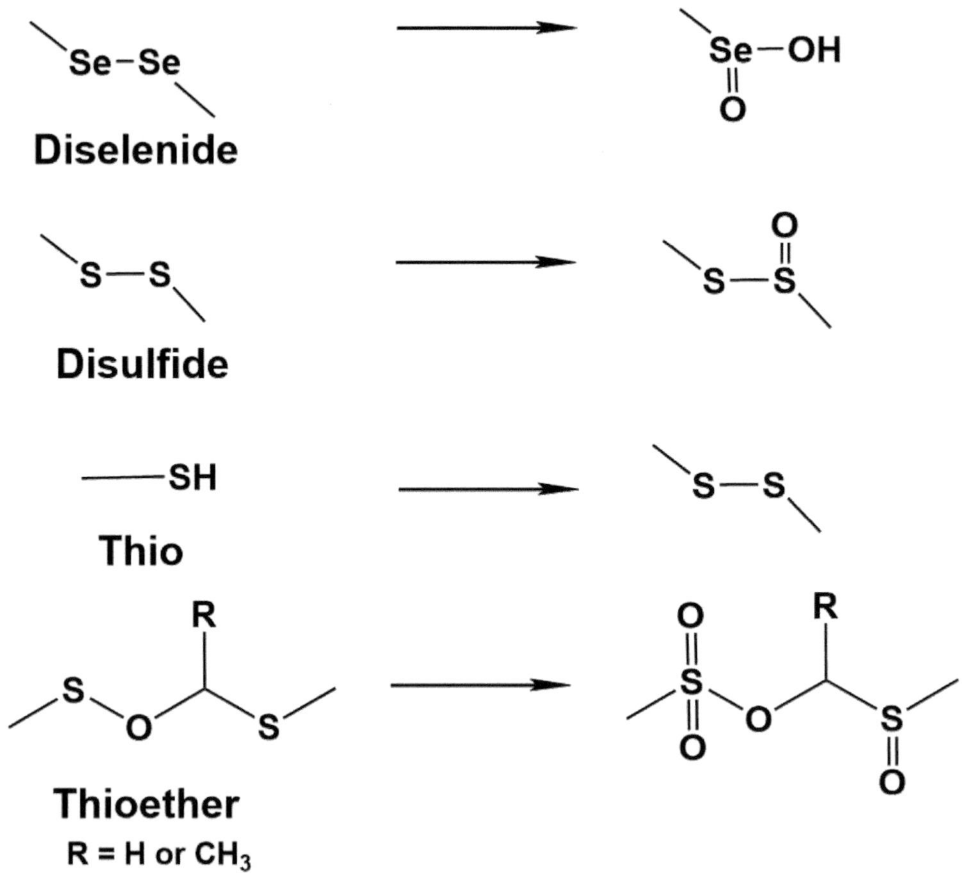

FIGURE 14.7 Reaction scheme of ROS-responsive bonds/groups.

asthma. The nanoparticles are based on chitosan and poly(ethylene glycol)methyl ether (mPEG). The drug release mechanism is GSH mediated as the GSH concentration is much higher at inflamed sites [23]. Similarly, pH/GSH sensitivity shell-crosslinked micelles were developed [24]. As shown in Fig. 14.9, poly(2-(diisopropylaminoethyl) methacrylate (PDPA) contributed to the pH-sensitivity of the micelles, and the crosslinking *via* disulfide bond-contained crosslinker led to GSH sensitivity.

14.4 Enzyme-responsive drug delivery systems

Enzyme-responsive drug delivery systems are beneficial for the sites of interest with increased accumulation of certain enzymes [2,21]. For example, enzymes that have been used as "targets" for cancer therapy include matrix metalloproteinases (MMPs; are related to nearly all human malignancies), cathepsin B (production and activity in cancer patients are increased), urokinase plasminogen activators (uPAs; are increased in a majority of cancer types), and phospholipase (is overexpressed in infectious diseases, inflammation, and peripheral areas of tumor invasion) [3,10,25]. Moreover, HIV-infected cells can exclusively express intracellular proteases (or kinases) [2].

Similar to other responsive drug delivery systems, novel enzyme-responsive platforms are mostly at the nanoscale, such as liposomes and nanoparticles. The systems have been widely used for applications such as cancer therapy, bacterial infection, and inflammatory disease treatment [3,26,27]. Now, let's look at some examples. Jinrong Peng *et al.* developed an MMP-responsive drug-dye-peptide nanoassembly for enhanced tumor targeting, penetration, and photochemoimmunotherapy. In this platform, near-infrared dye (IR820) was used as the carrier to induce the supramolecular assembly of chemodrugs (docetaxel [DTX]) to form nanoparticles and as a photosensitizer for photothermal therapy. A specially designed peptide with 27 amino acids units (CF27) and N'-bis(acryloyl)cystamine (BISS) was used to form a crosslinking network structure (between the acrylic groups of BISS and -SH of CF27) to coat the nanoparticles. Regarding the functionalities of CF27, one segment was designed to block the programmed

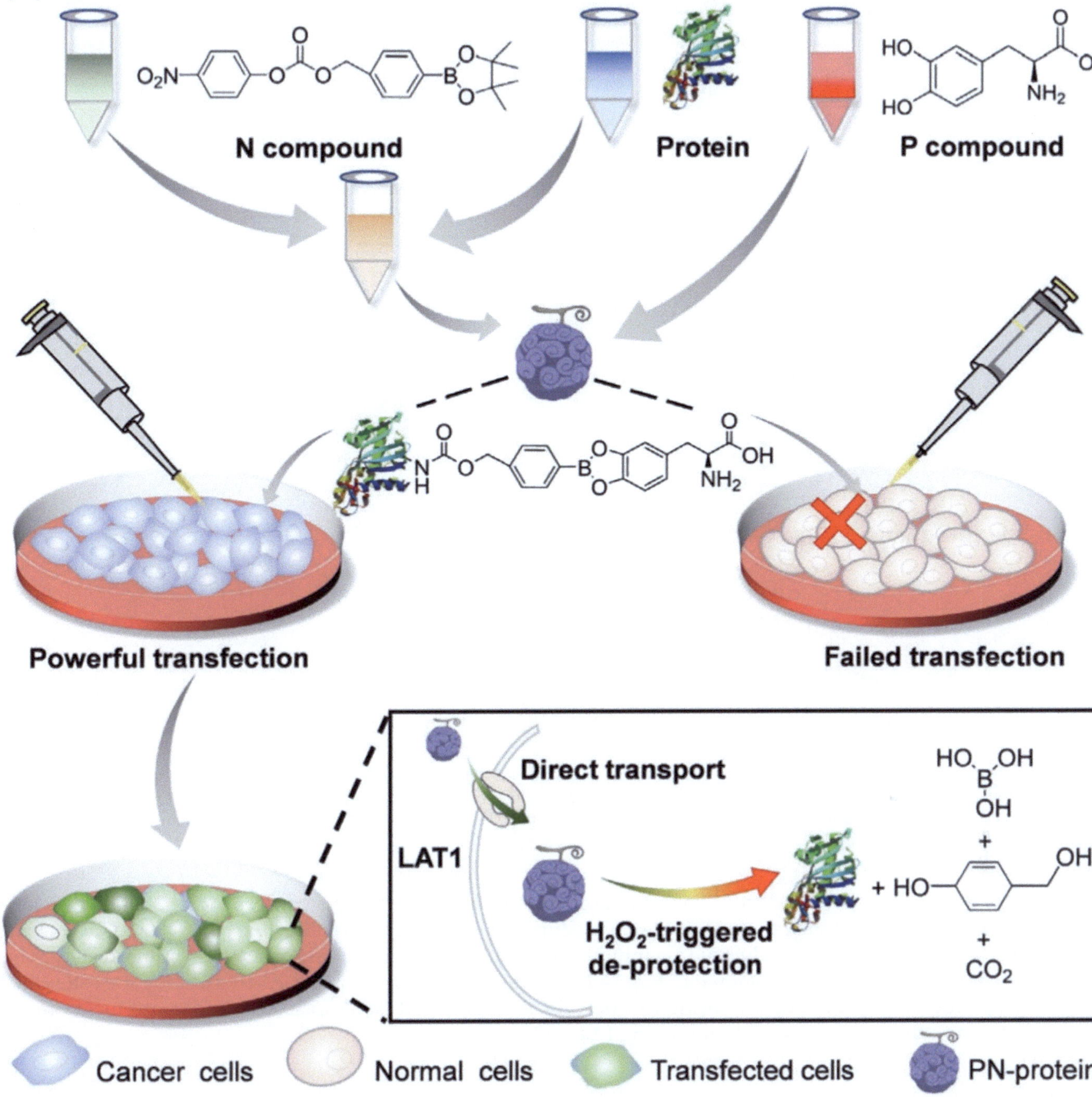

FIGURE 14.8 Schematic illustration showing the synthesis of pro-protein, LAT1-mediated direct transport across cancer cell membrane, and H_2O_2-triggered restoration of the native protein structure inside cells. *LAT1*, L-type amino acid transporter 1; *N compound*, 4-nitrophenyl,4-(4,4,5,5-tetramethyl-1,3,2-dioxaborolan-2-yl)benzyl carbonate; *P compound*, 3,4-dihydroxy-L-phenylalanine. *From Zhao, Z., et al.,* Endocytosis-independent and cancer-selective cytosolic protein delivery via reversible tagging with LAT1 substrate. *Adv Mater, 2022.* ***34****(35): p. e2110560, with permission from John Wiley & Sons, Inc.*

cell death-1/programmed cell death-ligand 1 (PD-1/PD-L1) to strengthen the immune response to tumor cells. Additionally, CF27 contains an MMP2-responsive segment (PLGVRG) and a nine–amino acid sequence (Lyp-1; CGNKRTRGC) for tumor targeting. At the same time, BISS is GSH responsive due to its disulfide bond (Fig. 14.10) [28]. Jingyi Rao *et al.* developed a polymer micelle system based on the azobenzene motif, which is azoreductase responsive. The system can be used for colonic-specific drug delivery due to the presence of azoreductase in the human intestine [29]. Recently, enzyme-responsive biomimetic solid lipid nanoparticles (SLNs) were

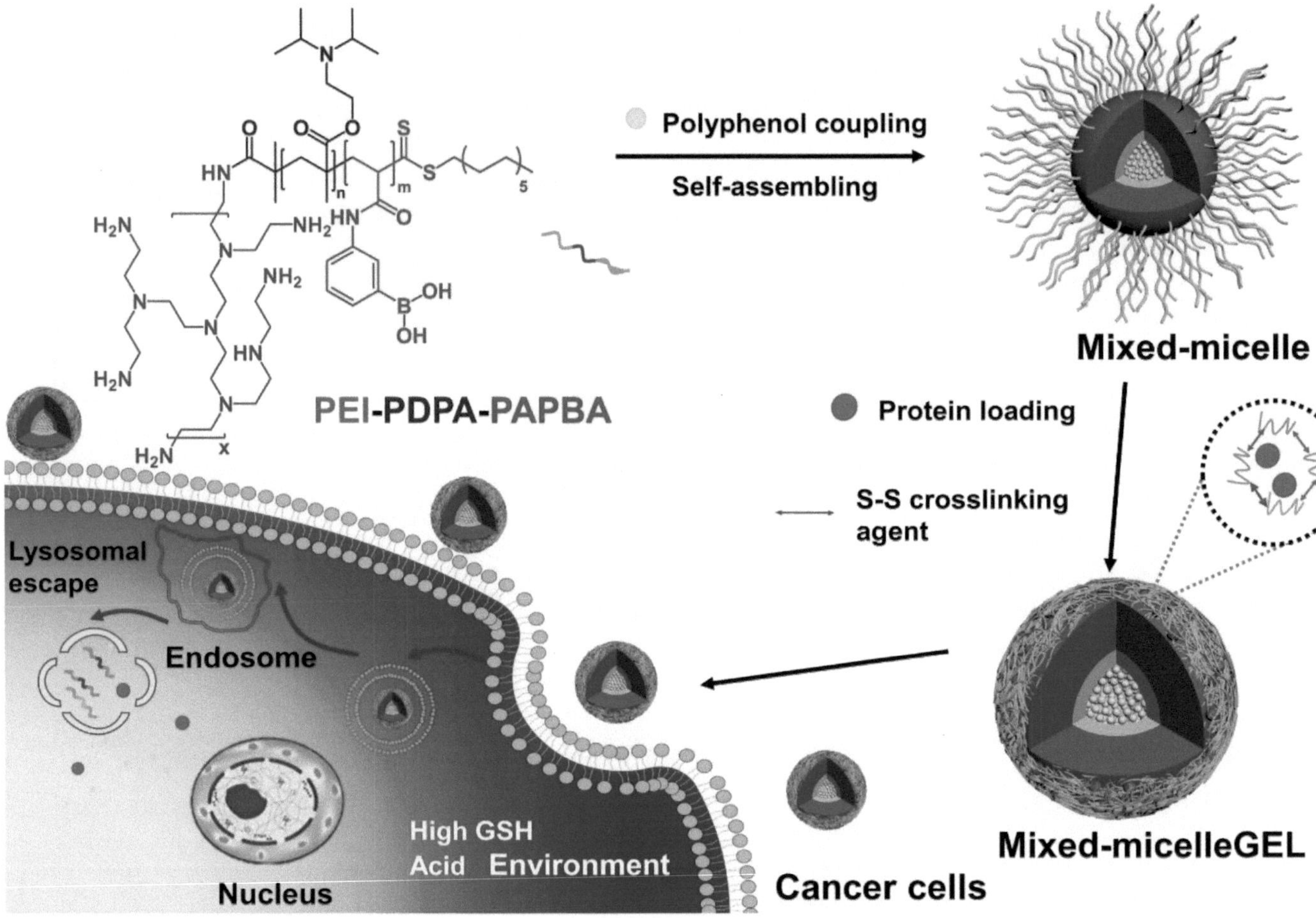

FIGURE 14.9 Schematic representation of the preparation of microgel from amphiphilic copolymers and their application for drug delivery in tumor treatment. *PAPBA*, Poly(3-acrylamido)phenylboronic acid; *PDPA*, poly(2-(diisopropylaminoethyl)methacrylate; *PEI*, polyethylenimine. *From Liu, Y., et al.,* Shell-crosslinked micelles with neighborhood effect and pH/GSH sensitivity for co-loading of protein and polyphenol drugs. *Colloids Surf. A: Physicochem Eng Aspects, 2023.* ***679****: p. 132512, with permission from Elsevier.*

developed for antibiotic delivery against hyaluronidase-secreting bacteria. The system was incorporated with vancomycin (VCM) and ascorbyl stearate (AS). Bacterial hyaluronidase (B-HAase) is critical for many extra- and intracellular functions. AS is a potent hyaluronidase inhibitor providing the enzyme responsiveness of the system. The working mechanism of the system is shown in Fig. 14.11—bacterial lipase hydrolyzes AS by cleaving the ester linkage and changes the structure of SLN, releasing vancomycin. In addition, SLNs, AS, ascorbic acid (a product from AS degradation), and other molecules could inhibit B-HAase [30].

14.5 External stimuli—based drug delivery systems

This section overlaps with Section 11.3 but focuses on the drug release due to the external stimuli rather than drug targeting. External stimuli are from outside the body and commonly used triggers are temperature, light, ultrasound, electric, and magnetic fields [3,10,21]. Thermoresponsive drug delivery systems are among the most investigated stimuli-responsive strategies and are governed by a nonlinear shaped property change of the drug carrier or at least one component. Generally, the system should be stable and retain the load and suddenly release the load with a locally elevated/reduced temperature [31]. Poly(*N*-isopropylacrylamide) (PNIPAM) and Pluronic polymers have been used for designing thermoresponsive drug delivery systems (Fig. 14.12). PNIPAM is composed of both hydrophilic amide groups and hydrophobic isopropyl side chains. Its lower critical solution temperature (LCST; minimal temperature required for the polymer to form a gel [from one-phase to two-phase status] [32]) is around 32°C —PNIPAM solutions take a sol state at room temperature and are transformed into a gel at body temperature

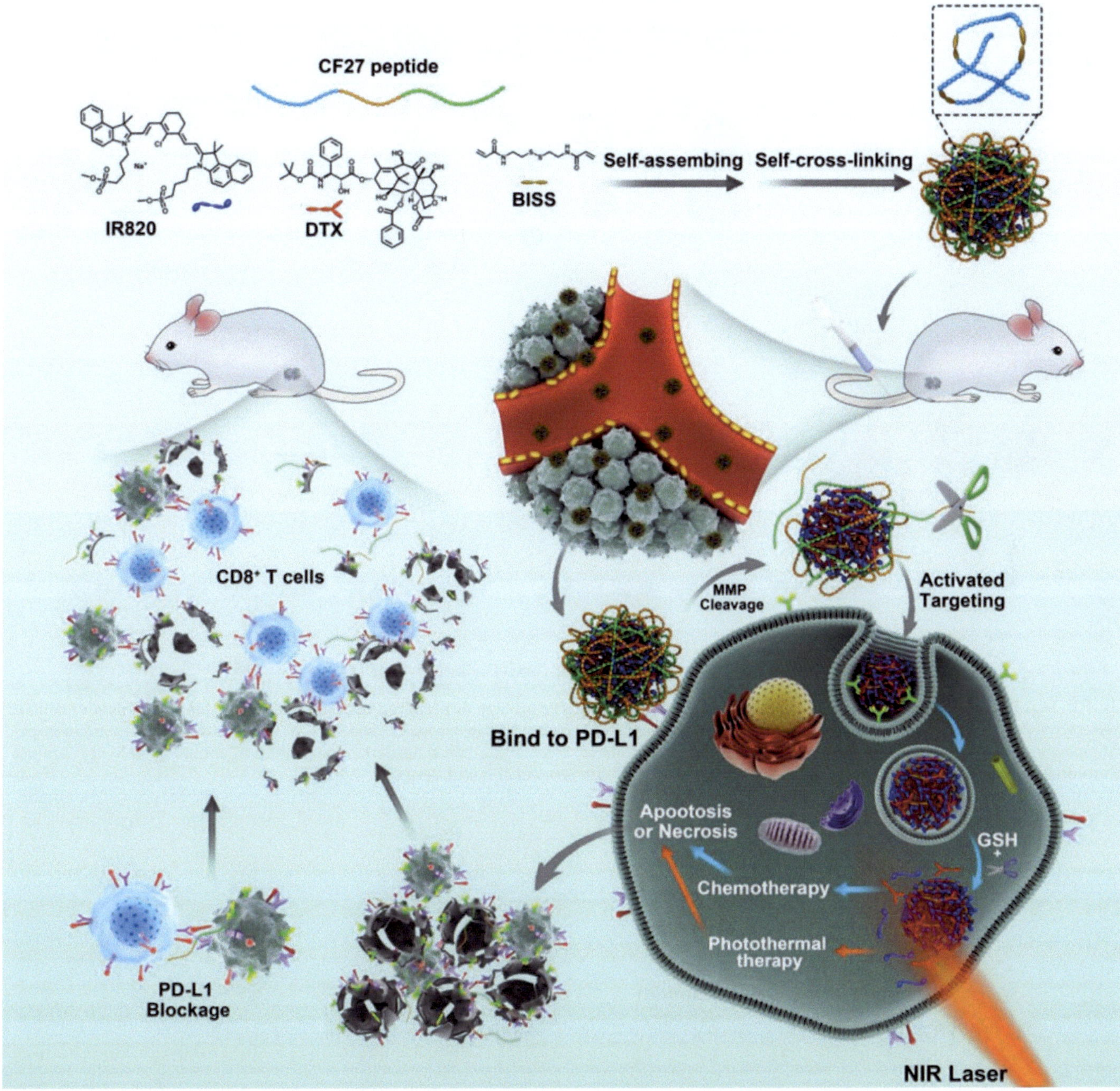

FIGURE 14.10 The supramolecular assembly and self-crosslinking formation of NIR dye/drug/peptide hybrid nanoparticles and their applications in versatile cancer combinatorial therapies. *DTX*, Docetaxel; *BISS*, *N′*-bis(acryloyl)cystamine; *PD-L1*, programmed cell death-ligand 1; *NIR*, near-infrared. *From Peng, J., et al.,* Tumor microenvironment responsive drug-dye-peptide nanoassembly for enhanced tumor-targeting, penetration, and photo-chemo-immunotherapy. *Adv. Funct. Mater, 2019.* ***29****(19): p. 1900004, with permission from John Wiley & Sons, Inc.*

(~ 37°C > LCST) [33]. Pluronic polymers, triblock copolymers, are poly(ethylene)oxide-poly(propylene)oxide-poly(ethylene)oxide (PEO-PPO-PEO) with hydrophilic PEO chains on the sides and a central hydrophobic PPO chain [34]. Pluronic F127 (PEO_{100}-PPO_{65}-PEO_{100}) is the most frequently used among Pluronic polymers. It forms micelles and becomes hydrogels above the critical micelle concentration (CMC) and lower critical solution temperature (LCST) (Fig. 14.13) [35,36]. There are many Pluronic F127–based nanoplatforms for controlled drug delivery, such as Pluronic F127-Chitosan nanocapsules [37]. The Pluronic F127-Chitosan nanocapsules were ~37 nm at 37°C and

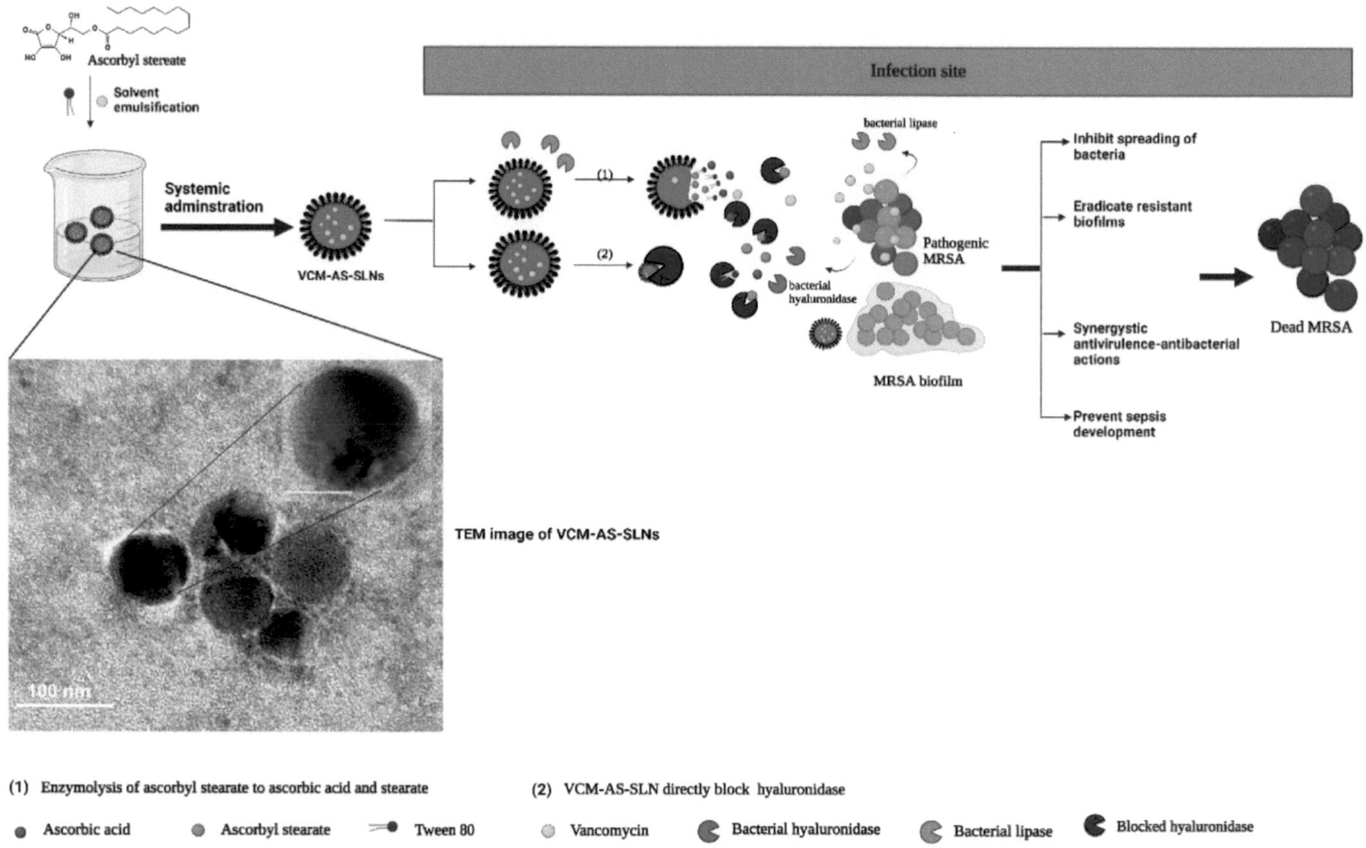

FIGURE 14.11 Schematic illustration of VCM-AS-SLNs preparation, TEM image of prepared nanoparticles and their mechanism of action. *AS*, Ascorbyl stearate; *SLNs*, solid lipid nanoparticles; *MRSA*, methicillin-resistant *Staphylococcus aureus*; TEM, transmission electron microscope; *VCM*, vancomycin. *From Mohammed, M., et al.,* Enzyme-responsive biomimetic solid lipid nanoparticles for antibiotic delivery against hyaluronidase-secreting bacteria. *Int. J. Pharm, 2023.* ***640****: p. 122967, with permission from Elsevier.*

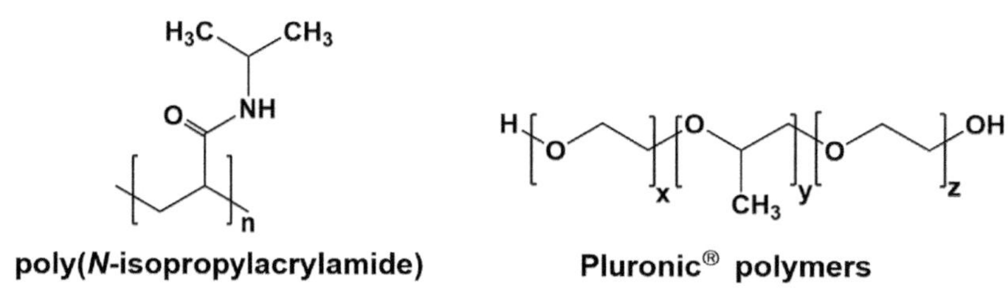

FIGURE 14.12 Chemical structures of poly(*N*-isopropylacrylamide) and Pluronic polymers.

~240 nm at 4°C. The responsiveness of the nanocapsules was successfully used for hydrophilic molecule encapsulation and controlled release (Fig. 14.14). Recently, a thermoresponsive nanoparticle-hydrogel composite based on Pluronic F127 and phycocyanin (PC) was developed for cancer therapy. Nanoparticles (DOX-UA NPs) were formed by self-assembly of doxorubicin (DOX) and ursolic acid (UA) and incorporated into the thermoresponsive hydrogel composed of Pluronic F127 and phycocyanin, which is a photosensitizer. UA can promote the tumor cells' response to DOX and PC can produce ROS when exposed to laser radiation (Fig. 14.15). The system displayed an exceptional tumor inhibition rate of 91.05% during the *in vivo* experiments [38]. ThermoDox, a thermosensitive liposome containing doxorubicin, is the most clinically advanced thermosensitive liposome formulation and has been evaluated through various clinical trials (please refer to Case Study VI) [39].

Regarding light as an external stimulus, light with wavelengths in the UV, visible, and near-infrared (NIR) ranges have been investigated. NIR light is of particular interest due to its high tissue penetration [3,21]. Light-responsive moieties have been incorporated into drug delivery systems including nitrobenzyl group, perylene, cardiogreen, and riboflavin chromophores [21]. Azobenzene, *O*-nitrobenzene, coumarin, and pyrene derivatives are commonly

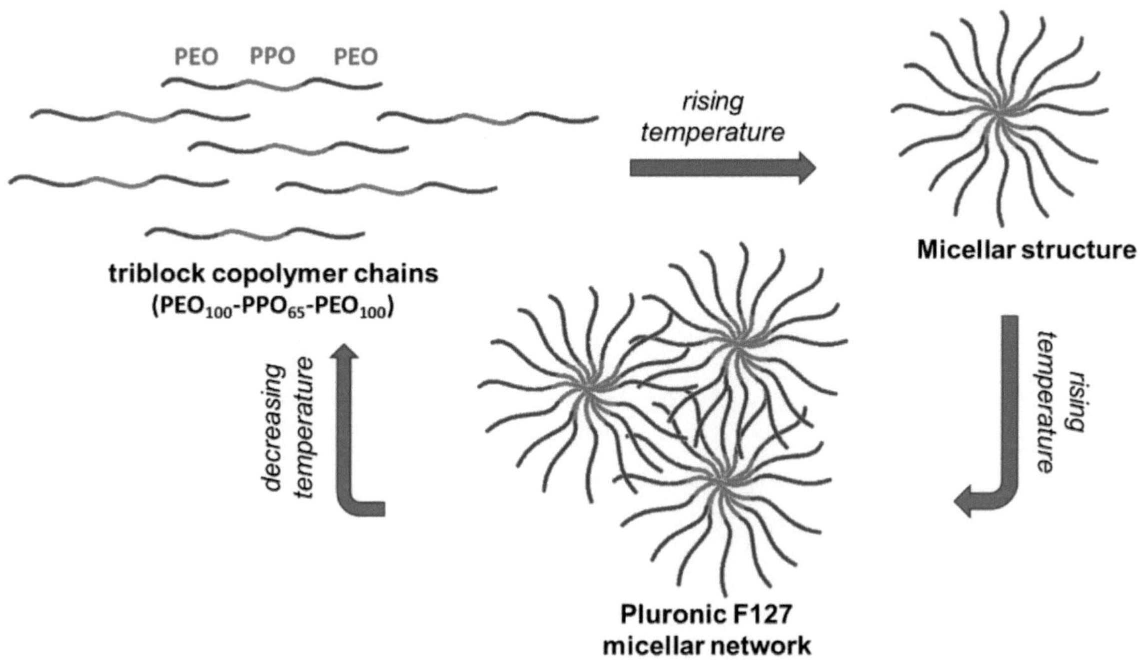

FIGURE 14.13 Schematic presentation of temperature-induced gelation for Pluronic F127. *From Lupu, A., et al.,* Self-healing of Pluronic; F127 hydrogels in the presence of various polysaccharides. *Gels, 2023.* ***9****(9): p. 719.*

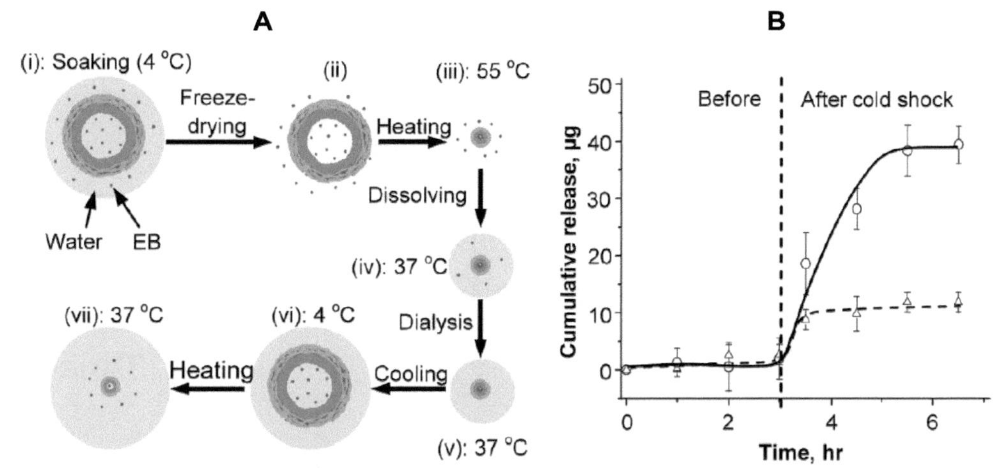

FIGURE 14.14 (A) Schematic illustration of the procedure for encapsulating (i–v) ethidium bromide (EB) in the Pluronic F127-chitosan nanocapsules and the cold shock treatment (v–vii) to achieve temperature-controlled release of the encapsulated EB and (B) cumulative release of EB encapsulated in the Pluronic F127-chitosan nanocapsules synthesized using either 30% *(circle)* or 10% *(triangle)* Pluronic F127 out of the nanocapsules into water in the 1 mL dialysis tube and further into the 45 mL deionized water outside the dialysis tube at 37°C before and after the cold shock treatment at 3 hr. *From Zhang, W., et al.,* Synthesis and characterization of thermally responsive Pluronic F127–chitosan nanocapsules for controlled release and intracellular delivery of small molecules. *ACS Nano, 2010.* ***4****(11): p. 6747-6759. Copyright (2010), American Chemical Society.*

used materials for constructing light-responsive drug delivery systems [10]. The different kinds of light response mechanisms for drug release are photocleavage, photoisomerization, photosensitization (e.g., ROS generation), and photocrosslinking [3,40]. Pedro Mena-Giraldo *et al.* developed photosensitive nanocarriers based on UV photosensitive n-succinyl chitosan amphiphilic copolymer (PNSC), and the drug is released through azobenzene isomerization (Figs. 14.16 and 11.14) [41].

Ultrasound offers various advantages in stimuli-responsive drug delivery systems—precise spatiotemporal control, safe, and deep tissue penetration [3,42]. The three main mechanisms for ultrasound energy-mediated drug release are heat generation, acoustic cavitation, and acoustic radiation [10]. Microbubbles are the most well-known

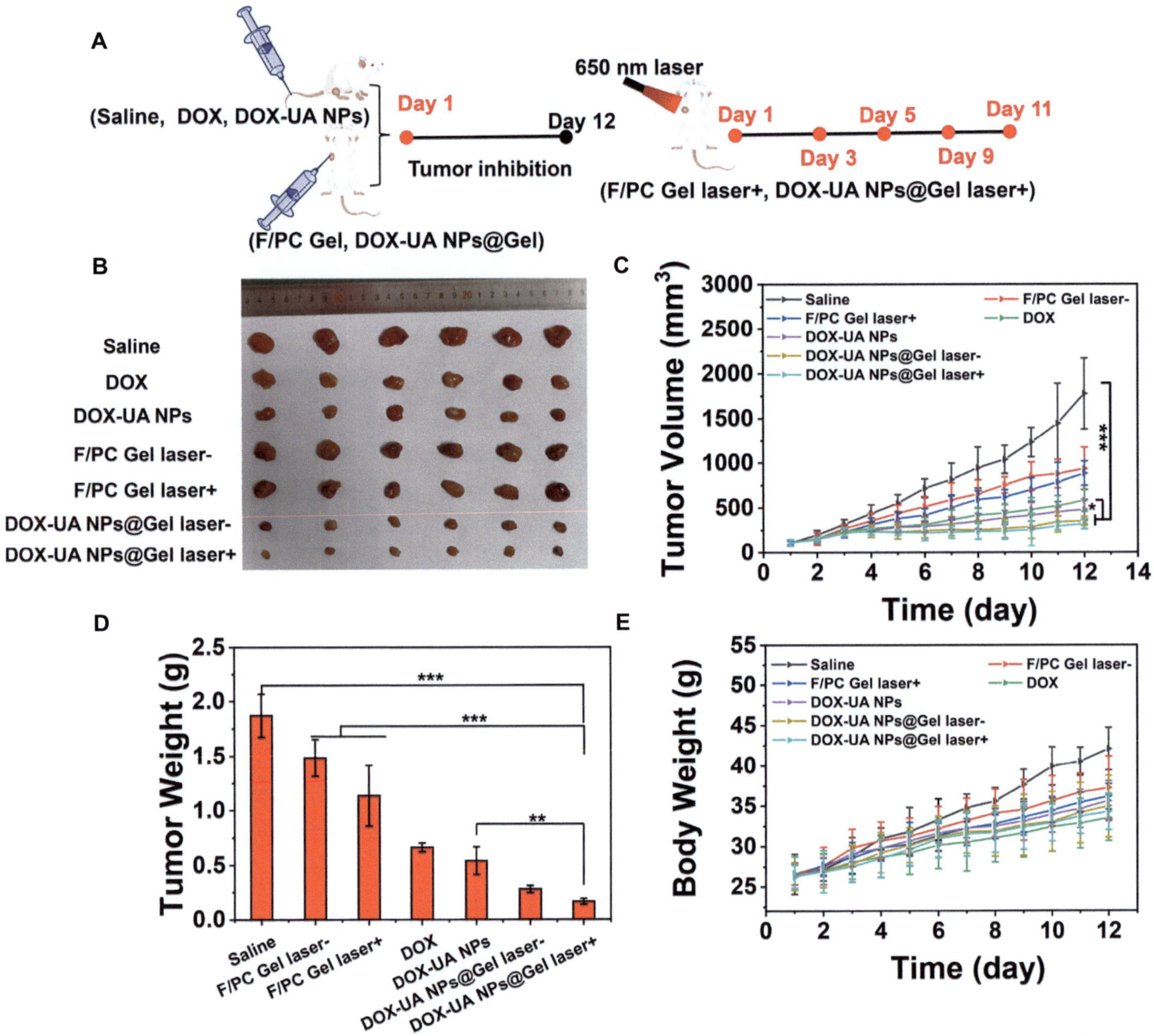

FIGURE 14.15 Schematic illustration of an *in vivo* experiment about tumor inhibition (A). Tumor mass images after 12 days of treatment (B). Tumor volume changes during treatment with various formulations for 12 days (C). The mean tumor weight at the end of the experiment (D). The weight change of mice over 12 days (E). *DOX*, Doxorubicin; *F*, Pluronic F127; *NP*, nanoparticle; *PC*, phycocyanin; *UA*, ursolic acid. *From Song, J., et al.,* Thermo-sensitive nanoparticle-hydrogel composite based on Pluronic F127 and phycocyanin for an enhanced chemo-photodynamic anti-tumor effect. *ACS Appl. Polym. Mater, 2023. 5(8): p. 6244-6254. Copyright (2023), American Chemical Society.*

ultrasound-responsive delivery systems. Nanobubble, micelles, and liposome-based novel systems have also been developed [43,44]. Ping Wei *et al.* developed ultrasound/pH-responsive polymersomes for cancer therapy. The polymersomes were prepared through self-assembly of poly(ethylene oxide)-*block*-poly(2-(diethylamino)ethyl methacrylate)-*stat*-poly(methoxyethyl methacrylate) [PEO-*b*-P(DEA-*stat*-MEMA)] where MEMA acted as the ultrasound-responsive segment [45]. It has been reported that the intrinsic ultrasound responsiveness of the nanoplatforms based on poly(ethylene oxide)-*b*-polymethacrylates block copolymer originates from their metastable states; both self-assembly temperature (T_s) and solvents for the self-assembly are two main regulating factors. And the higher the sonication temperature (T_u), the faster is the responsive rate [46].

High-intensity exogenous electric fields have the ability to directly affect the permeability of cellular membranes. Moreover, the electric field can trigger the drug release from electrically conductive polymers (e.g., polypyrrole

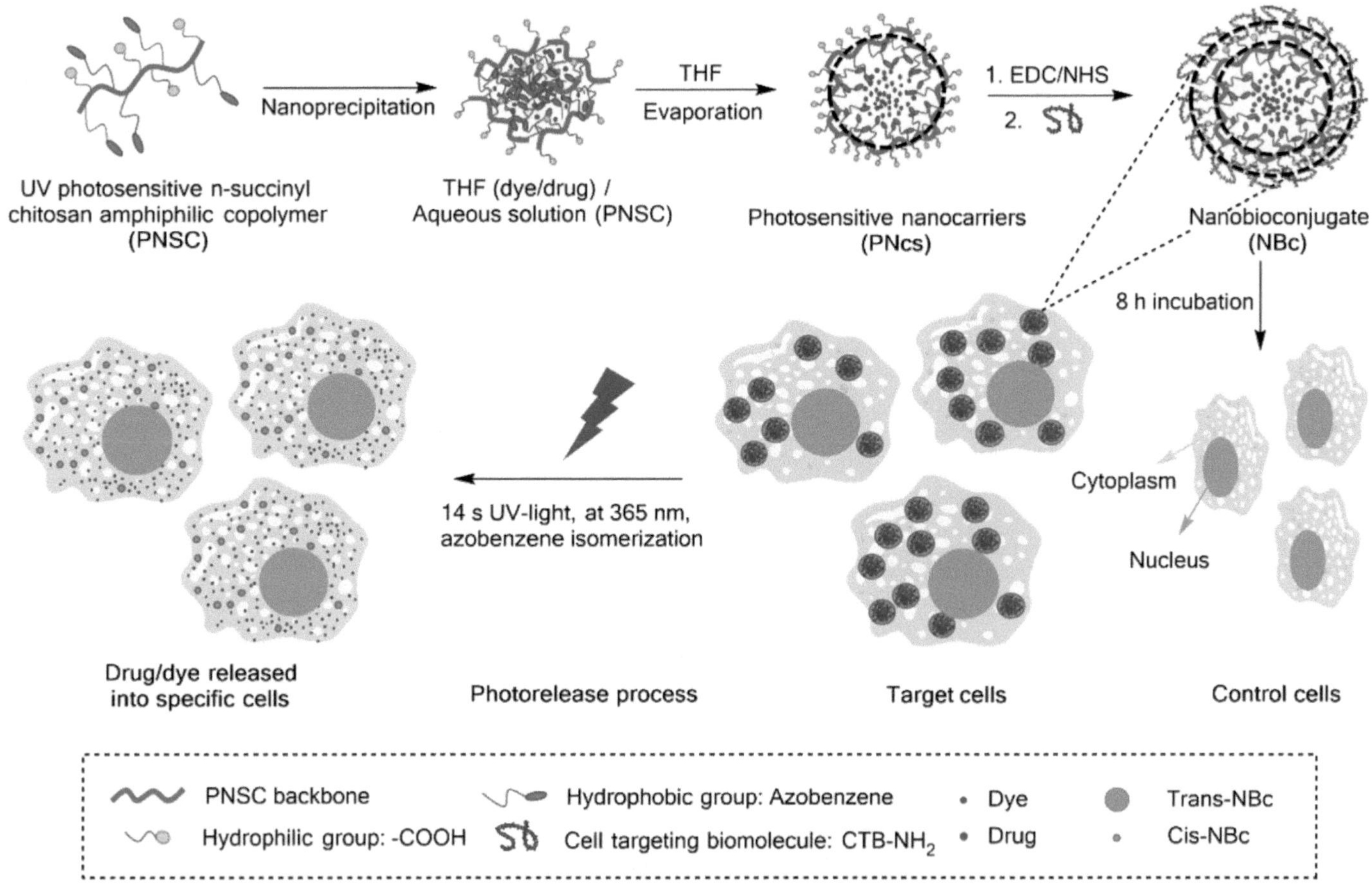

FIGURE 14.16 Schematic illustration of PNc synthesis, nanocarrier self-assembly, cargo co-encapsulation, and further functionalization with the CTB. Selective internalization of the resultant NBc and UV-light induced cargo release into cardiomyocytes by an isomerization process of the azobenzene photosensitive molecule-containing PNc. *CTB,* Cell-targeting biomolecule; *EDC/NHS,* 1-ethyl-3-(3- dimethylaminopropyl)carbodiimide/*N*-hydroxysuccinimide; *THF,* tetrahydrofuran. *From Mena-Giraldo, P., et al.,* Photosensitive nanocarriers for specific delivery of cargo into cells. *Sci. Rep, 2020.* ***10****(1): p. 2110.*

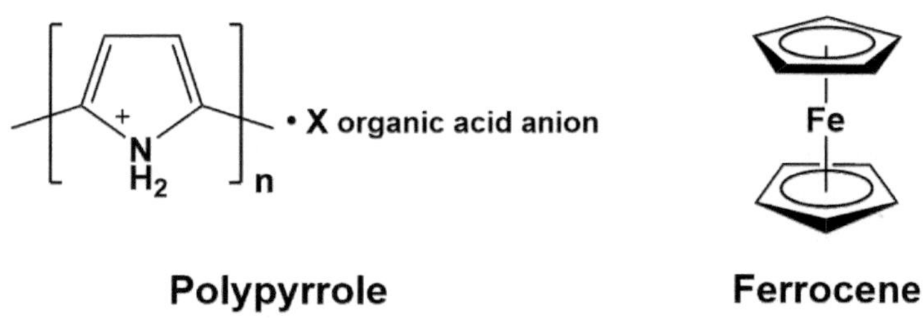

FIGURE 14.17 Chemical structure of polypyrrole and ferrocene.

(Fig. 14.17) and polyaniline), polymer composites, or fillers (e.g., carbon nanotubes) [3]. Novel electro-responsive systems including colloidal systems have been developed, such as micelles based on Pluronic F127 and D-α-tocopherol polyethylene glycol succinate (TPGS) conjugated with an electro-sensitive group ferrocene (change of hydrophobic Fc to hydrophilic Fc^{+} upon the application of current; Fig. 14.17) [47].

Magnetic-responsive drug delivery systems usually are composed of assembled paramagnetic and superparamagnetic nanoparticles, such as iron oxide, graphene hydrides, and zinc ferrite. These magnetic nanoparticles are commonly modified/encapsulated using polymers or lipids to improve their stability and cellular uptake. Moreover, superparamagnetic iron oxide nanoparticles have also been widely used as magnetic resonance imaging (MRI) contrast agents for diagnosis. When it comes to drug release, magnetic field–induced hyperthermia is commonly used [3,10,21]. For example, Guru Karthikeyan Thirunavukkarasu *et al.* encapsulated iron oxide

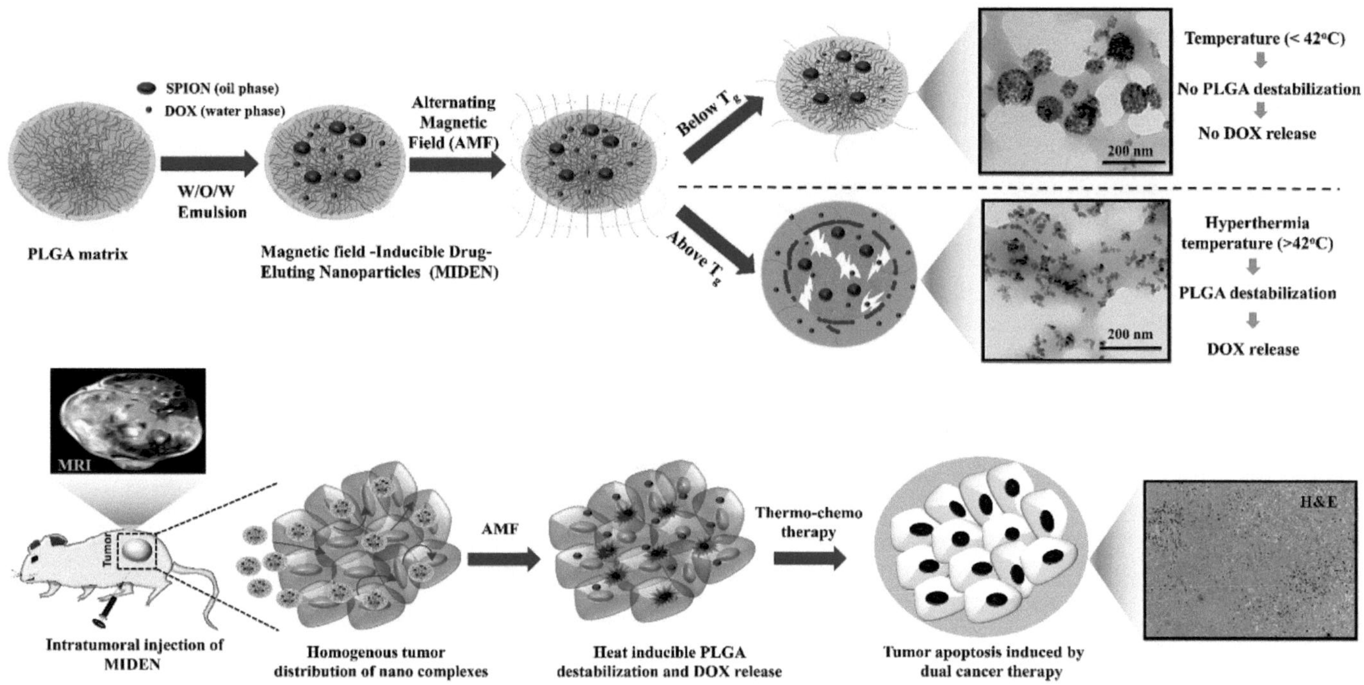

FIGURE 14.18 Schematic illustration showing the formation of magnetic field inducible drug-eluting nanoparticles and their application in image-guided thermochemotherapy. *DOX,* Doxorubicin; *PLGA,* poly(lactic-*co*-glycolic acid); T_g, glass transition temperature; *SPION,* superparamagnetic iron oxide nanoparticles; *W/O/W,* water-in-oil-in-water. *From Thirunavukkarasu, G.K., et al.,* Magnetic field-inducible drug-eluting nanoparticles for image-guided thermo-chemotherapy. *Biomat. J, 2018.* ***180****: p. 240-252, with permission from Elsevier.*

nanoparticles and doxorubicin in a temperature-responsive poly(lactic-*co*-glycolic acid) (PLGA) nanomatrix, and an external alternating magnetic field was used to generate heat above 42°C to change the PLGA matrix from glassy to rubbery state, releasing doxorubicin (Fig. 14.18) [48].

14.6 Design of stimuli-responsive drug delivery systems

When designing a stimuli-responsive drug delivery system, the delivery route should be considered first. For systemic delivery, targeting should be considered to increase the therapeutic efficacy while reducing the toxicity. Certain stimuli, such as magnetic fields, can also be used for targeting. More than one stimulus can be used. However, the manufacturing ability and cost should also be taken into consideration. Comparing external with internal stimuli, external stimuli-responsive systems must be exposed to an exogenously applied force, which poses various challenges such as compliance and penetration. The unique advantage of applying external stimuli is the drug release can be easily switched "on" or "off" [21]. Computer-aided approaches can also be utilized in designing stimuli-responsive systems [3]. Overall, stimuli-responsive drug delivery systems exhibit great promise; however, there are still a few challenges—stability (e.g., premature release of drug during storage) and heterogeneity of cell/tissue environments (variations in stimuli responsiveness) [21].

Case Study VI: ThermoDox: ups and downs

Lyso-thermosensitive liposomal doxorubicin (LTLD, ThermoDox), developed at Duke University, is the first heat-activated formulation of a liposomal drug carrier to be utilized in human clinical trials [49]. It was the lead program of Celsion (now Imunon)—a fully integrated oncology company focused on developing a portfolio of innovative cancer treatments [50]. The three design features of LTLD are the high drug-loading liposomal carrier,

Case Study VI: ThermoDox: ups and downs (*cont'd*)

long-enough circulation half-life, and thermal-responsive drug release (mild thermal warming - > 39.5°C) [49]. ThermoDox is composed of a lysolipid component (1-stearoyl-2-hydroxy-sn-glycero-3-phosphatidylcholine), 1,2-dipalmitoyl-*sn*-glycero-3-phosphocholine (DPPC), and *N*-(carbonyl-methoxypolyethyleneglycol2000)-1,2-distearoyl-*sn*-glycero-3-phosphoethanolamine (mPEG2000-DSPE) (Fig. CS 14.1) [51].

The first patient received the ThermoDox combined with the interventional oncology technique radiofrequency ablation (RFA), for the treatment of hepatocellular carcinoma, in 2005. And then it progressed to a phase III clinical trial (i.e., the "HEAT" trial) but failed to meet its endpoint for progression-free survival. Based on some of the promising findings from the HEAT trial, a new phase III trial (i.e., OPTIMA trial) started in 2014, which mandated a standardized heating protocol—a minimal RFA dwell time of 45 min [52]. The company announced the discontinuation of following patients and stated that "A single disappointing study does not mean an end to the future of ThermoDox" [53]. Moreover, the clinical study "PanDox: Targeted Doxorubicin in Pancreatic Tumors" was withdrawn due to the lack of recruitment [54]. Despite the setbacks, thermosensitive liposomes (TSLs) are still believed to be an effective component of cancer therapy [52]. For example, a clinical study, "A Pilot Study of ThermoDox and MR-HIFU for Treatment of Relapsed Solid Tumors," is currently recruiting. In this study, "Magnetic Resonance-Guided High Intensity Focused Ultrasound (MR-HIFU)" is for triggering doxorubicin release [55].

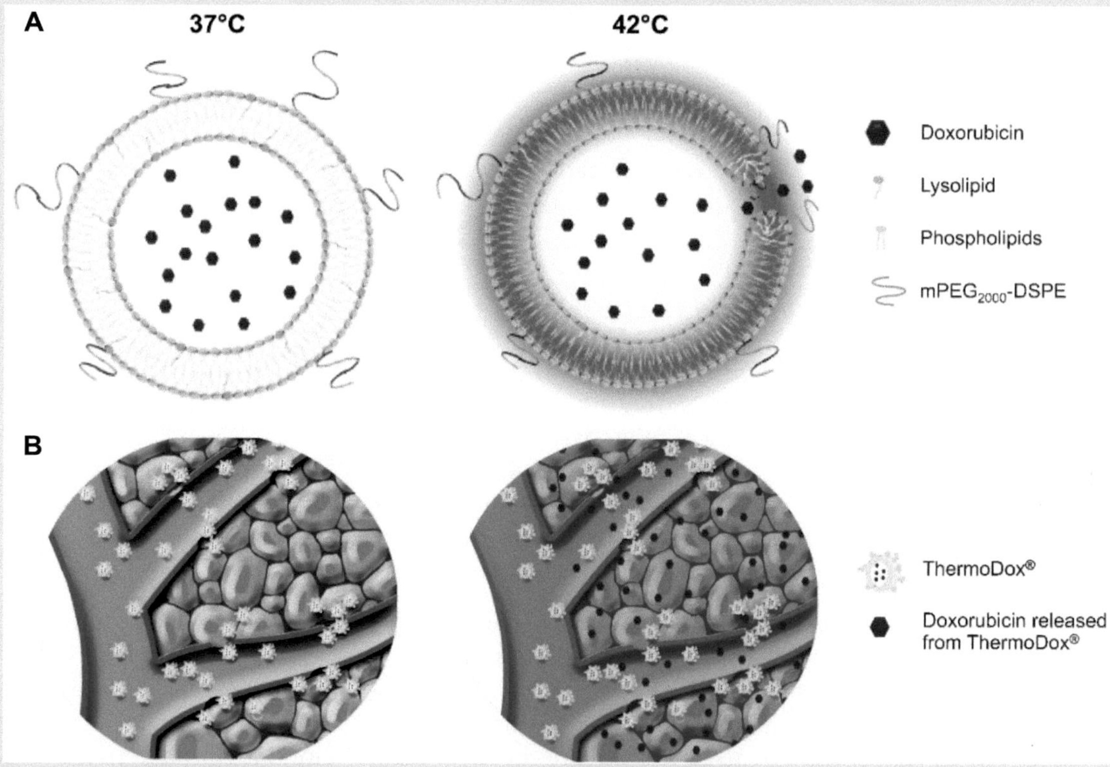

FIGURE CS 14.1 ThermoDox formulation and intravascular release. (A) Heating to the phase transition temperature of the lipid mixture that comprises the ThermoDox formulation (i.e., ~ 42°C) results in the formation of nanopores and an increase in lipid membrane permeability, yielding a burst release of the encapsulated agent. (B) Intravascular release of doxorubicin from ThermoDox is then followed by interstitial penetration of the free drug (doxorubicin). *From Dou, Y., K. Hynynen, and C. Allen,* To heat or not to heat: challenges with clinical translation of thermosensitive liposomes. *JCR, 2017.* ***249****: p. 63-73, with permission from Elsevier.*

Lab Activity VIII: Stimuli-responsive drug carriers

Stimuli-responsive micro/nanocarriers have been widely used in controlled/targeted drug delivery. The objectives of this experiment are to:

(1) Design the protocol for studying the stimuli-responsive microencapsulated drug release profiles.

(2) Understand how to calculate drug loading efficiency.
(3) Understand the importance of stimuli-responsive drug delivery systems from engineering and physiological views.

Background

Both alginate and pectin have been commonly used to design stimuli-responsive drug micro/nanocarriers, hydrogel systems in particular. Both alginate and pectin can be crosslinked to form hydrogels through their carboxyl groups using divalent cations (e.g., Ca^{2+}) and oligochitosan. The pH-responsiveness of the alginate/pectin hydrogels, stable at low pH conditions, is due to the protonation/deprotonation of the carboxyl groups [56–62]. Pectin-based systems can also be used to design enzyme-responsive systems due to the enzymatic activity of the colon [58,59].

Materials and Instruments

Sodium alginate solution (low viscosity; 2% (w/v)
LM pectin solution (3% w/v)
150 mmol/L $CaCl_2$ solution
Pepsin
Trypsin
Fluorescein isothiocyanate-dextran (FITC-dextran or other drug models)
Sodium chloride
Concentrated hydrochloric acid
Monobasic potassium phosphate
Sodium hydroxide
Encapsulator (or other setups)
UV spectrophotometer/plate reader
Digital microscope

Laboratory Procedure

I. *Prepare Simulated Gastric Fluid and Intestinal Fluid* [58]

1. Simulated gastric fluid: Dissolve 2 g sodium chloride and 3.2 g purified pepsin in sufficient DI water containing 7.0 mL of concentrated hydrochloric acid and make the final volume of 1000 mL (scale up or down as needed).
2. Simulated intestinal fluid: Dissolve 6.8 g of monobasic potassium phosphate in 250 mL of water, mix, and add 77 mL of 0.2 mol/L sodium hydroxide and 500 mL of water. Add 10 g of trypsin, mix, and adjust the resulting solution with either 0.2 mol/L sodium hydroxide or 0.2 mol/L hydrochloric acid to a pH of 6.8 ± 0.1. Dilute with DI water to 1000 mL (scale up or down as needed).

II. *Prepare Standard Curves of FITC-Dextran*

1. Prepared standard solutions of different concentrations.
   Note: The concentration range used to generate the standard curves should be determined first.
   Q1: What solutions should be used to make the standard curves of FITC-dextran?
2. Using the UV spectrophotometer or plate reader, measure the absorbance/fluorescence intensity of different FITC-dextran solutions. Record the results in Table LVIII.1.
   Q2: What wavelength should be used to measure the absorbance? How do you determine this?

TABLE LVIII.1 Absorbance/fluorescence intensity of FITC-dextran.

	Absorbance/fluorescence intensity		
Concentration	$CaCl_2$	Gastric	Intestinal

3. Make plots of concentration vs. absorbance/fluorescence intensity. Determine the slope, intercept, and R^2 value.

III. *Determination of Encapsulation Efficiency*

1. FITC-dextran encapsulation.

Note: Measure a certain amount of FITC-dextran for encapsulation and dissolve in the alginate or pectin solution (avoid vigorous mixing). Record the volume of the mixture (FITC-dextran in alginate or pectin) used during the encapsulation process (e.g., final FITC-dextran concentration of 1 mg/mL).

2. Quickly collect the microcapsules prepared. Determine the FITC-dextran absorbance/fluorescence intensity of the supernatant.

3. Use the standard curve (FITC-dextran in $CaCl_2$ solution) and the FITC-dextran fluorescence intensity of the supernatant to determine the amount of the unencapsulated (i.e., $Amount_{Unencapsulated} = Concentration_{FITC-Dextran\ of\ the\ supernatant} \times Volume_{CaCl_2\ solution\ used\ for\ encapsulation}$). Encapsulation efficiency can be calculated based on the equation:

$$Encapsulation\ efficiency = \frac{Amount_{Total} - Amount_{Unencapsulated}}{Amount_{Total}} \times 100\%,$$

where

$Amount_{Total} = Concentration_{FITC-Dextran\ of\ the\ mixture} \times Volume_{Mixture\ used\ for\ encapsulation}$ and the mixture refers to the FITC-dextran in alginate or pectin (step III.1).

IV. *Extended Encapsulated Drug Release Studies*

1. Divide the encapsulated FITC-dextran into different groups (based on the different kinds of release media and the number of lab teams).

2. Introduce the encapsulated FITC-dextran into different release media (i.e., stimulated gastric and intestinal fluids).

3. Place the suspension on a shaker (or manually shake gently and periodically). Monitor the absorbance/fluorescence intensity change of the supernatant at varying times. Record the data (Table LVIII.2), as well as the morphological changes of the microcapsule.

TABLE LVIII.2 Absorbance/fluorescence intensity of FITC-dextran concentration of supernatant at varying times.

Time (min)	Absorbance/fluorescence intensity	
	Gastric	Intestinal

4. (Optional) Percent of drug release (%R) can be calculated based on the equation:

$$\%R = \frac{Amount_{Released}}{Amount_{Total}} \times 100\%,$$

where

$$Amount_{Released} = Concentration_{FITC-Dextran\ of\ the\ release\ medium} \times Volume_{release\ medium} \text{ and } Amount_{Total}$$
$$= total\ amount\ of\ FITC - Dextran\ used\ for\ encapsulation \times \%\ of\ total\ encapsulated\ FITC - Dextran\ used\ in\ the\ release\ medium \times encapsulation\ efficiency.$$

Review and practice questions

1. What are commonly used internal stimuli?
2. What are commonly used external stimuli?
3. Provide an example of pH-responsive drug delivery systems.
4. Provide three examples of pH-responsive chemical bonds and their hydrolysates.
5. Provide an example of redox-responsive drug delivery systems.
6. Provide three examples of ROS-responsive chemical bonds/groups.
7. Provide an example of enzyme-responsive drug delivery systems.
8. Conduct a literature search and provide an example of hypoxia-responsive drug delivery systems.
9. Conduct a literature search and provide an example of glucose-responsive drug delivery systems.
10. Conduct a literature search and provide an example of ATP-responsive drug delivery systems.
11. Provide an example of external stimuli-responsive drug delivery systems.
12. Describe the temperature-induced gelation mechanism for Pluronic F127.
13. What are some of the general considerations when designing a stimuli-responsive drug delivery system?
14. What are the advantage(s) and disadvantage(s) of using external stimuli?
15. What are some of the challenges of utilizing stimuli-responsive drug delivery systems?

References

[1] Raza A, et al. Endogenous and exogenous stimuli-responsive drug delivery systems for programmed site-specific release. Molecules 2019;24(6):1117.
[2] Sun T, Jiang C. Stimuli-responsive drug delivery systems triggered by intracellular or subcellular microenvironments. Adv Drug Deliv Rev 2023;196:114773.
[3] Sun L, et al. Smart nanoparticles for cancer therapy. Signal Transduct Target Ther 2023;8(1):418.
[4] Yu J, et al. Stimuli-responsive delivery of therapeutics for diabetes treatment. Bioeng Transl Med 2016;1(3):323–37.
[5] Mu Y, et al. Advances in pH-responsive drug delivery systems. OpenNano 2021;5:100031.
[6] Gao W, Chan JM, Farokhzad OC. pH-responsive nanoparticles for drug delivery. Mol Pharm 2010;7(6):1913–20.
[7] Hao G, Xu ZP, Li L. Manipulating extracellular tumour pH: an effective target for cancer therapy. RSC Adv 2018;8(39):22182–92.
[8] Shinn J, et al. Smart pH-responsive nanomedicines for disease therapy. J Pharm Investig 2022;52(4):427–41.
[9] Ding H, et al. Preparation and application of pH-responsive drug delivery systems. J Control Release 2022;348:206–38.
[10] Singh A, Amiji M. Stimuli-responsive materials as intelligent drug delivery systems. Available from: https://www.sigmaaldrich.com/US/en/technical-documents/technical-article/materials-science-and-engineering/drug-delivery/stimuli-responsive-materials.
[11] Singh J, Nayak P. pH-responsive polymers for drug delivery: trends and opportunities. J Polym Sci 2023;61(22):2828–50.
[12] Bami MS, et al. pH-responsive drug delivery systems as intelligent carriers for targeted drug therapy: Brief history, properties, synthesis, mechanism and application. J Drug Deliv Sci Technol 2022;70:102987.
[13] Zhang H, et al. pH-sensitive O-carboxymethyl chitosan/sodium alginate nanohydrogel for enhanced oral delivery of insulin. Int J Biol Macromol 2022;223:433–45.
[14] Zhu H, et al. pH-responsive nanoparticles for delivery of paclitaxel to the injury site for inhibiting vascular restenosis. Pharmaceutics 2022;14(3):535.
[15] He W, et al. Preferential targeting cerebral ischemic lesions with cancer cell-inspired nanovehicle for ischemic stroke treatment. Nano Lett 2021;21(7):3033–43.
[16] Mollazadeh S, Mackiewicz M, Yazdimamaghani M. Recent advances in the redox-responsive drug delivery nanoplatforms: a chemical structure and physical property perspective. Mater Sci Eng C 2021;118:111536.
[17] Tao W, He Z. ROS-responsive drug delivery systems for biomedical applications. Asian J Pharm Sci 2018;13(2):101–12.
[18] Liang J, Liu B. ROS-responsive drug delivery systems. Bioeng Transl Med 2016;1(3):239–51.
[19] Jiang S, et al. Oxidation of protein disulfide bonds by singlet oxygen gives rise to glutathionylated proteins. Redox Biol 2021;38:101822.
[20] Vašková J, et al. Glutathione-related enzymes and proteins: a review. Molecules 2023;28(3):1447.
[21] Hughes KA, et al. Use of stimulatory responsive soft nanoparticles for intracellular drug delivery. Nano Res 2023;16(5):6974–90.
[22] Zhao Z, et al. Endocytosis-independent and cancer-selective cytosolic protein delivery via reversible tagging with LAT1 substrate. Adv Mater 2022;34(35):e2110560.
[23] Mariya GA, et al. Fabrication of chitosan-based redox-responsive polymeric nanoparticles: In-vitro and in-vivo evaluation for treating airway inflammation in asthma. J Drug Deliv Sci Technol 2023;84:104473.
[24] Liu Y, et al. Shell-crosslinked micelles with neighborhood effect and pH/GSH sensitivity for co-loading of protein and polyphenol drugs. Colloids Surf A 2023;679:132512.
[25] Shahriari M, et al. Enzyme responsive drug delivery systems in cancer treatment. J Control Release 2019;308:172–89.
[26] Dou Y, et al. Bioresponsive drug delivery systems for the treatment of inflammatory diseases. J Control Release 2020;327:641–66.
[27] Colilla M, Vallet-Regí M. Targeted stimuli-responsive mesoporous silica nanoparticles for bacterial infection treatment. Int J Mol Sci 2020;21(22):8605.
[28] Peng J, et al. Tumor microenvironment responsive drug-dye-peptide nanoassembly for enhanced tumor-targeting, penetration, and photo-chemo-immunotherapy. Adv Funct Mater 2019;29(19):1900004.

[29] Rao J, Khan A. Enzyme sensitive synthetic polymer micelles based on the azobenzene motif. J Am Chem Soc 2013;135(38):14056–9.
[30] Mohammed M, et al. Enzyme-responsive biomimetic solid lipid nanoparticles for antibiotic delivery against hyaluronidase-secreting bacteria. Int J Pharm 2023;640:122967.
[31] Mura S, Nicolas J, Couvreur P. Stimuli-responsive nanocarriers for drug delivery. Nat Mater 2013;12(11):991–1003.
[32] Zhang K, Xue K, Loh XJ. Thermo-responsive hydrogels: from recent progress to biomedical applications. Gels 2021;7(3):77.
[33] Xu X, et al. Poly(N-isopropylacrylamide)-based thermoresponsive composite hydrogels for biomedical applications. Polymers 2020;12(3):580.
[34] Naharros-Molinero A, et al. Direct and reverse pluronic micelles: design and characterization of promising drug delivery nanosystems. Pharmaceutics 2022;14(12):2628.
[35] Yap L-S, Yang M-C. Thermo-reversible injectable hydrogel composing of pluronic F127 and carboxymethyl hexanoyl chitosan for cell-encapsulation. Colloids Surf B Biointerfaces 2020;185:110606.
[36] Lupu A, et al. Self-healing of Pluronic; F127 hydrogels in the presence of various polysaccharides. Gels 2023;9(9):719.
[37] Zhang W, et al. Synthesis and characterization of thermally responsive Pluronic F127–chitosan nanocapsules for controlled release and intracellular delivery of small molecules. ACS Nano 2010;4(11):6747–59.
[38] Song J, et al. Thermo-sensitive nanoparticle-hydrogel composite based on Pluronic F127 and phycocyanin for an enhanced chemo-photodynamic antitumor effect. ACS Appl Polym Mater 2023;5(8):6244–54.
[39] Epp-Ducharme B, et al. Heat-activated nanomedicine formulation improves the anticancer potential of the HSP90 inhibitor luminespib in vitro. Sci Rep 2021;11(1):11103.
[40] Abdelmohsen HAM, Copeland NA, Hardy JG. Light-responsive biomaterials for ocular drug delivery. Drug Deliv Transl Res 2023;13(8): 2159–82.
[41] Mena-Giraldo P, et al. Photosensitive nanocarriers for specific delivery of cargo into cells. Sci Rep 2020;10(1):2110.
[42] Delaney LJ, et al. Making waves: how ultrasound-targeted drug delivery is changing pharmaceutical approaches. Mater Adv 2022;3(7): 3023–40.
[43] Cai X, et al. Ultrasound-responsive materials for drug/gene delivery. Front Pharmacol 2020;10:1650.
[44] Wei P, Cornel EJ, Du J. Ultrasound-responsive polymer-based drug delivery systems. Drug Deliv Transl Res 2021;11(4):1323–39.
[45] Wei P, et al. Ultrasound-responsive polymersomes capable of endosomal escape for efficient cancer therapy. J Control Release 2020;322:81–94.
[46] Yang B, Du J. On the origin and regulation of ultrasound responsiveness of block copolymer nanoparticles. Sci China Chem 2020;63(2): 272–81.
[47] Meng X-y, et al. Electro-responsive brain-targeting mixed micelles based on Pluronic F127 and d-α-tocopherol polyethylene glycol succinate–ferrocene. Colloids Surf A 2020;601:124986.
[48] Thirunavukkarasu GK, et al. Magnetic field-inducible drug-eluting nanoparticles for image-guided thermo-chemotherapy. Biomaterials 2018;180:240–52.
[49] Borys N, Dewhirst MW. Drug development of lyso-thermosensitive liposomal doxorubicin: Combining hyperthermia and thermosensitive drug delivery. Adv Drug Deliv Rev 2021;178:113985.
[50] Imunon. Celsion corporation announces issuance of new patent for ThermoDox®. Available from: https://investor.celsion.com/news-releases/news-release-details/celsion-corporation-announces-issuance-new-patent-thermodoxr.
[51] Dou Y, Hynynen K, Allen C. To heat or not to heat: challenges with clinical translation of thermosensitive liposomes. J Control Release 2017; 249:63–73.
[52] Regenold M, et al. Turning down the heat: the case for mild hyperthermia and thermosensitive liposomes. Nanomedicine 2022;40:102484.
[53] Imunon. Celsion corporation issues letter to stockholders. Available from: https://investor.celsion.com/news-releases/news-release-details/celsion-corporation-issues-letter-stockholders-0.
[54] https://classic.clinicaltrials.gov/ct2/show/NCT04852367?term=ThermoDox&draw=2&rank=4.
[55] https://classic.clinicaltrials.gov/ct2/show/NCT04791228?term=ThermoDox&draw=2&rank=7.
[56] Chai A, et al. Design of pectin-based hydrogel microspheres for targeted pulmonary delivery. Gels 2023;9(9):707.
[57] Zieman J, et al. Development of gelatin-coated hydrogel microspheres for novel bioink design: a crosslinker study. Pharmaceutics 2023;15(1): 90.
[58] Stealey S, et al. Calcium-oligochitosan-pectin microcarrier for colonic drug delivery. Pharm Dev Technol 2020;25(2):260–5.
[59] Zhang W, et al. Novel pectin-based carriers for colonic drug delivery. Pharm Dev Technol 2016;21(1):127–30.
[60] Zhang W, et al. Design of artificial red blood cells using polymeric hydrogel microcapsules: hydrogel stability improvement and polymer selection. Int J Artif Organs 2016;39(10):518–23.
[61] Das S. Pectin based multi-particulate carriers for colon-specific delivery of therapeutic agents. Int J Pharm 2021;605:120814.
[62] Abka-Khajouei R, et al. Structures, properties and applications of alginates. Mar Drugs 2022;20(6):364.

CHAPTER

15

Other drug delivery systems

Wujie Zhang

LEARNING OBJECTIVES

- To understand and interpret the mucoadhesive theories
- To understand and interpret different nebulization (soft mist formation) methods
- To differentiate different types of microrobots and discuss the design considerations of microrobots-based drug delivery systems
- To discuss different approaches of using cells as therapies, especially CAR-T therapy
- To explain the benefits of wireless on-demand drug delivery systems and the application of three-dimensional printing in drug delivery
- To discuss how artificial intelligence can transform the pharmaceutical industry, especially from drug delivery aspects

15.1 Mucoadhesive drug delivery systems

Mucoadhesion is commonly defined as the adhesion between two materials, at least one of which is a mucosal surface [1]. The mucous membranes (mucosae) are linings of mostly endodermal origin, covered in various types of epithelium, that are involved in absorption and secretion. Most mucous membranes secrete a sticky, thick fluid called mucus (secreted by goblet cells or specialized glands), which facilitates several barrier immune system functions and provides a moist environment for internal and semi-internal structures. The mucin glycoproteins are the most important structure-forming component of the mucus gel [2,3]. There are multiple mucoadhesion theories, which are summarized in Table 15.1. Generally, two steps in the adhesive process have been identified: contact (or wetting; correlated to wetting, electronic, adsorption, and mechanical theories) stage and consolidation stage (various physicochemical interactions occur to consolidate and strengthen the adhesive joint and involve the diffusion theory) (Fig. 15.1) [3,4].

The theory of mucoadhesion was introduced in the controlled drug delivery field in the early 1980s [5]. It is an effective approach to increase the residence time and hence the effectiveness of the drug delivery system [6]. Mucoadhesive drug delivery systems are intended for interacting and binding to the mucosal layer of the epithelium for localized, prolonged, and/or targeted drug delivery [7]. Polymeric systems are most commonly used for

Fundamentals and Design of Drug Delivery Systems
https://doi.org/10.1016/B978-0-443-23521-4.00015-1

TABLE 15.1 Mucoadhesion theories.

Theory	Mechanism
Wetting	It is primarily applied to liquid systems and involves the ability of a liquid to spread spontaneously onto a surface as a prerequisite for the development of adhesion. The contact angle can be used to indicate the affinity of a liquid for a surface.
Electronic	Electron transfer occurs across the adhesive interface and adhering surface forming an electrical double layer.
Diffusion	It describes that polymer chains from the bioadhesive interpenetrate into glycoprotein mucin chains and reach a sufficient depth within the opposite matrix to allow the formation of a semipermanent bond. The process is affected by chain lengths and mobilities.
Adsorption	It describes the surface forces acting between the chemical structures of the two surfaces, such as H-bonding, hydrophobic interactions, and van der Waals forces.
Fracture	It relates the adhesive strength to the forces required to separate the two involved surfaces after adhesion.
Mechanical	It considers adhesion due to the filling of irregularities, increasing the interfacial area available for interaction on a rough surface by a mucoadhesive liquid.

Data from several sources [3–5,7,8].

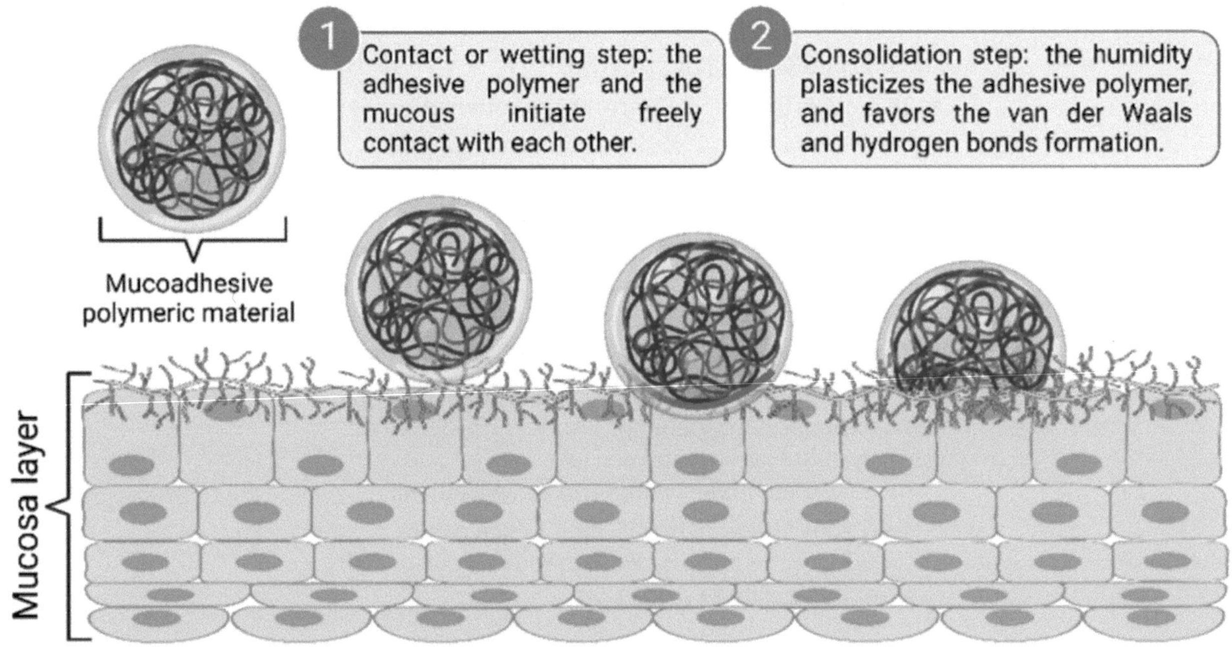

FIGURE 15.1 The mucoadhesive process—formation of mucoadhesive forces. *From de Lima, C.S.A., et al.,* Mucoadhesive polymers and their applications in drug delivery systems for the treatment of bladder cancer. *Gels, 2022. 8(9): p. 587; the original image was created with BioRender.com.*

designing mucoadhesion drug delivery systems. The properties that can affect the polymer/mucus adhesion include hydrophilicity, molecular weight, polymer chain length, viscosity, degree of crosslinking, spatial conformation, flexibility of the polymer chain, and charge/degree of ionization [1,5]. Examples of polymers used for mucoadhesive drug delivery are poly(acrylic acid), cellulose derivatives, chitosan, lectins, hyaluronic acid, gellan gum, alginate, pectin, starch, gelatin, poly(ethylene glycol), and poly(vinyl alcohol).

Lectins are found in various natural sources such as plants, animals, and microbes. They are protein or glycoprotein complexes that can selectively noncovalent bind to sugars due to their carbohydrate recognition domain within the polypeptide structure [9,10]. However, interactions of lectins can be specific to some particular cellular type or a specialized area [5]. The lectins-based mucoadhesive drug delivery systems are mostly specific. Glycoconjugates of different glycosylation patterns are usually expressed by different cell types, which favors distinct cells to interact specifically with different lectins [11]. For example, wheat germ agglutinin (WGA) (Fig. 15.2), a type of lectin, has been widely used for designing drug carriers. WGA binds directly to cell membranes by specifically recognizing *N*-acetylglucosamine and sialic acid residues on cell surfaces. A good example is WGA-liposomes with surface-grafted cyclodextrins as bioadhesive drug delivery nanocarriers (Fig. 15.3). The system showed significantly higher binding compared to the system without WGA (liposome-CD) as short as 1 minute [12].

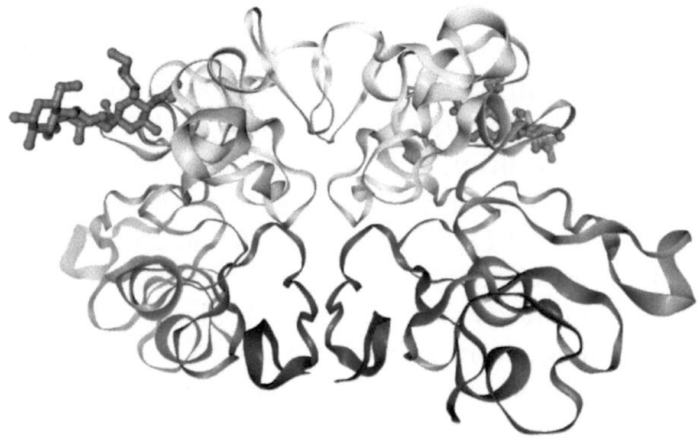

FIGURE 15.2 Structure of *N*-acetylneuraminyl-lactose-wheat germ agglutinin isolectin complexes. *Created with the PDB ID 1SUV and associated publication (Wright C. S. (1990).* 2·2 Å resolution structure analysis of two refined N-acetylneuraminyl-lactose—Wheat germ agglutinin isolectin complexes. *Journal of Molecular Biology, 215 (4), 635-651, https://doi.org/10.1016/S0022-2836(05)80174-3, NGL Viewer (AS Rose et al. (2018)* NGL viewer: web-based molecular graphics for large complexes. *Bioinformatics doi:10.1093/bioinformatics/bty419), and RCSB PDB.*

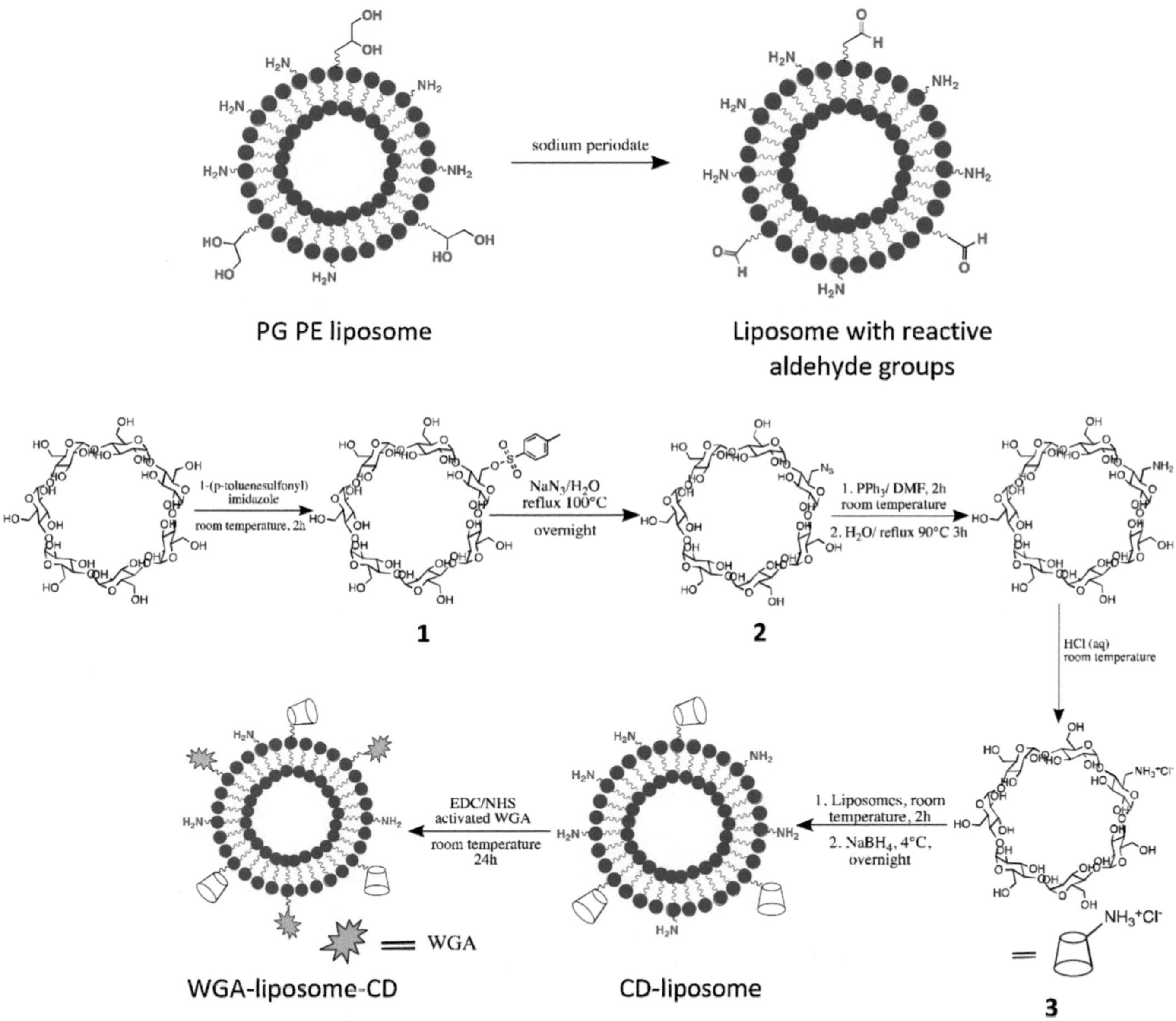

FIGURE 15.3 Synthetic route for the preparation of WGA-liposome-CD nanocarriers. *CD,* Cyclodextrin; *PE,* 1,2-dipalmitoleoyl-*sn*-glycero-3-phosphoethanolamine; *PG,* 1,2-dipalmitoyl-*sn*-glycero-3-phospho-(1′-rac-glycerol) (sodium salt); *WGA,* wheat germ agglutinin. *Adapted from Wijetunge, S.S., et al.,* Wheat germ agglutinin liposomes with surface grafted cyclodextrins as bioadhesive dual-drug delivery nanocarriers to treat oral cells. *Colloids Surf. B Biointerfaces, 2020.* ***185****: p. 110572, with permission from Elsevier.*

Chitosan and derivatives have also been widely used for designing mucoadhesive drug delivery systems. Chitosan, a cationic polymer, exhibits mucoadhesive properties *via* hydrogen and ionic bonds with mucin [7]. Among the derivatives, thiolated chitosan (through the immobilization of the thiol group on the chitosan polymeric chain) is one of the most extensively used and favored mucoadhesive polymers [13]. The primary amino group present in the glucosamine subunit of chitosan is a target for thiolation. The thiolation of chitosan can affect the hydroxy moieties. Different reagents can be used for thiolation—thioglycolic acid, cysteine, 2-iminothiolane (Traut's reagent), 4-mercaptobenzoic acid, and thioethyl amide [13,14]. Thiolated chitosan can interact with mucosal surfaces through the formation of disulfides with cysteine residues of mucins. This covalent bond formation is also responsible for the adhesion of thiolated chitosan to keratinous surfaces, which also displays a high cysteine content of 7% to 20% [14]. A recent study showed that 6-mercaptonicotinic acid (6-MNA) and L-cysteine-*S*—protected thiolated chitosan coatings (CS-Cys-MNA and CS-Cys-Cys) improved the solid lipid nanoparticles' retention on porcine intestinal mucosa by enabling a synergism of efficient mucus diffusion and strong mucoadhesion (Fig. 15.5) [15].

15.2 Micro nozzle technology-based drug delivery systems

Micro nozzle technology has been used for administering both liquid and powder formulations. Take soft mist inhalers for example; they use mechanical power to deliver inhalable drug aerosols in the form of a slow mist to patients. Different mechanisms are involved in soft mist formations (nebulization), such as colliding jets, and Rayleigh jets [16,17]. The colliding jet approach forces an aqueous drug formulation through a uniblock composed of filter structures, inlet and outlet channels, and exit nozzles. During the process, the solution is accelerated and split into two converging jets and the two opposing jets generated collide with each other, at a precisely set angle, creating a soft mist (Fig. 15.6b) [16,18,19]. The Rayleigh jet principle uses Rayleigh breakup theory to produce extruded jets resulting in the formation of a soft mist. This technology generally uses a chip with many uniform nozzles (holes) to mono-disperse droplets with each nozzle generating a Rayleigh jet. The droplet diameter is theoretically 1.95 times the nozzle diameter (Fig. 15.6c) [16,20].

Regarding the recent research progress, Head *et al.* developed lithographically patterned micro nozzles for controlling fluid flow profiles for drug delivery and *in vitro* imaging applications. In the study, micro nozzles were photolithographically integrated onto a microfluidic platform for tuning the fluid flow profile and depth of tissue penetration [21]. Last *et al.* reported a spring-actuated micro swirl nozzle for fast drug delivery to the lung. Swirl nozzles exploit a radial acceleration from a vortex in the outlet nozzle to form a circulating, thin liquid cone, which breaks up into droplets. The design could match propellant-containing inhalers in aerosolization time [22].

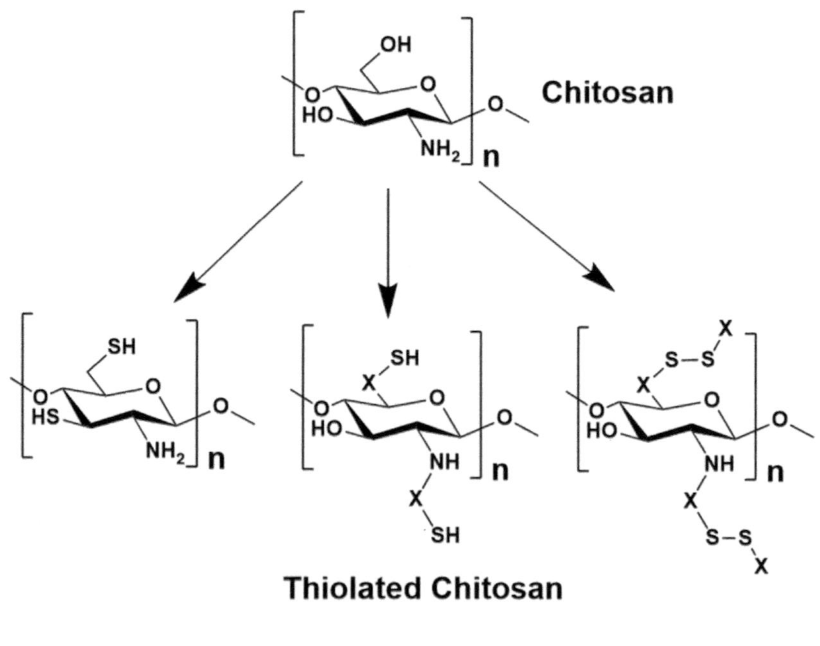

FIGURE 15.4 Structures of chitosan and thiolated chitosan. *Adapted from Federer, C., M. Kurpiers, and A. Bernkop-Schnürch,* Thiolated chitosans: a multi-talented class of polymers for various applications. *Biomacromolecules, 2021.* **22***(1): p. 24-56.*

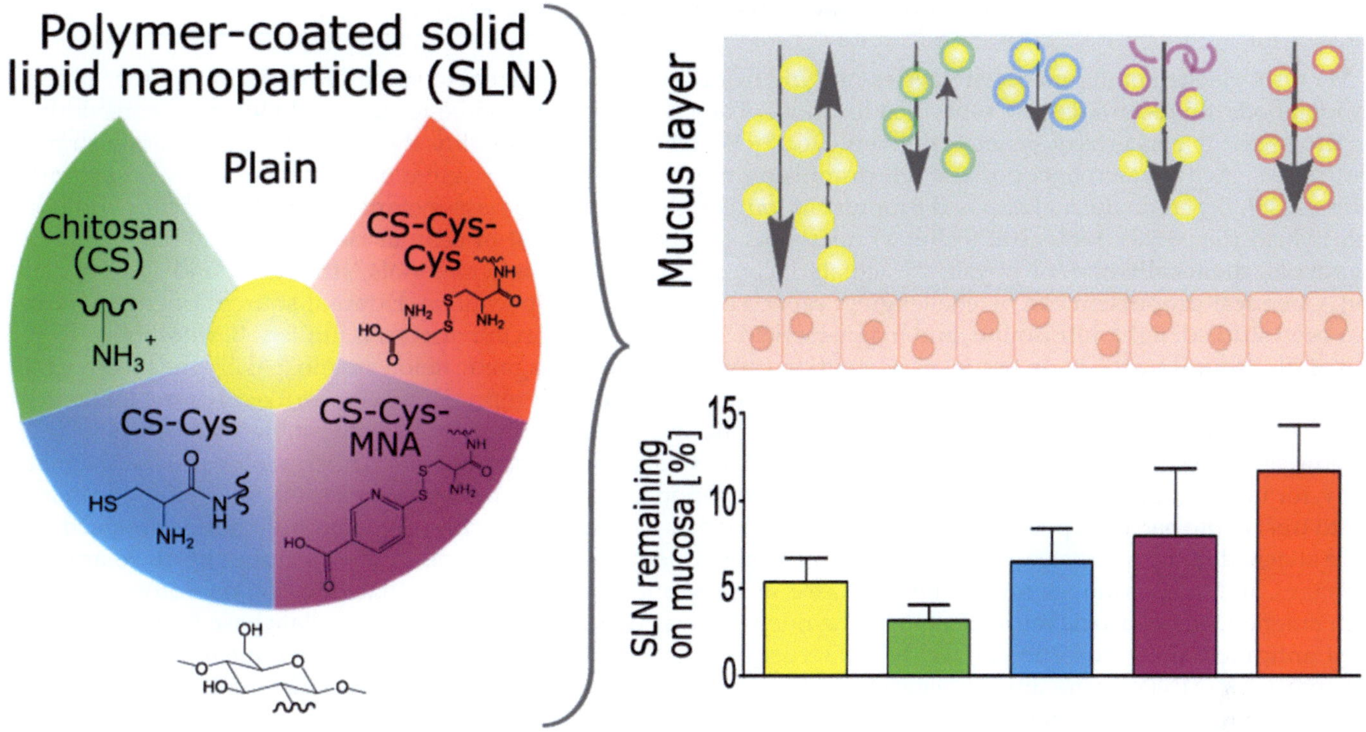

FIGURE 15.5 *In vitro* study of thiolated chitosan derivatives as mucoadhesive coating materials for solid lipid nanoparticles. *Cys*, Cysteine; *MNA*, mercaptonicotinic acid. *Adapted from Wibel, R., et al.,* In vitro investigation of thiolated chitosan derivatives as mucoadhesive coating materials for solid lipid nanoparticles. *Biomacromolecules, 2021.* ***22****(9): p. 3980-3991.*

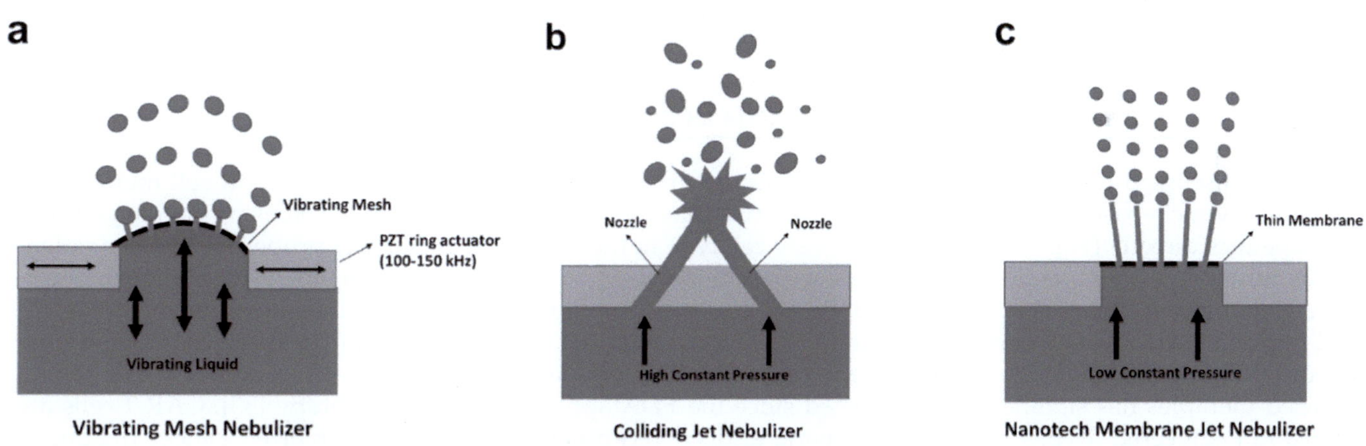

FIGURE 15.6 Different nebulization methods. (a) Vibrating mesh: a flexible mesh mounted on a ring actuator stretches and vibrates, thereby expelling droplets. (b) Colliding jet: two jets collide at a high velocity, herewith creating a Savart sheet that breaks up into small droplets. (c) Nanotech membrane (Rayleigh jet): at low pressure, the fluid is pushed through a thin nanotech membrane with pores, herewith creating a plurality of equally sized jets that subsequently break up in equally sized droplets. *Adapted from van Rijn, C.J.M., et al.,* Low energy nebulization preserves integrity of SARS-CoV-2 mRNA vaccines for respiratory delivery. *Sci Rep, 2023.* ***13****(1): p. 8851.*

A few companies have micro nozzle-based drug delivery systems. Here, let's look at some examples. Zeteo Biomedical LLC's ZTECH-L and ZTECH-P platforms incorporate a patented micro nozzle technology for specified volume and dispense characteristics (Case Study II, Chapter 4) [23]. Medspray owns various patents relating to the spray nozzle unit technology, which are based on plain orifice nozzles for generating Rayleigh jets [24]. Respimat Softmist Inhaler is the most widely used inhaler device. The drug solution is split into two jets that collide at a fixed angle by the nozzle (described at the beginning of this section) through the mechanical energy obtained by spring compression [16,25].

15.3 Microrobots-based drug delivery systems

Microrobots are small functional devices ranging from several nanometers to submillimeters in size that propel through body fluids and tissue to specified locations. They show great potential for targeted therapies, considering the drug toxicity concerns of systemic delivery [26,27]. Based on the functionality, there are active and passive transport robots. Active microbots possess self-propulsion mechanisms, while passive transport ones rely on external sources [28]. Based on the makeup and propulsion sources, there are three classes of microbots: biological, synthetic, and hybrid (Fig. 15.7). Biological (cellular) microbots exclusively consist of cellular components, while synthetic microbots, chemically and/or physically actuated, contain only man-made materials, structures, and components [29]. Chemical propulsion can be challenging, especially for *in vivo* applications. External sources of energy have also been studied: light, ultrasound, and magnetic field. Light penetration into tissues is limited. Besides the absorption of ultrasound by the body tissue, its navigation capability is low. Magnetic fields are most likely the most viable option for the navigation and actuation of microbots, at least in the near term. However, corrosion of magnetic material, such as iron, may be a concern [26]. Biohybrid microbots tend to be more biocompatible than others [30].

Now, let's look at some examples. First, in Section 11.3, we discussed a sperm-driven micromotor, guided magnetically, for targeted drug delivery. Zhang *et al.* designed nanoparticle-modified microbots for *in vivo* antibiotic delivery to treat acute bacterial pneumonia. The antibiotic-loaded neutrophil membrane-coated polymeric nanoparticles were attached to the microalgae (Fig. 15.8). The microbot systems showed fast speed, low clearance by alveolar macrophages, and long tissue retention time [31]. Lee *et al.* developed a magnetically actuated helical microrobot system with magnetic nanoparticle retrieval ability. The microbot was poly(ethylene glycol) diacrylate based with encapsulated anticancer drug doxorubicin; the helical structure was used to enhance the mobility of microbots. Magnetic nanoparticles (MNPs) were able to separate from the microbots using near-infrared as an external stimulus and retrieved to reduce their cytotoxicity to normal cells (Fig. 15.9) [32].

There are still a few remaining challenges/issues for the clinical translation of microbot-based drug delivery systems in addition to safety and biocompatibility considerations. For example, it may require many of them to reach the desired therapeutic effects. The scalability of microbots can be a main challenge, especially for those of high-order complexity. Besides tracking of microbots after implantation, the "elimination" of the microbots may also be necessary and should be taken into consideration during the design [26,29].

15.4 Engineered cells as drug delivery systems

We have discussed both (encapsulated) cells as living drug delivery systems (Chapter 7) and cell membrane/extracellular vesicle-based biomimetic drug delivery (Chapter 12). In this section, we focus on using engineered cells as therapeutics directly (Fig. 15.10). Although every cell type in the human body harbors properties that can potentially be turned into therapeutic use, engineering alterations in cellular function have enabled some of the highest-profile contemporary clinical successes. Cell-based therapies for humans were first introduced in the 1950s for blood-borne cancers through bone marrow transplantation, which set the foundation for the therapies using umbilical cord blood—derived hematopoietic stem cells and hematopoietic progenitor cells. Commercialization of cell-based therapies has significantly progressed since the FDA approval of CAR-T therapy [33]. CAR-T cells are genetically engineered T cells to display chimeric antigen receptors (CARs) for personalized cancer treatment. They recognize tumor antigens on their surface and induce downstream cytotoxic effects [29]. During CAR-T therapy, immune T cells from the patient are collected, engineered to create CAR-T cells, expanded, and infused back into the patient (Fig. 15.11) [29,34]. With the progress of synthetic biology, CAR-T therapies can be designed for control, flexibility, and specificity of cellular therapies (Fig. 15.12). For controllable CAR-T cells (Fig. 15.12a), an exogenous soluble ligand can switch ON and OFF CAR-T cells. A CAR fused with a ligand-induced degradation (LID) domain sequence can be used for improved control. For flexible CAR-T cells (Fig. 15.12b), CARs can be designed to target an adaptor molecule conjugated to an anti-tumor antigen. Selective CAR-T cells can be utilized to improve the specificity through AND gates, NOT gates, and combinatorial modules. As shown in Fig. 15.12c a NOT gate is used to prevent off-target and kill tumor cells exclusively expressing tumor-associated antigens (TAAs) [35].

Fig. 15.13 shows the cell therapy production process. Cell sources can be autologous, allogeneic, or xenogeneic. Upon modification and manufacturing following the cGMP guidelines, cellular products must be tested to ensure the product potency, sterility, viability, and purity/identity. There are still major challenges to successful cell-based treatments that are clinically and commercially viable. For example, a cell source needs to be identified

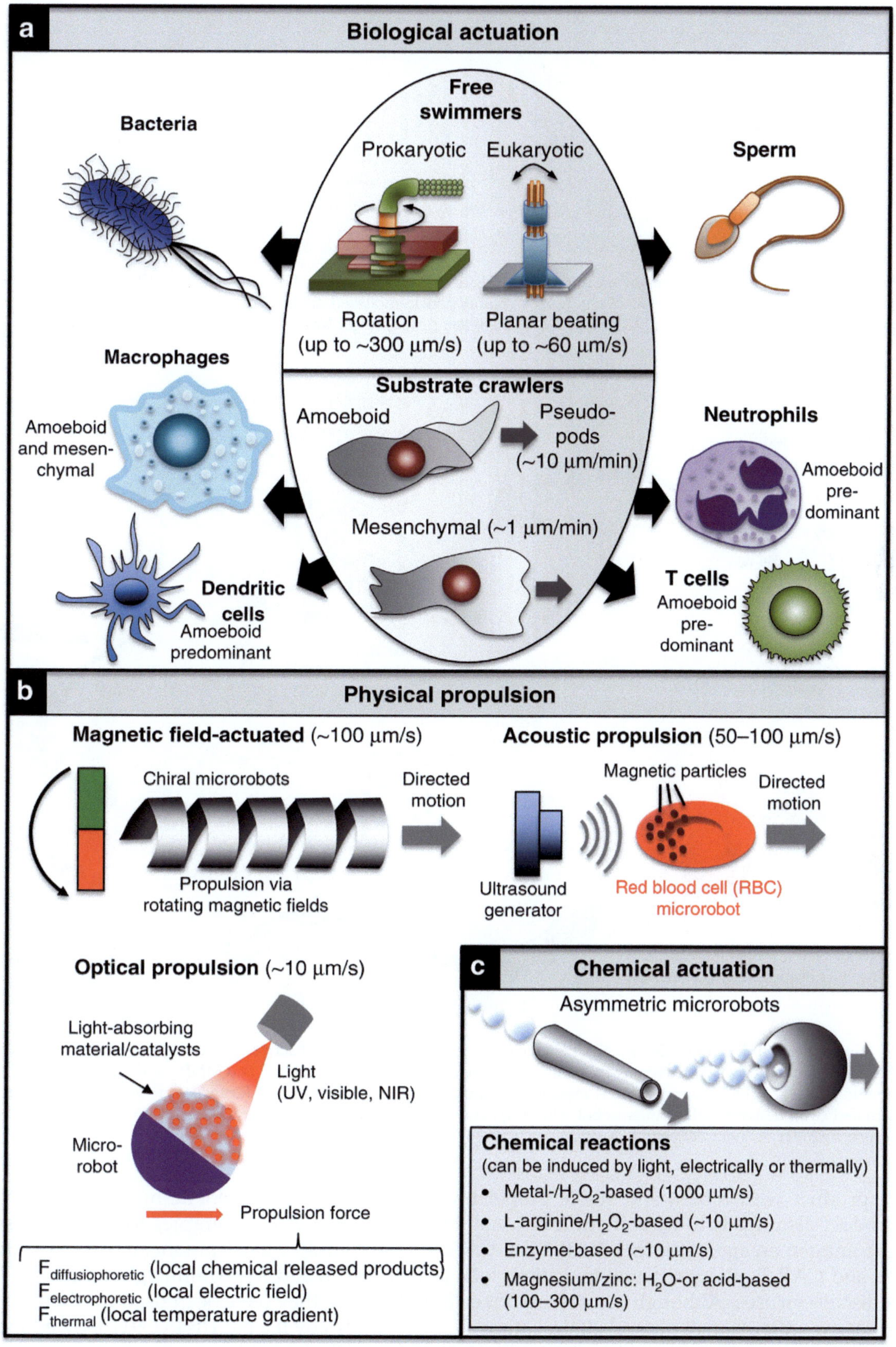

FIGURE 15.7 Mechanisms of actuation for microbots. Key examples for biological migration modes (a), physical propulsion (b), and chemical actuation (c). *Adapted from Schmidt, C.K., et al.,* Engineering microrobots for targeted cancer therapies from a medical perspective. *Nat Commun, 2020.* ***11****(1): p. 5618.*

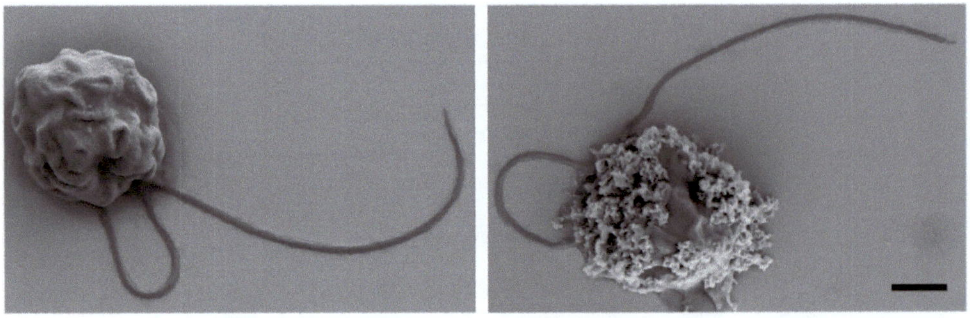

FIGURE 15.8 Pseudo-colored SEM images of an unmodified algae *(left)* and an algae-NP-robot *(right)*. *NP*, Nanoparticle; *SEM*, scanning electron microscopy. Scale bar, 2 μm. *Adapted from Zhang, F., et al.*, Nanoparticle-modified microrobots for in vivo antibiotic delivery to treat acute bacterial pneumonia. *Nat Mater, 2022.* ***21****(11): p. 1324-1332, with permission from Springer Nature.*

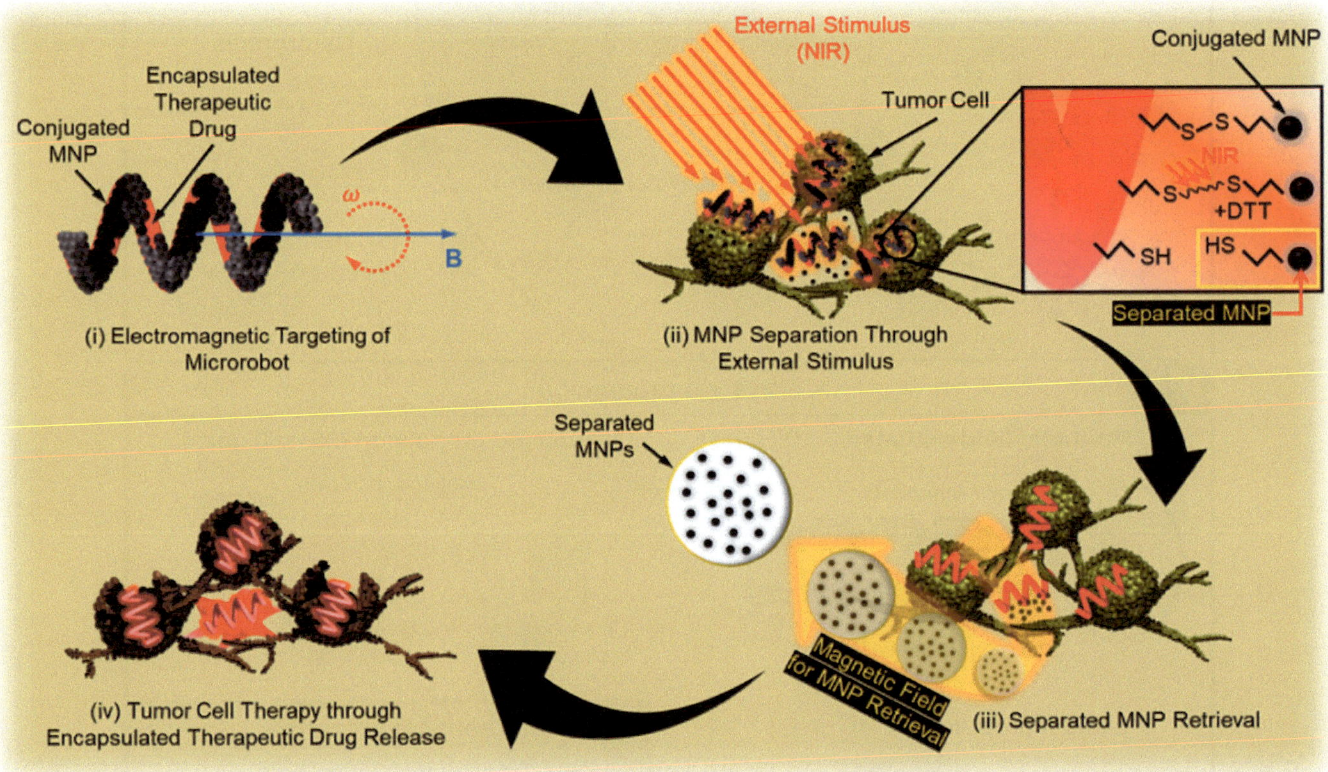

FIGURE 15.9 Concept of MNP retrievable helical-type microbot, showing the process of active electromagnetic targeting, NIR irradiation for external stimulus, MNP separation after weakening the conjugation between helical-type structure and MNPs, and separated MNP retrieval using a dynamic magnetic field. *DTT*, Dithiothreitol; *MNP*, magnetic nanoparticle; *NIR*, near-infrared. *Reproduced with permission from Lee, H., et al.*, Magnetically actuated drug delivery helical microrobot with magnetic nanoparticle retrieval ability. *ACS Appl. Mater. Interfaces, 2021.* ***13****(17): p. 19633-19647. Copyright (2021). American Chemical Society.*

that yields a product with robust and stable properties and is amenable to genetic manipulation. Moreover, a cell-based product also needs to exhibit sufficient viability [33]. Take CAR-T therapies for example, some of the limitations are antigen escape, off-target, CAR-T cell trafficking and infiltration, immunosuppressive tumor microenvironment, and CAR-T cell—associated toxicities (such as cytopenias and hypogammaglobulinemia) [33,36].

Last, let's discuss viruses. Although viruses are not cells technically, they have been used for therapies like engineered cells. For example, a small phase 3 clinical study (ClinicalTrials.gov ID: NCT04452591) showed that oncolytic viruses (engineered adenovirus; cretostimogene grenadenorepvec) eliminated tumors in 63.6% of 66 patients with bladder cancer that did not respond to mainline treatment [37—39].

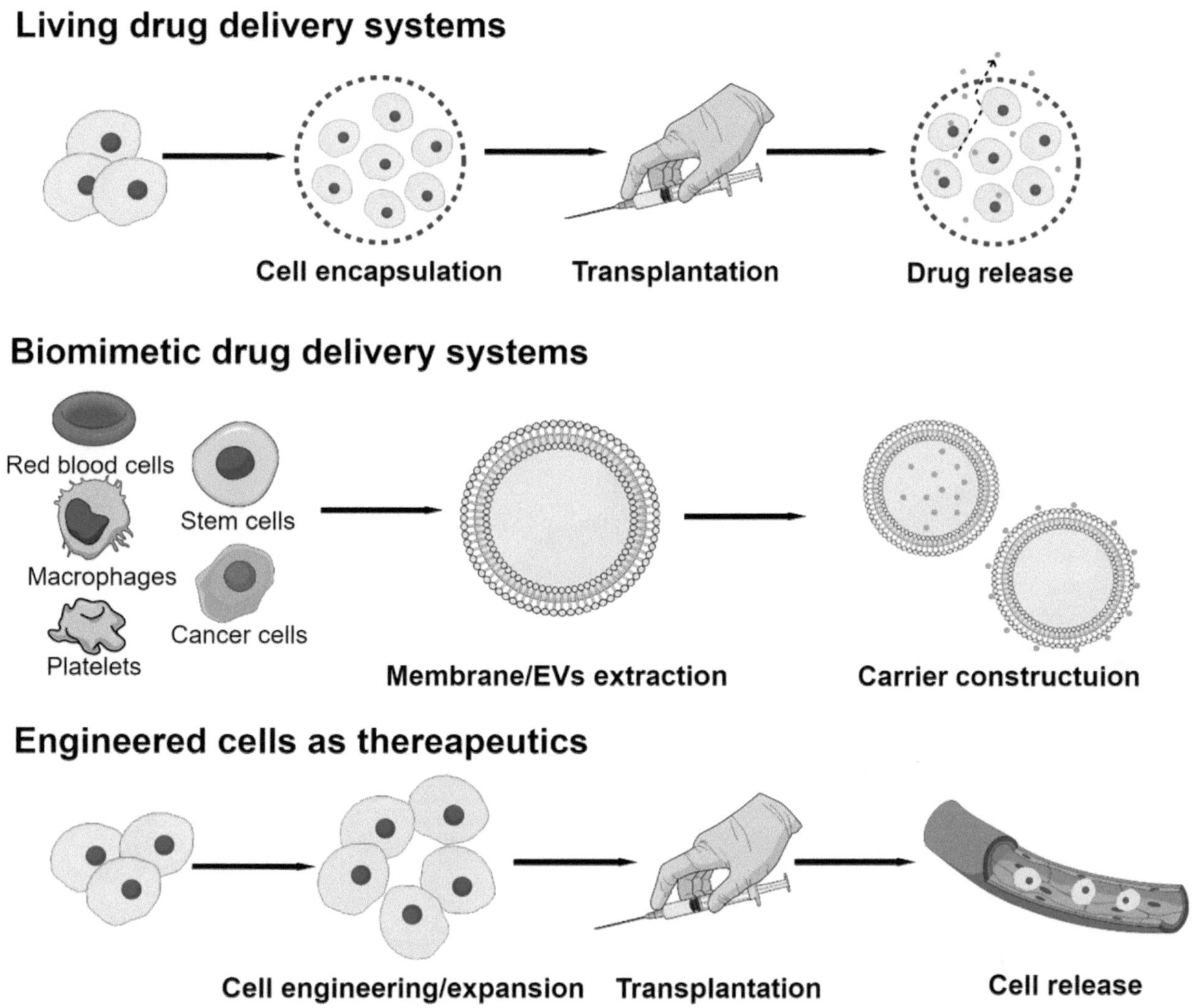

FIGURE 15.10 Different approaches to using cells for therapies. *EV*, Extracellular vesicle.

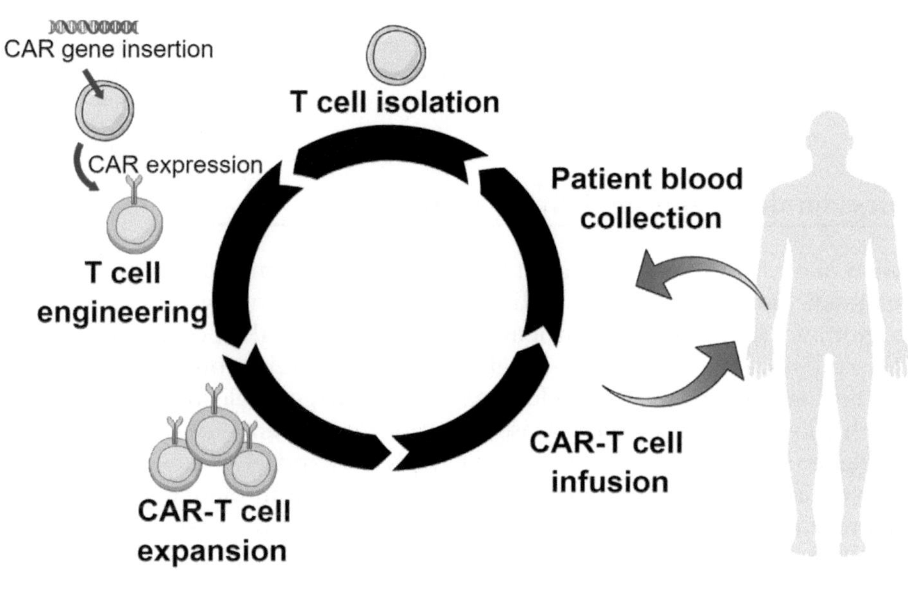

FIGURE 15.11 Process of CAR-T cell therapy. *CAR*, chimeric antigen receptor.

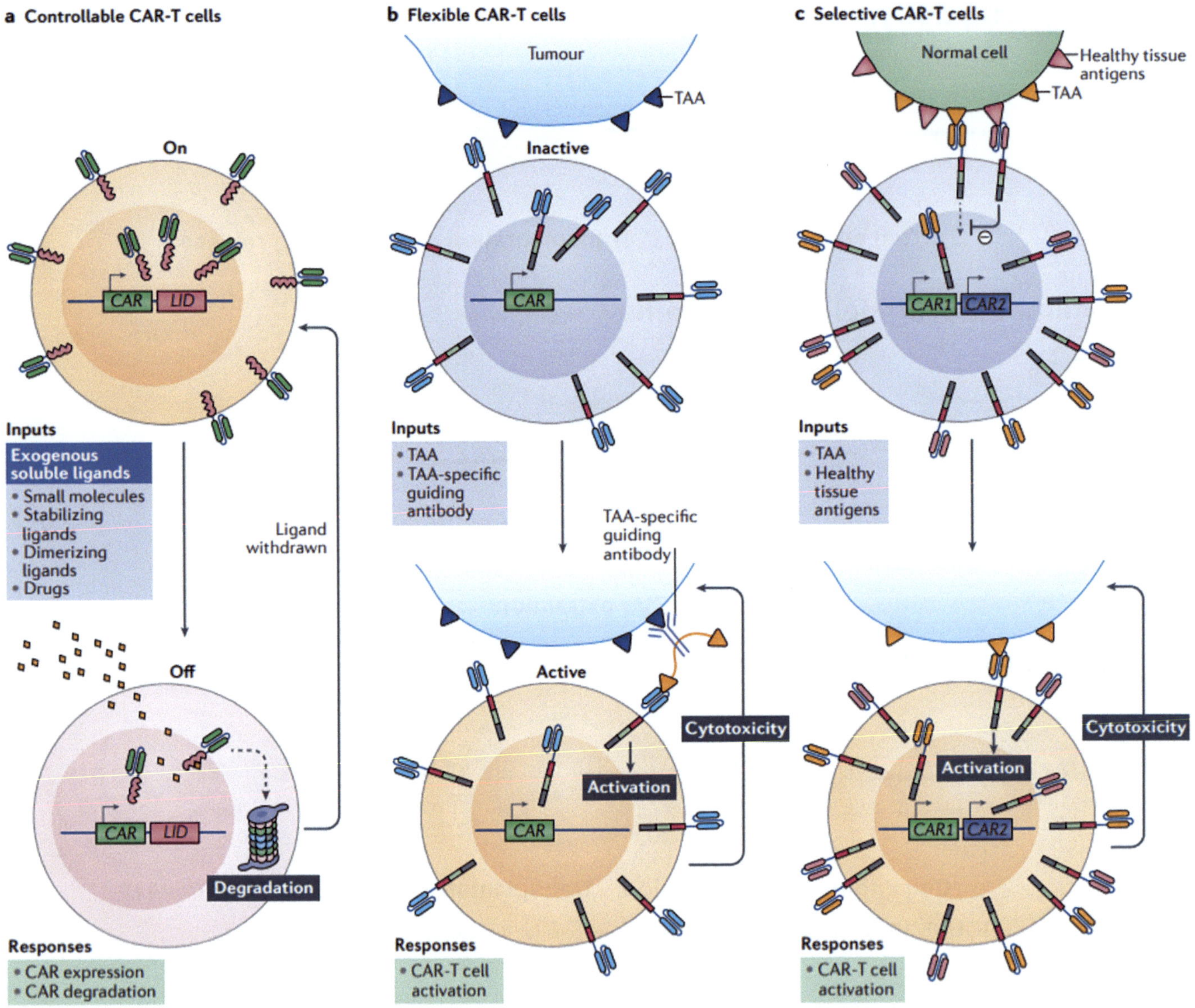

FIGURE 15.12 Human circulating CAR-T cell therapies with engineered genetic circuits. Circulating, engineered CAR-T cells can be designed for control (a), flexibility (b), and specificity (c) of cellular therapies. *CAR*, Chimeric antigen receptor; *LID*, ligand-induced degradation; *TAA*, tumor-associated antigen. *From Cubillos-Ruiz, A., et al.,* Engineering living therapeutics with synthetic biology. *Nat Rev Drug Discov, 2021.* ***20****(12): p. 941-960, with permission from Springer Nature.*

15.5 Wireless on-demand drug delivery systems

Wireless power transfer is the transmission of electrical power without wires and is based on technologies using time-varying electric, magnetic, or electromagnetic fields [40]. Various radiofrequency (RF) technologies are used for wireless power transmission. Near-field communication (NFC), in particular, is more efficient than other RF power transfers by inductive coupling between the coil in the device and the receiver coil [41]. Wireless on-demand drug delivery systems exploit exogenous stimuli, acoustic waves, electric fields, magnetic fields, and electromagnetic radiation to trigger drug carriers. This approach allows the controlled release of drugs with minimal off-target effects [42]. We have discussed exogenous stimuli-triggered drug delivery systems in Chapters 11 and 14. In this section, we will focus on wireless implantable drug delivery systems, such as an ultrasonically powered implantable potentiostat with bidirectional communication for programmable electrochemically controlled drug delivery. The system consisted of piezoelectric transducers for wireless power and data, an integrated circuit, and a drug delivery module containing drug-loaded electroresponsive nanoparticles [43].

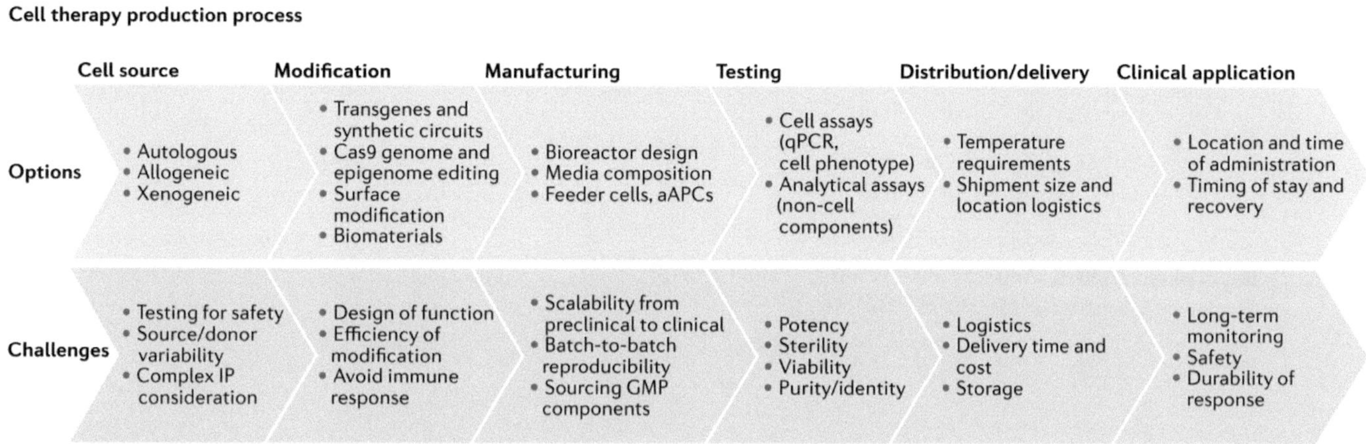

FIGURE 15.13 A cellular therapy process flow. *From Bashor, C.J., et al.,* Engineering the next generation of cell-based therapeutics. *Nat Rev Drug Discov, 2022.* ***21****(9): p. 655-675, with permission from Springer Nature.*

Recent progress of these systems is on the design of bioresorbable drug delivery devices that are wirelessly controlled to avoid the surgical procedures for extracting these systems after completion of the delivery function [44–46]. For example, Koo *et al.* developed a system with constituent materials that undergo complete bioresorption to eliminate device load from the patient after completing the final stage of the release process. Polybutanedithiol 1,3,5-triallyl-1,3,5-triazine-2,4,6(1H,3H,5H)-trione penteonic anhydride (PBTPA), a bioresorbable polyanhydride, was used as a substrate and a drug reservoir. The wireless power harvester relied on magnetic inductive coupling to an external transmission coil to produce an electrical bias between the Mg electrodes (one serves as an anode [i.e., gate, serving as the valve to an underlying reservoir] and the other one as the cathode). The harvesting unit consisted of an RF coil of Mg, an RF diode constructed using a silicon nanomembrane, and a parallel-plate capacitor (multilayer stack of $Mg/SiO_2/Mg$). *In vivo* testing indicated this system could be used for controlling blood glucose levels by timed delivery of insulin [44]. Huang *et al.* reported an implantable electronic delivery system based on bioresorbable microneedle devices that were activated wirelessly for electrostimulation and sustainable delivery of anti-inflammatory drugs. This fully bioresorbable design (IBMN) incorporated an RF wireless power transmission system and a drug-loaded microneedle structure (Fig. 15.14). Two layers of square-shaped Mg metallic coils were assembled with a poly(lactic-*co*-glycolic acid) dielectric interlayer for wireless power transmission as the antenna. A doped silicon diode connected the circuits and antenna to bring in the RF power wirelessly for electrostimulation. Mg was used because it is a commonly used metal in biodegradable devices, and a tungsten (W) coating was used due to its lower degradation rate compared to the e-beam evaporated Mg layer [47].

15.6 3D Printing-based drug delivery systems

Three-dimensional (3D) printing (or additive manufacturing [AM]) is a parallel design and manufacturing technology that integrates materials, structures, and functions [48]. It involves the laying down of successive layers of material to form 3D models [48]. 3D printing enables a fast and cheap design cycle for the preparation of personalized medicine. The 3D printing could also conquer the traditional manufacturing regimen of "one size fits all" by creating drug delivery systems for patients' requirements. And 3D printing can produce unique dosage forms and achieve more complex drug release profiles. The FDA approved the first and only 3D-printed (oral) drug in 2015 (levetiracetam [Spritam]), which supported the commercial feasibility of this technology [49]. Moreover, 3D printing can be used to design dosage forms during the early phases of drug development with a minimal investment of time, effort, and resources [48].

Now, let's look at some examples. Misra *et al.* 3D-printed multidrug-eluting stent from a graphene-nanoplatelet–doped biodegradable polymer composite. The stepwise process for developing this personalized coronary stent is shown in Fig. 15.15. Poly(ε-caprolactone) (PCL) was used as the matrix for 3D printing the cardiac stent and graphene nanoplatelets were used to increase the mechanical properties of the PCL matrix [50]. A recent case study demonstrated the foundational concepts for understanding the effects of critical formulation (drug and polymer loadings) and geometrical parameters (number of shell and septum layers and porosity) on the performance

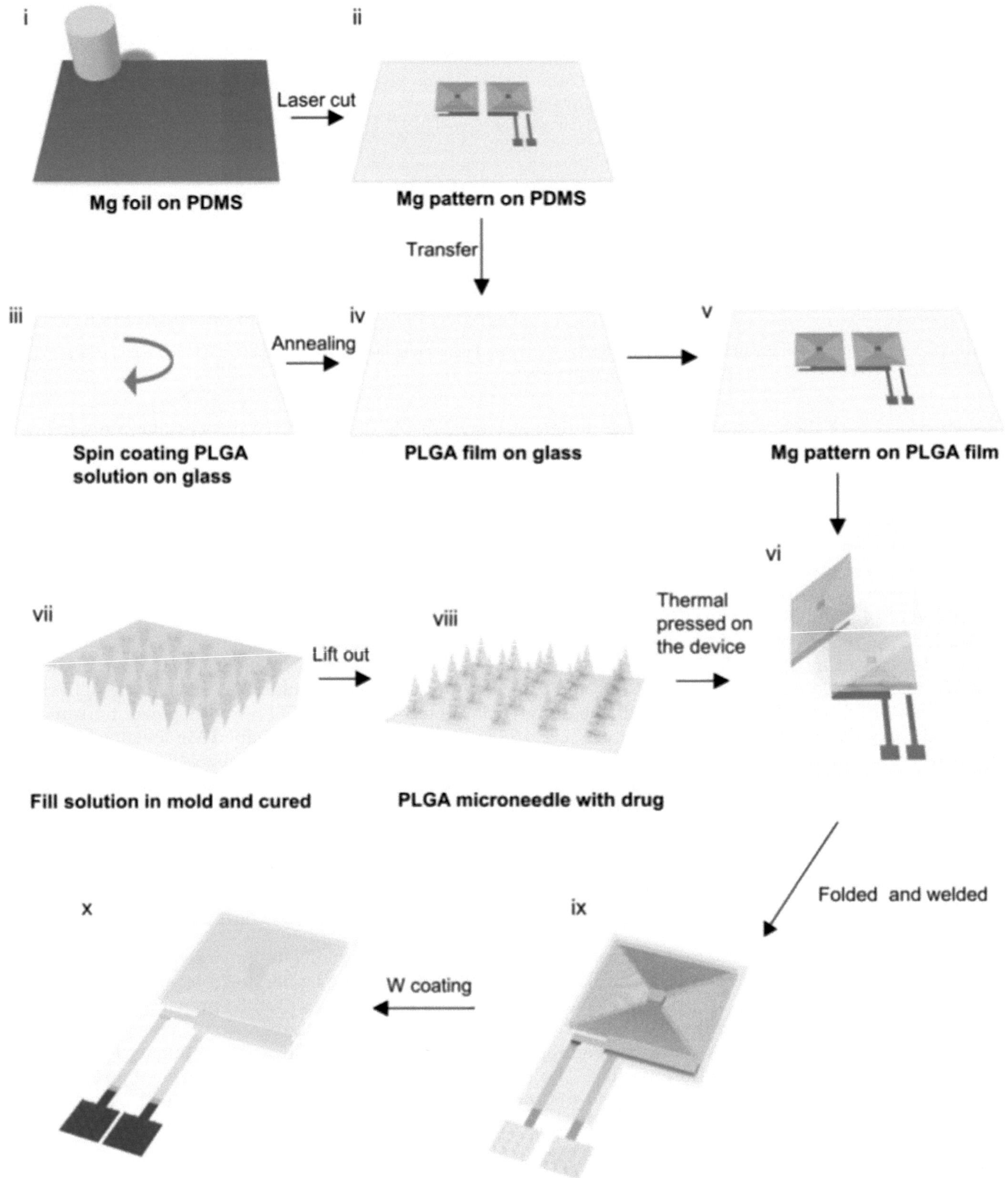

FIGURE 15.14 The fabrication process of the IBMN devices. *IBMN*, Implantable and bioresorbable microneedle; *Mg*, magnesium; *PDMS*, polydimethylsiloxane; *PLGA*, poly(lactic-*co*-glycolic acid); *W*, tungsten. *Reproduced with permission from Huang, Y., et al.*, Implantable electronic medicine enabled by bioresorbable microneedles for wireless electrotherapy and drug delivery. *Nano Lett, 2022.* **22***(14): p. 5944-5953. Copyright (2022). American Chemical Society.*

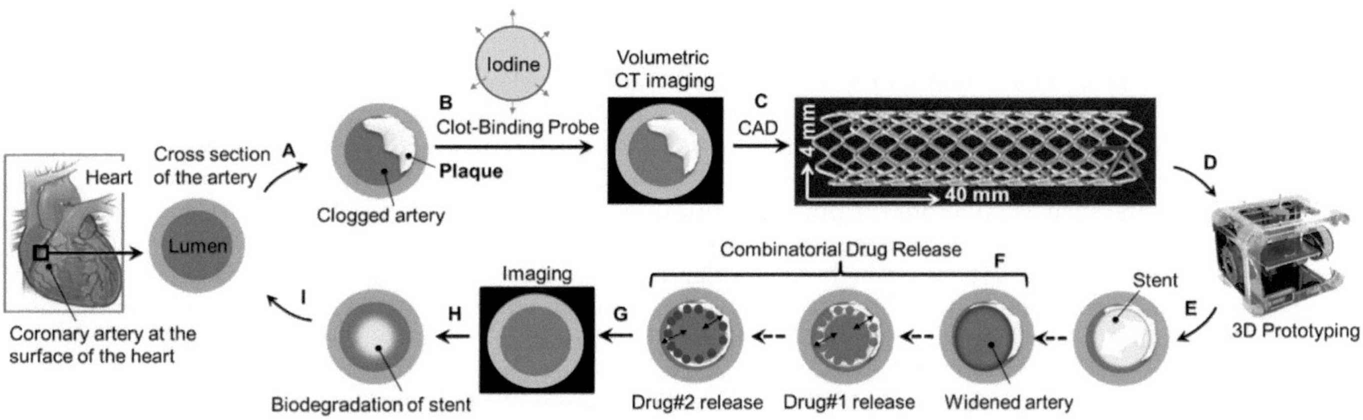

FIGURE 15.15 Stepwise process for developing a personalized coronary stent. (A) Cross section of the artery shown at the surface of the heart, plaque buildup is shown inside the lumen due to various factors. (B) Clot-binding (a fibrin-targeted iodinated) probe is administered to locate the blood clot. (C) Imaging information is transferred to computer-aided design (CAD) software to design a personalized stent. (D) PCL-GR polymer composite is used for fused deposition modeling additive manufacturing technique in a commercial 3D printing machine. (E) Prototyped stent is placed inside the artery. (F) Incorporation of two drugs for sequential release. (G) The healing process is further monitored by CT imaging. (H, I) Polymer gets biodegraded inside a widened artery. *CT*, Computed tomography; *GR*, graphene nanoplatelets; *PCL*, poly(ε-caprolactone). *From Misra, S.K., et al.*, 3D-printed multidrug-eluting stent from graphene-nanoplatelet-doped biodegradable polymer composite. *Adv Healthcare Mater, 2017. **6**(11): p. 1700008, with permission from John Wiley and Sons.*

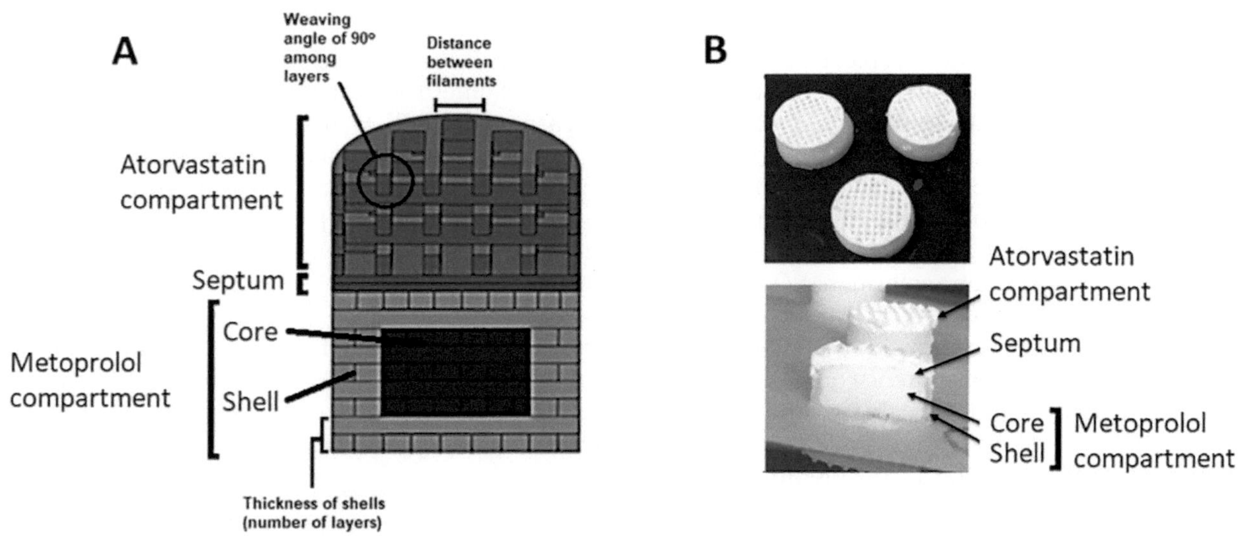

FIGURE 15.16 Design (A) and digital photograph (B) of the atorvastatin/metoprolol polypill. *Reproduced from Alayoubi, A., et al.*, Mechanistic understanding of the performance of personalized 3D-printed cardiovascular polypills: A case study of patient-centered therapy. *Int. J. Pharm, 2022. **617**: p. 121599, with permission from Elsevier.*

characteristics (drug strength, dosage uniformity, drug release, and breaking strength) of the cardiovascular polypills (i.e., a combination of cardiovascular medications taken in a single pill [51]) to meet the needs of individual patients. Atorvastatin and metoprolol were used as model drugs and the 3D printing technology utilized was pressure-assisted microextrusion. A geometric design with two separate compartments, separated by a septum, was developed to custom design independent release profiles for two drugs (Fig. 15.16). It was concluded that 3D printing provides the flexibility for tailoring the release of different drugs in the same dosage form for personalized therapy [52].

Overall, 3D printing in the pharmaceutical sector is still at an early stage. There are still major hurdles—concerns related to the regulatory issues, scalability, and cost-effectiveness. Looking forward, multimaterial printing and four-dimensional printing represent a new paradigm for AM technologies, which show great potential in addressing the unmet needs for personalized medicine. In particular, technological innovations can lead to the designing of a single printing device competent enough to produce multiple-release formulations [53,54].

15.7 Artificial intelligence (AI) in drug delivery

FDA's Center for Drug Evaluation and Research (CDER) defines AI as a branch of computer science, statistics, and engineering that uses algorithms or models that exhibit behaviors such as learning, making decisions, and making predictions. CDER has established a framework for the Regulatory Advanced Manufacturing Evaluation (FRAME) initiative to prepare a framework to support the adoption of advanced manufacturing that could benefit patients, such as AI. From the pharmaceutical manufacturing aspect, AI can assist in process optimization, process control, smart monitoring and maintenance, and continuous improvement [55]. Many pharmaceutical companies have collaborated with AI companies to develop tools for advancing the pharmaceutical industry [56]. AI has also begun to upend the drug discovery pipeline with several new compounds entering clinical trials [57]. Some of the key contributions of AI in drug discovery include target identification, virtual screening, structure-activity relationship modeling, *de novo* drug design, optimization of drug candidates, drug repurposing, and toxicity prediction [58]. In this section, we will focus on the application of AI in drug delivery.

Computational pharmaceutics and integration of AI and big data in the field of pharmaceutics, can analyze large datasets and predict drug behavior. By simulating drug formulation and delivery processes, computational pharmaceutics can accelerate the optimization of drug delivery systems including the prediction of drug release through formulations, patient-specific dosage formulation design, and the prediction of drug and drug delivery system behavior at various scales [58]. Take AI in drug delivery for infectious disease treatment, for example; the topics involved are drug development, drug resistance prediction, drug dosing optimization, drug combination selection, drug delivery system improvement, drug administration route design, drug pharmacokinetic profile characterization, and drug treatment outcome prediction (Fig. 15.18) [59]. Now, let's look at some examples. Nemati *et al.* studied the prediction of formulation parameters and drug release profiles from cochlear implant coatings fabricated as porous monolithic devices based on silicone rubber. As shown in Fig. 15.19, the effects of varying the rational function terms on the resulting curves for the cumulative amount of dexamethasone released at time *t* were studied, which revealed how each of the terms would affect the drug release profile [60]. Hsueh *et al.* used peptide engineering to impart melanin binding properties to peptide-drug conjugates to act as a sustained-release depot in the eye. The lead multifunctional peptide conjugated to brimonidine (an intraocular pressure lowering drug) reduced the intraocular pressure for up to 18 days after a single intracameral injection in rabbits [61]. Various AI tools and pipelines have been developed and can be used for designing drug delivery systems [62,63]. For example, BioTransformer 3.0 (https://biotransformer.ca/), ADMETlab 3.0 (https://admetlab3.scbdd.com/), and CYPstrate (https://nerdd.univie.ac.at/) are some public prediction tools [63].

Although AI shows great promise in transforming the pharmaceutical industry, there are a few limitations. Here are some examples: lack of transparency on how a model arrives at its prediction, limited availability of data (such as for a particular drug or population), biases and/or incompleteness in data, inability to incorporate new data or update the model, limited ability to account for variability, limited ability to capture the complex and dynamic biological system as a whole, and ethical considerations [58].

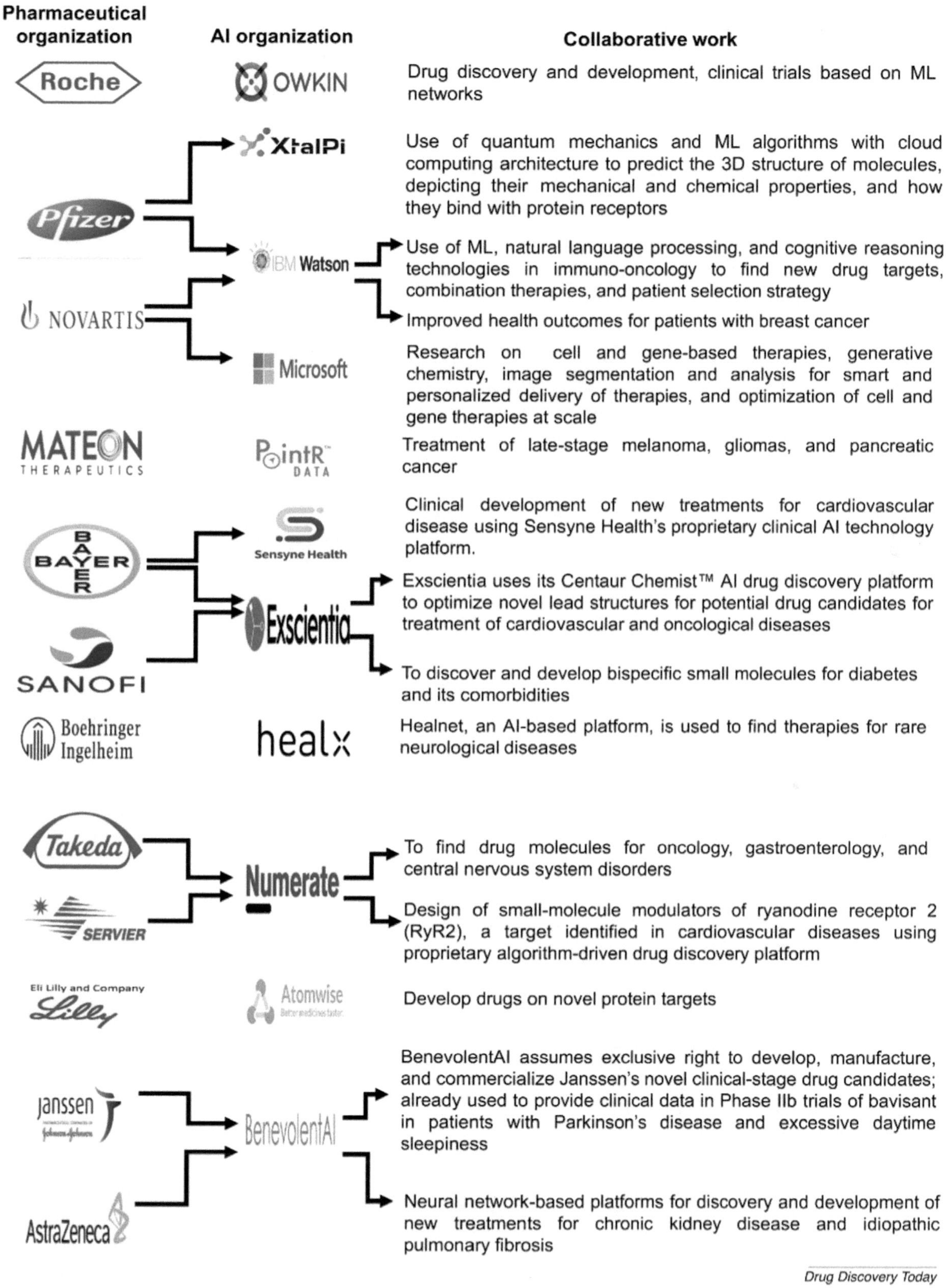

FIGURE 15.17 Leading pharmaceutical companies and their association with artificial intelligence (AI) organizations that are working in fields including oncology, cardiovascular diseases, and central nervous system disorders. *From Paul, D., et al.,* Artificial intelligence in drug discovery and development. *Drug Discov Today, 2021.* ***26****(1): p. 80-93, with permission from Elsevier.*

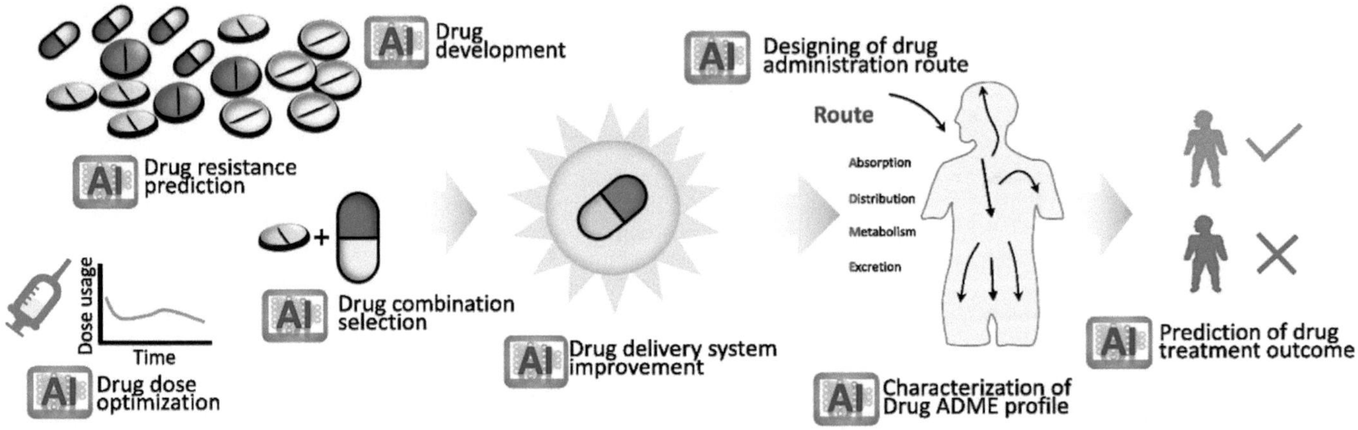

FIGURE 15.18 Current research and application of artificial intelligence (AI) in drug delivery for infectious disease treatment. *From He, S., L.G. Leanse, and Y. Feng,* Artificial intelligence and machine learning assisted drug delivery for effective treatment of infectious diseases. *Adv. Drug Deliv. Rev, 2021.* ***178****: p. 113922, with permission from Elsevier.*

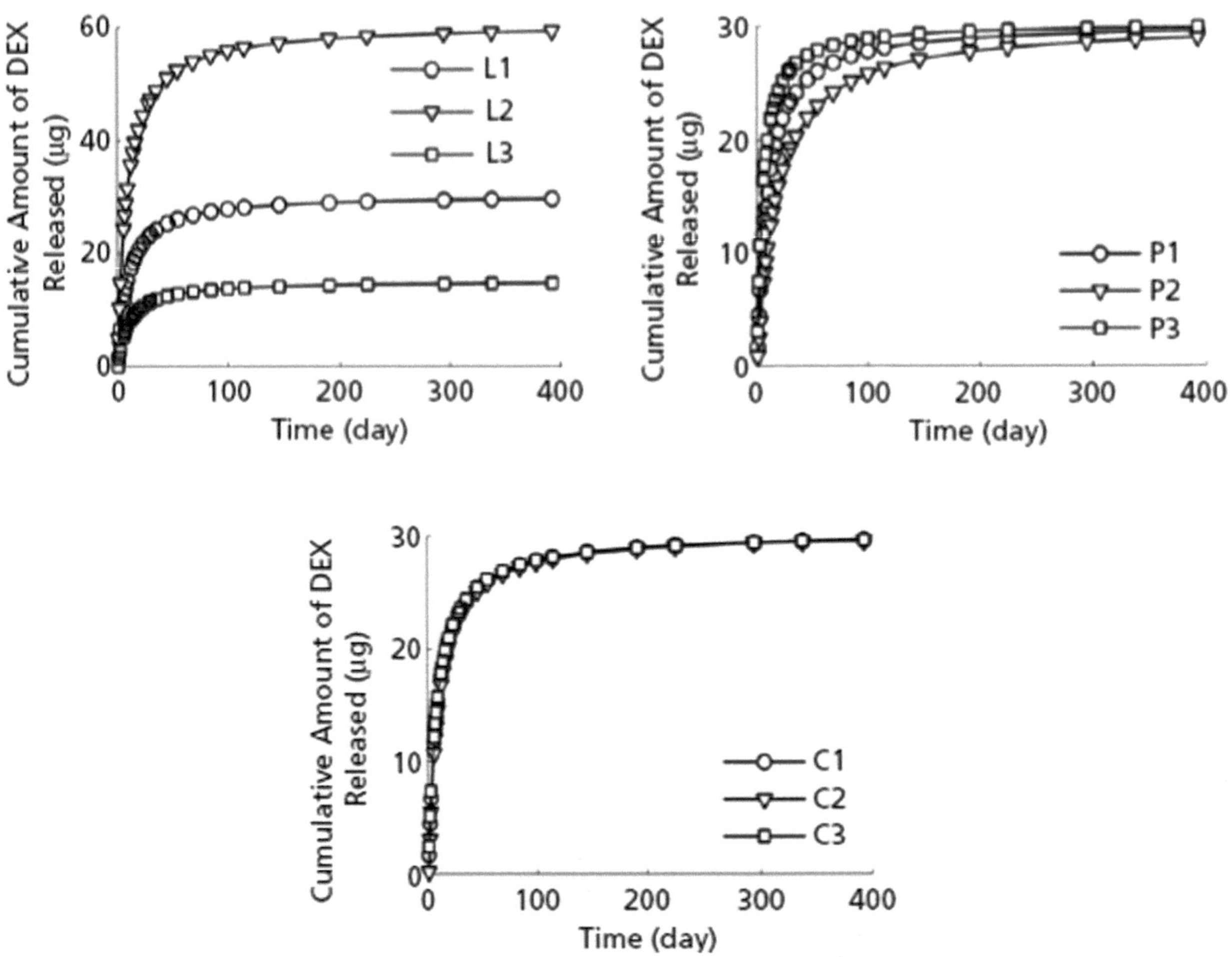

FIGURE 15.19 Effect of the rational function coefficients variation in three levels (30, 60, and 15 for L1 to L3; 8, 16, and 4 for P1 to P3, and −14, −28, and −7 for C1 to C3) on the predicted release profile of dexamethasone (DEX). *C*, Constant; *L*, coefficient relevant to loading percentage; *P*, parameter relevant to porogen content. *From Nemati, P., et al.,* Artificial neural networks for bilateral prediction of formulation parameters and drug release profiles from cochlear implant coatings fabricated as porous monolithic devices based on silicone rubber. *J. Pharm. Pharmacol, 2013.* ***66****(5): p. 624-638, with permission from Oxford University Press.*

Sample question 15.1

Sacubitril is a component of the FDA-approved prodrug product, Entresto (Chapter 5). Use the FAME 3 tool (https://nerdd.univie.ac.at/fame3/) [64,65] to predict its metabolism sites.

Answer: The predicted results are shown in Fig. 15.20. The prediction indicates that the C.4 atom is where a reaction catalyzed by a metabolic enzyme is initiated. This value also passed the decision threshold (FAMEscore of 0.6) [66]. The actual metabolism mechanism *in vivo* is deethylation by liver carboxylesterase 1 [67]. The first step of the mechanism of action of esterases is the nucleophilic attack at the carbonyl carbon [68]. Moreover, the GLORYx tool (https://nerdd.univie.ac.at/gloryx) [65,69] was used to predict the phases I and II metabolites. GLORYx incorporates the sites of metabolism and transforms the molecules into their potential metabolites using reaction rule sets [70]. As shown in Fig. 15.21, the drug (Sacubitrilat) is one of the most likely metabolites.

FAME 3 Output

Visualization:

To alternate between atoms and atom numbers, move the mouse cursor over the figure.

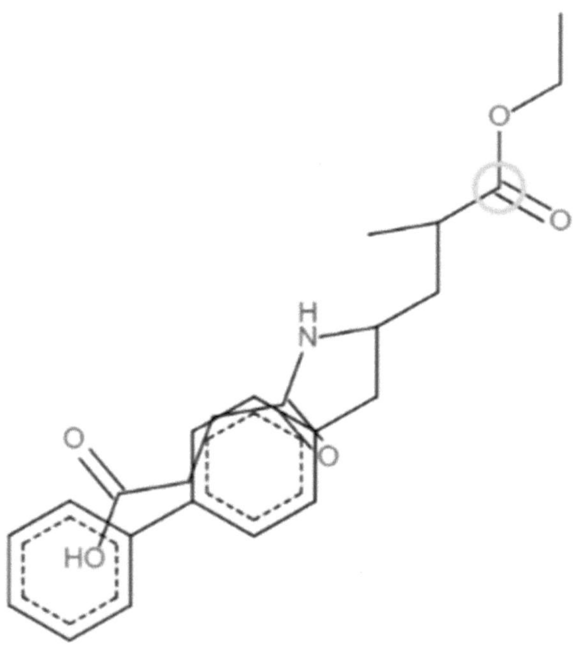

Model: P1+P2 (depth: 5)

Molecule mol_1

Atom	Probability	FAMEscore
C.4	**0.879**	**0.6**
O.30	0.387	0.548
C.28	0.33	0.535
C.27	0.259	0.571
C.18	0.172	0.778
C.24	0.16	0.613
C.10	0.126	0.606
C.2	0.088	0.572
C.6	0.072	0.625
C.7	0.064	0.607
N.23	0.048	0.588
C.26	0.044	0.553
C.1	0.032	0.549
C.19	0.028	0.783
C.17	0.028	0.783
O.3	0.028	0.566
C.22	0.024	0.608
C.12	0.024	0.608
C.9	0.024	0.668
C.21	0.024	0.627
C.13	0.024	0.627
C.20	0.02	0.733
C.16	0.02	0.733
O.25	0.012	0.611
C.8	0.012	0.596
C.11	0.004	0.614
O.29	0.0	0.544
C.15	0.0	0.629
C.14	0.0	0.62
O.5	0.0	0.612

FIGURE 15.20 Screenshot of the predicted results using FAME 3.

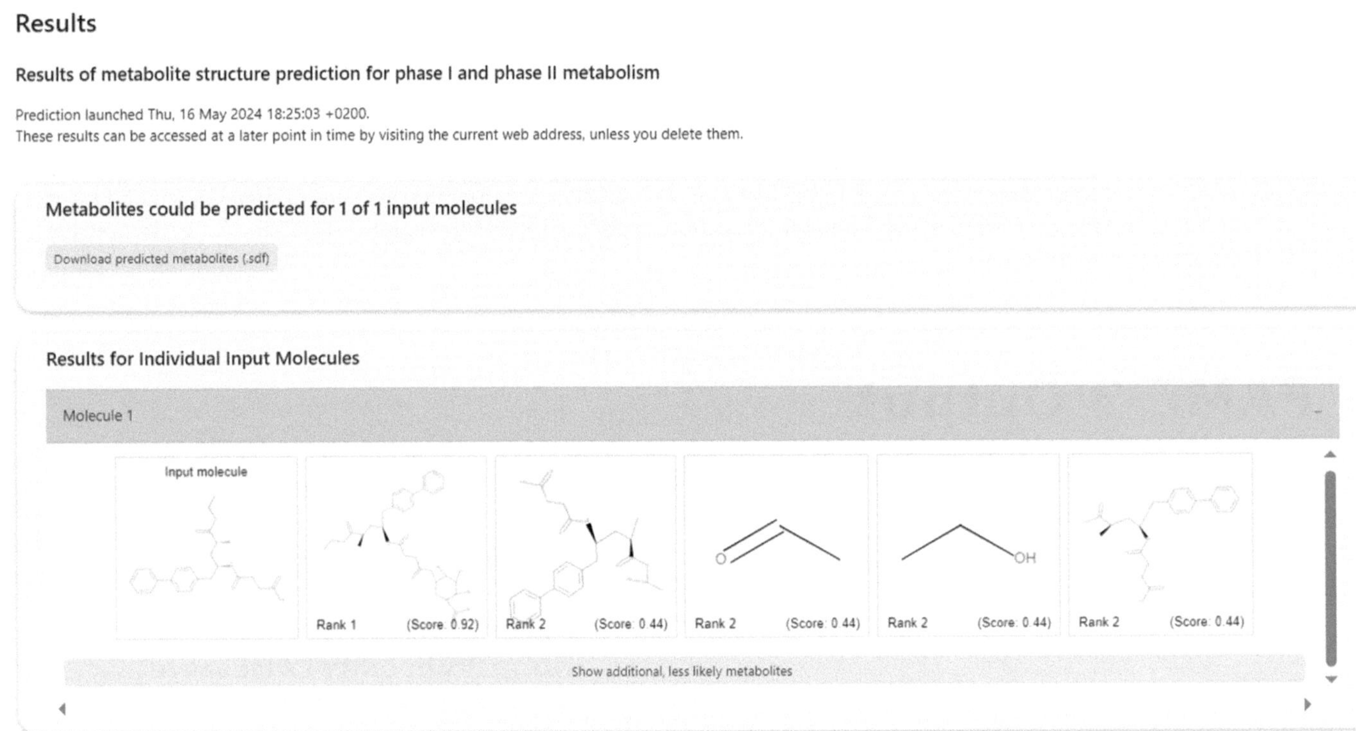
Results
Results of metabolite structure prediction for phase I and phase II metabolism
Prediction launched Thu, 16 May 2024 18:25:03 +0200.
These results can be accessed at a later point in time by visiting the current web address, unless you delete them.
Metabolites could be predicted for 1 of 1 input molecules
Download predicted metabolites (.sdf)
Results for Individual Input Molecules
Molecule 1
Input molecule
Rank 1 (Score 0.92)
Rank 2 (Score 0.44)
Rank 2 (Score 0.44)
Rank 2 (Score 0.44)
Rank 2 (Score 0.44)
OH
Show additional, less likely metabolites

FIGURE 15.21 Screenshot of the predicted metabolites using GLORYx.

Review and practice questions

1. What is mucoadhesion? And what are some of the mucoadhesion theories?
2. Why are lectins commonly used for designing mucoadhesion systems?
3. What are the different mechanisms of soft mist formations (nebulization)? And briefly describe them.
4. What are the different types of microrobots in drug delivery systems based on the make-up and propulsion sources?
5. What is the most viable option (external source of energy) for the navigation and actuation of microrobots?
6. Conduct a literature search and provide a recent example of microrobots-based drug delivery systems.
7. What are different approaches of using cells for therapies?
8. Describe the process of chimeric antigen receptor (CAR) T-cell therapy.
9. Describe the cellular therapy process flow (cell therapy production process).
10. What is the major benefit of using wireless on-demand drug delivery systems *in vivo*?
11. Conduct a literature search and provide a recent example of wireless on-demand drug delivery systems.
12. What are the benefits of three-dimensional (3D) printing-based drug delivery systems?
13. Conduct a literature search and provide a recent example of 3D printing–based drug delivery systems.
14. What are some of the key contributions of artificial intelligence (AI) in drug discovery?
15. How can AI, computation pharmaceutics, in particular, be applied in drug delivery?
16. Conduct a literature search and provide a recent example of the application of AI in drug delivery system design.
17. Prodrugs are controlled drug delivery systems with various benefits.
    a. Identify a commonly used drug.
    b. Design a prodrug based on the chosen drug.
    c. Compare their (drug vs prodrug) sites of metabolism using FAME 3 (https://nerdd.univie.ac.at/fame3/).
    d. Compare their metabolite structures (especially on whether the drug is a metabolite of your prodrug) using GLORYx (https://nerdd.univie.ac.at/gloryx/).

References

[1] Shaikh R, et al. Mucoadhesive drug delivery systems. J Pharm BioAllied Sci 2011;3(1):89–100.
[2] Skin and mucosae (surface barriers). Available from: https://med.libretexts.org/@go/page/7938
[3] Smart JD. The basics and underlying mechanisms of mucoadhesion. Adv Drug Deliv Rev 2005;57(11):1556–68.
[4] de Lima CSA, et al. Mucoadhesive polymers and their applications in drug delivery systems for the treatment of bladder cancer. Gels 2022; 8(9):587.
[5] Mansuri S, et al. Mucoadhesion: a promising approach in drug delivery system. React Funct Polym 2016;100:151–72.
[6] Thakur AK, Kaundle B, Singh I. Chapter 22 - mucoadhesive drug delivery systems in respiratory diseases. In: Dua K, et al., editors. Targeting chronic inflammatory lung diseases using advanced drug delivery systems. Academic Press; 2020. p. 475–91.
[7] Kulkarni R, Fanse S, Burgess DJ. Mucoadhesive drug delivery systems: a promising noninvasive approach to bioavailability enhancement. Part II: formulation considerations. Expet Opin Drug Deliv 2023;20(3):413–34.
[8] Komati S, et al. Mucoadhesive multiparticulate drug delivery systems: an extensive review of patents. Adv Pharm Bull 2019;9(4):521–38.
[9] Putri AP, et al. Alginate modification and lectin-conjugation approach to synthesize the mucoadhesive matrix. Appl Sci 2021;11(24):11818.
[10] Lavín de Juan L, et al. Pharmaceutical applications of lectins. J Drug Deliv Sci Technol 2017;42:126–33.
[11] Chettri D, et al. Lectins: biological significance to biotechnological application. Carbohydr Res 2021;506:108367.
[12] Wijetunge SS, et al. Wheat germ agglutinin liposomes with surface grafted cyclodextrins as bioadhesive dual-drug delivery nanocarriers to treat oral cells. Colloids Surf B Biointerfaces 2020;185:110572.
[13] Tekade M, et al. Chapter 13 - thiolated-chitosan: a novel mucoadhesive polymer for better-targeted drug delivery. In: Tekade RK, editor. Biomaterials and bionanotechnology. Academic Press; 2019. p. 459–93.
[14] Federer C, Kurpiers M, Bernkop-Schnürch A. Thiolated chitosans: a multi-talented class of polymers for various applications. Biomacromolecules 2021;22(1):24–56.
[15] Wibel R, et al. In vitro investigation of thiolated chitosan derivatives as mucoadhesive coating materials for solid lipid nanoparticles. Biomacromolecules 2021;22(9):3980–91.
[16] Komalla V, et al. Advances in soft mist inhalers. Expet Opin Drug Deliv 2023;20(8):1055–70.
[17] van Rijn CJM, et al. Low energy nebulization preserves integrity of SARS-CoV-2 mRNA vaccines for respiratory delivery. Sci Rep 2023;13(1): 8851.
[18] Dalby RN, Eicher J, Zierenberg B. Development of Respimat(®) Soft Mist™ inhaler and its clinical utility in respiratory disorders. Med Devices (Auckl) 2011;4:145–55.
[19] Dalby R, Spallek M, Voshaar T. A review of the development of Respimat® Soft Mist™ inhaler. Int J Pharm 2004;283(1):1–9.
[20] Munnik P, et al. In vivo performance testing of the novel Medspray wet aerosol inhaler. J Aerosol Med Pulm Drug Deliv 2009;22(4):317–21.
[21] Head T, Tokranova N, Cady NC. Lithographically patterned micro-nozzles for controlling fluid flow profiles for drug delivery and in vitro imaging applications. MRS Commun 2021;11(5):584–9.
[22] Last TS, Stemme G, Roxhed N. First micro swirl nozzle for fast drug delivery to the lung. In: 2021 IEEE 34th international conference on micro electro mechanical systems (MEMS); 2021. p. 22–5.
[23] Zeteo Biomedical LLC. Drug and biologic non-invasive delivery devices and primary containers. Available from: https://zeteobiomed.com/technology-devices/.
[24] Medspray. Technology. Available from: https://medspray.com/technology/.
[25] Jin W, et al. Three-dimensional simulation of impinging jet atomization of soft mist inhalers using the hybrid VOF-DPM model. Powder Technol 2022;407:117622.
[26] Nelson BJ, Pané S. Delivering drugs with microrobots. Science 2023;382(6675):1120–2.
[27] Zhang Y, et al. Micro/nanorobots for medical diagnosis and disease treatment. Micromachines 2022;13(5):648.
[28] Das T, Sultana S. Multifaceted applications of micro/nanorobots in pharmaceutical drug delivery systems: a comprehensive review. Future J Pharm Sci 2024;10(1):2.
[29] Schmidt CK, et al. Engineering microrobots for targeted cancer therapies from a medical perspective. Nat Commun 2020;11(1):5618.
[30] Xu Y, et al. Micro/nanorobots for precise drug delivery via targeted transport and triggered release: a review. Int J Pharm 2022;616:121551.
[31] Zhang F, et al. Nanoparticle-modified microrobots for in vivo antibiotic delivery to treat acute bacterial pneumonia. Nat Mater 2022;21(11): 1324–32.
[32] Lee H, et al. Magnetically actuated drug delivery helical microrobot with magnetic nanoparticle retrieval ability. ACS Appl Mater Interfaces 2021;13(17):19633–47.
[33] Bashor CJ, et al. Engineering the next generation of cell-based therapeutics. Nat Rev Drug Discov 2022;21(9):655–75.
[34] Ahmad A, Uddin S, Steinhoff M. CAR-T cell therapies: an overview of clinical studies supporting their approved use against acute lymphoblastic leukemia and large B-cell lymphomas. Int J Mol Sci 2020;21(11).
[35] Cubillos-Ruiz A, et al. Engineering living therapeutics with synthetic biology. Nat Rev Drug Discov 2021;20(12):941–60.
[36] Cappell KM, Kochenderfer JN. Long-term outcomes following CAR T cell therapy: what we know so far. Nat Rev Clin Oncol 2023;20(6): 359–71.
[37] Leslie M. Tumor-killing viruses score rare success in late-stage trial. Science 2023;382(6675):1101–2.
[38] Study of Cretostimogene given in patients with non-muscle invasive bladder cancer, unresponsive to bacillus-calmette-guerin *(BOND-003)*. Available from: https://clinicaltrials.gov/study/NCT04452591.
[39] CG Oncology. Mechanism of action. Available from: https://cgoncology.com/science/#moa.
[40] Bertos GA, Papadopoulos EG. Chapter six - upper-limb prosthetic devices. In: Segil J, editor. Handbook of biomechatronics. Academic Press; 2019. p. 177–240.
[41] Kim J. Chapter 13 - networks and near-field communication: up-close but far away. In: Godfrey A, Stuart S, editors. Digital health. Academic Press; 2021. p. 197–210.
[42] Mirvakili SM, Langer R. Wireless on-demand drug delivery. Nat Electron 2021;4(7):464–77.

[43] Wang ML, et al. A wireless implantable potentiostat for programmable electrochemical drug delivery. In: 2021 IEEE Biomedical Circuits and Systems Conference (BioCAS); 2021. p. 1–4.
[44] Koo J, et al. Wirelessly controlled, bioresorbable drug delivery device with active valves that exploit electrochemically triggered crevice corrosion. Sci Adv 2020;6(35):eabb1093.
[45] Lee CH, et al. Biological lipid membranes for on-demand, wireless drug delivery from thin, bioresorbable electronic implants. NPG Asia Mater 2015;7(11):e227–e227.
[46] Mariello M, Es I, Proctor CM. Soft and flexible bioelectronic micro-systems for electronically controlled drug delivery. Adv Healthc Mater 2024;13(24):2302969.
[47] Huang Y, et al. Implantable electronic medicine enabled by bioresorbable microneedles for wireless electrotherapy and drug delivery. Nano Lett 2022;22(14):5944–53.
[48] Beg S, et al. 3D printing for drug delivery and biomedical applications. Drug Discov Today 2020;25(9):1668–81.
[49] Bácskay I, et al. The evolution of the 3D-printed drug delivery systems: a review. Pharmaceutics 2022;14(7):1312.
[50] Misra SK, et al. 3D-printed multidrug-eluting stent from graphene-nanoplatelet-doped biodegradable polymer composite. Adv Healthc Mater 2017;6(11):1700008.
[51] Patel A, et al. Polypills for the prevention of cardiovascular disease: a framework for wider use. Nat Med 2022;28(2):226–9.
[52] Alayoubi A, et al. Mechanistic understanding of the performance of personalized 3D-printed cardiovascular polypills: A case study of patient-centered therapy. Int J Pharm 2022;617:121599.
[53] Wang J, et al. Emerging 3D printing technologies for drug delivery devices: current status and future perspective. Adv Drug Deliv Rev 2021; 174:294–316.
[54] Mohammed AA, et al. 3D Printing in medicine: Technology overview and drug delivery applications. Ann 3D Print Med 2021;4:100037.
[55] Fisher A. The future is the present: artificial intelligence in pharmaceutical manufacturing. Pharm Technol 2023;47(9):32–4.
[56] Paul D, et al. Artificial intelligence in drug discovery and development. Drug Discov Today 2021;26(1):80–93.
[57] Arnold C. Inside the nascent industry of AI-designed drugs. Nat Med 2023;29(6):1292–5.
[58] Vora LK, et al. Artificial Intelligence in pharmaceutical technology and drug delivery design. Pharmaceutics 2023;15(7):1916.
[59] He S, Leanse LG, Feng Y. Artificial intelligence and machine learning assisted drug delivery for effective treatment of infectious diseases. Adv Drug Deliv Rev 2021;178:113922.
[60] Nemati P, et al. Artificial neural networks for bilateral prediction of formulation parameters and drug release profiles from cochlear implant coatings fabricated as porous monolithic devices based on silicone rubber. J Pharm Pharmacol 2013;66(5):624–38.
[61] Hsueh HT, et al. Machine learning-driven multifunctional peptide engineering for sustained ocular drug delivery. Nat Commun 2023;14(1): 2509.
[62] Singh S, et al. Advances in artificial intelligence (AI)-assisted approaches in drug screening. Artif Intell Chem 2024;2(1):100039.
[63] Tran TTV, Tayara H, Chong KT. Artificial intelligence in drug metabolism and excretion prediction: recent advances, challenges, and future perspectives. Pharmaceutics 2023;15(4):1260.
[64] Šícho M, et al. FAME 3: predicting the sites of metabolism in synthetic compounds and natural products for phase 1 and phase 2 metabolic enzymes. J Chem Inf Model 2019;59(8):3400–12.
[65] Stork C, et al. NERDD: a web portal providing access to in silico tools for drug discovery. Bioinformatics 2019;36(4):1291–2.
[66] New E-Resource for Drug Discovery. About FAME 3. Available from: https://nerdd.univie.ac.at/fame3/about/.
[67] Najjar A, Karaman R. The prodrug approach in the era of drug design. Expet Opin Drug Deliv 2019;16(1):1–5.
[68] Barzkar N, et al. Marine bacterial esterases: emerging biocatalysts for industrial applications. Appl Biochem Biotechnol 2021;193(4):1187–214.
[69] de Bruyn Kops C, et al. GLORYx: prediction of the metabolites resulting from phase 1 and phase 2 biotransformations of xenobiotics. Chem Res Toxicol 2021;34(2):286–99.
[70] New E-Resource for Drug Discovery. About GLORYx. Available from: https://nerdd.univie.ac.at/gloryx/about/.

CHAPTER

16

Commercialization of controlled release products

Wujie Zhang

LEARNING OBJECTIVES

- To understand and implement the quality by design process
- To understand and describe the approval process of a controlled-release product
- To understand and explain the approaches of the Food and Drug Administration to making the drugs that treat serious diseases available as rapidly as possible
- To understand the differences between recalls, market withdrawals, and safety alerts

16.1 Implementation of quality by design, design of experiments, and process analytical technology

FDA defines quality as the suitability of either a drug substance or a drug product for its intended use (includes such attributes as identity, strength, and purity). Quality by design (QbD) is a systematic approach to development that begins with predefined objectives and emphasizes product and process understanding and process control, based on sound science and quality risk management [1]. Similarly, the European Medicines Agency (EMA) defines QbD as an approach that aims to ensure the quality of medicines by employing statistical, analytical and risk-management methodology in the design, development, and manufacturing of medicines [2].

QbD is one of the key elements of different pharmaceutical developments [3]. Fig. 16.1 shows a typical QbD scheme with QbD elements. Quality target product profile (QTPP) is a prospective summary of the quality characteristics of a drug product that ideally will be achieved to ensure the desired quality (e.g., delivery systems, drug release, and dosage strength[s]), taking into account safety and efficacy of the drug product. Critical quality attribute (CQA) is a physical, chemical, biological, or microbiological property or characteristic of an *output* material (intermediate or finished pharmaceutical product) that should be within an appropriate limit, range, or distribution to ensure the desired product quality. Critical material attributes (CMAs) include physical, chemical, biological, or microbiological properties or characteristics of an *input* material. Critical process parameters (CPPs) are controlled or monitored parameters, such as speed and temperature, whose variability significantly influences product quality [1,2,4–6]. Pharmaceutical products are frequently manufactured through a combination of unit operations. It is critical to perform the process evaluation on each unit operation or a combination of unit operations to determine CQAs,

Fundamentals and Design of Drug Delivery Systems
https://doi.org/10.1016/B978-0-443-23521-4.00016-3

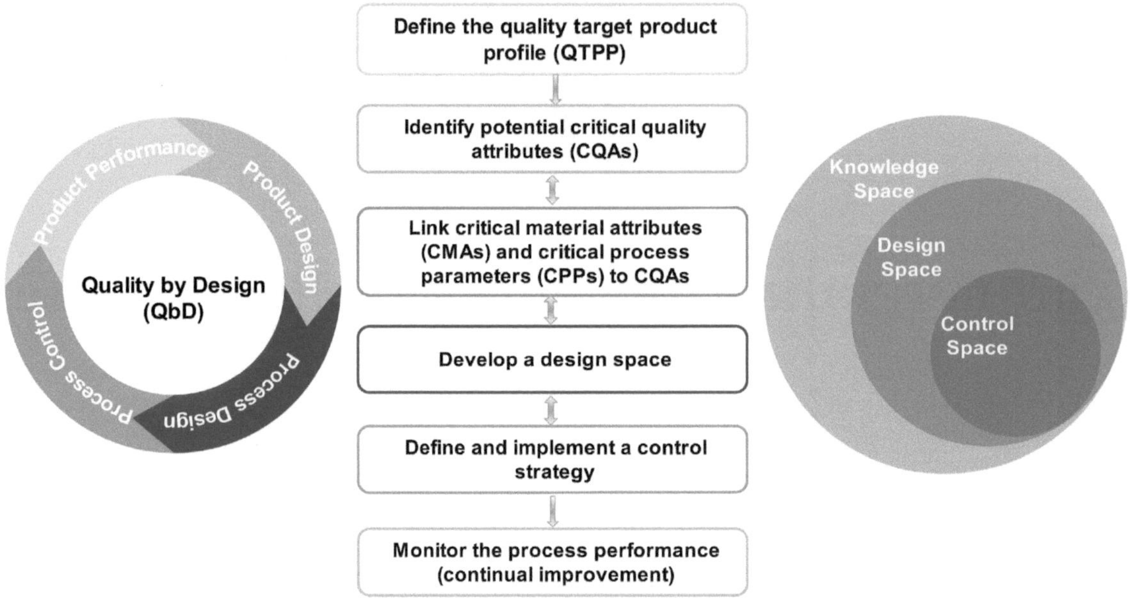

FIGURE 16.1 A typical quality by design scheme.

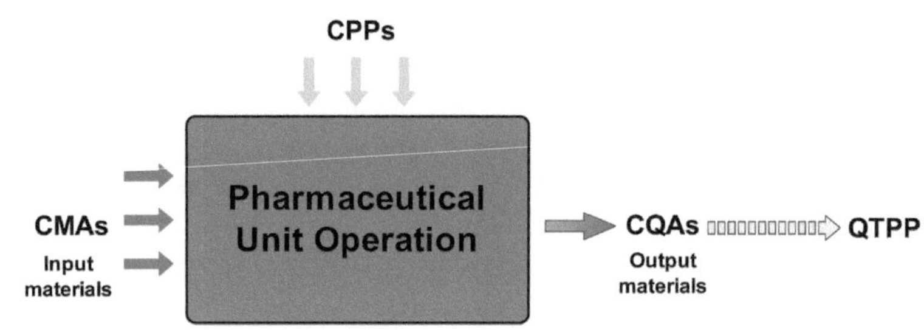

FIGURE. 16.2 Linking CMAs and CPPs to CQAs for a unit operation. *CMAs*, Critical material attributes; *CPPs*, critical process parameters, CQAs: critical quality attributes; *QTPP*, quality target product profile.

CMAs, and CPPs and link CMAs and CPPs to CQAs: CQAs = f (CMA_1, CMA_2, CMA_3, … CPP_1, CPP_2, CPP_3 …) (Fig. 16.2) [5]. Ishikawa (fishbone) diagrams can be used to identify potential variables that can have an impact on the desired quality attribute (Fig. 16.3).

Design space is the multidimensional combination and interaction of input variables (e.g., material attributes) and process parameters that have been demonstrated to provide assurance of quality. Design space is proposed by the applicant and is subject to regulatory assessment and approval. Parameter movements out of the design space would normally trigger a regulatory post–approval change process [1]. Design space may be scale and equipment dependent and justifications may be necessary such as due to scale-up (from laboratory to commercial scale) [5]. In simpler terms, design space is specific to a unit operation or a single manufacturing process and defines input variables and operating process parameters that are known to affect product quality and can be thought of as target settings for process development [7,8]. It can be described in terms of ranges of material attributes and process parameters, or through more complex mathematical relationships. It can also be described as a time-dependent function or as a combination of variables such as components of a multivariate model [1].

Design of experiments (DoE) is a tool for determining the relationship between the inputs and outputs of a process, which can help identify optimal conditions, CMAs, CPPs, and design space [4]. DoE can assist in the understanding of not only the effects of various factors but also the interactions among them [8]. The DoE methods that are commonly used to develop novel drug delivery systems include screening design (e.g., fractional factorial design) for identification of the potential significant variables through the use of a reduced number of experiments and *response surface methodology* (RSM) for subsequent identification of the critical level(s) of the most important

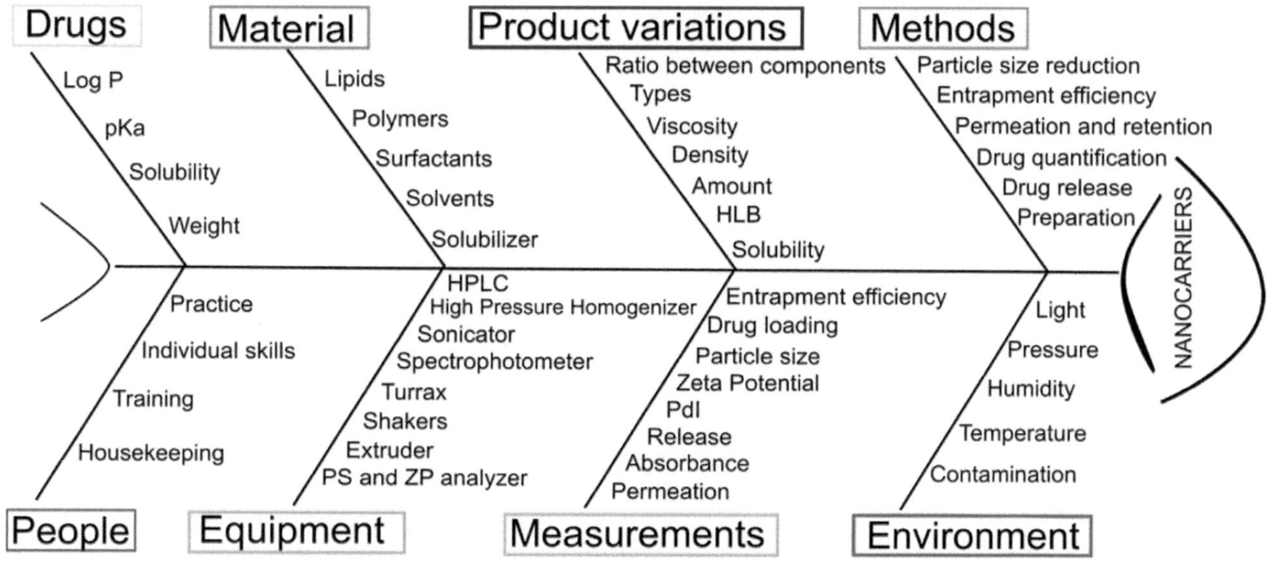

FIGURE. 16.3 Ishikawa diagram showing the main critical material attributes and critical process parameters that influence the critical quality attributes of drug nanocarriers. *From Tavares Luiz, M. et al.,* Design of experiments (DoE) to develop and to optimize nanoparticles as drug delivery systems. *Eur. J. Pharm. Biopharm, 2021.* ***165****: p. 127-148, with permission from Elsevier.*

factors and process optimization [9]. RSM is a statistical technique for modeling responses (response is a measurable product or process characteristic thought to be affected by experimental factors) *via* polynomial equations [10]. Box-Behnken design (BBD) is a commonly used RSM method in the pharmaceutical field. It relies on the combination of low, medium, and high levels (i.e., settings) of variables and requires a relatively small number of experimental runs, avoiding corner and star points (extreme combinations) [10]. Each factor has three levels, which are coded as +1, 0, and −1 and the total number of runs can be calculated using $2k(k-1)+C_0$ (k is the number of factors and C_0 is the center point [code 0 for all the factors]) (Fig. 16.4). For example, for a three-factor design with three center points, the total number of runs is 15 (Table 16.1). Usually, a second-order model is used in RSM:

$$Y=\beta_0+\sum_{i=1}^{k}(\beta_i X_i)+\sum_{i=1}^{k}(\beta_i X_i^2)+\sum_{i=1}^{k-1}\sum_{j>i}^{k}\left(\beta_{ij}X_iX_j\right),$$

where Y is the value of the response variable, β_0 is the intercept coefficient, the first β_i items are the linear coefficients, the second β_i items are the quadratic coefficients, and β_{ij} items are the coefficients of the interaction terms [11]. There are professional software such as Stat-Ease's Design Expert specifically designed for DoE.

Let's look at one example [12]. When producing a pectin-based hydrogel microsphere system for targeted pulmonary delivery using electrospray, four factors were identified: pectin percentage (70% to 90%), voltage (9 to 20 kV), flow rate (0.5 to 1.4 mL/h), and distance between the needle tip and aluminum foil sheet (5 to 20 cm). Take the pectin percentage for example; codes, 1, 0, and +1, represent 70%, 80%, and 90%, respectively. Using BBD, only 25 runs were necessary instead of 81 (4 factors and 3 levels; $3^4=81$). The two responses were size and morphology (quantified) (Fig. 16.5). Using Design Expert, the following equations were returned after inputting the actual experiment results:

$$Y_1=3.92-0.6923A-0.6302BD-0.6587B^2-2.08C^2-0.8762D^2$$

$$Y_2=4.54+1.75BD-1.75A^2+4.38C^2,$$

where Y_1 is size and Y_2 is morphology (uniformity). A, B, C, and D are the independent variables: pectin percentage, voltage, distance, and flow rate, separately. Both equations had high F values (8.11 and 16.46) and low p values (0.0003 and <0.0001), indicating both equations (models) were significant. The F value is the ratio of the model mean square to the appropriate mean square. The larger their ratio, the larger is the F value and the more likely that the variance contributed by the model is significantly larger than the random error. A low p value indicates the low probability that a large F value would occur due to noise [12,13]. Fig. 16.6 shows the impacts of the most significant interaction on microsphere size and uniformity.

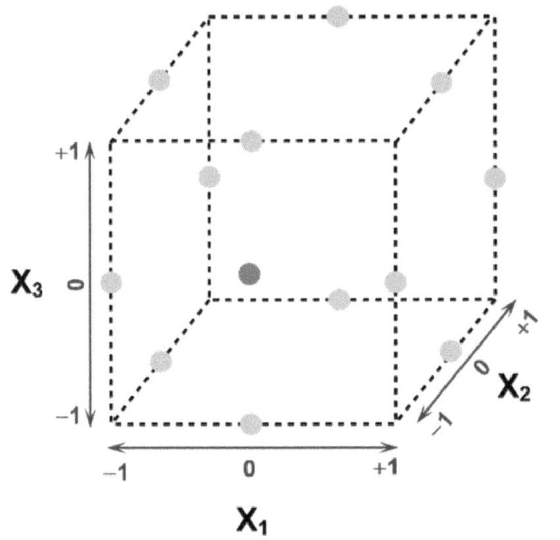

FIGURE. 16.4 Three-factor ($k = 3$) Box-Behnken design (BBD). *Yellow*, design points; *orange*, center point.

TABLE 16.1 Three-factor ($k = 3$) Box-Behnken design with three center points.

	Factor		
Run	X_1	X_2	X_3
1	+1	+1	0
2	+1	−1	0
3	−1	+1	0
4	−1	−1	0
5	+1	0	+1
6	+1	0	−1
7	−1	0	+1
8	−1	0	−1
9	0	+1	+1
10	0	+1	−1
11	0	−1	+1
12	0	−1	−1
13	0	0	0
14	0	0	0
15	0	0	0

Control strategy is a planned set of controls, derived from current product and process understanding that ensures performance and product quality. The controls can include parameters and attributes related to drug substance and drug product materials and components, facility and equipment operating conditions, in-process controls, finished product specifications, and the associated methods and frequency of monitoring and control [1]. There are three levels of control strategy: real-time automatic control plus flexible process parameters to respond to variability in the input material attributes (level 1), reduced end product testing plus flexible critical material attributes and critical process parameters within design space (level 2), and end product testing plus tightly constrained material attributes and process parameters (level 3). In practice, a hybrid approach combining levels 1 and 2 can be used [5]. The control strategy in QbD revolves around defining the process capability and CQA and is created to ensure the process is following the desired trajectory and that product quality consistently meets predefined specifications. Once the control strategy has been defined and implemented, appropriate monitoring of product quality needs to be performed to demonstrate that the designed process is capable of consistently delivering products of acceptable quality [8].

The application of process analytical technology (PAT) may be part of the control strategy to ensure the process remains within an established design space [5]. PAT is a system for designing, analyzing, and controlling manufacturing through timely measurements (i.e., during processing) of critical quality and performance attributes

Run	Factor 1 A:percent pectin 1	Factor 2 B:voltage kV	Factor 3 C:distance cm	Factor 4 D:flow rate mL/hr	Response 1 size micrometer	Response 2 morphology 1
1	70	14.5	12.5	1.4	5.429	1
2	70	14.5	5	0.95	1.389	9
3	80	9	12.5	1.4	1.478	8
4	80	14.5	20	0.5	1.256	8
5	70	14.5	20	0.95	1.374	8
6	90	9	12.5	0.95	3.124	3
7	90	20	12.5	0.95	2.143	1.5
8	80	9	20	0.95	1.404	9
9	80	20	20	0.95	1.415	8
10	90	14.5	5	0.95	1.472	9
11	80	20	12.5	0.5	3.578	1
12	90	14.5	12.5	0.5	1.262	6
13	90	14.5	20	0.95	1.337	8
14	80	20	12.5	1.4	1.367	8
15	70	14.5	12.5	0.5	3.47	1.5
16	80	9	5	0.95	1.39	8
17	80	14.5	12.5	0.95	3.743	3
18	80	20	5	0.95	1.284	9
19	70	20	12.5	0.95	3.626	1
20	90	14.5	12.5	1.4	2.978	2
21	70	9	12.5	0.95	5.336	1
22	80	14.5	5	0.5	1.174	8
23	80	14.5	5	1.4	1.236	8
24	80	9	12.5	0.5	1.168	8
25	80	14.5	20	1.4	1.177	8

FIGURE. 16.5 Screenshot of the experiment design and the results (recorded as two responses) using Design Expert.

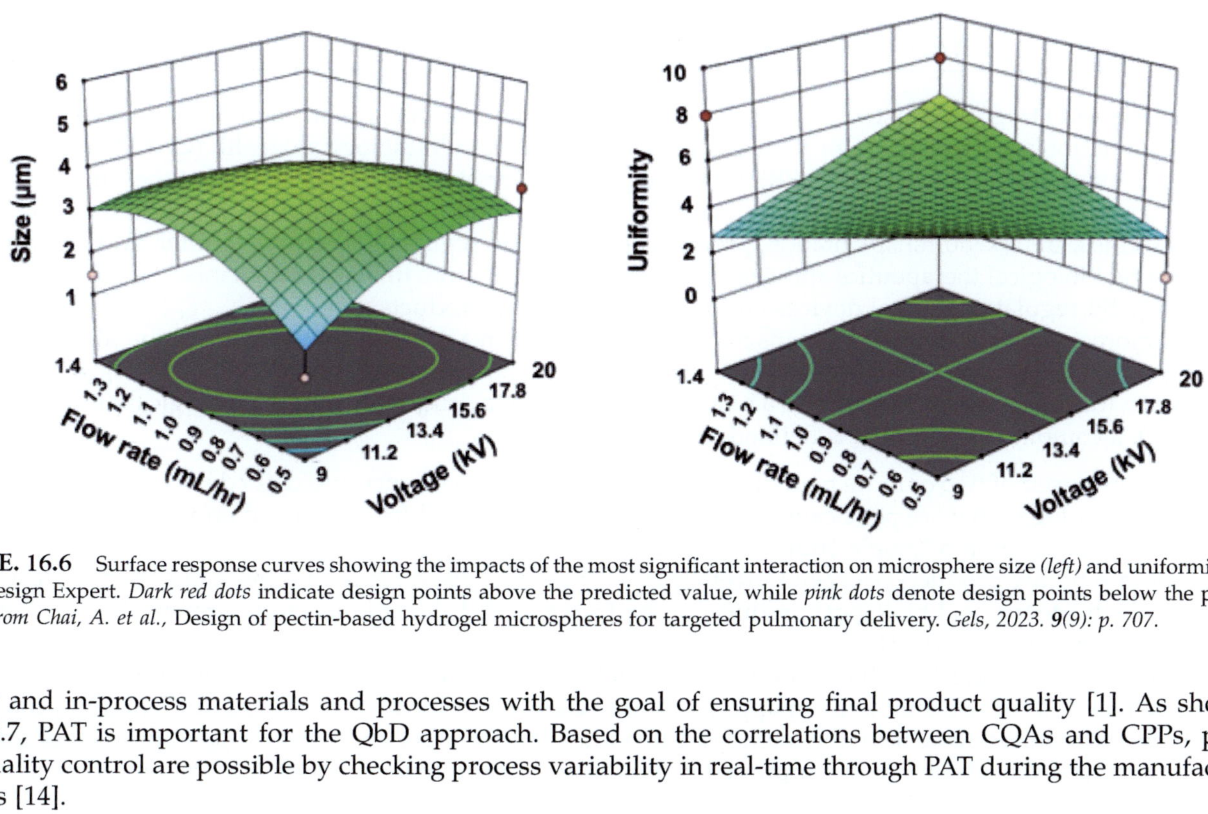

FIGURE. 16.6 Surface response curves showing the impacts of the most significant interaction on microsphere size *(left)* and uniformity *(right)* using Design Expert. *Dark red dots* indicate design points above the predicted value, while *pink dots* denote design points below the predicted value. *From Chai, A. et al.,* Design of pectin-based hydrogel microspheres for targeted pulmonary delivery. *Gels, 2023.* ***9****(9): p. 707.*

of raw and in-process materials and processes with the goal of ensuring final product quality [1]. As shown in Fig. 16.7, PAT is important for the QbD approach. Based on the correlations between CQAs and CPPs, process and quality control are possible by checking process variability in real-time through PAT during the manufacturing process [14].

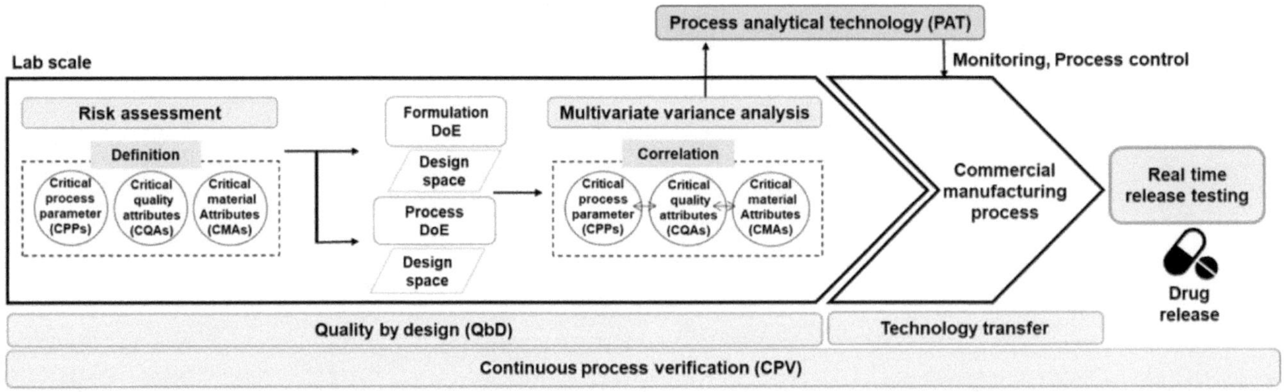

FIGURE. 16.7 Framework of process analytical technology (PAT) application in quality by design (QbD) approach. *DoE*, Design of experiments. *Adapted from Kim, E.J. et al.,* Process analytical technology tools for monitoring pharmaceutical unit operations: a control strategy for continuous process verification. *Pharmaceutics, 2021.* ***13****(6): p. 919.*

There are four key categories of PAT tools [15]:

(1) multivariate tools for design, data acquisition, and analysis;
(2) process analyzers;
(3) process control tools; and
(4) continuous improvement and knowledge management tools.

Simply, PAT tools are just one set of analytical techniques to consider when determining which analytics are appropriate for process and product understanding, monitoring, and control. Temperature, pressure, and flow measurements are not often considered PAT tools as these measurements have been routinely made for decades. Spectroscopic tools (e.g., near-infrared and Raman) are used for analytical specificity, and techniques such as chromatography and mass spectrometry have been used for process monitoring [16].

16.2 New drug development and approval process

The U.S. Food and Drug Administration (FDA) consists of nine center-level organizations including the Center for Biologicals Evaluation and Research (CBER), the Center for Devices and Radiological Health (CDRH), and the Center for Drug Evaluation and Research (CDER). CBER regulates a variety of different product types, including biologics such as allergenics, blood and blood products, cellular and gene therapies, tissue and tissue-based products, vaccines, and xenotransplantation products [17]. CDER regulates over-the-counter and prescription drugs, including biological therapeutics and generic drugs (drugs are more than just medicines; e.g., fluoride toothpaste) [18]. CDRH regulates medical devices and radiation-emitting products.

More and more novel drug delivery systems may contain more than a drug (drugs), that is, combination products. According to the FDA [19], a combination product is a product composed of any combination of a drug and a device; a biological product and a device; a drug and a biological product; or a drug, device, and a biological product. Under 21 CFR 3.2 (e), a combination product is defined to include:

1. A product comprised of two or more regulated components (i.e., drug/device, biologic/device, drug/biologic, or drug/device/biologic) that are physically, chemically, or otherwise combined or mixed and produced as a single entity [often referred to as a "single-entity" combination product];
2. Two or more separate products packaged together in a single package or as a unit and comprised of drug and device products, device and biological products, or biological and drug products [often referred to as a "co-packaged" combination product];
3. A drug, device, or biological product packaged separately that according to its investigational plan or proposed labeling is intended for use only with an approved individually specified drug, device, or biological product where both are required to achieve the intended use, indication, or effect and where, upon approval of the proposed product, the labeling of the approved product would need to be changed (e.g., to reflect a change in

intended use, dosage form, strength, route of administration, or significant change in dose) [often referred to as a "cross-labeled" combination product]; or

4. Any investigational drug, device, or biological product packaged separately that according to its proposed labeling is for use only with another individually specified investigational drug, device, or biological product where both are required to achieve the intended use, indication, or effect [another type of "cross-labeled" combination product].

The Office of Combination Products was established on December 24, 2004. One of its roles is to classify medical products as drugs, devices, biological products, or combination products and assign them to an FDA center for premarket review and regulation, particularly in cases where the product classification or assignment is unclear or in dispute [19,20]. It is highly encouraged for a sponsor to reach out to the FDA regarding the regulatory identity or classification of a product as a drug, device, biological product, or combination product, as the requirements and approval processes differ based on the product classification.

Here, let's start with the drug development and approval process. As shown in Fig. 16.8, there are five steps: discovery and development, preclinical research, clinical research, FDA review, and FDA postmarket safety monitoring [21]. When a drug is ready for clinical study, the drug's sponsor has to file an investigation new drug application (IND) with the FDA. All IND applications require three basic categories of information: data regarding preclinical animal and toxicological studies and any previous human experience with the drug, manufacturing information, and the clinical protocols for the study. There are three different types of IND applications: investigator IND, emergency use investigational new drug (EIND), and treatment IND [22]. The FDA review team has 30 days to review the original IND submission. While a clinical hold is rare, in most cases, the applicant is allowed to proceed with the proposed study if FDA is satisfied that the trial meets federal standards [23]. As shown in Table 16.2, there are different phases of clinical trials [22,23]. Phase 0 (exploratory) clinical trials represent the earliest, first-in-man use

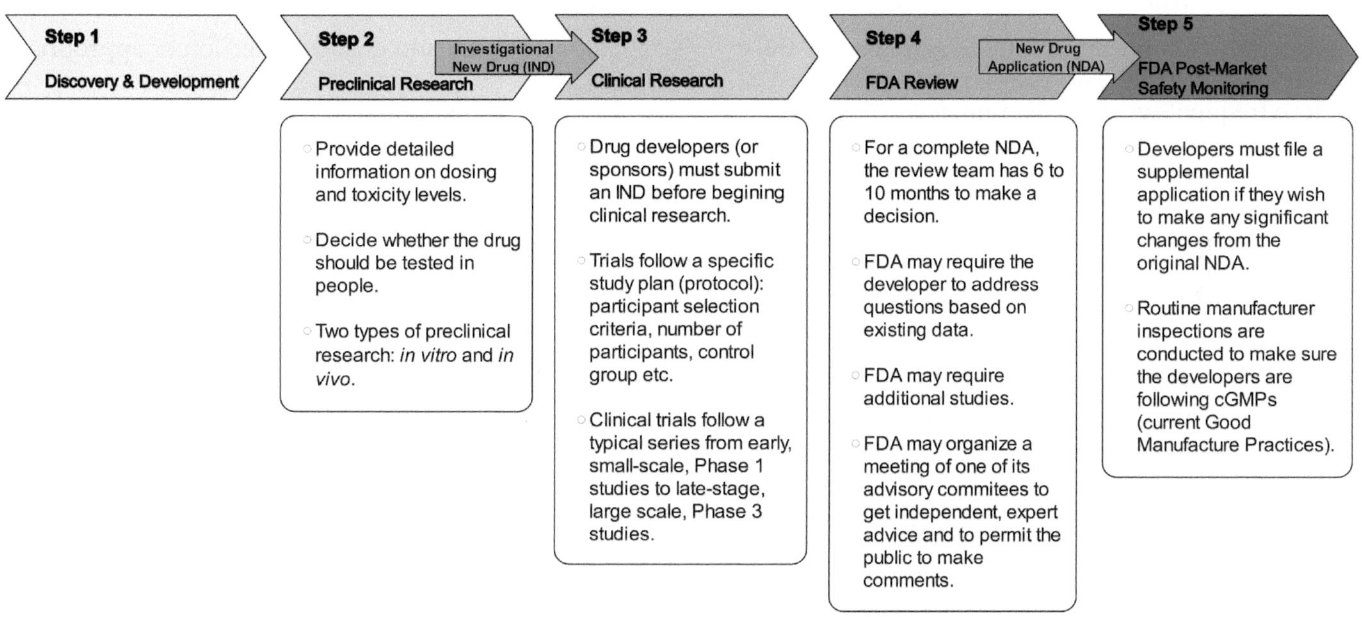

FIGURE. 16.8 FDA's drug development and approval process.

TABLE 16.2 Different phases of clinical trials.

Phase	Number of participants	Length	Purpose	Percentage of drugs move to the next phase
1	20-100	Several months	Safety and dosage	~ 70%
2	Several hundreds	Several months to 2 years	Efficacy and side effects	~ 33%
3	300-3000	1-4 years	Efficacy and monitoring of adverse reactions	~ 25% to 30%
4	Several thousands		Safety and efficacy	

of a proposed drug therapy and are conducted before the traditional dose escalation, safety, and tolerance studies that ordinarily initiate a clinical drug development program (with limited duration of dosing and no therapeutic and diagnostic intent). Phase 0 clinical trials require submission of an exploratory IND followed by a full IND [22,24]. Phase 4 trials are carried out once the drug has been approved by the FDA during the postmarket safety monitoring [23]. However, there is concern regarding the small sample size for phase 4 trials with safety surveillance as a main task [25].

Moreover, the FDA has developed four distinct and successful approaches to making the drugs that treat serious diseases (e.g., AIDS, Alzheimer, heart failure, and cancer) available as rapidly as possible: priority review, breakthrough therapy, accelerated approval, and fast track [26]. However, there are concerns with the global consequences of the accelerated approval of drugs. For example, most cancer drugs granted accelerated approval did not demonstrate benefit in overall survival or quality of life within 5 years of accelerated approval [27,28]. In 2023, the FDA issued draft guidance offering several possible solutions to improve oncology clinical trials for accelerated approval but these might also have limitations [29,30].

Fast track. Fast track is a process designed to facilitate the development and expedite the review of drugs to treat serious conditions and fill an unmet medical need. Filling an unmet medical need is defined as providing a therapy where none exists or providing a therapy that may be potentially better than available therapy. If there are available therapies, a fast-track drug must show some advantage over available therapy, such as:

- Showing superior effectiveness, effect on serious outcomes, or improved effect on serious outcomes
- Avoiding serious side effects of an available therapy
- Improving the diagnosis of a serious condition where early diagnosis results in an improved outcome
- Decreasing a clinically significant toxicity of an available therapy that is common and causes discontinuation of treatment
- Ability to address emerging or anticipated public health need

A drug that receives *fast track* designation is eligible for some or all of the following:

- More frequent meetings with FDA to discuss the drug's development plan and ensure collection of appropriate data needed to support drug approval
- More frequent written communication from FDA about such things as the design of the proposed clinical trials and use of biomarkers
- Eligibility for *accelerated approval and priority review*, if relevant criteria are met
- *Rolling review*, which means that a drug company can submit completed sections of its Biologic License Application (BLA) or New Drug Application (NDA) for review by FDA, rather than waiting until every section of the NDA is completed before the entire application can be reviewed. BLA or NDA review usually does not begin until the drug company has submitted the entire application to the FDA

Fast track designation must be requested by the drug company. The request can be initiated at any time during the drug development process. The FDA will review the request and make a decision within sixty days based on whether the drug fills an unmet medical need in a serious condition [31].

Breakthrough therapy. Breakthrough therapy designation is a process designed to expedite the development and review of drugs that are intended to treat a serious condition and preliminary clinical evidence indicates that the drug may demonstrate substantial improvement over available therapy on a clinically significant endpoint(s). To determine whether the improvement over available therapy is substantial is a matter of judgment and depends on both the magnitude of the treatment effect, which could include the duration of the effect and the importance of the observed clinical outcome. In general, the preliminary clinical evidence should show a clear advantage over available therapy. For purposes of breakthrough therapy designation, a clinically significant endpoint generally refers to an endpoint that measures an effect on irreversible morbidity or mortality (IMM) or on symptoms that represent serious consequences of the disease. A clinically significant endpoint can also refer to findings that suggest an effect on IMM or serious symptoms, including:

- An effect on an established surrogate endpoint
- An effect on a surrogate endpoint or intermediate clinical endpoint considered reasonably likely to predict a clinical benefit (i.e., the accelerated approval standard)
- An effect on a pharmacodynamic biomarker(s) that does not meet criteria for an acceptable surrogate endpoint, but strongly suggests the potential for a clinically meaningful effect on the underlying disease

- A significantly improved safety profile compared to available therapy (e.g., less dose-limiting toxicity for an oncology agent), with evidence of similar efficacy

A drug that receives *breakthrough therapy* designation is eligible for all fast-track designation features. *Breakthrough therapy* designation is requested by the drug company. Ideally, a breakthrough therapy designation request should be received by the FDA no later than the end-of-phase-2 meetings if any of the features of the designation are to be obtained. The FDA will respond to breakthrough therapy designation requests within 60 days of receipt of the request [32].

Accelerated approval. In 1992, the FDA instituted the *accelerated approval* regulations. These regulations allowed drugs for serious conditions that filled an unmet medical need to be approved based on a surrogate endpoint. Using a surrogate endpoint enabled the FDA to approve these drugs faster. In 2012, Congress passed the Food and Drug Administration Safety Innovations Act (FDASIA). Section 901 of FDASIA amends the Federal Food, Drug, and Cosmetic Act (FD&C Act) to allow the FDA to base accelerated approval for drugs for serious conditions that fill an unmet medical need on whether the drug has an effect on a surrogate or an intermediate clinical endpoint. A surrogate endpoint used for accelerated approval is a marker—a laboratory measurement, radiographic image, physical sign or other measure that is thought to predict clinical benefit—but is not itself a measure of clinical benefit. Likewise, an intermediate clinical endpoint is a measure of a therapeutic effect that is considered reasonably likely to predict the clinical benefit of a drug, such as an effect on irreversible morbidity and mortality [33].

Priority review. In 1992, under the Prescription Drug User Fee Act (PDUFA), the FDA agreed to specific goals for improving the drug review time and created a two-tiered system of review times – *standard review* and *priority review.* A *priority review* designation means the FDA's goal is to take action on an application within 6 months (compared to 10 months under standard review). A *priority review* designation will direct overall attention and resources to the evaluation of applications for drugs that, if approved, would be significant improvements in the safety or effectiveness of the treatment, diagnosis, or prevention of serious conditions when compared to standard applications. The FDA decides on the review designation for every application. However, an applicant may expressly request priority review as described in the Guidance for Industry Expedited Programs for Serious Conditions – Drugs and Biologics. It does not affect the length of the clinical trial period. The FDA informs the applicant of a Priority Review designation within 60 days of the receipt of the original BLA, NDA, or efficacy supplement. Designation of a drug as "Priority" does not alter the scientific/medical standard for approval or the quality of evidence necessary [34].

Additionally, the Orphan Drug Act (ODA) was enacted in 1983 to stimulate the development of drugs and biologics for rare diseases or conditions. The ODA primarily defined a rare disease or condition as one that affects fewer than 200,000 people in the United States [35]. The FDA has authority to grant *orphan drug* designation to a drug or biological product to prevent, diagnose or treat a rare disease or condition. Sponsors seeking *orphan drug* designation for a drug must submit a request for designation to the agency. Sponsors requesting designation of the same drug for the same rare disease or condition as a previously designated product must submit their own data and information to support their designation request. *Orphan drug* designation is a separate process from seeking approval or licensing. Drugs for rare diseases go through the same rigorous scientific review process as any other drug for approval or licensing [36]. Recent analysis has shown a dramatic rise in overall orphan designations leading to an increased number of approvals for drugs and biologics designed specifically for diagnosing, preventing, and treating rare diseases with the top three therapeutic areas being oncology, neurology, and infectious diseases [37].

Regarding the device development process, there are also five steps: device discovery and concept, preclinical research-prototype, pathway to approval, FDA review, and FDA post-market safety monitoring. Under the risk-based device classification system for medical devices, Class I (low risk of illness or injury) devices are mostly exempted from premarket submission [38]. Most Class II (moderate risk) devices undergo a premarket notification process (PMN; 501[k]), which does not require stringent clinical evidence. Class III (significant risk) devices mostly require premarket approval (PMA). However, if a Class III device only has minor changes from an already approved device (i.e., predicate) and it is generally approved through the PMN process. Generally, Level I or II evidence is required to obtain FDA approval of most new Class III devices (an investigational device exemption (IDE) is required for premarket clinical trials). Most new devices that do not have predicates and are automatically placed as Class III have to go through the PMA process. However, a sponsor can submit 513(g) application to reclassify the device if it is of low to moderate risk (i.e., *de novo* device). Last, the humanitarian device exemption (HED) is for humanitarian use devices (HUD) which are expected to treat or diagnose conditions that affect fewer than 4,000 individuals in the United States annually [39]. The FDA medical device approval pathway is summarized in Fig. 16.9.

When it comes to biologics, a biologics license application (BLA) is required for biological products subject to licensure under the Public Health Service (PHS) Act. There are many similarities between NDA and BLA.

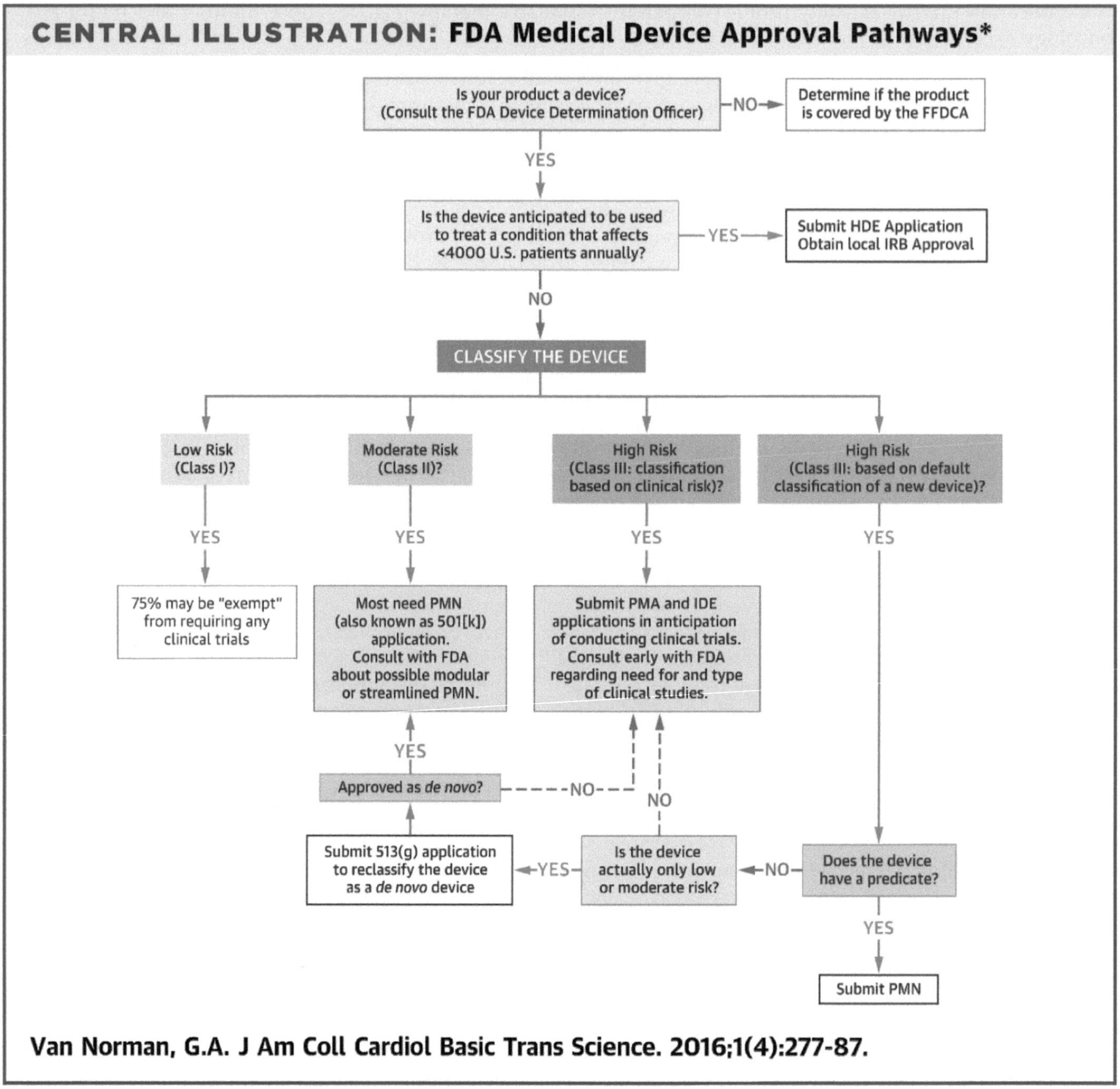

FIGURE. 16.9 FDA's medical device approval pathway. *Adapted from Van Norman, G.A.,* Drugs, devices, and the FDA: Part 2: an overview of approval processes: FDA approval of medical devices. *JACC: Basic to Translational Science, 2016.* **1***(4): p. 277-287, with permission from Elsevier.*

However, BLAs (the majority of submissions are assigned to CBER) have more regulations related to the manufacturing facility [40].

Now, let's examine the drug and device approval processes in the European Union (EU). Similar to those of the FDA, clinical trials require pre-authorization (from one or more states of the EU) for the use of the drug and progress through sequential studies. Upon clinical trials, there are four pathways for drug approval: centralized process (controlled through the European Medicines Agency (EMA); for designated drugs [41]), national process (a single EU state), mutual recognition (approved in one EU state and obtain marketing authorization in another EU member state), and decentralized procedure (simultaneous application in multiple EU states) [42]. Regarding medical devices, with the adoption of the EU Medical Device Regulation (MDR; which took effect in May 2021), EU regulations are much closer match to those of the FDA. Under MDR, there are five classes of devices (from low to high risks): I (nonsterile or no measuring function), I (sterile and a measuring function), IIa, IIb, and III. Class IIb and III devices require extensive technical documentation and risk evaluation during the conformity assessments with notified bodies (organizations designated by EU countries to assess the conformity of certain products before they can be placed on the market) involving at least two audits [43,44].

16.3 Recalls, market withdrawals, and safety alerts

According to the FDA [45], recalls are actions taken by a firm to remove a product from the market, which may be conducted on a firm's own initiative, by FDA request, or by FDA order under statutory authority. Based on the likelihood and severity of the adverse health consequences, there are classes (I, II, and III) of recall. Class I recall is a situation in which there is a reasonable probability that the use of or exposure to a violative product will cause serious adverse health consequences or death; while Class III recall describes a situation in which use or exposure to a violative product is not likely to cause adverse health consequences. FDA's role in a recall is to oversee a company's recall strategy, assess the adequacy of the company's action and classify the recall [46]. Market withdrawal occurs when a product has a minor violation that would not be subject to FDA legal action, such as tampering without evidence of manufacturing or distribution problems. The firm removes the product from the market or corrects the violation. A medical device safety alert is issued in situations where a medical device may present an unreasonable risk of substantial harm. Recalls, market withdrawals, and safety alerts can be accessed at https://www.fda.gov/safety/recalls-market-withdrawals-safety-alerts and https://datadashboard.fda.gov/ora/cd/recalls.htm. Additionally, there is *MedWatch*, which is the FDA's medical product safety reporting program for health professionals. Among all the recall product types, the devices category has the highest number of recall events (Fig. 16.10) [47].

Similarly, the EU's European Medicines Agency [48,49] has a classification of recalls with regard to the relative health hazard associated with the use of or exposure to the recalled (defective medicinal; i.e., not of the correct quality) product with Class I defects that are potentially life-threatening. The other two classes of defects could cause illnesses or mistreatment (Class II) or may not pose a significant hazard to health, but withdrawal may be initiated for other reasons (Class III).

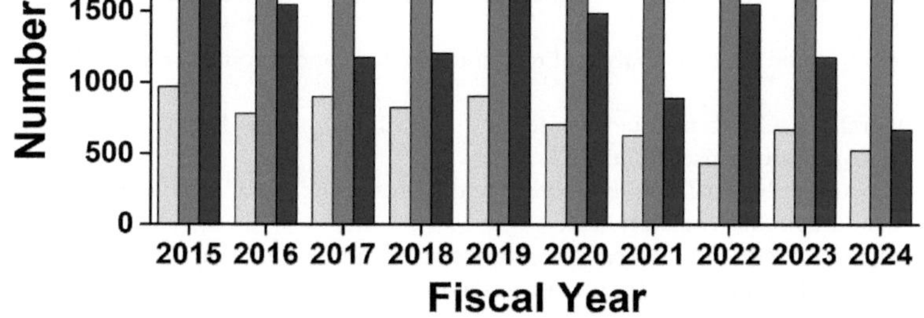

FIGURE. 16.10 Statistics of FDA recalls based on product types. *From FDA* Recalls. *Available from: https://datadashboard.fda.gov/ora/cd/recalls.htm.*

Review and practice questions

1. What is a typical QbD scheme?
2. What are CMAs, CPPs, and CPAs? And how are they linked?
3. Conduct a literature search and find one article with an Ishikawa (fishbone) diagram. Draw an Ishikawa diagram based on the information from the literature and compare it to the one within the literature.
4. What is a design space?
5. Based on the Box-Behnken model, what is the total number of runs for a four-factor design with 3 center points?
6. Show the list (like Table 16.1) of runs from question 5.
7. What is process analytical technology (PAT)? What are the four key categories of PAT tools?
8. What is a typical drug development and approval process?
9. Compare different phases of clinical trials.
10. What are fast track, breakthrough therapy, accelerated approval, and priority review?
11. What are the four drug approval pathways in the European Union?
12. Visit the FDA's recalls, withdrawals, and safety alerts website (https://www.fda.gov/safety/recalls-market-withdrawals-safety-alerts), and find one product that utilizes the engineered drug delivery approach.

References

[1] U.S. Food and Drug Administration. Guidance for industry Q8(R2) pharmaceutical development. Available from: https://www.fda.gov/media/71535/download.
[2] European Medicines Agency. Quality by design. Available from: https://www.ema.europa.eu/en/human-regulatory-overview/research-development/quality-design.
[3] Pallagi E, et al. New aspects of developing a dry powder inhalation formulation applying the quality-by-design approach. Int J Pharm 2016;511(1):151–60.
[4] Zhang L, Mao S. Application of quality by design in the current drug development. Asian J Pharm Sci 2017;12(1):1–8.
[5] Yu LX, et al. Understanding pharmaceutical quality by design. AAPS J 2014;16(4):771–83.
[6] Ter Horst JP, et al. Implementation of quality by design (QbD) principles in regulatory dossiers of medicinal products in the European Union (EU) between 2014 and 2019. Ther Innov Regul Sci 2021;55(3):583–90.
[7] Gurba-Bryśkiewicz L, et al. Quality by design (QbD) and design of experiments (DOE) as a strategy for tuning lipid nanoparticle formulations for RNA delivery. Biomedicines 2023;11(10):2752.
[8] Rathore AS. Quality by design (QbD)-based process development for purification of a biotherapeutic. Trends Biotechnol 2016;34(5):358–70.
[9] Tavares Luiz M, et al. Design of experiments (DoE) to develop and to optimize nanoparticles as drug delivery systems. Eur J Pharm Biopharm 2021;165:127–48.
[10] Mahmoud BS, McConville C. Box–Behnken design of experiments of polycaprolactone nanoparticles loaded with irinotecan hydrochloride. Pharmaceutics 2023;15(4):1271.
[11] Cherwin A, et al. Design of a novel oxygen therapeutic using polymeric hydrogel microcapsules mimicking red blood cells. Pharmaceutics 2019;11(11):583.
[12] Chai A, et al. Design of pectin-based hydrogel microspheres for targeted pulmonary delivery. Gels 2023;9(9):707.
[13] Anderson MJ, Whitcomb PJ. DOE simplified: practical Tools for effective experimentation. 3rd ed. Productivity Press; 2015.
[14] Kim EJ, et al. Process analytical technology tools for monitoring pharmaceutical unit operations: a control strategy for continuous process verification. Pharmaceutics 2021;13(6):919.
[15] U.S. Food and Drug Administration. Guidance for industry PAT — a framework for innovative pharmaceutical development, manufacturing, and quality assurance. Available from: https://www.fda.gov/media/71012/download#:~:text=The%20scientific%2C%20risk-based%20framework%20outlined%20in%20this%20guidance%2C,efficiency%20in%20pharmaceutical%20development%2C%20manufacturing%2C%20and%20quality%20assurance.
[16] Chanda A, et al. Industry perspectives on process analytical technology: tools and applications in API development. Org Process Res Dev 2015;19(1):63–83.
[17] U.S. Food and Drug Administration. CBER product jurisdiction. Available from: https://www.fda.gov/about-fda/center-biologics-evaluation-and-research-cber/cber-product-jurisdiction.
[18] U.S. Food and Drug Administration. Center for Drug Evaluation and Research (CDER). Available from: https://www.fda.gov/about-fda/fda-organization/center-drug-evaluation-and-research-cder.
[19] U.S. Food and Drug Administration. Frequently asked questions about combination products. Available from: https://www.fda.gov/combination-products/about-combination-products/frequently-asked-questions-about-combination-products#:~:text=What%20is%20a%20combination%20product%3F%20What%20are%20some,Products%20How%20are%20combination%20products%20assigned%20for%20review%3F.
[20] U.S. Food and Drug Administration. Office of combination products. Available from: https://www.fda.gov/about-fda/office-chief-medical-officer/office-combination-products.
[21] U.S. Food and Drug Administration. The drug development process. Available from: https://www.fda.gov/patients/learn-about-drug-and-device-approvals/drug-development-process#:~:text=Discovery%20and%20Development%20Research%20for%20a%20new%20drug,to%20make%20sure%20they%20are%20safe%20and%20effective.

[22] Van Norman GA. Drugs, devices, and the FDA: part 1: an overview of approval processes for drugs. JACC Basic Transl Sci 2016;1(3):170–9.
[23] U.S. Food and Drug Administration. Step 3: clinical research. Available from: https://www.fda.gov/patients/drug-development-process/step-3-clinical-research#:~:text=Before%20a%20clinical%20trial%20begins%2C%20researchers%20review%20prior,studies%20to%20late-stage%2C%20large%20scale%2C%20Phase%203%20studies.
[24] U.S. Food and Drug Administration. Exploratory IND studies. Available from: https://www.fda.gov/regulatory-information/search-fda-guidance-documents/exploratory-ind-studies.
[25] Xinji Z, et al. Overview of phase IV clinical trials for postmarket drug safety surveillance: a status report from the ClinicalTrials.gov registry. BMJ Open 2016;6(11):e010643.
[26] U.S. Food and drug administration. Fast track, breakthrough therapy, accelerated approval, priority review. Available from: https://www.fda.gov/patients/learn-about-drug-and-device-approvals/fast-track-breakthrough-therapy-accelerated-approval-priority-review.
[27] Akhade A, Sirohi B, Gyawali B. Global consequences of the US FDA's accelerated approval of cancer drugs. Lancet Oncol 2022;23(2):201–3.
[28] Liu ITT, Kesselheim AS, Cliff ERS. Clinical benefit and regulatory outcomes of cancer drugs receiving accelerated approval. JAMA 2024;331(17):1471–9.
[29] U.S. Food and Drug Administration. FDA issues draft guidance aimed at improving oncology clinical trials for accelerated approval. Available from: https://www.fda.gov/news-events/press-announcements/fda-issues-draft-guidance-aimed-improving-oncology-clinical-trials-accelerated-approval.
[30] Benjamin DJ, Lythgoe MP. The FDA's latest draft guidance on accelerated approvals — one step forward, two steps back? Nat Rev Clin Oncol 2023;20(9):577–8.
[31] U.S. Food and Drug Administration. Fast track. Available from: https://www.fda.gov/patients/fast-track-breakthrough-therapy-accelerated-approval-priority-review/fast-track#:~:text=Fast%20track%20is%20a%20process%20designed%20to%20facilitate,Track%20addresses%20a%20broad%20range%20of%20serious%20conditions.
[32] U.S. Food and Drug Administration. Breakthrough therapy. Available from: https://www.fda.gov/patients/fast-track-breakthrough-therapy-accelerated-approval-priority-review/breakthrough-therapy#:~:text=Breakthrough%20Therapy%20designation%20is%20a%20process%20designed%20to,improvement%20over%20available%20therapy%20on%20a%20clinically%20significan.
[33] U.S. Food and Drug Administration. Accelerated approval. Available from: https://www.fda.gov/drugs/nda-and-bla-approvals/accelerated-approval-program#:~:text=The%20FDA%20instituted%20its%20Accelerated%20Approval%20Program%20to,unmet%20medical%20need%20based%20on%20a%20surrogate%20endpoint.
[34] U.S. Food and Drug Administration. Priority review. Available from: https://www.fda.gov/patients/fast-track-breakthrough-therapy-accelerated-approval-priority-review/priority-review#:~:text=A%20Priority%20Review%20designation%20means%20FDA%E2%80%99s%20goal%20is,months%20%28compared%20to%2010%20months%20under%20standard%20review%29.
[35] Miller KL, et al. Drugs and biologics receiving FDA orphan drug designation: an analysis of the most frequently designated products and their repositioning strategies. Expert Opin Orphan Drugs 2021;9(11–12):265–72.
[36] U.S. Food and Drug Administration. Designating an orphan product: drugs and biological products. Available from: https://www.fda.gov/industry/medical-products-rare-diseases-and-conditions/designating-orphan-product-drugs-and-biological-products#:~:text=Supporting%20the%20development%20and%20evaluation%20of%20new%20treatments,diagnose%20or%20treat%20a%20rare%20disease%20or%20condition.
[37] Miller KL, Fermaglich LJ, Maynard J. Using four decades of FDA orphan drug designations to describe trends in rare disease drug development: substantial growth seen in development of drugs for rare oncologic, neurologic, and pediatric-onset diseases. Orphanet J Rare Dis 2021;16(1):265.
[38] U.S. Food and Drug Administration. The device development process. Available from: https://www.fda.gov/patients/learn-about-drug-and-device-approvals/device-development-process.
[39] Van Norman GA. Drugs, Devices, and the FDA: Part 2: an overview of approval processes: fda approval of medical devices. JACC Basic Transl Sci 2016;1(4):277–87.
[40] U.S. Food and Drug Administration. Types of applications. Available from: https://www.fda.gov/drugs/how-drugs-are-developed-and-approved/types-applications.
[41] European Medicines Agency. Authorisation of medicines. Available from: https://www.ema.europa.eu/en/about-us/what-we-do/authorisation-medicines.
[42] Van Norman GA. Drugs and devices: comparison of European and U.S. approval processes. JACC Basic Transl Sci 2016;1(5):399–412.
[43] Celegence. FDA vs EU MDR – medical device approvals. Available from: https://www.celegence.com/medical-device-approvals-fda-vs-eu-mdr/.
[44] European Commission. Notified bodies. Available from: https://single-market-economy.ec.europa.eu/single-market/goods/building-blocks/notified-bodies_en.
[45] U.S. Food and Drug Administration. Recalls background and definitions. Available from: https://www.fda.gov/safety/industry-guidance-recalls/recalls-background-and-definitions?os=firetv%3Fno_journeys%3DtruekjUHL2Zj&ref=app#:~:text=Recalls%20are%20actions%20taken%20by%20a%20firm%20to,request%2C%20or%20by%20FDA%20order%20under%20statutory%20authority.
[46] U.S. Food and Drug Administration. FDA's role in drug recalls. Available from: https://www.fda.gov/drugs/drug-recalls/fdas-role-drug-recalls#:~:text=FDA%E2%80%99s%20role%20in%20a%20recall%20is%20to%20oversee,announced%20on%20FDA.gov%20or%20in%20the%20news%20media.
[47] U.S. Food and Drug Administration. Recalls. Available from: https://datadashboard.fda.gov/ora/cd/recalls.htm.
[48] European Medicines Agency. Standard operating procedure for dealing with reports of defective medicinal products. Available from: https://www.ema.europa.eu/en/documents/sop/standard-operating-procedure-dealing-reports-defective-medicinal-products_en.pdf.
[49] European Medicines Agency. Quality defects and recalls. Available from: https://www.ema.europa.eu/en/human-regulatory-overview/post-authorisation/compliance-post-authorisation/quality-defects-recalls.

Using ImageJ as a tool to analyze and process biological images

Running ImageJ

Open the program. This will bring up a toolbar (not a window).

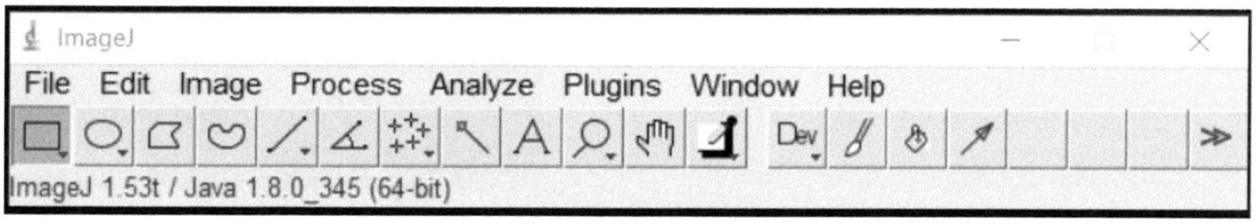

To open an image, go to **File-Open**. The program allows you to open several images at the same time, so you can collect data on one image and apply it to another. You can also open files from a series by using **File-Import-Image Sequence**. Select the folder including all the images you want to process at the same time and then type in a file name. ImageJ will then create a **stack** for you of the data.

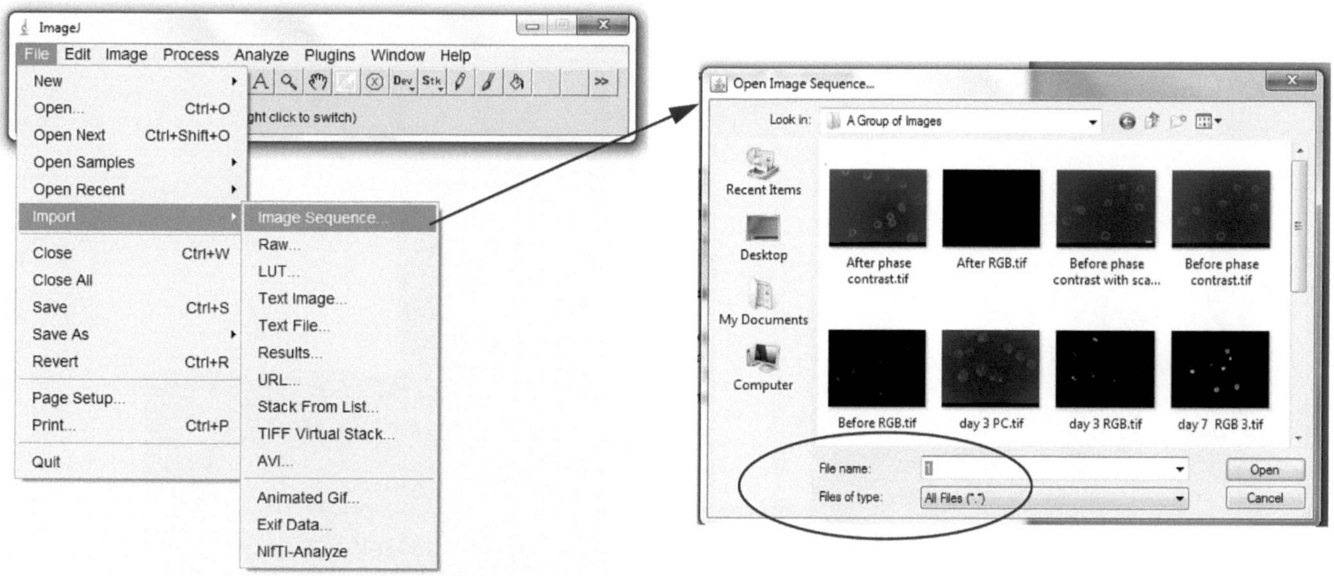

Using a scale in one image to make measurements and add a scale bar to another

Open two images, one showing your scale and the other showing your sample. This procedure only works if both images were obtained at identical resolutions using the same objective. Do not alter the size of either image prior to performing this analysis (other than zooming; see below).

First, calibrate the scale. Select the Line button on the toolbar. On your scale image, carefully draw a line that spans a known distance. Note: your accuracy will improve the longer you make this line. Select **Analyze-Set Scale**. In the "Known Distance" box, enter the actual distance of line. In the "Unit of Length" box, enter the corresponding unit (e.g., micrometer). Select the Global option, and hit OK. From that point on, all measurements you make will be in that unit.

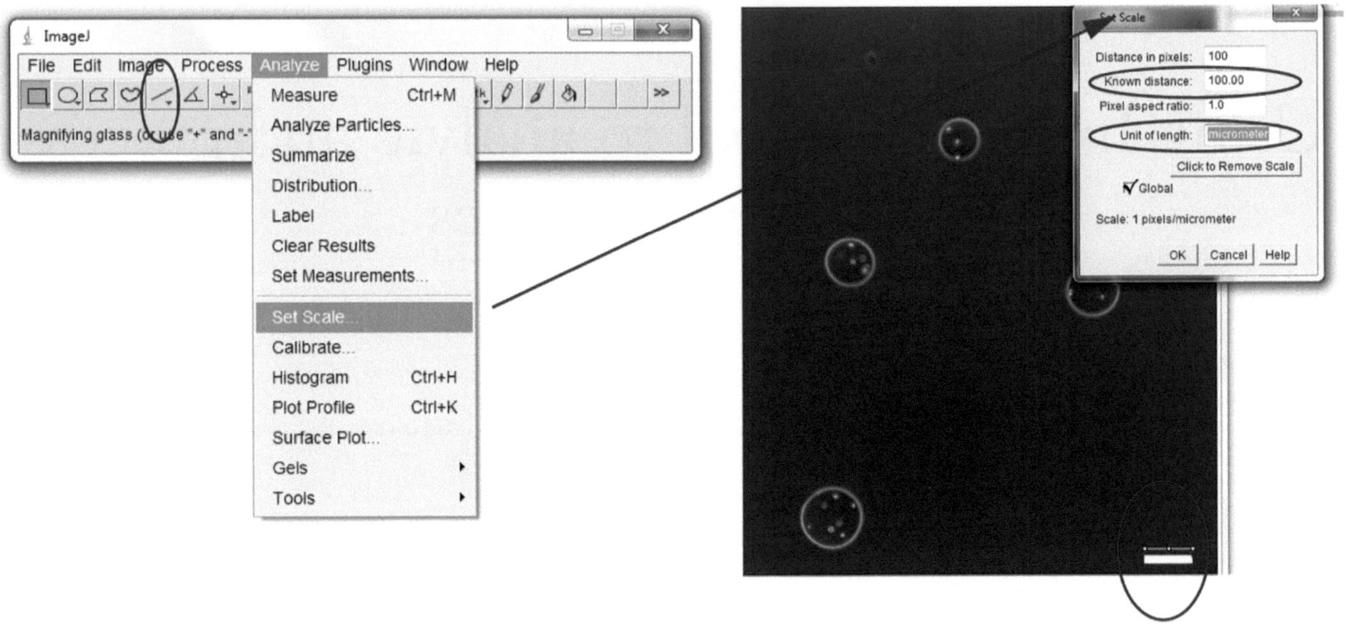

At this point, length measurements can be made in the sample image following the procedure above. Results will be shown in the "Results" window. *It's a good idea to make sure your scale was set accurately by performing a test measurement somewhere else on the scale image.*

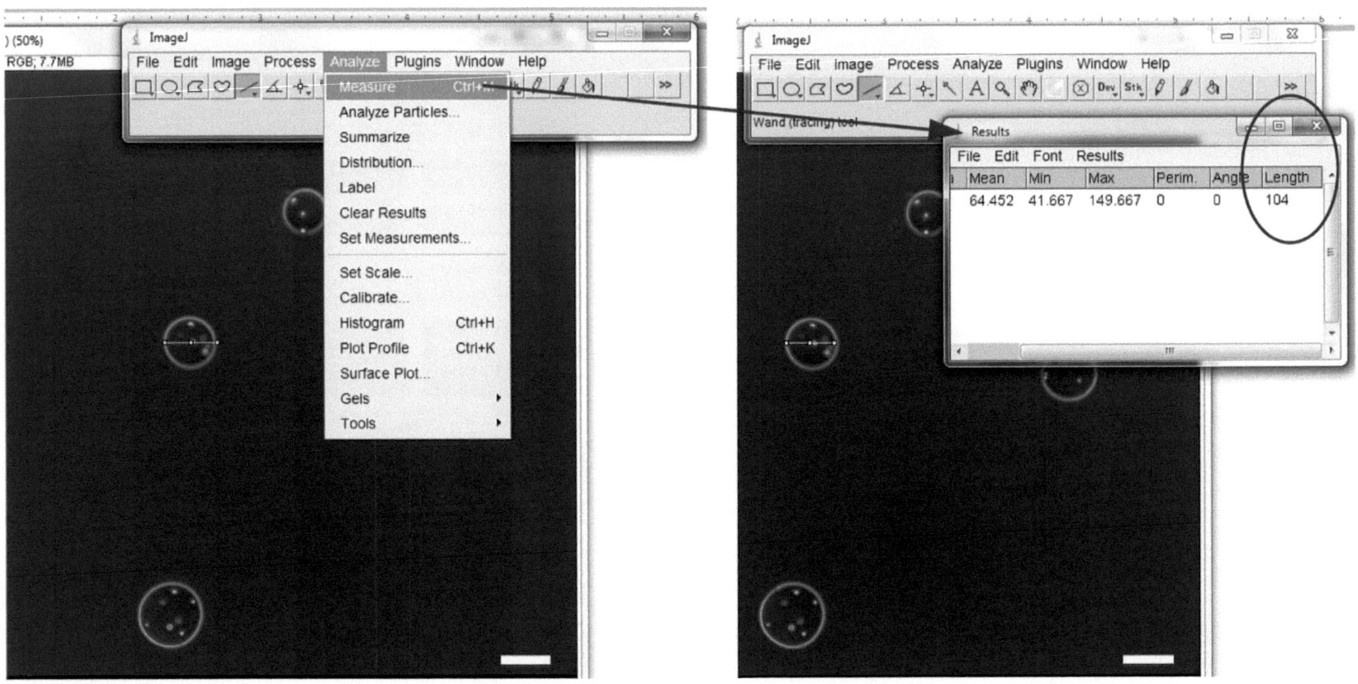

To add a scale bar to the sample image, select this image. Then, select **Analyze-Tools-Scale Bar**. You can choose the length of the scale bar, where it will be placed in the image, and how it will appear.

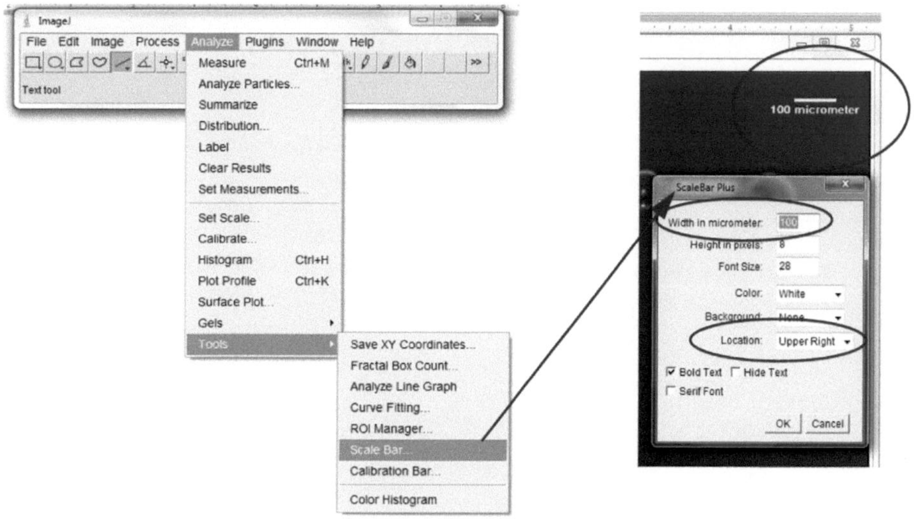

Further Help

You can get more information on how to use ImageJ at http://rsb.info.nih.gov/ij/docs/index.html.

Derivation of Higuchi equation [1-4]

The scenario is the release of the drug from an ointment film into the skin. The skin acts as a perfect sink, and the drug diffusion through the ointment base is rate-limiting. Other assumptions are that the diffusion coefficient (D) does not change, the initial drug concentration (C_0) is much higher than its solubility C_s, the drug is initially evenly distributed, the size of the drug molecules is much smaller than the film thickness, the dissolution of the drug is much faster than the drug diffusion, and the ointment base does not change with time with negligible edge effects. The theoretical drug concentration profile is shown in Fig. AB.1. The drug concentration in the partially extracted region containing dissolved drug is assumed to be linear (i.e., pseudo—steady state assumption).

The shaded area (*blue*) corresponds to the cumulative amount of drug release divided by the surface area (A) of the ointment film exposed to the skin (the figure shows only a cross-section of the ointment film). Hence,

$$\frac{M_t}{A} = h\frac{(C_0 - C_s) + C_0}{2} = h\left(C_0 - \frac{C_s}{2}\right)$$

$$\frac{dM}{A} = (h + dh)\frac{(C_0 - C_s) + C_0}{2} - h\frac{(C_0 - C_s) + C_0}{2} = dh\frac{(C_0 - C_s) + C_0}{2} = dh\left(C_0 - \frac{C_s}{2}\right).$$

Professor Higuchi foresaw that Fick's law can also be written as:

$$\frac{dM}{dt} = \frac{DC_s}{h}$$

$$dM = A\frac{DC_s}{h}dt,$$

where D is the diffusion coefficient.

Now, we get

$$Adh\left(C_0 - \frac{C_s}{2}\right) = A\frac{DC_s}{h}dt$$

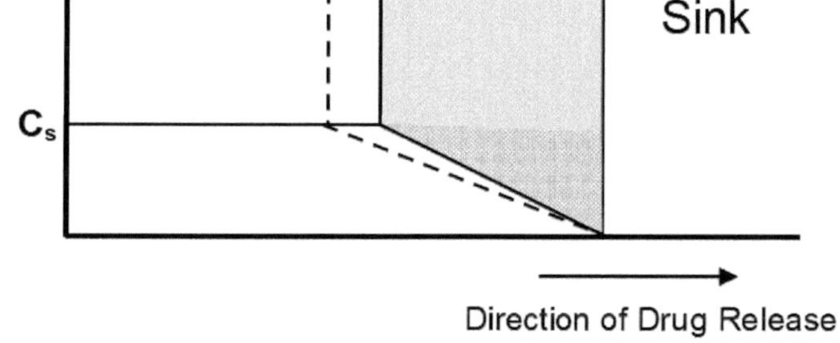

FIGURE. AB.1 Theoretical drug concentration profiles at times t (*solid line*) and $t + dt$ (*dashed line*). *h*, Distance of the front that separates ointment free of nondissolved drug excess from ointment still containing nondissolved drug excess; *dh*, distance that front moves inward during the time interval *dt*.

$$dh\left(C_0-\frac{C_s}{2}\right)=\frac{DC_s}{h}dt$$

$$hdh\frac{\left(C_0-\frac{C_s}{2}\right)}{DC_s}=dt$$

then integrate

$$\frac{\left(C_0-\frac{C_s}{2}\right)}{DC_s}\int hdh=\int dt$$

$$\frac{\left(C_0-\frac{C_s}{2}\right)}{DC_s}\times\frac{h^2}{2}=t$$

$$h^2=\frac{2DC_st}{\left(C_0-\frac{C_s}{2}\right)}$$

$$h=\sqrt{\frac{2DC_st}{\left(C_0-\frac{C_s}{2}\right)}}.$$

Finally, go back to the first equation:

$$\frac{M_t}{A}=h\left(C_0-\frac{C_s}{2}\right)$$

$$M_t=Ah\left(C_0-\frac{C_s}{2}\right)=A\sqrt{\frac{2DC_st}{\left(C_0-\frac{C_s}{2}\right)}}\left(C_0-\frac{C_s}{2}\right)=A\sqrt{2DC_st\left(C_0-\frac{C_s}{2}\right)}$$

In general, C_0 is much greater than C_s. As a result,

$$M_t=A\sqrt{2DC_st\left(C_0-\frac{C_s}{2}\right)}\approx A\sqrt{2DC_0C_st}.$$

References

[1] Siepmann J, Peppas NA. Higuchi equation: Derivation, applications, use and misuse. *Int J Pharm* 2011;418(1):6–12.
[2] Higuchi T. Rate of release of medicaments from ointment bases containing drugs in suspension. *J Pharm Sci* 1961;50(10):874–5.
[3] Elmas A, et al. Mathematical modelling of drug release. *RESM* 2020;6(4):327–50.
[4] Lee PI. Modeling of drug release from matrix systems involving moving boundaries: Approximate analytical solutions. *Int J Pharm* 2011;418(1): 18–27.

Index

Note: Page numbers followed by *f* indicate figures, *t* indicate tables, and *b* indicate boxes.